W9-BLS-762

CLINICAL CARE

in the Rheumatic Diseases

Second Edition

LAURA ROBBINS, DSW, EDITOR

CAROL S. BURCKHARDT, RN, PhD, ASSOCIATE EDITOR

MARIAN T. HANNAN, MPH, DSc, ASSOCIATE EDITOR

RAPHAEL J. DeHORATIUS, MD, CONSULTING EDITOR

Published by the Association of Rheumatology Health Professionals
A Division of the American College of Rheumatology
1800 Century Plaza
Suite 250
Atlanta, Georgia 30345-4300

Library of Congress Control Number: 2001090004
ISBN: 0-9654316-1-4

The information and the views and opinions contained in this publication are those of the authors and unless clearly specified, do not represent the views or opinions of the American College of Rheumatology. The American College of Rheumatology does not endorse, approve, guarantee or warrant any particular technique or therapy or product, method of instruction or recommendation contained in this publication.

Copyright 2001 by the American College of Rheumatology, Atlanta, Georgia.

Published by the American College of Rheumatology, Atlanta, Georgia. All rights reserved. No part of this book may be reproduced, stored in a retrieval system, or transmitted in any form or by any means, electronic, mechanical, photocopying, recording, or otherwise, without written permission of the publisher. Printed in the United States of America by Cadmus Journal Service, Richmond, Virginia.

Managing Editor: Elizabeth E. Axtell
Manuscript Editor: Cynthia M. Kahn
Editorial Assistant: Melissa Basso
Executive Director, Association of Rheumatology Health Professionals: David M. Haag

Authors

Saralynn Allaire, ScD, CRC
Boston University School of Medicine
Boston, MA

Roy D. Altman, MD
University of Miami School of Medicine
Miami, FL

Diana Anderson, PhD
Rheumatology Research Intnl
Dallas, TX

Ann Aspnes, BA
Duke University Medical School
Durham, NC

Basia Belza, PhD, RN
University of Washington
Seattle, WA

David Borenstein, MD
George Washington Univ Med Center
Washington, DC

Michele L. Boutaugh, BSN, MPH
Arthritis Foundation
Atlanta, GA

Teresa J. Brady, PhD, LP, OTR
Centers Dis Control Prevention
Atlanta, GA

D.J. Brower, BA
Temple Univ Sch Podiatric Med
Philadelphia, PA

Carol S. Burckhardt, RN, PhD
Oregon University Health Sciences Center
Portland, OR

David S. Caldwell, MD
Duke University Medical School
Durham, NC

Leigh F. Callahan, PhD
University of North Carolina
Chapel Hill, NC

A. Betts Carpenter, MD, PhD
Marshall University School of Medicine
Huntington, WV

Diane M. Erlandson, RN, MS, MPH
U.S. Dept of Health and Human Services
Boston, MA

Judith Falconer, PhD, MPH, OTR/L
Northwestern University
Evanston, IL

Robert G. Frank, PhD
University of Florida
Gainesville, FL

Sandy B. Ganz, PT, MS, GCS
Amsterdam Nursing Home
New York, NY

Marcin Gornisiewicz, MD
University of Alabama at Birmingham
Birmingham, AL

Kristofer J. Hagglund, PhD
University of Missouri at Columbia
Columbia, MO

Marian T. Hannan, DSc
Harvard Med Sch Div on Aging
Boston, MA

Pamela B. Harrell, OTR, CHT
Nashville, TN

Donna J. Hawley, EdD, RN
Wichita State University
Wichita, KS

Karen W. Hayes, PhD, PT
Northwestern University Medical School
Chicago, IL

Antoine Helewa, PT, MSc (epid)
University of Western Ontario
Kearney, ON, Canada

Howard J. Hillstrom, PhD
Temple Univ Sch Podiatric Medicine
Philadelphia, PA

Francis J. Keefe, PhD
Duke University Medical School
Durham, NC

Sharon L. Kolasinski, MD
Univ Pennsylvania Sch Med
Philadelphia, PA

H. Lemont, DPM
Temple Univ Sch Podiatric Med
Philadelphia, PA

Kathleen S. Lewis, RN, CMP, LPC
Celebrate Life
Decatur, GA

Christopher Lorish, PhD
University of Alabama School of Medicine
Birmingham, AL

Carlos J. Lozada, MD
University of Miami School of Medicine
Miami, FL

K.T. Mahan, DPM, MS
Temple Univ Sch Podiatric Med
Philadelphia, PA

Maren Lawson Mahowald, MD
University of Minnesota Medical School
Minneapolis, MN

Michael J. Maricic, MD
Southern Arizona VA Health Care Sys
Tucson, AZ

James McGuire, DPM, PT
Temple Univ Sch Podiatric Med
Philadelphia, PA

Donald R. Miller, PharmD
North Dakota State University
Fargo, ND

Marian A. Minor, PT, PhD
University of Missouri
Columbia, MO

Carolee Moncur, PT, PhD
University of Utah
Salt Lake City, UT

Larry W. Moreland, MD
University of Alabama at Birmingham
Birmingham, AL

Lisa A. Nichols, MSN, RN, CCRA
Novartis Pharmaceuticals
Bellevue, NE

Jill Noaker Luck, OTR/L
Univ Penn Med Center, St. Margaret
Pittsburgh, PA

Stephen A. Paget, MD, FACP, FACR
Hospital for Special Surgery
New York, NY

Jerry C. Parker, PhD
Truman Memorial Veterans Hospital
Columbia, MO

Rosalind Ramsey-Goldman, MD, DrPH
Northwestern University Medical School
Chicago, IL

Michael A. Rapoff, PhD
University of Kansas Medical Center
Kansas City, KS

Laura Ray, MA, MLS
Cleveland State University
Seven Hills, OH

Antonio J. Reginato, MD
Cooper University Medical Center
Camden, NJ

Anthony M. Reginato, MD, PhD
Massachusetts General Hospital
Boston, MA

Cheryl Riegger-Krugh, ScD, PT
Univ Colorado Health Sci Center
Denver, CO

Laura Robbins, DSW, MSW
Hospital for Special Surgery
New York, NY

Kathleen M. Schiaffino, PhD
Fordham University
Bronx, NY

H. Ralph Schumacher, Jr., MD
Veterans Administration Medical Center
Philadalphia, PA

Karen L. Smarr, MA
Truman Memorial Veterans Hospital
Columbia, MO

Barbara Stokes, PT
The Arthritis Society
Ottawa, ON, Canada

Janalee Taylor, RN, MSN
Childrens Hospital Medical Center
Cincinatti, OH

Gigi Viellion, RN, ONC
Beth Israel Medical Center
New York, NY

Stephen T. Wegener, PhD
Johns Hopkins University
Baltimore, MD

Mark H. Wener, MD, FACR
University of Washington
Seattle, WA

Marie D. Westby, BSc, PT
Mary Pack Arthritis Program
Vancouver, BC, Canada

Kendrick Whitney, DPM
Temple Univ Sch Podiatric Med
Philadelphia, PA

Gail E. Wright, PhD
Truman Memorial Veterans Hospital
Columbia, MO

Contributors

The following individuals made publication of *Clinical Care in the Rheumatic Diseases,* 2nd Edition, possible by participating in the editorial process or serving as chapter reviewers. Contributors of illustrations are identified in figure legends.

John Allegrante, PhD
Diana Anderson, PhD
Balu Athreya, MD
Judy Bautch, PhD, RN
Laurence Bradley, PhD
Bruce Clark, BPT
Sharon Clark, PhD, RN
Daniel Clauw, MD
Diane Dolan, RN
David Felson, MD
Liana Fraenkel, MD
Eric Gall, MD
Vickie Gall, PT, MEd
Don Goldenberg, MD
Andrew Guiccone, PhD, PT, FAPTA
Scott Hasson, EdD, PT
Charles Helmick, MD
Carol Henderson, PhD, RD

Marc Hochberg, MD, MPH
Gary Hoffman, MD
Roberta Horton, MSW, ACSW
Dennis Janisse, C Ped
Dorothy Johnson, DNSc, FNP
Kim Jones, RNC, MN
Patricia Katz, PhD
Kimberly Kimpton, PT
John Klippel, MD
David Krebs, PT, PhD
Hollis Krug, MD
Michael LaValley, PhD
Marc Mahowald, PhD
Ray Marks, MD
Timothy McAlindon, MD
Carolyn McGrory, MS, RN
Perry Nicassio, PhD
Jill Noaker Luck, OTR/L, CHT

Jim O'Dell, MD
Carol Oatis, PhD, PT
Murray Passo, MD
Cheryl Riegger-Krugh, ScD, PT
Paul Romain, MD
I. Jon Russel, MD
Rodney Rutowski, MSW
Robert Simms, MD
Lee Simon, MD
Judy Sotosky, MEd, PT
Terence Starz, MD
Stephen Wegener, PhD
James Williams, MD
David Wofsy, MD
Terri Wolfe, OTR/L, CHT
Ed Yelin, PhD

Table of Contents

Foreword

Rheumatic and musculoskeletal conditions are the most prevalent chronic conditions in the United States, affecting more than 37 million Americans (1). As the population continues to grow in age and number, the Centers for Disease Control and Prevention estimates that nearly 60 million people will be affected by rheumatic diseases by the year 2020 (2). Not only are rheumatic diseases highly prevalent, they can have a profound impact on the physical and psychological function, productivity, and quality of life of affected individuals and their families, as well as having a major economic impact on society.

Health professionals, rheumatologists, and primary care providers need resources that allow them to keep pace with the latest in the management of the rheumatic diseases. This second edition of *Clinical Care in the Rheumatic Diseases* is designed to meet that need. Developed and written by leaders in the field of rheumatology who represent a variety of clinical disciplines, this text emphasizes the biologic, psychological, functional, and sociologic factors that interact to form our understanding of the causes of and treatments for rheumatic diseases.

Clinical Care in the Rheumatic Diseases will be of value to providers for several reasons. This text provides a single source of information for the comprehensive management of rheumatic diseases. Because of the interdisciplinary nature of the authors and content, this text has the potential to be shared and valued by providers and trainees across the health science disciplines. Building on the success of the previous edition, the editors have attempted to keep pace with the dynamic and ever-changing field of health care. Since the publication of the first edition, not only have several new treatments and diagnostic modalities become widely available, but the use of the Internet as a source of information has also become the norm. Chapters have been updated or completely revised to reflect these changes and new chapters have been added specifically to address major practice changes.

The American College of Rheumatology (ACR) is the largest professional organization of physicians, scientists, and health professionals devoted to the study and treatment of the rheumatic diseases (www.rheumatology.org). ACR members maintain a strong commitment to research and education, advancing the understanding of the rheumatic diseases, and discovering new therapies. The Association of Rheumatology Health Professionals (ARHP) is a division of the ACR, whose professional membership is made up of individuals from various disciplines including nursing, physical therapy, occupational therapy, social work, psychology, health services research, and others.

Clinical Care in the Rheumatic Diseases represents a major educational endeavor by the ARHP and is an example of how members of this organization view their commitment as premier providers in the care of people with rheumatic disease. This text is one of a number of ARHP educational initiatives (such as the journal *Arthritis Care and Research*, national scientific meetings, and the ARHP slide collection) that the organization currently offers.

In keeping with ACR's commitment to serving the needs of its members and the greater rheumatology community, this text provides the most up-to-date information on clinical care. By providing this information, we hope to improve the quality of care of individuals with rheumatic diseases. We commend the volunteer authors and reviewers, the ARHP staff, and most especially, editor Laura Robbins, DSW; associate editors Carol S. Burckhardt, PhD, RN, and Marian T. Hannan, MPH, DSc; and consulting editor Raphael J. DeHoratius, MD, for their significant role in this contribution to the field.

Basia Belza, PhD, RN
President
Association of Rheumatology Health Professionals

Michael E. Weinblatt, MD
President
American College of Rheumatology

1. Lawrence RC, Helmick CG, Arnett FC, Deyo RA, Felson DT, Giannini EH, et al. Estimates of the prevalence of arthritis and selected musculoskeletal disorders in the United States. Arthritis Rheum 1998;41:778–99.
2. Centers for Disease Control and Prevention. Arthritis prevalence and activity limitations–United States, 1990. MMWR 1994;43:433–8.

Introduction

What an exciting time to be part of *Clinical Care in the Rheumatic Diseases,* 2nd Edition! A plethora of new knowledge since the first edition—from new therapeutic treatments and genetic coding to unprecedented developments in understanding the way patients cope and efficacious interventions aimed at enhancing quality of life—is now available. Like its predecessor, this edition strives to be the premier source of information for all multidisciplinary health professionals who diagnose and treat patients with rheumatic diseases. The cover illustration has been expanded, building upon the foundations and blueprint that were established by the rheumatology community in the first edition. The globe symbolizes the vast world of health care, and the computer, the link to technology that connects the health care community to each other and to patients with rheumatic diseases. Through technology, all clinicians, those who are in the specialty of rheumatology as well as those who are not, have access to state-of-the-art information that broadens the possibility for all clinicians to affect the lives of the more than 43 million people with some form of rheumatic or musculoskeletal disease.

Following the precedent set in the first edition, the text of *Clinical Care in the Rheumatic Diseases,* 2nd Edition is unique in two ways. First, it continues to go beyond the medical model to embrace the biopsychosocial model of health care, emphasizing the interdependence of biologic, psychological, and social factors in determining the course and outcome of disease (1). Second, this edition presents clinical information to the wide professional community responsible for the care of patients with rheumatic diseases: professionals in medicine, nursing, physical and occupational therapy, pharmacy, education, health services, and behavioral and social science. Its utility as a training tool for students in these professions should prove invaluable.

To accomplish these ambitious goals, the 2nd edition of the text has been expanded to 44 chapters, divided into 6 sections that relate to clinical care of patients with rheumatic diseases and their concerns. Section A, Clinical Foundations, lays the groundwork for understanding the musculoskeletal system, the epidemiology of rheumatic diseases, basic immunology, inflammation, and genetics. It also presents the most recent data on the impact and burden of rheumatic diseases on society. The chapter on human development expands issues of disease impact on the psychological stages of development from childhood to adulthood.

The second section, Diagnosis and Assessment, includes the necessary components of a patient evaluation. It incorporates information on history and physical assessment, diagnostic testing, psychosocial assessment, and social and cultural assessment. A new chapter has been added to this section to provide the patient's perspective. To be truly multidisciplinary, the editors felt it would be remiss not to include the patient's point of view in the process of diagnosis and treatment. The chapters on health status and outcome measures provide the clinician with tools to enhance patient care, and those on evidence-based medicine and decision making address issues of efficacy and cost effectiveness.

In the third section, Common Rheumatic Diseases, there is a disease-specific approach to clinical care. The new chapters, added to reflect the current spectrum of prevalent musculoskeletal diseases, include information on osteoporosis, fibromyalgia, and polymyalgia rheumatica.

The next section, Clinical Interventions, has been expanded to 12 chapters that span the options available to clinicians in the management of rheumatic diseases. The chapters on patient education, cognitive behavioral interventions, rest and exercise, physical modalities, splinting of the hand, enhancing functional ability, foot management and ambulatory aids, and pre- and post-surgical management of the hip and knee have been updated to reflect advances in these areas of care. As well, the explosion of new therapeutic agents for treatment of the rheumatic diseases is reflected in the chapter on pharmacologic interventions. New chapters have been added to address the growing knowledge in the areas of shoulder disorders and low back and neck pain. The complementary and alternative treatments chapter presents current knowledge in this burgeoning field with an openness to evaluation of what is known and what is not, so that clinicians and patients can make informed decisions.

The next section, Problem-Focused Management, presents management options for the clinician based on patients' symptoms. Each chapter in this section has been updated to include state-of-the art information that addresses issues of pain, fatigue, sleep disturbance, mood disorders, deconditioning, adherence, and work disability.

The text concludes with a section on Clinician Resources. Here the editors have added two new chapters vital to the provision of good patient care. One chapter provides a user's guide to the World Wide Web so that the clinician can obtain information relevant to the many aspects of clinical care. The second chapter provides links to organizations and other web-based resources for those readers wanting information to expand their knowledge and assist their patients.

The second edition of this text is a testimony to the philosophical commitment to a multidisciplinary approach to patient care that embodies the relationship between the Association of Rheumatology Health Professionals (ARHP) and the American College of Rheumatology (ACR). One professional alone cannot provide the best patient care. Likewise, one person alone cannot produce a comprehensive text. The associate and consulting editors provided invaluable insight, time, and professionalism to this publication. Drs. Marian T. Hannan and Carol Burckhardt, associate editors, gave generously of their time, scholarly criticism, and problem-solving skills. Dr. Ralph DeHoratius, consulting editor, provided medical perspective and guidance. More than 60 authors and 50 reviewers contributed their knowledge and expertise to produce an updated, clear, and concise text.

Julie Epps, former ARHP Executive Director, and current Vice President of Education for ACR, supported the 2nd edition project proposal and helped launch its production. David Haag, ARHP's current Executive Director, embraced the text as one of his first projects, and worked with the editors to ensure a quality product. Manuscript editor Cynthia Kahn is a master, and helped to put the pieces together so the text was greater than the sum of the parts. Beth Axtell, who came to the project midway as Managing Editor, was a savior, and her editorial talents further refined each chapter.

Deep gratitude is due to the staff and faculty at the Hospital for Special Surgery (HSS) in New York City for their support, focus, and time spent to produce the best text possible. Keeping track of numerous iterations of chapters, communicating with authors, ARHP staff, and the associate and consulting editors would not have been feasible without the unwavering assistance and dedication of Melissa Basso, a former colleague in the Education Division at HSS and my editorial assistant for the text.

Many people made this publication possible. It takes many people, working as a team, to provide quality care to people with rheumatic disease. Teamwork in rheumatic disease care is a strong theme in our professional lives and served as part of the blueprint for the first edition. *Clinical Care in the Rheu-*

matic Diseases, 2nd Edition builds upon and enhances the original blueprint. Like the World Wide Web, this text provides access to information the clinician may need, linking experts throughout the rheumatology community to community-based health care providers. The blueprint has been altered due to gains in the field over the past few years, but the goal remains the same—to touch the lives of and improve the care for the millions of people with rheumatic diseases.

Laura Robbins, DSW, Editor
Clinical Care in the Rheumatic Diseases, 2nd Edition
New York, NY

1. Wegener ST. Introduction. In: Wegener ST, Belza BL, Gall EP, editors. Clinical Care in the Rheumatic Diseases. Atlanta: American College of Rheumatology. p. vii

SECTION A: CLINICAL FOUNDATIONS

Musculoskeletal Systems

CAROLEE MONCUR, PT, PhD

To appreciate the impact of rheumatic disease on the musculoskeletal system, it is important to have some understanding of the anatomic characteristics and biomechanical responses of the tissues at risk for developing arthritis. Muscles, bones, cartilage, tendons, ligaments, aponeuroses, and fascia are all dynamic tissues important to the integrity, stability, and mobility of the musculoskeletal system. This chapter presents a brief overview of these structures.

JOINTS

Joints are concerned with differential growth (1), with the transmission of tensile, shear, compressive, and torsion forces (2), and with a wide variety of movements (3). The dominant function at any given time depends on the location of the joint and age of the individual (4). The scientific study of the functional topography and unique anatomy of each joint is called *arthrology*.

Classification schemes for joints range from simple to more complex systems; the more complex are used by specialists to evaluate the intricacies of human movement. For this review, joints can be assigned to one of two categories: synarthroses or diarthroses. Synarthrodial joints are solid, nonsynovial joints. They are grouped either as fibrous joints or cartilaginous joints depending on their mode of ossification. Synarthroses are found in the cranial junctions, epiphyseal plates, and various midline joints of the body such as the symphysis pubis (4).

Diarthrodial or Synovial Joints

Diarthrodial or synovial joints are of primary interest in joint pathology. Each articular surface is composed of specialized hyaline cartilage strongly adherent to the underlying subchondral bone. On the outer surface, the cartilage is macroscopically smooth and free to be lubricated. This provides a near frictionless surface over which to move in concert with another articular surface. A classification scheme for diarthrodial joints is presented in Figure 1.

A typical example of the characteristics of the knee synovial joint is shown in Figure 2. Characteristic structures include 2 bones linked by a fibrous capsule that may have intrinsic ligamentous thickenings to support the joint, a layer of synovial membrane deep to the fibrous capsule, an articular disc and/or meniscus not covered by the synovial membrane, a

Surface Shape	Surface Topology
plane = gliding joints spheroid = ball and socket or enarthrosis ellipsoid = condyloid ginglymus = hinge bicondylar = double condyloid trochoid = pivot sellar = saddle joint	simple (concave and convex surfaces) compound (concave and convex surfaces) sellar (concave and convex surfaces)
Axes of Movement	**Joint Mechanics**
uniaxial biaxial triaxial polyaxial	Movements are related to the concept of the mechanical axis of a bone. Movements are all resolvable as rotations around one, two or three orthogonal axes, i.e., possessing 1-3 degrees of freedom of motion.
Types of Movement	**Types of Movement**
Translation Angulation Rotation Circumduction Examples: flexion/extension abduction/adduction pronation/supination elevation/depression protraction/retraction isometric (neuromuscular) stabilizing (mechanical: close-packing)	Terms refer to one mobile articular surface moving relative to its fixed partner: **Spin**: pure rotation of a surface around its mechanical axis. Two varieties of spin: pure and impure. **Roll**: tips of mechanical axis move end over end. **Slide**: tips of mechanical axis trace a translatory path (like ice on ice).
Fundamental Joint Positions	
Loose Packed: controlled free mobility Close Packed: position of functional rigidity	

Figure 1. Classification of diarthrodial joints.

fibrocartilage labrum (as in the case of the hip), fat pads, and a vascular, neural, and lymphatic supply.

Joint Capsule. The joint capsule ensheathes the 2 ends of the bone. Because the fibrous layer of the joint capsule blends with the periosteum of the bones, meeting some distance away from the articulating ends, it does not impede movement. The fibrous layer is composed of relatively inelastic sheets of white collagen fibers, which contributes to joint stability. Blood vessels and nerves perforate the layer, and occasionally gaps are present.

Ligaments of the joint represent cord-like thickenings of parallel collagen bundles formed intrinsically in the fibrous layer of the capsule. They may be separated from the capsule by bursae formed from outpouchings of the synovial lining. Ligaments are pliant and structured to resist excessive or abnormal movements of the joints; they yield very little to tension. Reflex neural mechanisms protect the ligament from excessive tension and stretch (5). In some joints, such as the

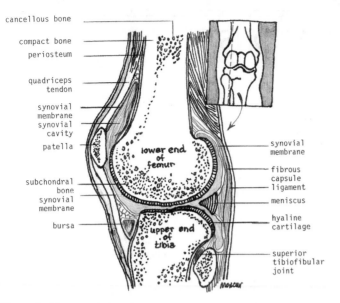

Figure 2. Characteristics of a diarthrodial joint as depicted by the knee joint.

knee, the intrinsic ligamentous properties are critical to the arthrokinematics of the joint.

Synovial Membrane. The synovial membrane or *synovium* lines the joint everywhere, with the exception of the articular cartilage. The inner surface of the membrane is usually smooth and glistening, and it may be folded into numerous processes called *villi*. Synovium is abundantly supplied with blood vessels, nerves, and lymphatics (4), and it produces synovial fluid and provides immunologic protection. Synovial tissues are capable of rapid and complete repair when injured or surgically removed (6,7).

Blood Vessels and Lymphatics. Synovial joints have a relatively rich blood supply. The branches of arteries to a joint commonly supply 3 structures: the epiphysis, the joint capsule, and the synovium. Arteriovenous anastomoses are formed in these joints, but their significance has not yet been determined. Due to the enriched vasculature of the synovial membrane, injury to the joint may allow blood to escape into the joint space and mix with the synovial fluid (4,7).

Nerve Supply. Hilton's law (8), the fundamental statement regarding the nerve supply to joints, postulates that the nerve trunks supplying joint musculature furnish innervation to skin over the muscle and to the tissues of the joint. Arrays of afferent receptors are found in and near the articular capsule. These provide information regarding the position, movement, and stresses that act on the joint. At least 4 types of receptors have been identified (9). Type I endings (Ruffini type) are found in the superficial layers of the fibrous capsule and are slowly adapting mechanoreceptors. They provide awareness of joint position and movement, particularly in terms of postural control. Type II endings (Pacinian type) occur in small groups in the deeper structures of the joint capsule. They are rapidly adapting, low-threshold mechanoreceptors that are sensitive to movement and pressure changes within the joint capsule. Type III endings (Golgi type) are identical to neurotendinous organs in structure and function and are found in the articular ligaments of the joint. They appear to be high-threshold, slowly adapting receptors that prevent excessive tension and stress on the joint by reflex inhibition of the adjacent musculature. Type

IV endings are free terminals of myelinated and nonmyelinated fibers located in the articular capsule, the adjacent fat pads, and around the blood vessels of the synovial layer. These endings are high-threshold, slowly adapting receptors that seem to respond to excessive motion or injury. They may provide a basis for articular pain (9).

Articular Cartilage. Healthy hyaline cartilage is a specialized connective tissue characterized by considerable extracellular matrix composed mainly of proteoglycans, collagen, glycoproteins, other proteins (such as chondronectin and anchorin CII), and water. Proteoglycans are hydrophilic and give compressive strength to the cartilage, while collagen functions to provide shape and tensile strength. Chondrocytes are responsible for the homeostasis of the extracellular matrix of articular cartilage. Located at a distance from blood vessels, chondrocytes receive their nutrition via diffusion or convection through the matrix. This arrangement has led to the common understanding that hyaline cartilage is avascular and receives nutrients from the synovial fluid during the movement and loading of the joint. Hyaline cartilage is also aneural. Collagen, proteoglycans, other proteins, and glycoproteins represent about 20% of the tissue wet weight; water and inorganic salts constitute the remainder. Maintenance of the water content is critical to the continued resilience and function of the cartilage in terms of joint nutrition and lubrication (4,7,10,11).

Synovial Fluid and Lubrication. Synovial fluid is produced by the cells lining the intima of the synovia and is found in the joint space, within bursae, and in tendon sheaths. It provides a liquid environment for joint surfaces; nutrition to chondrocytes, articular discs, and menisci; and lubrication and reduction of erosion of the joint surfaces and structures. Because synovium has a rich vascular supply that is fenestrated (has openings), diffusion between the plasma and interstitial spaces can occur. A delicate balance exists between the exchange rate of plasma and synovial fluid particularly in the medical and rehabilitative treatment of the inflammatory arthritides. Severe impairment of this process can create ischemia, effusion, and increased intraarticular temperature (12).

Joint lubrication is an intricate process. Proposed models have followed engineering physics and attempted to equate the human joint with a hydrodynamic function. Considerable data have shown that the human joint is more remarkable than any hydrodynamic system and that the coefficient of friction is very low in a healthy joint (13). The coefficient of friction is defined as a measure of the energy required to move the joint in proportion to the energy available to do the work of moving the joint. That synovial joints possess a highly effective lubrication system is widely appreciated; however, the mechanics are less well understood. Current descriptions include a component called *boundary layer lubrication* and a second component referred to as *hydrodynamic lubrication* (11,14–16).

Boundary layer lubrication occurs as a result of a proposed small glycoprotein called lubricin. This substance appears to bind to the weight-bearing surface and facilitate the intrinsic arthrokinematics of the joint, while providing protection against wear. Lubricin is a synovium-derived molecule that binds to articular cartilage and retains molecules of water. These properties contribute to joint stability as well as lubrication of the joint (16).

Hydrodynamic lubrication seems to contribute to the low friction of the joint during motion. The theory is that load-induced compression of hyaline cartilage will force interstitial fluid to flow laterally to an unloaded surface where it exudes over the surface of the cartilage, thus generating a cushioning layer of fluid when the joint is further loaded. This may reduce the shearing stresses and friction between the joint surfaces (11,14–16).

Reaction of Articular Cartilage to Injury. The response of articular cartilage to injury depends on the type and extent of injury. Synovial joints can develop at least 3 types of articular cartilage defects: 1) age-related superficial fibrillation, 2) cartilage degeneration due to osteoarthritis, and 3) focal chondral and osteochondral defects (17). Superficial cartilage fibrillation occurs in joints with increasing age; however, individuals do not usually experience symptoms or have difficulty with joint function. There does not appear to be a progressive loss of articular cartilage (18). In contrast, the joint degeneration that leads to osteoarthritis consists of a progressive loss of proteoglycans, and hence water, resulting in a loss of compressibility that leads to remodeling and sclerosis of articular cartilage. As the cartilage attempts to repair itself, remodeling and sclerosis of subchondral bone, and in some cases, the formation of subchondral bone cysts and marginal osteophytes, may occur (19). Focal articular cartilage and osteochondral defects appear to result most commonly from trauma. They occur in adolescents and young adults, and some of these individuals may experience joint pain, effusions, and mechanical dysfunction.

Trauma can result in 3 types of articular cartilage injury: chondral damage without visible tissue disruption, disruption of articular cartilage alone, and disruption of articular cartilage and the underlying subchondral bone (20,21). Injury can cause alterations in the matrix of the articular cartilage that may include a decrease in proteoglycan concentration and possible disruption of the collagen framework (22). If the loss of matrix proteoglycans does not exceed what chondrocytes are able to produce, then the matrix can be restored. However, the collagen meshwork needs to remain intact and enough viable chondrocytes must be present (20,21,23). Without a healthy matrix, the chondrocyte can be exposed to excessive loads, and tissue degeneration occurs (12).

Acute or repetitive trauma can cause focal mechanical disruption of articular cartilage including fissures, chondral flaps or tears, and loss of a cartilage segment. The response of articular cartilage to this type of injury is limited by the lack of blood vessels and cells that can repair significant tissue defects (20,21,23). Chondrocytes respond to tissue injury by proliferation and synthesis of the matrix near the injury. The new matrix and proliferating cells may be unable to fill the defect, and soon after the injury the attempt to heal ceases (18).

If the injury extends into the subchondral bone, hemorrhage and fibrin clot formation occur and the inflammatory response is activated. Vascular invasion and migration of undifferentiated cells into the clot is stimulated, and within 2 weeks of injury some of these cells assume the rounded form of chondrocytes. These cells produce regions of hyaline-like cartilage in the chondral and bone portion of the defect. The repaired chondral tissue typically has a composition and structure intermediate between hyaline and fibrocartilage; it rarely, if ever, has the elaborate structure of normal articular cartilage. Occasionally the repaired cartilage persists unchanged or progressively remodels to form a functional joint surface, but in most large subchondral injuries the chondral repair tissue begins to show degeneration within a year (18).

Intraarticular Menisci. Not all diarthrodial joints have menisci; however, when present, menisci differentiate into fibrocartilage during embryonic development. Menisci may have a free inner border (as in the knee joint) or they may traverse the joint, dividing it into 2 separate synovial cavities (as in the sternoclavicular joint). The functions of intraarticular fibrocartilage may include absorbing shock, improving fit between articulating surfaces, improving the mechanics of movement, checking translatory motions of joints, deploying weight over a large surface, and dissipating the synovial fluid throughout the joint space (4).

Surface Shape and Topology. Some synovial joints have 2 articulating surfaces forming simple articulations. In this case, one surface is convex in shape and the other is concave, as in the metacarpophalangeal (MCP) joint. Joints such as the elbow are compound articulations, because there are 2 convex surfaces (capitulum and trochlea) that articulate with 2 concave surfaces (radius and ulna). Furthermore, in the elbow the circumference of the convex radial head articulates with the concave radial notch of the ulna. Joints such as the knee, which contain an intracapsular disc or meniscus, are complex articulations (4).

The general shape of synovial joints has been classified into 7 different categories (Figure 1). *Plane or gliding joints* are articulations between almost flat surfaces, such as between the carpal or tarsal bones. *Ginglymi or hinge joints* resemble a hinge and are restricted to one plane of motion, as demonstrated by the interphalangeal joints. *Trochoid or pivot joints* are also uniaxial; however, these rotate around a longitudinal axis, as in the case of the radial head and ulnar notch, or the atlas around the dens of the axis. *Bicondylar joints* such as the knee have 2 convex condyles that articulate with 2 concave surfaces. *Ellipsoid joints* are oval and convex. They articulate with an elliptical concave surface, as in the radiocarpal or MCP joints. *Sellar or saddle joints* are concavoconvex surfaces, meaning that both a convex and a concave surface are found on the articulating surfaces. The carpometacarpal joint of the thumb is an example of a sellar joint. *Spheroidal or ball and socket joints* are formed by a spherical surface directed into a cup-like articulating surface, as seen in the hip and shoulder joints (3,4).

TENDONS, LIGAMENTS, APONEUROSES, AND FASCIA

Tendons

Tendons, which attach muscles to bones or aponeuroses, are largely composed of collagen fibers. They are somewhat flexible, resist overstretching, and are white due to their low density of vascular supply. The anatomic sites where tendons attach to bone are called *entheses*. At these locations the collagen fibers of the tendon have undergone a transition to fibrocartilage and become continuous with the Sharpey's fibers of the bone. Sharpey's fibers serve as anchorage for tendons, ligaments, and the periodontal membranes of the teeth by becoming buried in bones (7). Entheses can become inflamed in the spondylarthropathies.

The blood supply to tendons is sparsely provided by small arterioles that run parallel to the adjacent musculature and intercommunicate freely. Vena communicantes and lymphatic vessels accompany these arterioles. Although the metabolism of tendinous tissue is low, it increases in reaction to injury or insult. Repair is almost exclusively due to proliferation of fibroblasts associated with collagen fibers (4,7). Tendons severed in accidents heal very well with proper surgical management and rehabilitation.

The nerve supply to tendons appears to be mostly afferents, and there is no clear evidence of vasomotor control. Specialized neurotendinous endings called Golgi tendon organs exist in tendons, particularly at the myotendinous junction.

Bursae are present where tendons are deflected around bones or pass under a retinaculum near a joint. The bursa is a simple, flattened sac of synovial membrane supported by dense regular connective tissue. It decreases friction by allowing complete freedom of movement over a limited range. Each bursa contains a lubricating film of synovial fluid. Most bursae occur between tendons and bones, tendons and ligaments, or between tendons.

Tendon synovial sheaths occur where tendons would otherwise rub against bone or other friction-generating surfaces. They are arranged in a closed double-walled cylinder, separated by a thin film of synovial fluid. The inner sheath attaches to and encloses the tendon. The external layer attaches to the neighboring connective tissue structures, allowing the surfaces to glide easily past one another in healthy tissues.

The tendon's primary function is to attach muscle to bone and to transmit tensile loads from muscle to bone during joint movement. The tendon guides the muscle belly to maintain optimal distance from the joint center during movement. Viscoelastic properties give tendons a tensile strength that is greater than necessary during normal movement. The tensile strength is similar to that of bone—about half that of steel. A tendon of 1 cm² cross-sectional area can support 600–1,000 kg of weight.

During muscle contraction, tendons become elastic and can have considerable contractile energy transferred to them during movement (24). During normal activity, a tendon is subjected to less than one-fourth of its ultimate capacity to handle tension (25). Aging, disease, trauma, medications, mobilization or immobilization, and pregnancy are a few of the factors that can affect the ability of both tendons and ligaments to accomplish their tensile responsibilities.

Ligaments

Ligaments attach one bone to another and are often thickenings of the joint capsule. Like tendons, ligaments are dense, regular connective tissues of parallel arranged collagenous tissue that are sparsely vascularized. Ligaments also undergo transition into fibrocartilage and attach to the bone, forming an enthesis.

The collagen arrangement in ligaments is aligned parallel and straight, restricting elongation and lending stability and protection from abnormal motion or force. A minor amount of elasticity is present in the collagen fibers of ligaments, which allows some deformation and then return of the fiber to the original position. Excessive or prolonged elongation may impair the ability of the ligament to return to its original position, thus compromising joint stability.

Aponeuroses

Aponeuroses are flat sheets of densely arranged collagen fibers showing a surface iridescence when newly exposed. Aponeuroses usually consist of several layers, with the fasciculi of fibers arranged parallel within one layer but inclined in a different direction in subsequent layers. Typical examples are the aponeurosis forming the sheath of the rectus abdominis muscle and the iliotibial band of the thigh. Smaller aponeuroses are found in the palm of the hand and on the plantar surface of the foot. The aponeurosis of the rectus sheath houses the muscle and serves as a midline attachment for the other abdominal musculature. The iliotibial band lends support laterally to the integrity of the hip and the knee. The palmar aponeurosis is important to the arches of the hand; similarly, the plantar aponeurosis is important to the bony arches of the foot.

Fascia

Fascia can describe a variety of connective tissues large enough to be seen with the unaided eye. Typically, fascia forms the enveloping fibers of muscles, nerves, and tendons, and sheaths between whole muscles, viscera, and skin. Superficial fascia is found deep to the dermis and serves as an insulator. It also connects the skin to deeper structures. It sometimes contains muscle fibers, for example the muscles of facial expression. It is distinct and of variable thickness over the anterior abdominal wall, the limbs, and the perineum. Fascia tends to be thinnest over the hands and feet, at the side of the neck, around the anus, and especially over the penis and scrotum. It is particularly dense in the scalp, the palms, and the soles.

Deep fascia forms intermuscular septa that separate muscles or groups of muscles while connecting extensively to bone. The crural fascia of the leg is an example. Sometimes the deep fascia becomes specialized into localized transverse thickenings and is attached at both ends to local bony prominences. An example is the transverse carpal ligament that helps form the carpal tunnel.

BONE

The skeletal system provides a rigid framework for support and weight bearing. In addition, it forms a lever system to which muscles attach and provides smooth, polished surfaces for joints. Other functions include protection for vulnerable viscera; formation of hematopoietic tissue for production of erythrocytes, granular leukocytes and platelets; and storage of calcium, phosphorus, magnesium, and sodium.

Cells and the Intercellular Substance of Bone

In order to appreciate how bone develops, it is important to understand the duties and functions of the cells and intercellular substance of bone. Bone is a living tissue. Modeling and remodeling occurs in healthy bone and requires healthy cells and a healthy environment. Osteogenic (bone-producing) cells lie on the deep layers of the periosteum and endosteum of bone. The periosteal membrane covers the outer surface of the bone, except where there is hyaline cartilage. Comprising an outer fibrous coat and an inner cellular coat of osteogenic cells, this membrane is highly vascularized with vessels that enter and leave the nutrient foramen of the bone. Myelinated and nonmyelinated neural fibers accompany the arteries, some of which are nociceptors.

The endosteum lines the inner spaces of the marrow cavity, spaces of cancellous bone, and the canals of compact bone. Large multinucleated cells called *osteoclasts* are scattered along the inner layer of these membranes and function to resorb bone. During growth, the osteoclasts of the endosteum widen the marrow cavity. After growth, the endosteum becomes a resting membrane unless a fracture or change in hormonal levels occur, requiring an increase of osteoclast production.

Osteoblasts, derived from osteogenic cells, synthesize and secrete the organic matrix of bone around their cell processes to form canaliculi and future osteons (the basic unit of bone, also known as a Haversian system). When mature, osteoblasts become osteocytes that reside in the lacunae of bone and maintain bone metabolism. Their cell junctions with other osteocytes appear to maintain the integrity of the bone matrix, which is composed of collagen fibers and amorphous ground substance containing water, glycoproteins, and inorganic materials of calcium, phosphate, fluoride, magnesium, and sodium (4,7).

Bone Remodeling and Healing

Remodeling of bone occurs in response to change in type or amount of physical stresses (or to the lack of them), healing fractures, or rheumatic disease. The phenomenon of bone deposited in sites subjected to stress and reabsorbed in sites where there is little stress is known as Wolff's law. This is exemplified by marked cortical thickening on the concave side of a curved bone. The trabeculae align along the lines of weight-bearing stress in the internal architecture of the bone.

Bone healing consists of several phases that occur concurrently: inflammation, soft callus formation, hard callus formation, and remodeling. Soft and hard callus formation is equivalent to the proliferative phase of wound healing. *Soft callus* is the term given to soft, collagenous, revascularizing, osteogenic tissue that unites the bone fragments and from which bone regenerates. In primary bone healing, new Haversian systems or osteons are regenerated across the site of the fracture. Osteoclasts assemble at ends of the Haversian canals near the fracture site forming spearheads or cutting cones, which advance at a rate of 50–80 μm per day across the fracture, enlarging the canals as they advance. These are closely followed by osteoblasts, which form new Haversian systems in the enlarged canals and cross the fracture site to link bone fragments. The entire process takes about 5 or 6 weeks; however, any major surgical intervention increases the trauma to the tissues and may prolong the healing process (4,7). Excessive motion at the site or an infection may also prolong healing.

Comparison of Cartilage and Bone

Like cartilage, bone consists of cells and an organic intercellular matrix, which in turn consists of collagen fibers embedded in an amorphous component. The osteocytes of bone, like the chondrocytes of cartilage, live in lacunae within a matrix. Just as a cartilage structure is covered with *perichondrium*, the outer surface of a bone is covered with a membrane called *periosteum*. Finally, bone tissue, like cartilage, develops from a mesenchymal model (4).

Unlike cartilage, however, bone is a highly vascular, living, constantly changing, and mineralized connective tissue. It is remarkable for its hardness, resilience, characteristic growth mechanisms, regenerative capacity, and its stone-like resistance to bending during weight bearing. While all bone consists of cells embedded in an amorphous and fibrous organic matrix permeated by inorganic bone salts, its fine structure varies widely with age, site, and natural history. Thus, bone may develop either by the direct transformation of condensed mesenchyme, or it may be preceded by a cartilaginous model, later replaced by bone. The inorganic matrix may exist as irregular, dense masses with scattered bone cells, or it may be arranged as a series of thin sheets (lamellae) in a variety of patterns, with intervening rows of bone cells. Both lamellar and nonlamellar bone often develops as minute rough cylindrical masses or *osteons*, each with a central vascular canal.

Bone nutrition differs from that of cartilage. If the lacunae in which osteocytes live were solidly calcified, no diffusion of nutrients could occur. The osteocytes would die just as chondrocytes die if the matrix surrounding them becomes calcified. Microscopic evidence shows that osteocytes in calcified bone are connected to each other and to a canal, or to some other surface where there is tissue fluid, by what appears as fine lines. These lines, called *canaliculi*, are tiny tubular passageways through the calcified matrix. They contain tissue fluid and hair-like cytoplasmic processes of osteocytes that connect osteocytes together. Canaliculi provide the means for nutrients to reach osteocytes, thus keeping them alive within a calcified matrix (7).

SKELETAL MUSCLE

Muscle fibers are the cellular units of skeletal muscle and are bound by a plasma membrane called the *sarcolemma*. This membrane encloses numerous nuclei and a large amount of cytoplasm called *sarcoplasm*. Groupings of muscle fibers (fasciculi) can vary in size and pattern depending on the individual muscle. Connective tissue sheaths surround different components of the muscle, including the delicate network between muscle fibers termed the *endomysium*; a stronger *perimysium* ensheathing individual fascicles of muscle fibers; and *epimysium*, which encases the entire muscle and is continuous with the perimysium and the connective tissue external to the muscle.

Skeletal muscles vary considerably in size, shape, fascicular architecture, type of fiber, and attachment to bone. Each muscle is composed of numerous longitudinal cylindrical myofibrils, which provide range, direction, velocity, and force of action appropriate to the particular joint. Myofilaments of actin and myosin are located on the myofibrils, forming serial units called *sarcomeres* visible only with an electron microscope. Sarcomeres are considered the functional unit of skeletal muscle.

Contraction and Relaxation

Much has been written on the contraction of skeletal muscle. Individual muscle fibers demonstrate differences in their rates of contraction, development of tension, and susceptibility to fatigue. All of these are characteristics that classify muscle fibers according to the type of metabolic and contractile properties they display (26–28). Three fiber types have been identified: type I, slow-twitch oxidative fibers; type IIA, fast-twitch oxidative-glycolytic fibers; and type IIB, fast-twitch glycolytic fibers. Type I fibers are characterized by a relatively slow contraction time and have a high potential for aerobic activity. Very difficult to fatigue, type I fibers are capable of prolonged, low intensity work. Myoglobin content is high in these fibers, giving the muscle a distinct red color.

Type IIA muscle fibers have a fast contraction time, providing a moderately well developed capacity to do both aerobic and anaerobic work. Possessing a well developed blood supply, they can maintain contractile activity for relatively long periods as long as the rate of activity does not exceed the ability of the fiber to utilize adenosine triphosphate (ATP). Once exceeded, the muscle will fatigue. Myoglobin content is fairly high in this muscle type; therefore, it is often classified as red muscle.

Type IIB fibers contain very little myoglobin and are often referred to as white muscle. These fibers rely primarily upon glycolytic (anaerobic) activity for ATP production. Very few capillaries appear in the vicinity of these fibers. While type IIB fibers can produce energy rapidly, they fatigue quickly as their high rate of ATP utilization depletes the glycogen needed for their metabolism. These large muscles can produce considerable tension for a short period of time before they fatigue (26–28).

Researchers have demonstrated that the innervation to the muscle fiber determines the type it will become; thus, each motor unit innervates a single type of muscle fiber. The fiber composition of a muscle depends on the function of that muscle. The soleus muscle of the calf is an example of a muscle with a high percentage of type I fibers, which are necessary in a postural muscle. Muscles that perform both endurance and strength activities are generally composed of a mixture of the 3 fiber types. Controversy exists as to whether fiber types are genetically determined.

The most widely held theory of muscle contraction is the sliding filament theory proposed by Huxley et al (29) and refined by others (30,31). As proposed, muscle contraction requires the sarcomere to actively shorten due to the relative movement of the actin and myosin filaments past one another in response to a variety of stimuli. Wilkie (32) described the activity of the actin and myosin during muscle contraction to be "similar to a man pulling on a rope hand over hand."

Once the motor neuron has initiated an action potential along the sarcolemma, an orderly sequence of events occurs. From the sarcolemma, the action potential proceeds through the T-tubule system to the sarcoplasmic reticulum, resulting in the release of calcium into the sarcoplasm. Calcium concentrations increase, causing release of actin. This allows actin and myosin cross-linkages or bridges to proceed, leading to shortening of the myofilaments. Shortening continues until the calcium source is actively pumped back into the sarcoplasmic reticulum, thus breaking the cross-linkages between actin and myosin and allowing the muscle to relax. Both contraction and relaxation of the muscle are active processes.

Energy Metabolism

Energy for cross-linkage between actin and myosin is provided in the form of hydrolysis of ATP to diphosphate ($ADP+P_1$) by an ATPase. The splitting of ATP releases energy for the mechanical work of moving the actin filaments along the myosin filaments. Once ATP is hydrolyzed, the remaining ADP and free phosphate leave the binding site on the myosin. ATP provides the energy required to release a contraction of the myofilaments. The muscle relaxes when new ATP is bound

to the myosin, promptly disassociating actin from myosin by breaking the cross-linkage. Absence of ATP would result in permanent bonding between actin and myosin as seen in rigor mortis.

JOINT MECHANICS AND MOVEMENT

A classification scheme for the shape of synovial joints is shown in Figure 1. Movement of joints is often taken for granted and the complexity for accomplishing movement not consciously considered. Kinesiology and biomechanics have become intricate and complex sciences made more intriguing when a joint has been affected by a rheumatic disease. The study of the structure, function, and movement of joints is called *arthrokinesiology.*

Fundamental Joint Positions

Joint surfaces are capable of becoming fully congruent with each other at some point in the movement of the joint. At this juncture, the soft tissues around the joint become elongated, tense, and slightly stretched. One example occurs during full extension of the knee and is called the *close-packed position* of the knee. No further intrinsic motion can occur and an excessive external force applied to the knee may disrupt tissues. Close-packing is the terminal limiting position of the joint; any further attempt to increase motion will be resisted by reflex protective contraction of the associated muscles around the joint. Excessive close-packing can cause deformation of the ligaments and joint structures, including the articular cartilage.

When the joint capsule is lax and the articular surfaces are not congruent, the joint is said to be in the *loose-packed position.* In mid-position of the range of motion, capsules are lax enough that an external force to the knee may allow separation of the bony surfaces. This concept is the basis for using mobilization techniques to increase the motion of a joint following knee surgery, for example. Furthermore, the loose-packed position allows normal movement to occur in joints. Thus, loose-packed positions are important for joint mobility, while close-packed positions are necessary for joint stability (3,4).

Kinematics

The study of the motion within the joint or between bones is called *kinematics,* without regard for the force that caused the motion. *Osteokinematics* is a subcategory of kinematics that describes the motion of a rotating bone around an axis that is oriented perpendicular to the path of the moving bone. An example of osteokinematics would be a description of the relationship between the femur and the tibia when the knee is flexed or extended. Another way of describing the osteokinematics of bone is by linkages. An open kinematic chain describes the relationship of a moving distal bone to a proximal stable bone (foot and tibia moving on a stable femur). A closed kinematic chain describes the relationship of a proximal moving bone to a distal stable bone (foot and tibia fixed on the floor and femur moving).

Arthrokinematics describes the motions occurring within the joint or between joint surfaces. In the case of the knee, the femoral condyles, tibial plateaus, and patella are related to each other during these motions. Because the femoral condyles are smooth and rounded, whereas the tibial plateaus are more flattened with a meniscus on each, the arthrokinematics of the motions of flexion and extension require the bones to slide, spin, and roll. These intricate movements require the joint to be in loose-packed position.

Kinetics

Kinetics comprises the unique science of biomechanics and describes the forces and torques necessary to cause the joint to move. Active forces are generally produced by muscle contraction. Passive forces may be generated by the intrinsic structures of the joint such as the joint capsule, ligaments, or other connective tissues. When evaluating joint motion kinetically, consideration must be given to the ability of the muscle to produce force, the integrity of bone and joint structures, the amount of work the muscle can generate, and the power or rate at which the muscle can perform the work. External forces such as gravity, body weight, and general health of the person should also be considered.

Types of Movement

There are a variety of descriptions of the movement of joints (Figure 1); however, most joint movement could be considered to be translation, angulation, rotation, and circumduction. *Translation* (gliding) is sliding without rotation or angulation of the bone. It is a common arthrokinematic motion, which is frequently combined with other motions such as a spin or rolling on the joint surfaces. *Angulation* describes an osteokinematic movement of bones as seen in flexion/extension or abduction/adduction. *Rotation* is used to describe rotation around the longitudinal axis of a bone, as seen in pronation/supination of the forearm or internal/external rotation of the glenohumeral joint. *Circumduction* is commonly ascribed to ball and socket joints that circumscribe their movements in the shape of a cone, combining all of the above motions (3,4).

Axes of Movement

The type and shape of the synovial joint dictate the axes of movement. Axes of movement are usually perpendicular to the moving bone. However, bones have mechanical axes that run perpendicular to the articular center and allow the bone to rotate or spin in such movements as supination and pronation. Uniaxial joints commonly move in one plane of motion (sagittal, frontal, horizontal) such as flexion and extension; biaxial joints move in 2 planes such as flexion/extension and abduction/adduction; triaxial joints move in 3 planes of motion such as flexion/extension, abduction/adduction, and internal/external rotation; and multi- or polyaxial joints are capable of moving in all planes of motion, usually resulting in circumduction (4).

SUMMARY

Successful management of the joint impairment caused by rheumatic diseases can be enhanced if the health provider appreciates fully the intricate nature of the structures of the musculoskeletal system. Beyond the effects of rheumatic disease on the musculoskeletal system, considerations should also be given to the effects of age, medications, exercise history, and environment in which the person with arthritis must function. Understanding human movement involves integrating the knowledge of the anatomy, biomechanics, and arthrokinesiology of the musculoskeletal system; the attributes of the specific rheumatic disease and its impact on these structures; and an appreciation of the personal performance attributes and attitudes of the person with arthritis.

REFERENCES

1. Larsen WJ. Development of the limbs. In: Larsen WJ, editor. Human embryology. New York: Churchill-Livingstone; 1993. p. 281–307.
2. Viidik A. Biomechanics and functional adaptation of tendons and joint ligaments. In: Evans FG, editor. Studies on the anatomy and function of bones and joints. Berlin: Springer-Verlag; 1966. p. 17–39.
3. Norkin C, LeVange P. Biomechanics. In Norkin C, LeVange P, editors. Joint structure and function: a comprehensive analysis. Philadelphia: FA Davis; 1992. p. 3–51.
4. Williams PL, Bannister LH, Berry MM, Collins P, Dussek JE, Dyson M, et al. Skeletal system. In: Williams PL, Warwick R, Dyson M, Bannister LH, editors. Gray's anatomy. 38th ed. Edinburgh: Churchill-Livingstone; 1995. p. 425–736.
5. Smith JW. Muscular control of the arches of the foot in standing: an electromyographic assessment. J Anat 1954;88:152–63.
6. Key JA. The reformation of synovial membrane in knees of rabbits after synovectomy. J Bone Joint Surg 1925;7:793–813.
7. Ham AW, Cormack DH. Histophysiology of cartilage, bone and joints. Philadelphia: JB Lippincott; 1979.
8. Hilton J. Lecture VII. In: Jacobson WHA, editor. On rest and pain: a course of lectures on the influence of mechanical and physiological rest in the treatment of accidents and surgical diseases, and the diagnostic value of pain. New York: William Wood; 1879. p. 96.
9. Wyke B. The neurology of joints: a review of general principles. Clin Rheum Dis 1981;7:223–39.
10. Myers ER, Mow VC. Biomechanics of cartilage and its response to biomechanical stimuli. In Hall BK, editor. Cartilage. Vol. 1. Structure, function and biochemistry. New York: Academic Press; 1983. p. 313–41.
11. Mow VC, Proctor CS, Kelly MA. Biomechanics of articular cartilage. In: Nordin M, Frankel VH, editors. Basic biomechanics of the musculoskeletal system. 2nd ed. Philadelphia: Lea & Febiger; 1989. p. 5–8.
12. Simkin PA. The musculoskeletal system. A. Joints. In: Schumacher HR, Klippel JH, Koopman WF, editors. Primer on the rheumatic diseases. 10th ed. Atlanta: Arthritis Foundation; 1993. p. 5–8.
13. Charnley J. The lubrication of animal joints. In: Proceedings of the Symposium on Biomechanics. London: Institution of Mechanical Engineers; 1959. p. 12–9.
14. McCutcheon CW. Boundary lubrication by synovial fluid: demonstration and possible osmotic explanation. Fed Proc 1966;25:1061–8.
15. Swann DA, Radin EL, Hendren RB. The lubrication of articular cartilage by synovial fluid glycoproteins [abstract]. Arthritis Rheum 1979;22:665–6.
16. Swann DA, Silver FH, Slayter HS, Stafford W, Shore E. The molecular structure and lubricating activity of lubricin isolated from bovine and human synovial fluids. Biochem J 1985;225:195–201.
17. Mankin JH, Buckwalter JA. Restoring the osteoarthritis joint. J Bone Joint Surg Am 1996;78:1–2.
18. Buckwalter JA. Articular cartilage: injuries and potential for healing. J Orthop Sports Phys Ther 1998;28:192–202.
19. Buckwalter JA, Mankin HJ. Articular cartilage. II. Degeneration and osteoarthrosis, repair, regeneration and transplantation. J Bone Joint Surg Am 1997;79:612–32.
20. Buckwalter JA, Rosenberg LA, Hunziker EB. Articular cartilage: composition, structure, response to injury, and methods of facilitation of repair. In: Ewing JW, editor. Articular cartilage and knee joint: basic science and arthroscopy. New York: Raven Press; 1996. p. 19–56.
21. Buckwalter JA, Rosenberg LC, Coutts R, Hunziker E, Reddi AH, Mow AC. Articular cartilage: injury and repair. In: Woo SL, Buckwalter JA, editors. Injury and repair of the musculoskeletal soft tissue. Park Ridge (IL): American Academy of Orthopaedic Surgeons Symposium; 1988. p. 83–96.

22. Buckwalter JA. Mechanical injuries of articular cartilage. In: Finerman G, editor. Biology and biomechanics of the traumatized synovial joint: the knee as a model. Rosemont (IL): American Academy of Orthopaedic Surgions Symposium; 1992. p. 83–96.

23. Buckwalter JA, Mow VC. Cartilage repair in osteoarthritis. In: Moskowitz RW, Howell DS, Goldberg VM, Mankin HJ, editors. Osteoarthritis: diagnosis, medical and surgical management. Philadelphia: WB Saunders; 1992. p. 71–107.

24. Carlstedt CA, Nordin M. Biomechanics of tendons and ligaments. In: Nordin M, Frankel VH, editors. Basic biomechanics of the musculoskeletal system. 2nd ed. Philadelphia: Lea & Febiger; 1989. p. 59–74.

25. Kear M, Smith RN. A method for recording tendon strain in sheep during locomotion. Acta Orthop Scand 1975;46:896–905.

26. Astrand P-O, Rodahl K. Textbook of work physiology: physiological basis for exercise. 2nd ed. New York: McGraw Hill; 1977.

27. Engel WK. Fiber-type nomenclature of human skeletal muscle for histochemical purposes. Neurology 1974;25:344–8.

28. Huxley AF. Muscular contraction. J Physiol 1974;243:1–43.

29. Huxley AF, Huxley HE. Organizers of a discussion of the physical and chemical basis of muscular contraction. Proc R Soc Lond B Biol Sci 1964;160:433–7.

30. Huxley HE. The mechanism of muscular contraction. Science 1969;164: 1356–66.

31. Weber A, Murray JM. Molecular control mechanisms in muscular contraction. Physiol Rev 1973;53:612–73.

32. Wilkie DR. The mechanical properties of muscle. Br Med Bull 1956;12: 177–82.

Additional Recommended Reading

Kelley WN. Textbook of rheumatology. 4th ed. Philadelphia: Saunders; 1993.

Klippel JH, Dieppe P. Rheumatology. St. Louis, London: Mosby; 1994.

Williams PK. Gray's anatomy: the anatomical basis of medicine and surgery. 38th ed. New York: Churchill-Livingstone; 1995.

CHAPTER 2

Epidemiology of Rheumatic Diseases

MARIAN T. HANNAN, DSc

Rheumatic disorders affect more than 37 million Americans and include over 100 different conditions (1–3). Nearly one-third of adults in the United States have signs or symptoms of arthritis (2), and arthritis is cited as the leading cause of disability in US adults (4). In fact, rheumatic disease is the main reason why adults over age 65 visit a physician. *Epidemiology*, the study of the occurrence of disease in populations and of factors that may cause disease, provides the tools to understand the impact and potential causes of rheumatic diseases.

Epidemiologic studies may provide prevalence estimates for a population, or information on the scope of the problem, although they also examine risk factors, leading to inferences on causality and allowing insight into disease biology or modification of risk factors. This chapter reviews current epidemiologic knowledge on incidence and prevalence rates as well as findings from epidemiologic studies for osteoarthritis, rheumatoid arthritis, gout, fibromyalgia, osteoporosis, systemic lupus erythematosus, juvenile rheumatoid arthritis, and ankylosing spondylitis.

PATTERNS OF RHEUMATIC DISEASE

Rheumatic and musculoskeletal conditions are the most prevalent chronic conditions in the US, reported by nearly 15% of the population (2,5). The musculoskeletal regions most often affected are the knees, hips, hands, lower back, and neck. Although the primary cause for most rheumatic diseases remains unknown, age and gender clearly play a role. More than two-thirds of those affected by rheumatic disease are women (3). Rheumatic diseases affect all age groups, although typically the prevalence is highest among the elderly. In 1990 the CDC reported that the average annual prevalence of self-reported arthritis increased linearly with age, showing rates higher in women at all ages compared to men (5). In an analysis of rankings of chronic medical conditions in the US, arthritis was the most common condition in both women (544.1 per 1,000) and men (382.6 per 1,000) over age 65 years, followed in ranking by high blood pressure and hearing impairment (6).

Rheumatic diseases are associated with more disability, impairment, and job loss among older workers than any other disease (2,4,6) (see also Chapter 42, Work Disability). These figures and the overall impact of the rheumatic diseases are cause for current and future concern. As the population continues to age and grow in number, the CDC estimates that by the year 2020 nearly 60 million people will be affected by rheumatic diseases (5).

OSTEOARTHRITIS

Osteoarthritis (OA) is the most common rheumatic disease as well as the most common painful and disabling joint disorder. It may be defined in epidemiologic studies using either radiographic criteria or clinical criteria that incorporate radiographs, pain symptoms, and clinical signs; however, concordance between these different definitions is poor (7–10). Figure 1 shows the discordance between 3 definitions of arthritis; note in particular that symptomatic knee pain often does not correlate with radiographic changes, and, among the subjects with radiographic knee changes, only half also reported knee pain (10). It is important to examine the criteria for definitions when studying or reporting OA findings, particularly when mild disease is included. Definitions of OA in epidemiologic studies typically include both symptomatic and radiographic aspects. In hips and knees, severe radiographic disease is very likely to produce symptoms that are often disabling (7,8,11).

Clinical signs of osteoarthritis include slowly developing joint pain, aching, and stiffness with limitation of motion. Radiographic signs include osteophytes, joint space narrowing, and sclerosis. Two US population surveys estimate that 37% of adults have some degree of radiographic OA, with roughly one-quarter of those having moderate or severe disease (7–9). Women are at least twice as likely to be affected as men. While symptomatic onset typically occurs after age 45, pathologic evidence of OA is almost universal in elderly persons and clinical signs are common.

The weight-bearing lower extremity joints and hand joints are typically affected by OA. The distribution of joints appears to differ by race. African Americans have a higher age-adjusted prevalence of knee OA than whites, and yet no difference is seen at the hip or hand joints (7,9,12). Recent data from the Johnson County OA study do not support a race difference in prevalence of knee OA; however, increased severity in knee OA in African Americans was noted (13). European Caucasians have been reported to have a higher prevalence of hip OA than African or Jamaican blacks, a fact often attributed to a higher rate of developmental hip disorders among Europeans.

Although much is known of the prevalence of OA, relatively little is known of the incidence and progression in populations. Data from the population-based Framingham Study showed that women's incidence of knee OA was 1.7 times higher than the rate for men (14). Among elderly participants, 2% developed incident radiographic knee OA each year, while about 4% per year experienced progressive knee OA. Incidence of hand OA based on data from the Baltimore Longitudinal Study of Aging as well as the Tecumseh Study also showed approximately 4% increase per year (7).

Several risk factors for osteoarthritis have been implicated by epidemiologic studies (Table 1). Incidence is known to

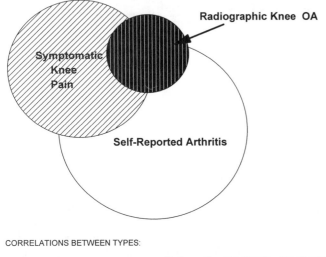

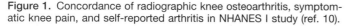

CORRELATIONS BETWEEN TYPES:

	Radiographic	Symptomatic	Any site arthritis
Radiographic knee changes (n = 319)	100%	47%	61%
Symptomatic knee pain (n = 1,004)	15%	100%	59%
Arthritis at any site (n = 1,762)	11%	34%	100%

Figure 1. Concordance of radiographic knee osteoarthritis, symptomatic knee pain, and self-reported arthritis in NHANES I study (ref. 10).

increase with advancing age, especially in women after age 45. Both prevalence and incidence of OA are higher in women (2,3,8,9). OA occurs not only most frequently in women but also with greater severity (2,3), including a larger number of involved joints and more frequent reports of morning stiffness, joint swelling, and pain at night (3,9). Women also have a much higher proportion of Heberden's nodes, or swelling of the distal interphalangeal joints of the hands, generally thought to be influenced by heredity (7). The causes of OA are probably multifactorial, such that the risk factors for OA in all joints are probably not the same, even if the biology of OA is the same (8,9).

Obesity is the second strongest risk factor for OA (7–9,12), especially in women and especially for knee involvement. Studies have shown that obesity precedes the development of OA (7,8), while weight loss lowers the risk of knee OA (15). How obesity causes OA is unknown. Some suggest increased joint loading due to weight, but obesity may also be associated with hand OA where there is no increased joint loading. Mechanical loading also does not explain the obesity association. It may be that obesity, through its association with increased bone density, causes stiff subchondral bone. Alterna-

Table 1. Risk factors for osteoarthritis (OA).

Known
  Age
  Female sex
  Obesity
  Major joint injury (trauma)
  Repeated overuse (especially occupational)
  Knee bending or lifting (knee OA)
  Heredity (Heberden's nodes)
  Prior inflammatory disease
  Developmental abnormality
Suspected or unconfirmed
  Heredity
  High bone mass
  Lack of estrogen replacement therapy
  Early hysterectomy/surgical menopause

Table 2. Occupations associated with increased rates of osteoarthritis.

	Joints involved
Cotton mill workers	Fingers—interphalangeal joints
Miners	Knees, spine
Jackhammer operators	Elbows, wrists, metacarpophalangeal joints
Farmers	Hips
Shipyard/dock workers	Knees, fingers
Ballet dancers	Ankles, feet

tively, obesity may reflect some metabolic effect in women that affects joints throughout the body.

Occupational knee bending and physical demands have been implicated as a risk factor for both clinical and radiographic knee OA (8,12,16,17). Major joint injury, common in sports and certain occupational activities, is a well-established risk factor (Table 2). Repetitive joint overuse is associated with OA and is considered by some as an extension of joint injury, especially in certain occupations. Many studies support the notion that OA is related to prolonged occupational overuse (7–9,18), including increased severity of OA in the dominant hand. Individuals with jobs requiring repetitive knee bending had more than twice the rate of knee OA compared to those with jobs not requiring such activity, even after controlling for known risk factors (12,17). Most epidemiologic studies show no association between sports activities and OA once major joint injury is accounted for in the analysis. For example, runners have no increased risk of knee or hip OA or joint instability (7,9). Early studies suggesting an association were probably confounded by the role played by joint injury.

Risk factors that are suspected but not proven include heritability, high bone mass, and absence of estrogen replacement therapy. Heberden's nodes are well-known for their sex-linked inheritance pattern, yet other anatomic sites are less clear. Heritability was implicated in a study describing early onset of severe generalized OA in 2 families with an abnormality in the type II procollagen gene, suggesting a genetic predisposition related to cartilage disorders (7,9). Genetic factors—perhaps associated with a major recessive gene—may account for a substantial number of hand and hip OA cases and, to a lesser extent, knee OA cases (19,20).

OA is thought to be inversely related to osteoporosis or low bone mineral density (BMD). However, several large studies have shown that increased BMD was only related to certain features of knee OA, notably knee osteophytosis, and not more severe knee OA (21,22). Finally, the relation between osteoarthritis and estrogen replacement therapy is unclear. Several studies report no increase in rates of osteoarthritis with estrogen replacement therapy, and further show a possible protective effect for women using postmenopausal estrogens for at least 4 years (23–25). Studies also report an association between OA and surgical menopause, possibly due to loss of estrogen. While these studies suggest a possible protective effect of estrogen, the extent to which these data are confounded by the overall healthy status of self-selected estrogen users is unclear.

Vitamin D deficiency has been recently reported to be associated with a 3-fold increased risk of knee OA (26) and similar risk for hip OA (27) in elderly populations. Lane et al also found mild acetabular dysplasia to be a risk factor for incident hip OA (28). In addition, major developmental abnormalities are known to contribute to early or premature hip OA (1,7–9).

RHEUMATOID ARTHRITIS

Rheumatoid arthritis (RA) is a chronic inflammatory disease of unknown cause and one of the more disabling rheumatic diseases. Prevalence definitions rely on the American College of Rheumatology (ACR) criteria for RA: morning stiffness for at least one hour, soft-tissue swelling of 3 or more joints, soft-tissue swelling of hand joints, symmetric arthritis, rheumatoid nodules, serum rheumatoid factor positive, and typical radiographic changes in the hand and wrist (7,9). The annual incidence is between 20 and 40 cases per 100,000 adults, with onset typically occurring between ages 20 and 45. Prevalence is about 0.8% in most white U.S. or European adult populations (2,7); American Indian populations have much higher prevalence rates. The two major risk factors for RA are increased age and female sex. Although it can occur at any age, both the incidence and prevalence of RA increase with age, and are 2 to 4 times higher in women compared to men at all ages (2,9,29). A recent report from the Mayo Clinic indicates a possible secular decline in the incidence and prevalence of RA in their population (29). Their findings lend support to the idea of a host–environment interaction in the pathogenesis of RA.

Genetic and hormonal factors are suspected to play a role in the development of RA, including oral contraceptive use and estrogen loss. Genetic factors may account for up to 30% of susceptibility. Family studies of first-degree relatives show a 3- to 4-fold higher risk of RA than those not related (7,9). However, most people closely related to someone with RA do not develop the disease, implying that penetrance is relatively low. Some genetic susceptibility is due to the shared epitope, an identical genetic sequence in the HLA type II region found in a large percentage of persons with RA.

The influence of hormonal factors is suggested by the following observations: RA is more common in women than men; up to 75% of RA cases in women remit during pregnancy and flare is likely after pregnancy; and in several case series, men with RA had low circulating testosterone levels (3,7,9). Despite the suggested hormonal link, the role of oral contraceptives as well as postmenopausal estrogens remains unclear. A large British cohort study of women using oral contraceptives found lower rates of RA, but other studies found no association (3,9). Similarly, a study of postmenopausal estrogen use reported that it protected against RA, while this finding was not confirmed in 2 other large studies (3,7,9).

GOUT

Gout is a common rheumatic disorder in middle-aged and older men, although elderly women also develop this disease, which is characterized by acute arthritis with deposits of crystals, an acute inflammatory response with elevated uric acid, and severe pain. The most common site for gout is the base of the big toe, followed by the ankle, heel, midfoot, and knee. Although gout is up to 2.5-fold more common in men than women (7), it also is associated with age, increasing in incidence and prevalence with age in both men and women (9). Prevalence rates per 1,000 range from 28.5 in men to 3.9 in women in the

Framingham Study (7,9). Others have reported a prevalence rate for gout of 8.4 per 1,000 in the U.S. in 1998. For individuals aged 45–64 years, the prevalence was 26.3 per 1,000 for men and 8.1 for women, while those aged 65 and older had rates of 44.1 per 1,000 for men and 18.2 for women (2). Incidence of gout follows a similar distribution, with males at greater risk than females in all age groups. In the U.K., incidence rates per 1,000 were reported in 1990 as 2.1 for men and 0.7 for women, while incidence rates in the Framingham Study were 1.6 for men and 0.2 for women (7).

In addition to male gender, risk factors include sustained hyperuricemia, obesity, diuretic use, and high alcohol intake (9), while cardiovascular disease is suspected to be related to gout. Clinical and population-based studies have implicated obesity with onset of gout, independent of uric acid levels. Several cohort and case–control studies (7) have shown a 3-fold increased risk for gout in those with hypertension, which went away after controlling for diuretic use. Alcohol intake, particularly beer intake, has been linked to occurrence of gout because it increases purine metabolism, producing more uric acid. Cardiovascular disease is suspected to be linked to gout, but the relation remains unclear (9). Lead intake (dietary and occupational), while rare now, is strongly related to gout, as reported in studies of moonshine liquor and of occupations formerly exposed to high levels of lead (plumbers, painters, and shipbuilders).

FIBROMYALGIA

Fibromyalgia is second only to OA in frequency in most clinical rheumatology practices (3,9). Clinical features include diffuse pain, stiffness, fatigue, and nonrestorative sleep with apparently normal laboratory tests and radiographs. In 1990 the ACR developed diagnostic criteria defined as "widespread pain in all four quadrants of the body for at least three months, and tenderness in at least 11 of 18 specified tender points" (7,9). A population-based study of Swedish adults aged 50–70 years reported prevalence of 1% or about double the rate of RA for this age group (3,9). A community-based prevalence study in Wichita, Kansas (30) found a prevalence of 3.7% in women and 0.5% in men. Prevalence was strongly age-related, increasing to 4.0% for women and men over age 60. While the typical clinical presentation is a woman between the ages of 25 and 45, the mean age of the Wichita study subjects with fibromyalgia was 59 years.

There are no known risk factors for fibromyalgia aside from the age and sex patterns reported in community-based samples and demographics seen in clinical patients. Common associations include major depression, sleep disturbance, and trauma injuring the neck or lower back. Fibromyalgia is difficult to study because case definitions depend on pain, a difficult entity to quantify and define. Nevertheless, roughly a third of patients implicate trauma as leading to symptom onset, one-third identify a viral illness, and one-third have no clear preceding factor (7,9). At this point there is no clear understanding of the condition, its possible causes, or potential prevention.

OSTEOPOROSIS

Osteoporosis is characterized by low bone mineral density (BMD) and enhanced bone fragility, which increase the risk of

Table 3. Risk factors for osteoporosis.

Known
  Age
  Female sex
  White or Asian ethnicity
  Hormonal factors, menstrual factors (oophorectomy, amenorrhea,
    hypogonadism)
  Low body weight
  Cigarette smoking
  Heredity factors
  Immobility
  Alcohol abuse
  Corticosteroid use
  Family history of fracture
Suspected or unconfirmed
  Lack of physical activity
  High caffeine intake
  Low calcium intake
  Low vitamin D levels

fracture. It is a common disorder in women over age 50 and is often diagnosed after a relatively atraumatic fracture. Osteoporosis accounts for at least 1.5 million fractures annually in the U.S. (3,7,9). The most common sites of osteoporotic fracture are the hip, wrist, and vertebrae. An estimated 15% of women will fracture their hip, and, of women who survive to age 85, one-third will have fractured their hip. Half of those who have a hip fracture are unable to walk independently again, and such fractures lead to 15–20% excess mortality rate.

Risk factors for osteoporosis are listed in Table 3. The incidence of osteoporosis dramatically increases with age. Women are affected nearly 5 times more often than men (3,7,9,31). Although osteoporosis also occurs in men, their loss of bone and of sex hormones occurs at a much lower rate, thus symptoms (i.e., fractures) show up later in life.

Abundant research indicates that estrogen deficiency due to menopause causes bone loss and fracture, and that estrogen replacement therapy prevents or slows the increased risk (3,7,9), even in elderly women (32). Loss of estrogen, including premature menopause in women and gonadal failure in men, is a major cause of bone loss. Excessive exercise leading to amenorrhea in younger women also causes low BMD and osteoporosis. Low weight and thin body build are additional risk factors for osteoporosis, perhaps mediated by estrogen mechanisms. Increased weight is associated with increased BMD and higher estrogen levels after menopause, thus further protecting against bone loss. In addition, fat may protect against fracture by cushioning a fall and absorbing the impact.

Immobility is a suspected risk factor for osteoporosis because decreased weight bearing increases bone resorption. Patients confined to bed lose 4% of bone mass each month and are at increased risk for fracture (3). Factors thought to be implicated in osteoporosis include a family history of fracture, genetic factors related to attainment of peak bone mass, smoking, and caffeine consumption (3,7,9). Other risk factors include decreased physical activity, low calcium intake, alcohol abuse, low vitamin D levels, excessive amounts of thyroid replacement drugs, corticosteroids, certain diuretics, and anticoagulants.

SYSTEMIC LUPUS ERYTHEMATOSUS

Systemic lupus erythematosus (SLE, lupus) is characterized by the presence of multiple autoantibodies that take part in immune-mediated tissue injury, damaging joints, blood, kidneys, skin, and the central nervous system. Symptoms may include skin rash, fever, weakness, fatigue, or weight loss. Common clinical features include joint pain, muscle aches, swollen glands, lack of appetite, and nausea as well as irregular menstrual periods. SLE is a relatively uncommon disease with estimated prevalence rates ranging from 15 to 52 cases per 100,000 adults (7,9). It affects women 8–10 times more often than men, particularly women ages 20–35 (3,7). Age-specific prevalence in women aged 15–64 years is about 100 per 100,000 in whites and 400 per 100,000 in African Americans (7). Lupus occurs more frequently in African Americans; Filipino women, in addition to American Indian, Hispanic, Puerto Rican, and perhaps Chinese women, may have an increased risk of developing SLE compared to whites (7). Several studies have reported a secular increase in the incidence of SLE; however, part of this increase is certainly due to the now widespread use of serologic testing to identify SLE cases. Annual incidence of SLE is estimated at 2–8 cases per 100,000 (7,9).

Lupus may be influenced both by hormonal factors and by genetic predisposition. Women have a higher incidence and prevalence than men, and in most clinical series women account for 90% of SLE cases. The onset of SLE in women between the ages of 15 and 45 is well documented, and this female propensity is not seen in children or in elders (3,7). The female:male ratio in prevalence and incidence ranges from 5:1 to 10:1, to a high of approximately 15:1 in one large series (7,9). In addition to female sex, black race is a major risk factor for both incident disease and poor outcome in SLE studies, including kidney failure, infection, and mortality (7,33). Hormonal factors are implicated by the great sex differential in SLE as well as the facts that women with lupus are at increased risk of miscarriage and that onset of lupus frequently occurs at menarche or during pregnancy (7,9,34,35). Several small studies report abnormalities in estrogen metabolism in lupus patients of both sexes compared to controls. The abnormalities produced stronger estrogen effects that lasted longer with weaker androgenic effects, particularly in women. Oral contraceptive use has been suspected as a triggering agent; however, a number of case–control studies reported no association (7,9). SLE tends to worsen during late pregnancy and in the immediate postpartum period.

Available evidence supports a genetic predisposition to SLE. About 10% of patients report having an affected first-degree relative, and concordance is greater in monozygotic compared to dizygotic twins (7,9). Yet, while family studies report higher rates of disease, autoantibodies are increased not only in first-degree relative of SLE patients but also in nonrelated individuals sharing the same household. In addition, certain drugs or chemical compounds are thought to induce idiopathic lupus. Despite speculation that hair dyes and infectious agents may be related to SLE, recent studies report no association (36).

JUVENILE RHEUMATOID ARTHRITIS

Juvenile rheumatoid arthritis (JRA) is a chronic synovial inflammation of unknown cause with onset prior to age 16. It contains several subsets. Polyarticular seropositive JRA ("true" RA beginning in childhood) comprises about 40% of JRA, with girls affected twice as often as boys. The risk factors for seropositive polyarticular JRA closely resemble adult-onset RA. Pauciarticular JRA accounts for an additional 40% of JRA and affects 4 or fewer joints within the first 6 months of symptom onset. The onset before age 6 is primarily in females, whereas disease at an older age occurs mainly in males, often with a positive family history for spondylarthropathy. Still's disease is a systemic form of the disease, comprising 20% of JRA with an equal ratio of boys to girls. Whether the subgroups arise from different causes or varying responses to a common cause is not known (37). Estimated prevalence ranges from 200 per 100,000 for girls to 30 per 100,000 for boys, and affects 60,000 to 200,000 children in the U.S. (9). Prevalence of JRA appears to be 7 times higher in girls than boys, and the prevalence is comparable between blacks and whites. Peak incidence occurs at 1–2 years of age (7,37). Incidence data are limited but appear to range from 2.2 to 14 per 100,000 (7,9).

Relatively little is known of risk factors for JRA, other than the age and sex patterns noted above. Heritability is suspected in the occurrence of JRA, as the disease shows higher concordance rates among monozygotic (44%) than dizygotic (4%) twins, yet JRA rarely occurs in the same family. Familial aggregation and several reports of HLA associations with different clinical subsets of JRA also lend further support to the presence of genetic predisposition. Both rubella virus and Lyme disease infections have been suggested as possible triggering agents, but the role for infectious agents remains unclear (7,9).

ANKYLOSING SPONDYLITIS

Ankylosing spondylitis (AS) is an arthritis of the sacroiliac joints and spine with the primary pathologic site of inflammation at the insertion of ligaments and capsules into bone. Inflammation may cause the vertebrae to grow bony bridges that lead to fusion with adjacent vertebrae. AS usually has an insidious onset and affects individuals between ages 16 and 35; roughly 5% of spondylitis starts in adolescence. The prevalence of AS is 0.1–1% of the adult U.S. population (7,9), although the 1% figure is thought to be high. Prevalence estimates for women previously were reported to be 70 per 100,000 or nearly two-thirds lower than the rate for men (190 per 100,000) (7). Ankylosing spondylitis is predominantly a male disease with a male:female ratio of 4:1. Although recent medical texts suggest a male tendency for more severe disease, most also note that ankylosing spondylitis in women may be underdiagnosed (3,7,9). African Americans have prevalence rates that are approximately one-fourth the rate of whites; however, prevalence is higher in certain American Indian populations, such as the Haida and Pima Indians (7,9). There are few incidence studies of AS, but data from Rochester, Minnesota report an age-adjusted incidence rate of 12 per 100,000 in men and 3 per 100,000 in women.

Prevalence is highly correlated with variation in the frequency of the histocompatibility antigen, HLA–B27 for both men and women. While people with this marker do not always develop AS, they are more likely to develop the disease than those without HLA–B27. The frequency of HLA–B27 in persons with AS ranges from 88% to 96%, compared with 4–8% in controls (7). Familial aggregation of ankylosing spondylitis is well known, and the genetic disposition is further supported by twin studies. In addition, some have suggested that a trigger (e.g., infectious agents or environmental agents such as *Klebsiella* bacterium) may be important in the development of ankylosing spondylitis (7,9).

OTHER RHEUMATIC DISEASES

Other rheumatic diseases are not covered due to space limitations, however several references provide excellent coverage of their epidemiologic aspects (7–9). These include Lyme disease, systemic sclerosis or scleroderma, myopathies, giant cell arteritis and other vasculitides, and conditions such as low back pain.

FUTURE RESEARCH

Much of the clinical work in rheumatology has focused appropriately on treatment and symptom relief. Yet in order to understand occurrence of rheumatologic diseases and suggest preventive measures, more information is needed about risk factors and possible interactions. The primary cause for most rheumatic diseases remains unknown. Etiologic investigations need to be woven increasingly around the interrelationships of risk factors, particularly genetic, immunologic, environmental, and endocrinologic factors. The high rate of certain rheumatic diseases in certain epidemiologic subsets needs to be examined for etiologic components. Population-based longitudinal studies are needed to provide information on underserved populations such as African Americans and the elderly.

Epidemiology is a science that shows patterns of disease, allowing a focus on causality and perhaps insight into intervention. An estimated 22.8 million women are affected with arthritis and rheumatic conditions, and 4.6 million limit their activities because of rheumatic disease (38). In addition, the prevalence of these conditions is projected to increase 21% by the year 2020. While certain rheumatic diseases have garnered a reasonably large body of knowledge, major knowledge gaps exist. More information is needed on long-term outcomes, natural history, incidence, preservation of function, use of biomarkers to intervene earlier in the disease process, and the safety (and perhaps protective effects) of common hormone interventions such as oral contraceptives and estrogen replacement by women. Epidemiologic studies continue to examine clinical groups of patients and populations for explanatory risk factors to determine the occurrence and patterns seen in the rheumatic diseases. These studies, especially when linked to basic science research, may yield insights into disease etiology. Clinical intervention beyond pain relief is a goal still in the future for many rheumatic diseases.

Findings from epidemiologic studies of rheumatic diseases may be used to describe which subgroups are most affected by rheumatic diseases and to plan treatments and public health efforts. Risk factors for rheumatic diseases must be examined to seek clues as to etiology and primary interventions. Possible explanations for risk factor differences must be developed. Definitive work is needed on the detection of risk factors as well as evaluation of the impact of rheumatic disease and possible personal interventions.

REFERENCES

1. Kelsey JL. Epidemiology of musculoskeletal disorders. New York: Oxford University Press; 1982.
2. Lawrence RC, Helmick CG, Arnett FC, Deyo RA, Felson DT, Giannini EH, et al. Estimates of the prevalence of arthritis and selected musculoskeletal disorders in the United States. Arthritis Rheum 1998;41:778–99.
3. Hannan MT. Epidemiologic perspectives on women and arthritis: an overview. Arthritis Care Res 1996;9:424–34.
4. Centers for Disease Control and Prevention. Prevalence of disabilities and associated health conditions among adults, U.S., 1999. MMWR Morb Mortal Wkly Rep 2000;50:120–5.
5. Centers for Disease Control and Prevention. Arthritis prevalence and activity limitations–United States, 1990. MMWR Morb Mortal Wkly Rep 1994;43:433–8.
6. Verbrugge L, Patrick D. Seven chronic conditions: their impact on US adults' activity levels and use of medical services. Am J Public Health 1994;85:173–81.
7. Silman AJ, Hochberg MC. Epidemiology of the rheumatic diseases. New York: Oxford University Press; 1993.
8. Felson DT, Lawrence RC, Dieppe PA, Hirsch R, Helmick CG, Jordan JM, et al. Osteoarthritis: new insights. Part 1. The disease and its risk factors. Ann Intern Med 2000;133:635–46.
9. Hochberg MC, editor. Epidemiology of the rheumatic diseases. Rheum Dis Clin North Am 1990;16:499–781.
10. Hannan MT, Pincus T, Felson DT. Analysis of the discordance between radiographic changes and knee pain in osteoarthritis of the knee. J Rheumatol 2000;27:1513–8.
11. Felson DT, Zhang Y. An update on the epidemiology of knee and hip osteoarthritis with a view to prevention [review]. Arthritis Rheum 1998;41:1343–55.
12. Anderson J, Felson DT. Factors associated with knee osteoarthritis (OA) in the HANES I survey, evidence for an association with overweight, race and physical demands of work. Am J Epidemiol 1988;128:179–89.
13. Clark AG, Jordan JM, Vilim V, Renner JB, Dragomir AD, Luta G, et al. Serum cartilage oligomeric matrix protein reflects osteoarthritis presence and severity: the Johnston County Osteoarthritis Project. Arthritis Rheum 1999;42:2356–64.
14. Felson DT, Zhang Y, Hannan MT, Naimark A, Weissman BN, Aliabadi P, et al. The incidence and natural history of knee osteoarthritis in the elderly: the Framingham Osteoarthritis Study. Arthritis Rheum 1995;38:1500–5.
15. Felson DT, Zhang Y, Anthony JM, Naimark A, Anderson JJ. Weight loss reduces the risk of symptomatic knee osteoarthritis in women: the Framingham Study. Ann Intern Med 1992;116:535–9.
16. Cooper C, McAlindon T, Coggon D, Egger P, Dieppe P. Occupational activity and OA of the knee. Ann Rheum Dis 1994;53:90–3.
17. Felson DT, Hannan MT, Naimark A, Berkeley J, Gordon G, Wilson PWF, et al. Occupational physical demands, knee bending and knee osteoarthritis: results from the Framingham Study. J Rheumatol 1991;18:1587–92.
18. Lawrence JS. Rheumatism in cotton operatives. Br J Ind Med 1961;18:270–6.
19. Felson DT, Couropmitree NN, Chaisson CE, Hannan MT, Zhang Y, McAlindon TE, et al. Evidence for a Mendelian gene in a segregation analysis of generalized radiographic osteoarthritis: the Framingham Study. Arthritis Rheum 1998;41:1064–71.
20. Spector TD, Cicuttini F, Baker J, Loughlin J, Hart D. Genetic influences on osteoarthritis in women: a twin study. BMJ 1996;312:940–3.
21. Hannan MT, Anderson JJ, Zhang Y, Levy D, Felson DT. Bone mineral density and knee osteoarthritis in elderly men and women: the Framingham Study. Arthritis Rheum 1993;36:1671–80.
22. Nevitt MC, Lane NE, Scott JC, Hochberg MC, Pressman AR, Genant HK, et al. Radiographic osteoarthritis of the hip and bone mineral density. Arthritis Rheum 1995;38:907–16.
23. Hannan MT, Felson DT, Anderson JJ, Naimark A, Kannel WB. Estrogen use and radiographic osteoarthritis of the knee in women: the Framingham Osteoarthritis study. Arthritis Rheum 1990;33:525–32.
24. Nevitt MC, Cummings SR, Lane NE, Hochberg MC, Scott JC, Pressman AR, et al, Study of Osteoporotic Fractures Research Group. Association of estrogen replacement therapy with the risk of osteoarthritis of the hip in elderly white women. Arch Intern Med 1996;156:2073–80.
25. Zhang Y, McAlindon TE, Hannan MT, Chaisson CE, Klein R, Wilson PWF, et al. Estrogen replacement therapy and worsening of radiographic knee osteoarthritis: the Framingham Study. Arthritis Rheum 1998;41:1867–73.
26. McAlindon TE, Felson DT, Zhang Y, Hannan MT, Aliabadi P, Weissman B, et al. Relation of dietary intake and serum levels of vitamin D to progression of osteoarthritis of the knee among participants in the Framingham Study. Ann Intern Med 1996;125:353–9.
27. Lane NE, Gore LR, Cummings SR, Hochberg MC, Scott JC, Williams EN, et al, The Study of Osteoporotic Fractures Research Group. Serum vitamin D levels and incident changes of radiographic hip osteoarthritis: a longitudinal study. Arthritis Rheum 1999;42:854–60.
28. Lane NE, Lin P, Christiansen L, Gore LR, Williams EN, Hochberg MC, et al. Association of mild acetabular dysplasia with an increased risk of incident hip osteoarthritis in elderly white women: the study of osteoporotic fractures. Arthritis Rheum 2000;43:400–4.
29. Gabriel SE, Crowson CS, O'Fallon WM. The epidemiology of rheumatoid arthritis in Rochester, Minnesota, 1955–1985. Arthritis Rheum 1999;42:415–20.
30. Wolfe F, Ross K, Anderson J, Russell IJ, Hebert L. The prevalence and characteristics of fibromyalgia in the general population. Arthritis Rheum 1995;38:19–28.
31. Kleerekoper M, Avioli LV. Evaluation and treatment of postmenopausal osteoporosis. In: Favus MJ, editor. Primer on the metabolic bone diseases and disorders of mineral metabolism. 2nd ed. New York: Raven Press; 1993. p. 223–9.
32. Felson DT, Zhang Y, Hannan MT, Kiel DP, Wilson PW, Anderson JJ. The effect of postmenopausal estrogen therapy on bone density in elderly women. N Engl J Med 1993;329:1141–6.
33. McAlindon TE, Giannotta L, Taub N, D'Cruz D, Hughes G. Environmental factors predicting nephritis in SLE. Ann Rheum Dis 1993;52:720–4.
34. Petri M, Allbritton J. Fetal outcome of lupus pregnancy: a retrospective case-control study of the Hopkins lupus cohort. J Rheumatol 1993;20:650–6.
35. Lahita RG. Sex hormones and systemic lupus erythematosus. Rheum Dis Clin North Am 2000;26:951–68.
36. Hess EV, Farhey Y. Epidemiology, genetics, etiology and environmental relationships of systemic lupus erythematosus. Curr Opin Rheumatol 1994;6:474–80.
37. Cassidy JT. Juvenile rheumatoid arthritis. In: Kelley WM, Harris ED, Ruddy S, Sledge CB, editors. Textbook of rheumatology. 3rd ed. Philadelphia: WB Saunders; 1989. p. 1289–311.
38. Helmick CG, Lawrence RC, Pollard RA, Lloyd E, Heyse SP. Arthritis and other rheumatic conditions: who is affected now, who will be affected later? Arthritis Care Res 1995;8:203–11.

CHAPTER 3

Immunology, Inflammation, and Genetics

A. BETTS CARPENTER, MD, PhD

The immune system is a complex system crucial to our survival. It provides our primary defense against any foreign substances. Immunity may be thought of as innate or acquired. Innate immunity does not require previous exposure and involves phagocytic cells, natural physical barriers, and a special group of lymphocytes, termed *natural killer* (NK) cells. Acquired immunity has great specificity, requiring previous exposure to foreign pathogens, and involves lymphocytes. When referring to the immune system, one is usually referring to acquired (specific) immunity; however, in this review, components of both innate and acquired immunity will be discussed.

The specific immune system is divided into 2 parts: humoral and cellular, which relate to the response of distinct types of lymphocytes. *Humoral* responses are mediated by B lymphocytes, and they produce specific antibodies whose function is to neutralize foreign substances known as *antigens*. Antibody-mediated responses can be transferred from one individual to another by serum or plasma. Humoral immunity is predominantly concerned with protection against bacterial pathogens. *Cellular* responses are mediated by T lymphocytes, which produce soluble factors for the immune response. Cellular responses are transferred via cells, and are mainly involved with immunity against fungi, parasites, and intracellular bacteria (1–3).

CELLS OF THE IMMUNE SYSTEM

B Lymphocytes

B lymphocytes make up a major cell population vital to the immune system (1–4). They respond to extracellular antigens of many different types: proteins, lipids, nucleic acids, and others. The major mediators are known as B lymphocytes, because they are a product of an organ in the chicken, the Bursa of Fabricius. This organ is unique to the chicken; however, the mammalian equivalent is the bone marrow. B lymphocytes are the sole producers of proteins called immunoglobulins, which are termed *antibodies* when produced in response to a specific antigen. B lymphocytes have antigen-binding surface membrane receptors with the same specificity as the immunoglobulin that they secrete.

There are 5 major classes of immunoglobulins: IgM, IgG, IgA, IgE, and IgD. All immunoglobulins consist of at least 2 heavy chains (with a molecular weight of 50,000–70,000) and 2 light chains (with a molecular weight of 23,000) that form a basic Y shape (Figure 1). Each chain is composed of a *constant region*, in which the amino acids are relatively unchanged between different molecules, and a *variable region*, which is composed of different amino acids between different molecules. Within the variable region, there are areas with much

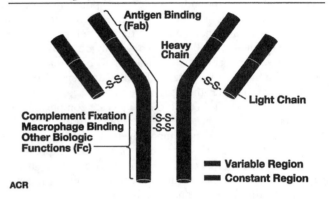

Figure 1. Antibody structure. Reprinted from the Clinical Slide Collection on the Rheumatic Diseases, copyright 1995 by the American College of Rheumatology.

variability of amino acids, the *hypervariable region*. These areas are responsible for the antigen-binding specificity of each immunoglobulin. The variable or "V" end of the molecule is where the antigen-binding specificity is located; this area is alternatively termed the Fab (fragment antigen-binding) region. The straight end of the molecule is composed exclusively of the constant region and is involved in other activities of the immune system, such as binding complement. It is termed the Fc region. Various inflammatory cells have Fc receptors that can bind immunoglobulin via their Fc end, which can facilitate phagocytosis of foreign particles.

Each of the 5 classes of immunoglobulins has distinctive characteristics. IgM is the largest immunoglobulin, with 5 unit immunoglobulin molecules. Its primary task is to respond to antigen on initial exposure. IgG is the most prevalent immunoglobulin in the serum, and it responds mostly to antigen on secondary exposure. IgA is predominantly produced by submucosal lymphocytes. This immunoglobulin provides protection at mucosal surfaces and is highly concentrated in tears, saliva, bronchial secretions, breast milk, intestinal fluids, and other body fluids. IgE mainly responds to allergens and is important in response to parasitic infections. IgD has the lowest concentration in the serum, is important mainly as a cell surface immunoglobulin, and has a role in differentiation of B cells.

Upon first exposure to an antigen, a resting B cell—with the help of T lymphocytes—responds by proliferating and differentiating into an activated B cell, which can produce antibodies to bind and neutralize specific antigens. With this first exposure (primary response), the major immunoglobulin produced is IgM; during subsequent responses, IgG is the predominant

15

immunoglobulin secreted. At the initial antigen exposure, there are several paths of differentiation the B cell can take. It may become an activated B cell, which can go on to an end stage of development, the plasma cell. These cells are chiefly found in organ sites, where they represent constitutive producers of antibodies. Alternatively, some B cells differentiate to form memory cells that allow the immune system to remember and respond quickly to antigen upon repeat exposure. These cells are responsible for the long-term efficacy of vaccines.

T Cells

T lymphocytes are the other major cell population of the specific immune system (1–4). They are initially produced in the bone marrow and then complete their development in the thymus, thus the term T cells. They provide vital defense against viruses, intracellular bacteria, fungi, protozoa, and tumor cells. In contrast to B cells, T cells can respond only to peptides, and only after they have been processed by antigen-presenting cells (APC). In addition, T cells are complexed with protein products of the major histocompatibility complex (MHC), a complex of genes important in the immune system (as described later in this chapter). The T cell expresses a protein on its surface that can bind antigen (cell surface antigen receptor). This is similar to the cell surface antigen receptor expressed on the B cell. B and T cells cannot be differentiated by microscopy. They must be identified by cell surface protein receptors, which in turn can be identified by their reactivity with monoclonal antibodies.

To simplify the many cellular subpopulations, each population has been given a CD (cluster of differentiation) designation followed by a number. All mature T cells are CD3 antigen positive, thus T cells are alternatively referred to as CD3 cells. The major T cell subpopulations are helper cells (CD4) and cytotoxic cells (CD8). Both CD4 and CD8 cells are crucial in the body's defense against infectious agents. The role of CD4 cells is especially highlighted in acquired immunodeficiency syndrome, where depleted CD4 cells cause a profound immunodeficiency. CD8 cells have an important role in lysis of virally infected cells and in killing of tumor cells. T cells do not produce antibodies. They produce soluble factors termed *cytokines*, which are important mediators of these cells.

Phagocytic Cells

The major phagocytes are monocytes/macrophages and neutrophils (2,5). *Monocytes* circulate in the peripheral blood; once they home to the tissues, they are termed *macrophages*, or histiocytes. In the tissue, multiple histiocytes coalesce to become giant cells. Macrophages in different body sites have different designations: Kuppfer cells (liver), alveolar macrophages (lungs), glial cells (brain). Mononuclear phagocytes are involved in mediating cellular responses, especially pathogenic responses to intracellular organisms such as mycobacterium. They are also important phagocytic cells. Many microbes, such as encapsulated bacteria, do not readily bind to the surface of phagocytes for engulfment. However, upon coating with substances such as products of the complement system and immunoglobulins, the particles are recognized as foreign and can bind to the Fc portion of the immunoglobulin molecule and/or complement receptors on the macrophage cell surface. This process, called opsonization, facilitates the process of phagocytosis. Macrophages also function in cell-to-cell interactions as APCs. Along with the protein products of the MHC, macrophages process and express protein antigen to T lymphocytes. Macrophages also produce cytokines, which effect cell interactions and recruit inflammatory cells to sites of injury.

Neutrophils are the other major phagocytic cells (2,6). They comprise the major population of white cells in the peripheral blood (up to 80%). Neutrophils are formed in the bone marrow from myelocytic precursors and are terminally differentiated, living only 1–2 days after reaching the peripheral blood. They have a multi-lobed nucleus and a variety of storage cytoplasmic granules containing digestive enzymes that break down phagocytized particles. Neutrophils provide one of the first lines of defense against foreign invaders, and they are one of the first cell populations present in tissues with an acute infection. They mediate their effects via phagocytosis or release of granules, either intracellularly or extracellularly.

Natural Killer Cells

Natural killer cells are a population of cells distinct from T or B cells (7,8). They have large cytoplasmic granules and are thus called large-granular lymphocytes. These cells are able to kill tumor cells and virally infected cells. In contrast to the tumor-cell killing by cytotoxic CD8+ T cells, killing mediated by NK cells does not require previous exposure or products of the MHC. In addition, NK cells can interact with antibody-coated tumor cells and kill them in a process termed *antibody-dependent cellular cytotoxicity*. The exact role of NK cells in normal immunity has not been unequivocally established. Rare individuals with a deficiency of NK cells have been shown to develop severe viral infections.

SOLUBLE MEDIATORS OF THE IMMUNE SYSTEM

Cytokines are soluble mediators produced by a variety of cell types (1–3,9). Most of these substances are produced in very small amounts and act either on adjacent cells or the cell that produced them. However, some act on distant cells and tissues. Cytokines have a wide variety of effects on many cellular functions and cell populations. Their major roles include mediating effects induced by infectious agents, regulating lymphocyte growth, stimulating growth of precursor cell populations, and mediating inflammatory reactions. One major group of cytokines are the interleukins (IL), which are presently numbered IL-1–18. Some additional cytokines include tumor necrosis factor (TNF), T cell transforming factor, and interferons. Only some of the cytokines with special relevance to the rheumatic diseases will be discussed.

Interleukin-1 (IL-1) and TNF are 2 cytokines that differ structurally but have very similar physiologic effects. IL-1 can be produced by essentially all nucleated cells, but most predominantly by macrophages and activated T cells. Both IL-1 and TNF are important co-stimulators in the antigen-induced activation of T cells. They are important mediators of inflammatory responses. In addition, they cause fever; thus they are endogenous pyrogens. Both of these cytokines act on hepatocytes to induce the synthesis of plasma proteins termed *acute phase reactants*, which are increased in infection, neoplasia, burns, and trauma. Multiple proteins can be increased in an acute phase reaction, including the third component of complement (C3), C-reactive protein, serum amyloid protein, and haptoglobin. These proteins can be measured by laboratory tests to determine whether a patient is undergoing an inflammatory response. IL-1 and TNF affect cells important in rheumatic disease. These cytokines can cause bone loss, affect joint cartilage, and cause changes to the tissues in the joint (1–3,10).

TNF has an important role in the pathogenesis of rheumatoid arthritis (RA) (10). The application of this basic information to clinical practice is highlighted in the development of new drugs (etanercept, infliximab) that block TNF, thus dampening the inflammatory response. These TNF inhibitors have been FDA-approved and are being used to treat both adults and children with RA and other rheumatic diseases (10–15) (see also Chapter 25, Pharmacologic Interventions in the 21st Century). Another recently approved drug, leflunomide, is an inhibitor of pyrimidine synthesis. This drug blocks T cell proliferation and thus can affect cytokine production (16). It has also been shown to induce clinical improvement in RA.

Interleukin-2 is a crucial growth factor for T cells. Activated T cells produce IL-2, which then acts on the same cell that produced it to further stimulate its growth. It also stimulates the growth of nearby cells. IL-2 has been utilized to grow T cells in the laboratory, furthering our knowledge of cellular interactions. It has also been used therapeutically in some cancers.

Interleukin-6 is produced by monocytes/macrophages and other tissue cells in response to IL-1 and TNF. It has two major effects. It stimulates hepatocytes to increase the production of fibrinogen, which causes red blood cells to stack. An increase in this protein is measured by the erythrocyte sedimentation rate (ESR) test, frequently used in patients with rheumatic disease to assess inflammation and follow their disease course. In addition, IL-6 acts as a B cell growth factor.

THE COMPLEMENT SYSTEM

The complement system, a complex group of serum proteins, is important to both natural and acquired immunity (1,2). It is a cascade system of approximately 25 serum proteins, including the regulatory proteins, that are normally inactive. Upon activation, they sequentially mediate a number of biologic effects. The main actions of the complement system are as follows: 1) mediate lysis of antibody-coated targets, such as bacteria, viruses, cells, and others; 2) act as mediators of inflammation via recruitment of inflammatory cells and cellular products to the sites of inflammation; and 3) aid in removal of foreign pathogens by increasing the efficiency of phagocytosis through opsonization.

The complement system is divided into 2 pathways: the classical (discovered first) and the alternative. There are 3 key proteins that are unique to each pathway, along with a number of proteins common to both. C3 is a crucial component in both pathways. The classical pathway only interacts with IgG and IgM when they are complexed with antigen to form an immune complex. The unique classical pathway components, C1, C2, and C4, are sequentially activated and then interact with C3 to form a complex that interacts with the common terminal components of the system (C5–C9). The classical complement pathway is a major effector mechanism of humoral immunity

because it allows the destruction of antibody-coated microbes and the recruitment of inflammatory cells to sites of inflammation.

The alternative pathway is also important as part of the innate or natural immune system, allowing complement to interact directly on the surface of the molecule without the requirement for antigen-antibody complexes. Proteins unique to the alternative pathway include factors B, D, H, I, and properdin. The end result of activation of either pathway is the formation of the membrane attack complex (MAC). This mediates cell lysis by intercalating into the lipid bilayer membrane and forming lytic pores, which allow the passage of water into the cell and cause subsequent cell lysis.

In addition to direct destruction of cell targets by the MAC, complement split products cause a variety of effects. C5a and C3a are anaphylatoxins that cause release of histamine from mast cells and smooth muscle contraction. In addition, C5a attracts and activates neutrophils. C3b bound to the surface of microorganisms binds to receptors on macrophages and neutrophils and promotes phagocytosis. Complement also enhances solubilization and clearance of immune complexes by interacting with the formation of immune complexes and enhancing clearance by phagocytic cells.

A deficiency of complement can lead to increased or decreased patterns of complement activation. There are a variety of genetic deficiencies of various complement components, commonly the early pathway proteins, C2 and C4. Over 50% of the patients with deficiencies of C2 and C4 have systemic lupus erythematosus (SLE). C2 and/or C4 deficiencies may lead to altered clearance of immune complexes and immune complex disease characteristic of SLE. In addition, in patients without an inherited complement deficiency, there can be alterations in the normal levels of complement. In the presence of activation by a persistent infection or an autoimmune disease such as SLE, there can be persistent activation of the complement system, resulting in low serum levels. Generally, the serum levels of C3 and C4 correlate with disease activity and they are monitored in patients with SLE.

INFLAMMATION

Inflammation is the response of the body to injured tissues (1–3,17), characterized by the movement of vascular fluid and cells from the vessels into the extravascular spaces. The inflammatory response is a complex process initiated by a variety of foreign insults (e.g., microbes, altered cells, and foreign particles), and involving a variety of cells and soluble inflammatory mediators. It can be acute or chronic. Acute inflammation often occurs as the initial response to highly virulent organisms and tissue injury, and it is characterized by a cellular infiltrate primarily of neutrophils. A chronic inflammatory response occurs later (usually as a response to a persistent and/or intracellular organism), and it is characterized by an infiltrate of primarily lymphocytes, plasma cells, and macrophages.

The local signs of inflammation were originally described by Celsus in the second century AD as rubor (redness), calor (heat), tumor (swelling), and dolor (pain). In response to an inciting noxious agent that causes tissue injury, the capillary and postcapillary venules containing the inflammatory cells respond to the injury. There is a disruption of the endothelial

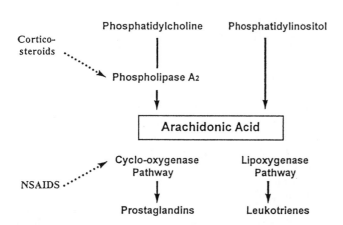

Figure 2. Arachidonic acid pathway. NSAIDS = nonsteroidal antiinflammatory drugs.

cells lining the vessel walls, thus allowing movement of fluid and cells into the extravascular spaces and to the site of injury. The inflammatory cells (neutrophils, platelets, mast cells, eosinophils, basophils, and lymphocytes) release mediators with a myriad of effects, including an increase in vascular permeability, recruitment of additional cells, contraction of smooth muscle, and release of additional mediators. Thus, from the initial injurious stimuli, the body responds with a cascade of events.

The inflammatory response usually resolves the noxious assault and restores the tissues to normal physiologic integrity and functioning. However, in a number of pathological situations, tissue injury results from the inflammatory response. The inflammatory response may become chronic due to characteristics of the inciting agent (persistent, intracellular) or to factors in the host, or both.

A variety of inflammatory mediators are released from the infiltrating cells during the inflammatory response. Some are preformed and in cytoplasmic granules, and some are formed from the metabolism of membrane phospholipids, such as prostaglandins and leukotrienes. In addition, cytokines are released from infiltrating macrophages or lymphocytes, and complement split products are produced from the activation of the complement system.

Arachidonic acid (AA), a 20-carbon fatty acid, is the central compound in the generation of prostaglandins and leukotrienes (Figure 2). It is created during the inflammatory process from membrane phospholipids in 2 ways. It can be generated from membrane phosphatidylinositol via cleavage by phospholipase C to diacylglycerol, followed by the generation of arachidonic acid from diacylglycerol by the action of diacylglycerol lipase. Alternatively, phosphatidylcholine is acted upon by phospholipase A2 to generate AA directly. From this point, AA can proceed either by the cyclooxygenase pathway to prostaglandins/thromboxanes or via the lipoxygenase pathway to leukotrienes. Prostaglandins and leukotrienes have diverse proinflammatory actions, including chemotaxis, smooth-muscle constriction, and vasoactive properties. Corticosteroids act as antiinflammatory agents by inducing an inhibitor of phospholipase A2, thus inhibiting the formation of AA. Nonsteroidal antiinflammatory drugs (NSAIDs) directly inhibit the cyclooxygenase pathway, thus inhibiting the formation of prostaglandins and thromboxanes.

There are 2 distinct enzymes involved in the cyclooxygenase pathway, cyclooxygenase 1 (COX-1) and cyclooxygenase 2 (COX-2). Conventional NSAIDs inhibit both of these enzymes. Gastrointestinal toxicity common with NSAID therapy is mediated primarily by inhibition of the COX-1 form of the enzyme. Recently 2 selective COX-2 inhibitors, celecoxib and rofecoxib, have been approved by the FDA. These drugs offer comparable analgesic and antiinflammatory effects with fewer gastrointestinal side effects than nonspecific COX inhibitors (18). They have been widely used to treat many rheumatologic diseases, including osteoarthritis, RA, SLE, and others.

Inflammatory responses that result in tissue injury are termed *hypersensitivity reactions*. These include allergic reactions, antigen–antibody reactions that are cytotoxic, immune complex reactions, and cell-mediated responses. The response most relevant to rheumatic disease is the immune complex reaction, which involves immune complexes that deposit in the tissue. Complement is activated and neutrophils are attracted to the site of deposition, causing local damage. Tissue injury occurs primarily from the resultant inflammatory reaction. The antigen may be exogenous or endogenous (an autoantigen). This immune mechanism is responsible for much of the tissue destruction seen in SLE.

HUMAN HISTOCOMPATIBILITY COMPLEX

The human MHC is a group of closely related genes on human chromosome 6, which encodes proteins important in the immune system (19–21). The protein products of these loci are called human leukocyte antigens (HLA). The gene products are highly polymorphic, meaning that there are many alleles or forms of the genes in different individuals. This system was first discovered in graft rejection. It is vital to the functioning of the immune system and crucial to the interaction of T cells, because MHC products are markers of "self" for T cells. The MHC contains 2 sets of genes coding for cell surface antigens, which are divided into Class I and Class II. Class I antigens are expressed on the surface of all nucleated cells. T cells only respond to antigens that are noncovalently bound to MHC gene products. CD8 cytolytic T cells will only respond to antigen when they are complexed with Class I antigens. Class II antigens have a more limited cell distribution: B cells, macrophages, and dendritic cells. CD4 T cells can only react to antigens complexed with Class II molecules. Clinically, the MHC is important in transplantation, platelet transfusions, and associations with disease. Traditional HLA typing is performed using serologic tests that examine the HLA proteins expressed on the cell surface.

There are a variety of diseases—mostly autoimmune—associated with the MHC. The strongest association is with a Class I HLA-B antigen, HLA-B27, which is associated with ankylosing spondylitis. HLA-B27 is also associated with Reiter's syndrome; however, the association is not as strong. While more than 90% of Caucasian patients with ankylosing spondylitis have HLA-B27, only a small percentage of individuals with HLA-27 actually have ankylosing spondylitis. The remainder of disease associations are with Class II antigens, primarily with the HLA-D/DR antigens. Associations with various rheumatic diseases are listed in Table 1. The

Table 1. Association of human leukocyte antigens with rheumatic diseases.*

Disease	HLA antigen	Relative risk
AS	HLA-B27	69–90
RS	HLA-B27	37
RA	HLA-DR4	2.7–6
SS	HLA-DR2	5.2–9.7
	HLA-DR3	3.6
SLE	HLA-DR2	2.3
	HLA-DR3	2.5–5.8

* Data compiled from references 1–3,19–21. AS = ankylosing spondylitis; RS = Reiter's syndrome; RA = rheumatoid arthritis; SS = Sjögren's syndrome; SLE = systemic lupus erythematosus.

significance of an HLA disease association is generally expressed as a relative risk, which is the risk of an individual with the particular HLA type of developing the disease, as compared with the risk for an individual without the antigen. For example, an individual with HLA-B27 is 90 times more likely than someone who is HLA-B27 negative to develop ankylosing spondylitis. The relative risks listed in Table 1 are reported as a range of figures representing data from numerous studies.

Molecular methods are now available to perform DNA typing on patients with a particular HLA type (20,21). Using this technique, the actual DNA sequence that makes up a particular HLA specificity can be examined. For example, DNA typing of HLA-DR4 has led to the identification of a common amino acid sequence among RA patients, termed the "rheumatoid epitope" (22). In contrast to the traditional serologic methods, DNA typing allows examination of the actual components of the patient's DNA, and both copies of the gene can be examined. Studies have shown that patients who receive 2 copies of the rheumatoid epitope (one from each parent) have more severe disease (20). While routine DNA typing of patients with rheumatic diseases is controversial, as additional information is gained, this type of testing could become part of routine clinical practice.

When examining the association of HLA and disease, there are several caveats. First, HLA disease associations are neither sufficient nor necessary for the development of a particular disease. Autoimmune disease causation is multifactorial and involves HLA genes, non-HLA genes, and environmental factors. For example, a mouse model of lupus found more than 20 non-HLA genes important in disease susceptibility, while in human lupus, 9 non-HLA loci have been linked to disease development (21,22). Association with a particular HLA antigen may not be with the gene itself, but the actual disease-associated gene could be a non-HLA locus that is closely linked to the MHC. It must be emphasized that possession of a particular HLA allele is not diagnostic of a particular disease; it simply means that an individual has an increased risk for developing a particular disease. Many of the HLA associations are epidemiologic data from large groups of individuals, and they may not significantly affect individual patients. With the mapping of the human genome and the explosion of our knowledge of genetics, information that is more definitive will be available in the next decade.

AUTOIMMUNITY

Autoimmunity is defined as pathologic changes that occur due to the immune reaction against autologous antigens (1–3,23),

representing a loss of self-tolerance. *Tolerance*, or the unresponsiveness of the immune response to antigens, occurs both peripherally and centrally. Central tolerance occurs in immature lymphocytes in the thymus and bone marrow. Immature lymphocytes, which can recognize self, "see" these antigens in the thymus and bone marrow and are deleted or inactivated. Peripheral tolerance occurs in mature lymphocytes that "see" self-antigen in peripheral tissues. It provides for maintenance of self-tolerance for clones that escape destruction in the thymus or bone marrow, which is important for tolerance to tissue-specific self-antigens not found in the generative organs.

If tolerance is present, then how does autoimmunity occur? There are many theories to explain autoimmune disease. One explanation relates to changes in lymphocytes. Individuals may have autoreactive B cells, but without self-reactive CD4 T cells to provide help to these B cells, no immune response can occur. Because most of the potentially self-reactive T cells have been deleted or rendered inactive, these cells must be "tricked" into providing help to the self-responsive B cells. This process can occur via stimulation with microbial antigens that cross-react with self-antigens. Another mechanism of autoimmunity involves the widespread activation of previously unresponsive self-reactive lymphocytes by substances that stimulate many clones of lymphocytes—so-called polyclonal activators. Substances such as lipopolysaccharides from gram-negative bacteria are polyclonal activators. In addition, tissue injury and inflammation can lead to autoimmunity by causing the release of normally sequestered self-antigens, which are seen as foreign upon release. There can be alterations of self antigens by either a microbial agent or by injury or inflammation, so that they are recognized as foreign. As discussed in the section on the HLA system, a variety of genetic factors play a role in the autoimmune system. In summary, there is no single theory that explains all autoimmune diseases. In most situations, it is likely a complex interplay between environmental factors, including exposure to microbial antigens in a genetically susceptible host, that determines the development of autoimmune disease.

Autoimmune diseases may be classified as organ specific or non-organ specific, depending on whether the response is primarily against antigen localized to one or a limited number of organs, or whether the autoimmune reaction is directed against many tissues of the body. Common targets of organ specific autoimmune responses include the thyroid, adrenals, stomach, and pancreas. The non-organ specific reactions include rheumatic diseases that involve primarily the skin, joints, kidney, and muscle. However, this classification is not absolute; within each group, there is considerable overlap.

Many rheumatic diseases are characterized by detectable circulating levels of autoantibodies that are useful in diagnosis, following disease activity, and in prognosis (23–25). For example, the presence of antibody against double stranded DNA (anti-DNA) in SLE is used both for initial diagnosis and for following disease activity. Anti-DNA immune complexes may be deposited along the glomerular basement membrane in the kidney and along the dermal–epidermal junction in the skin. They are believed to be an important factor in the pathology of SLE (24). Another common autoantibody is rheumatoid factor (RF), which is an IgM antibody directed against the IgG molecule (25). Although present in approximately 75% of patients with RA, RF does not establish the diagnosis of RA. Nearly 25% of patients who fulfill the criteria for RA do not have RF, while RF can be present in patients with no joint disease. The exact role of RF in the pathogenesis of RA has not been clearly established (25). While RF can be detected in the synovial fluid from RA joints, and cells producing RF can be found in synovial tissue, the majority of cells in the synovial tissue are not plasma cells but CD4 helper T cells. More studies are needed to define the role of RF in the pathogenesis of RA.

Caution should be used when evaluating the role of autoantibodies in disease states. The presence of autoantibodies does not mean that autoimmune disease is present. Low levels of autoantibodies are found in many normal individuals. Even when high levels of autoantibodies are found to be associated with disease, they may not necessarily have a pathogenic role. We know that age, sex, and genetics have an effect on autoantibodies. Many studies show that autoantibodies increase as we age. In addition, autoimmune disease is more common in women. Furthermore, our genetic background has an important effect on autoantibody production. For example, clinically normal relatives of patients with SLE have a greater number of positive autoantibodies than the general population. This knowledge should not dampen enthusiasm for evaluating autoantibodies, but they must be evaluated in the proper light.

REFERENCES

1. Abbas AK, Lichtman AH, Pober JS. Cellular and molecular immunology. 4th ed. Philadelphia: WB Saunders; 2000.
2. Stites DP, Terr AI, Parslow TG. Basic and clinical immunology. 8th ed. Norwalk, CT: Appleton and Lange; 1994.
3. Roitt I, Brostoff J, Male D. Immunology. 3rd ed. Chicago: Mosby; 1993.
4. Ikuta K, Uchida N, Friedman J, Weissman IL. Lymphocyte development from stem cells. Annu Rev Immunol 1992;10:759–83.
5. Johnston RB Jr. Current concepts: immunology. Monocytes and macrophages. N Engl J Med 1988;318:747–52.
6. Lehrer RI, Ganz T, Selsted ME, Babior BM, Curnutte JT. Neutrophils and host defense. Ann Intern Med 1988;109:127–42.
7. Trinchieri G. Biology of natural killer cells. Adv Immunol 1989;47:187–376.
8. Herberman RB, Reynolds CW, Ortaldo JR. Mechanism of cytotoxicity by natural killer (NK) cells. Annu Rev Immunol 1986;4:651–80.
9. Arai KI, Lee F, Miyajima A, Miyatake S, Arai N, Yokota T. Cytokines: coordinators of immune and inflammatory responses. Annu Rev Biochem 1990;59:783–836.
10. Choy E, Panayi GS. Cytokine pathways and joint inflammation in rheumatoid arthritis. N Engl J Med 2001;344:907–16.
11. Pisetsky DS. Tumor necrosis factor blockers in rheumatoid arthritis. N Engl J Med 2000;342:810–1.
12. Luong BT, Chong BS, Lowder DM. Treatment options for rheumatoid arthritis celecoxib, leflunomide, etanercept and infliximab. Ann Pharmacother 2000;34:743–60.
13. Maini R, St Clair EW, Breedveld F, Furst D, Kalden J, Weisman M, et al. Infliximab (chimeric antitumour necrosis factor α monoclonal antibody) versus placebo in rheumatoid arthritis patients receiving concomitant methotrexate: a randomised phase III trial. Lancet 1999;354:1932–9.
14. Weinblatt ME, Kremer JM, Bankhurst AD, Bulpitt KJ, Fleischmann RM, Fox RI, et al. A trial of etanercept, a recombinant tumor necrosis factor receptor:Fc fusion protein, in patients with rheumatoid arthritis receiving methotrexate. N Engl J Med 1999;340:253–9.
15. Brandt J, Haibel H, Cornely D, Golder W, Gonzalez J, Reddig J, et al. Successful treatment of active ankylosing spondylitis with the anti-tumor necrosis factor α monoclonal antibody infliximab. Arthritis Rheum 2000; 43:1346–52.
16. Tugwell P, Wells G, Strand V, Maetzel A, Bombardier C, Crawford B, et al. Clinical improvement as reflected in measures of function and health-related quality of life following treatment with leflunomide compared with methotrexate in patients with rheumatoid arthritis: sensitivity and relative efficiency to detect a treatment effect in a twelve-month, placebo controlled trial. Leflunomide Rheumatoid Arthritis Investigators Group. Arthritis Rheum 2000;43:506–14.
17. Cotran RS, Kumar V, Collins T. Robbins pathologic basis of disease. 6th ed. Philadelphia: WB Saunders; 1998. p. 50–88.
18. Everts B, Wahrborg P, Hedner T. Cox-2-specific inhibitors – the emergence of a new class of analgesic and anti-inflammatory drugs. Clin Rheumatol 2000;19:331–43.
19. Salazar M, Yunis EJ. MHC: Gene structure and function. In: Frank MM, Austen KF, Claman HN, Unanue ER, editors. Samter's immunologic diseases. 5th ed. Boston: Little, Brown; 1995. p. 101–16.
20. Reveille JD. The genetic contribution to the pathogenesis of rheumatoid arthritis. Curr Opin Rheumatol 1998;10:187–200.
21. Vyse TJ, Kotzin BL. Genetic susceptibility to systemic lupus erythematosus. Annu Rev Immunol 1998;16:261–92.
22. Gregersen PK, Silver J, Winchester RJ. The shared epitope hypothesis. An approach to understanding the molecular genetics of susceptibility to rheumatoid arthritis. Arthritis Rheum 1987;30:1205–13.
23. Naparstek Y, Plotz PH. The role of autoantibodies in autoimmune diseases. Annu Rev Immunol 1993;11:79–104.
24. Kotzin BL, O'Dell JR. Systemic lupus erythematosus. In: Frank MM, Austen KF, Claman HN, Unanue ER, editors. Samter's immunologic diseases. 5th ed. Boston: Little, Brown; 1995. p. 667–98.
25. Winchester R. Rheumatoid arthritis. In: Frank MM, Austen KF, Claman HN, Unanue ER, editors. Samter's immunologic diseases. 5th ed. Boston: Little, Brown; 1995. p. 699–758.

Additional Recommended Reading

Abbas A, Lichtman AH, Pober JS: Cellular and Molecular Immunology. Fourth Edition. Philadelphia, WB Saunders, 2000.
Roitt I, Brostoff J, Male D: Immunology. Fifth Edition. London, England, Mosby, 1998.

Impact and Economic Burden on Society

LEIGH F. CALLAHAN, PhD

Rheumatic disease and musculoskeletal conditions are the most prevalent chronic conditions in the United States and a leading cause of disability (1–3). The physical, social, psychological, and economic consequences associated with rheumatic diseases are enormous (1,4,5) and have a significant impact on the individuals with disease, families, and society at large. Some of the effects are easily translated into economic terms, such as lost wages and medical care costs, but many, such as pain, the inability to enjoy leisure activities, or reductions in housekeeping activities, are not easily estimated in monetary costs.

ACTIVITY AND ROLE LIMITATIONS

Over 7 million Americans are significantly limited in their ability to participate in their main daily activities, such as going to work or school, housekeeping, or performing other activities, as a result of arthritis (2). The prevalence of arthritis-related disability is expected to rise to an estimated 11.6 million individuals by the year 2020. Risk factors associated with arthritis-related disability include older age, female gender, higher body mass index, lower levels of formal education, and lower income levels (2,6). Seven percent of individuals aged 55–64, 10% aged 65–74, 13% aged 75–84, and 19% over age 85 report activity limitations due to arthritis (Figure 1) (6).

When the rank and prevalence of chronic conditions causing disability among adults in the US in 1999 were analyzed, arthritis was the leading cause of disability (Table 1) (5). Disability was assessed using 8 measures: 1) ability to perform functional activities; 2) activities of daily living (ADL); 3) instrumental ADL (IADL); 4) presence of selected impairments; 5) use of assistive aids; 6) limitation in the ability to work around the house; 7) limitation in the ability to work at a job or business; or 8) receiving federal benefits on the basis of an inability to work. An estimated 44.1 million adults reported one or more conditions they believed to be associated with their disability. Of those individuals, 17.5% reported arthritis or rheumatism as being associated with their disability (Table 1).

Individuals with arthritis were more likely to report some functional limitation (arthritis only 37%, arthritis plus other conditions 56%) compared with individuals without arthritis (1 other chronic condition 22%, multiple other chronic conditions 42%) (7). This pattern of higher limitation rates among individuals with arthritis compared with individuals without arthritis was evident among all physical activities evaluated (7).

Older women with arthritis have more difficulty performing personal care (ADL) and household management (IADL) activities than men, and the difference increases with advancing age (8). In addition, arthritis is the most prevalent chronic condition reported by older people who are chronically homebound (9), which is a predictor of nursing home use.

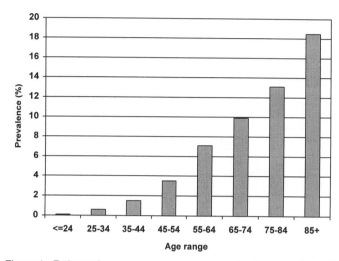

Figure 1. Estimated average annual prevalence of self-reported activity limitations attributed to arthritis and other rheumatic conditions by age. (Data adapted from the National Health Interview Survey (NHIS), United States, 1989–1991, presented in ref. 6.)

Rheumatic diseases also negatively affect family role functioning and the person with the condition (10). Role limitations associated with rheumatic disease include significant reductions in the amount of time individuals spend engaging in activities such as shopping, visiting the bank and supermarket, homemaking, interacting with friends and family, or participating in hobbies (1,10,11). Functional status has been shown to be the most important determinant of household work performance (10).

Table 1. Prevalence of chronic conditions causing disability in the United States in 1999 (data from ref. 5).

	Percentage of all disability
Arthritis or rheumatism	17.5
Back or spine problem	16.5
Heart trouble	7.8
Lung or respiratory trouble	4.7
Deafness or serious trouble hearing	4.4
Stiffness or deformity of limb	4.2
Diabetes	3.4
Blindness or other visual impairment	3.3
Stroke	2.8
Hypertension	1.7
Head or spinal cord injury	1.1
Paralysis of any kind	0.8
Alcohol- or drug-related problem or disorder	0.5
Cerebral palsy	0.3

PSYCHOLOGICAL CONSEQUENCES

The psychological impact of rheumatic disease has been documented in terms of depression, anxiety, learned helplessness, coping strategies, cognitive changes, and self-efficacy (1). Higher levels of psychological distress are noted in individuals with rheumatic disease than in the general population in most studies. Levels of distress reported in the rheumatic disease patients are comparable to levels noted in individuals with other chronic conditions (12). Higher levels of psychological distress in individuals with rheumatic disease have also been noted to be associated with poorer status on clinical outcome variables, as well as with increased health services utilization (13).

Research efforts on depressive symptoms and disorders have focused on osteoarthritis (OA), rheumatoid arthritis (RA), fibromyalgia, and systemic lupus erythematosus (12). Although depressive symptoms and disorders are more common among clinical samples of individuals with rheumatic disease than in the general population, the majority of individuals with rheumatic disease do not report increased depression. Among persons with RA, the loss of valued activities and the self-perception of the ability to do activities also are strongly correlated with psychological status (11).

ECONOMIC IMPACT

In addition to the significant impact rheumatic disease has on activity and role limitations and psychological consequences, there are enormous costs associated with rheumatic disease, including direct costs, indirect costs, and intangible costs (14). *Direct costs* accrue when people receive medical care, such as hospitalizations, medications, physician visits, and diagnostic tests. Expenditures for other items such as adaptations to the home environment and transportation costs to visit health care providers are also included as direct costs, but it is often difficult to estimate these expenditures accurately. *Indirect costs* are usually calculated as the costs due to lost wages from a reduction or cessation in work. *Intangible costs* are the costs of individuals foregoing the activities they and society value. These include the costs associated with a decline in functional capacity, increased pain, and reduced quality of life. Most comprehensive studies of the national cost of illness are restricted to only direct and indirect costs due to the difficulty of assessing intangible costs in population-based studies.

Comprehensive studies of the economic cost of musculoskeletal disease suggest that the total costs of these conditions are equivalent to 2.5% of the Gross National Product (GNP) (1). In 1995 dollars, the estimated total economic impact of musculoskeletal conditions on the US economy was $214.9 billion (Figure 2) (4). Of the total, direct costs accounted for 41% and indirect costs accounted for 59%. For all types of arthritis, the total costs were $82.5 billion, 38% of the total cost of all musculoskeletal conditions (Figure 2) (4).

The estimated direct costs of medical care for all forms of arthritis totaled $21.7 billion (Figure 2). The largest percentage of direct costs was expenditures for nursing home care, $12.7 billion (59%) (Table 2). Hospital inpatient care totaled $3.1 billion, or 14% of direct costs. According to the National Hospital Discharge Survey, patients hospitalized for arthritis account for approximately 2.6 million days of care (4). Ad-

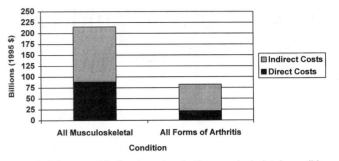
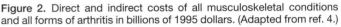

Figure 2. Direct and indirect costs of all musculoskeletal conditions and all forms of arthritis in billions of 1995 dollars. (Adapted from ref. 4.)

ministration and physician outpatient costs were the next largest contributors to direct costs, $1.2 billion and $1.1 billion, respectively (each approximately 5% of direct costs) (Table 2).

The magnitude of the estimated indirect costs due to arthritis in 1995 dollars was $60.8 billion or 74% of the total costs (Figure 2) (4). As noted in previous studies, the indirect costs are almost 3 times greater than the direct costs (1). This estimate would be even larger if the costs attributed to loss of homemaking functions could be more easily determined. Also, older women have lower labor force participation rates, resulting in lower estimates of economic impact.

The costs of rheumatic disease extend far beyond the direct medical care costs and the indirect costs associated with work loss. Intangible costs include pain, psychological distress, changes in family structure, limitations in instrumental and nurturant activities, and changes in appearance resulting from deformity (1,15). It is impossible to put a price on losses such as a grandparent not being able to play with a grandchild.

The economic costs of RA have been examined in studies of clinical populations and a few population-based studies (16). Although the clinical studies cannot be compared directly due to costing methods, some trends can be noted (16). With the exception of one study, the majority of direct costs of RA are due to hospitalizations. Although only a small percentage of patients are hospitalized and most patients receive outpatient treatment and medications, the costs of medications, diagnostic tests, and physician visits reflect less than 50% of the total direct costs of care for patients with RA (16).

As demonstrated for all rheumatic diseases, the indirect costs of RA, primarily from lost wages, are 3–4 times higher than direct costs (16). And, although the indirect cost estimates of RA are substantial, they are an underestimate of the true indirect costs. The human capital approach to estimating indirect costs tends to underestimate the work loss or disability days of older individuals and females. Homemaker costs are

Table 2. Direct costs of medical care for all forms of arthritis in millions of 1995 dollars (data from ref. 4).

Type of costs	Direct costs ($ millions)
Hospital inpatient	3,146
Hospital outpatient	485
Physician inpatient	76
Physician outpatient	1,099
Other practitioners	165
Drugs	184
Nursing home care	12,704
Prepayment/administration	1,152
Non-health sector	2,679

Table 3. Determinants of work disability in individuals with rheumatic disease.

Societal level
    Economic conditions
    Attitudinal barriers
    Architectural barriers
    Available jobs
    Employer practices
    Disability pension plan characteristics
Individual level
    Work autonomy
    Social factors
    Disease factors

estimated using the wages of housecleaners and day care workers, not teachers or counselors.

WORK DISABILITY

The capacity of individuals with rheumatic diseases to work is significantly affected (17–20). Rheumatic disease is the leading cause of work loss and the second leading cause of work disability payments (20,21) (see also Chapter 42, Work Disability). In two of the most prevalent rheumatic conditions, OA and RA, many studies have documented significant work disability (15,21). For example, substantial earnings losses and work disability have been noted in individuals younger than age 65 with asymmetric oligoarthritis, a surrogate for OA (18), and approximately one-half of the patients with RA who are working at the onset of disease become work disabled (20).

Determinants of work disability in individuals with rheumatic disease exist at both the societal and the individual level (21) (Table 3). Risk factors on a societal level include economic conditions, attitudinal and architectural barriers, types of jobs available, employer practices, and the characteristics of disability pension plans (21). Individual-level determinants include work autonomy, social factors, and disease factors (19,21).

POLICY IMPLICATIONS

The impact of rheumatic diseases in terms of economic, functional, social, and psychological consequences is enormous. Long-term consequences include medical costs, lost wages due to frequent work disability and reductions in work capacity, reductions in activities of importance and role functions, psychological distress, and social dislocation. Economic consequences are probably underestimated with current costing methods but even with underestimations are substantial.

Given the significant impact of rheumatic diseases, they should receive considerable attention from a societal as well as clinical perspective. These burdens will increase dramatically in the near future underscoring the need for a coordinated public health approach. In 1998, a consortium of national organizations produced "The National Arthritis Action Plan: A Public Health Strategy," which is a comprehensive and ambitious plan for addressing arthritis (22). The plan is based on a growing recognition that public health must shift its emphasis to diseases that reduce quality of life even as we add years to life. Mounting evidence suggests that arthritis can be addressed effectively at all 3 levels of the prevention spectrum—primary,

secondary, and tertiary (15). For example, primary prevention of OA is now feasible through weight control and injury prevention. Secondary prevention of RA appears achievable through early diagnosis and aggressive treatment, and tertiary prevention of the negative effects of arthritis can be achieved through self-management classes (15,22).

The National Arthritis Action Plan, the incorporation of arthritis-specific objectives in Healthy People 2010, and the launch of the Decade of Bone and Joint Disease in the year 2000 should further enhance society's understanding of the burden of rheumatic disease. Health professionals should familiarize themselves with these public health activities in rheumatic diseases.

REFERENCES

1. Yelin E, Callahan LF, The National Arthritis Data Work Group. The economic cost and social and psychological impact of musculoskeletal conditions. Arthritis Rheum 1995;38:1351–62.
2. Centers for Disease Control and Prevention. Arthritis prevalence and activity limitations–United States, 1990. MMWR Morb Mortal Wkly Rep 1994;43:433–8.
3. Centers for Disease Control and Prevention. Health-related quality of life among adults with arthritis–behavioral risk factor surveillance system, 11 States, 1996-1998. MMWR Morb Mortal Wkly Rep 2000;49:366–9.
4. Praemer A, Furner S, Rice D. Musculoskeletal conditions in the United States. 2nd ed. Rosemont (IL): American Academy of Orthopaedic Surgeons; 1999.
5. Centers for Disease Control and Prevention. Prevalence of disabilities and associated health conditions among adults–United States, 1999. MMWR Morb Mortal Wkly Rep 2001;50:120–5.
6. Helmick CG, Lawrence RC, Pollard RA, Lloyd E, Heyse SP, The National Arthritis Data Work Group. Arthritis and other rheumatic conditions: who is affected now, who will be affected later? Arthritis Care Res 1995; 8:203–11.
7. Dunlop DD, Manheim LM, Song J, Chang RW. Arthritis prevalence and activity limitations in older adults. Arthritis Rheum 2001;44:212–21.
8. Verbrugge LM. Women, men, and osteoarthritis. Arthritis Care Res 1995; 8:212–20.
9. Hughes SL, Dunlop D. The prevalence and impact of arthritis in older persons. Arthritis Care Res 1995;8:257–64.
10. Reisine ST. Arthritis and the family. Arthritis Care Res 1995;8:265–71.
11. Katz PP, Yelin EH. Life activities of persons with rheumatoid arthritis with and without depressive symptoms. Arthritis Care Res 1994;7:69–77.
12. DeVellis BM. Depression in rheumatological diseases. Baillieres Clin Rheumatol 1993;7:241–57.
13. Hawley DJ, Wolfe F. Anxiety and depression in patients with rheumatoid arthritis: a prospective study of 400 patients. J Rheumatol 1988;15:932–41.
14. Hall J, Mooney G. What every doctor should know about economics. Part 1. The benefits of costing. Med J Aust 1990;152:29–31.
15. Callahan LF. Impact of rheumatic disease on society. In: Wegener ST, Belza BL, Gall EP, editors. Clinical care in the rheumatic diseases. Atlanta: American College of Rheumatology; 1996. p. 209–13.
16. Callahan LF. Health economics. In: Firestein GS, Panayi GS, Wollheim FA, editors. Rheumatoid arthritis: frontiers in pathogenesis and treatment. Oxford (UK): Oxford University Press; 2000. p. 443–9.
17. Yelin E. Arthritis: the cumulative impact of a common chronic condition. Arthritis Rheum 1992;35:489–97.
18. Pincus T, Mitchell JM, Burkhauser RV. Substantial work disability and earnings losses in individuals less than age 65 with osteoarthritis: comparisons with rheumatoid arthritis. J Clin Epidemiol 1989;42:449–57.
19. Yelin EH, Henke CJ, Epstein WV. Work disability among persons with musculoskeletal conditions. Arthritis Rheum 1986;29:1322–33.
20. Yelin EH. Work disability and rheumatoid arthritis. In: Wolfe F, Pincus T, editors. Rheumatoid arthritis: pathogenesis, assessment, outcome, and treatment. New York: Marcel Dekker; 1994. p. 26–71.
21. Allaire SH. Work disability. In: Wegener ST, Belza BL, Gall EP, editors. Clinical care in the rheumatic diseases. Atlanta: American College of Rheumatology; 1996. p. 141–5.
22. Meenan RF, Callahan LF, Helmick CG. The National Arthritis Action Plan: a public health strategy for a looming epidemic [editorial]. Arthritis Care Res 1999;12:79–81.

Human Development in Rheumatic Diseases

KATHLEEN M. SCHIAFFINO, PhD

For many people the word *arthritis* conjures up an image of grandparents with the minor aches and pains inevitably associated with aging. Osteoarthritis, the most common form of arthritis, does tend to occur in old age, but the reality is that rheumatic disease can be found at every stage of life. Although sometimes mild, rheumatic disease can also severely limit individuals' activities and affect their ability to perform the life tasks before them. This chapter will examine the potential psychosocial impact of rheumatic disease at all ages from the perspective of developmental psychology.

THEORETICAL APPROACHES TO NORMAL DEVELOPMENT

Erikson's theory of psychosocial development (1) through the life cycle emphasizes the development of adaptive strengths through the ongoing balancing of competing predispositions. The opposing forces that create this dynamic balance are essential to adaptation and growth; the over-development of one aspect at the expense of the other contributes to adjustment difficulties. Erikson identified 8 key conflicts that commonly influence development at specific stages of life and play a role throughout the life span. At each new stage, and with each change in circumstance, earlier conflicts must be re-integrated to accommodate the new circumstances. Thus, these conflicts do not represent independent processes as much as themes that are perpetually intertwined over the life cycle.

According to Erikson, infancy is the time for balancing the opposing predispositions of *trust versus mistrust*. A basic sense of trust emerges from confidence in the predictability of one's world. The move from infant to toddler introduces the individual to the next 2 life stage tasks: *autonomy versus shame/doubt* and *initiative versus guilt*. The balance between autonomy and shame/doubt results in the capacity to exercise free choice as well as self-restraint; it emerges out of early exploration of the child's environment, which is encouraged by the parent and which contributes to feelings of independence and confidence. Initiative develops in response to pleasurable accomplishment in socially and culturally approved activities—from play activities arise a set of idealized goals and a sense of purpose.

The school-age child is confronted with the task of balancing *industriousness versus inferiority*, resulting in an adaptive sense of competence and mastery. With adolescence comes the need to balance *identity versus identity confusion*, when young adults struggle with the question of "Who am I?" in an effort to develop a coherent sense of self.

Critical to the development of adult relationships is the resolution of the conflict involving *intimacy versus isolation*. Only after establishing a sense of identity is the young adult ready for intimacy that finds expression in sharing and caring about another person without losing a sense of self. Resolution of this conflict results in a capacity for love and selective intimacy, and prepares the adult for the next developmental task of *generativity versus stagnation and self-absorption*. Generativity refers to procreation, productivity, and creativity; successful resolution of this stage is associated with the adaptive capacity for care in relation to family and society. Typically, resolution of this stage means becoming involved in something outside of oneself, such as work, family, or volunteer activities, while maintaining good self-care practices.

The final task at the end of the life cycle concerns the development of wisdom through the balance of *integrity versus despair*. This involves the ability to take stock of one's life; recognize successes, failures, and missed opportunities; and make sense of this all without succumbing to feelings of failure and despair.

Like Erikson, others have proposed a theory of developmental tasks based on the assumption that certain tasks arise at certain periods in an individual's life and that success in handling one task influences the likelihood of success in handling future tasks (2). For example, 8 age-specific developmental tasks for the adolescent period have been suggested: accepting one's body, adopting a masculine or feminine social role, developing close relationships with friends, preparing for an occupational career, preparing for romantic relationships, achieving emotional independence from parents, establishing values to live by, and striving for social responsibility (3).

Others have considered human development from the perspective of specific skills and/or specific life stages. Piaget's theory of cognitive development (4) focuses on the child's development of adaptive structures to deal with changing environmental demands. Development results from the use of the complementary processes of assimilation and accommodation. *Assimilation* refers to the process of responding to new experiences or stimuli by modifying them to conform to pre-existing "schema" or cognitive processes. *Accommodation*, on the other hand, results in changes in cognitive frameworks to fit new experiences (5). The process of accommodation allows for growth and change over time and for response to new experiences.

Theories delineating the development of self-concept in children and adolescents provide support for the notion of domain-specific self-worth and global self-worth. According to one theory (6), children age 8 or older have the ability to assess themselves in 5 separate domains: scholastic competence, athletic competence, social competence, physical appearance, and behavior. These evaluations can be quite different from each other and different also from an evaluation of overall global self-worth.

More recent theoretical approaches have reflected a life span developmental perspective that views development as taking place at multiple levels and assumes that these levels continuously influence each other (7). The levels considered in life span models include the biological, dyadic, family, community, and cultural. The multiple levels at which development takes place are known as *embeddedness,* and the ability of each of these levels to influence the other levels is *dynamic interactionism* (8).

Life span developmental theories underscore the fact that development involves the following: 1) normative age-related processes (things that occur at specific ages, such as puberty); 2) normative history-related processes (things that influence normal development for almost everyone at a given time, such as computers in schools and dual-career families); and, 3) non-normative life events, such as accidents, illness, or divorce (9). Included within this last set of experiences would be events that are perceived by the individual, and possibly by the larger social system, as non-normative events in that they "should not be happening to me now." Because of lay representations of arthritis, a diagnosis of rheumatic disease is commonly seen as non-normative for all but the older patient. This sense of arthritis as normal for the older person and not normal in middle adulthood or childhood can contribute to problems in adjustment.

IMPACT OF RHEUMATIC DISEASE ACROSS THE LIFE SPAN

The diagnosis of rheumatic disease at various life stages can be expected to have at least some impact on developmental tasks occurring at that stage. The following sections will provide some research evidence regarding the impact of rheumatic disease across the life span.

Infancy and Preschool

More than 160,000 children in this country have been diagnosed with juvenile rheumatoid arthritis (10). The potential impact of this diagnosis on a young person and his/her family is clear. At a time when an infant is ideally surrounded by a supportive, predictable, and nurturing environment, the infant with juvenile arthritis may be presented with inexplicable pain; unpredictable failures when attempting to learn the most basic skills such as rolling over, sitting up, standing, and walking; and parents and family members who are overprotective. Even more difficult are those situations in which the toddler, either unaware of or oblivious to pain and limitations, makes forays into the world of independence and initiative and is greeted with negative reactions from loved ones that might engender shame, doubt, or guilt.

Research on the experience of pain in children has long been controversial. It was traditionally thought that children either do not experience pain or somehow perceive pain as less distressing than their adult counterparts (11). More recently, it has been acknowledged that children do experience pain and that the pain perception is modulated by a variety of psychological and socioenvironmental factors (12). It is now generally conceded that family resources (such as psychological functioning and tangible resources) predict adjustment in the child

with arthritis, and that many families adjust quite well after an initial period of adaptation (12). The coping efforts of parent and child do not occur in a vacuum, however. These families are embedded in a larger social context, including medical professionals, child care professionals, and community. The parents' understanding of how to help their child is a function of other messages, which are often mixed. The challenge facing the rheumatology professional working with infants and toddlers diagnosed with juvenile arthritis is to help the family help the child master developmental tasks.

Primary School and Pre-adolescence

The task of the school-age, pre-adolescent child is to develop a realistic sense of competence based on activities both in and out of school. At this stage, the role of larger, social structures can have a strong impact on a young person's sense of mastery. School systems unresponsive to the limitations that the youngster is confronting, or resentful of demands on their own limited resources, can contribute to a sense of hopelessness, helplessness, and futility in the student.

Children with juvenile arthritis may experience such school-related problems as impaired mobility, late arrival, difficulties moving from class to class on time, poor stamina, difficulties with fine and gross motor skills, difficulties with medication, and need for physical therapy, among others (13,14). These children miss 25% more days of school than do children with other chronic illnesses and 300% more than children with acute illnesses (14). Because the pain and fatigue experienced by the youngster often are not visible to others, and because symptoms can be highly variable even within a given day, the child may encounter skepticism from both classmates and teachers. The health professional working with grade school patients may find that the education system plays a key role in successful treatment.

Studies that examined the contribution to adjustment of age at onset, on the one hand, and duration of illness, on the other, have resulted in conflicting findings. It has been suggested that younger children are less able to appreciate the burdens of treatment regimens associated with chronic illness and, therefore, experience less emotional distress (15). There is also some reason to believe that coping and adjustment problems are more common during the early stages of illness. It is in these early stages that the child must come to understand his or her illness and its impact. Perceptions of stigma associated with chronic illness have been found to be associated with lower self-esteem in children (16), as have perceptions of physical appearance (17).

Adolescence and Young Adulthood

With adolescence come efforts to define identity; these efforts are commonly associated with a need to rebel against the rules of parents, teachers, and other authority figures (18). The adolescent with juvenile arthritis may be willing to sacrifice control of the illness for control of his/her life. Adolescent rebellion may be pursued on the playing field of arthritis management, and the young person may become unexpectedly recalcitrant. It has been reported that restrictions associated with juvenile arthritis are least during preschool age and increase through adolescence, when the forced dependency on parents can significantly affect adjustment (19).

A crucial task for the young adult with arthritis is determining how to incorporate this illness within an overall sense of identity. At a time when being different from one's peers is hardly a preferred state of affairs, the adolescent may take any risk just to "fit in." A particular difficulty for the adolescent with arthritis is that medications to control the disease can contribute to puberty-onset delays and related growth difficulties. This assault on sexual development may seriously challenge the adolescent's efforts to define a sense of self (20). The rheumatology professional must help the young patient balance personal independence with treatment adherence. A crucial part of this challenge involves helping parents let go of treatment management and helping the young adult comfortably take charge.

Midlife

Although there are more than 100 different types of adult rheumatic disease, the most common are osteoarthritis (OA), rheumatoid arthritis (RA), fibromyalgia, systemic lupus erythematosus, and ankylosing spondylitis. It is ironic that, with the exception of OA, these other rheumatic diseases often begin between the ages of 25 and 40. For most adults confronting the middle of their lives, the specter of chronic illness is hardly considered normative. Nevertheless, these and other chronic illnesses tend to strike at precisely the time when people are beginning jobs, relationships, and families. The identity and sense of competence formed at earlier stages may be seriously threatened; both the individual and his/her social system may be more or less able to make the accommodations demanded by the illness.

Research examining the impact of RA has shown that pain is associated with higher levels of stress and depression among patients, and that these problems can have negative consequences for patients' families and for other members of their social networks (21). The impact on family functioning includes increased frequency of arguments with marital partners and increased sexual problems. According to some research in patients with RA (22), 28–36% of spouses report frustration with the physical limitations of their partners, and 21% expressed concern over the future of the marriage as a result of health problems.

Rheumatic disease can affect the new mother's ability to parent, as well as her ability to perform in valued professional roles. One of the few studies examining the impact of a parent's RA on healthy children found that the children had fewer social resources and a heightened vulnerability to stress (23). Interviews with mothers who had RA revealed a tendency to rely on children to do for themselves (or for Mom) many of the things that mothers usually do, from tying shoelaces to making beds.

The struggle with new limitations is accompanied by a struggle to incorporate this new "patient identity" into one's overall identity in a meaningful and acceptable way. Lupus patients who were unable to resolve this conflict, and who clung instead to their cherished "me before lupus" identity, experienced greater amounts of depression (24).

Women with rheumatic disease, like their healthier counterparts, report high levels of psychological demands both at paid work and family work; autonomy was important in reducing family demands, and social support reduced the effects of work demands (25). It is important to define disability not only in terms of paid work but also in terms of family responsibilities and unpaid activities (26).

Studies have examined factors that appear to mediate the relationship between disease severity and psychological functioning, and have found that cognitive variables such as a perception of control or self-efficacy, as well as a sense of mastery or competence, contribute to better psychological status. Feelings of helplessness and hopelessness contribute to poorer adjustment (21,27). These cognitive components are consistent with life tasks identified by Erikson, and demonstrate the need to revisit these issues throughout the life span.

Health professionals should help the adult patient prioritize more important roles and goals and communicate which parts of the self are most worth protecting and preserving. At the same time, the professional should look for indications that this patient has high self-efficacy regarding his or her ability to manage the illness. In the absence of this ability, the process of sharing responsibility for treatment decisions will need to proceed more slowly.

Retirement and Older Adulthood

Because arthritis is thought of by many as "normal" in older adults, its impact on development would seem to be less. However, this stereotype of old age has negative consequences, causing some individuals to restrict their activities in ways that may not be necessary. Patient and practitioner may jointly conclude that slowing down is normal and necessary at this stage of life. Retirement among individuals with arthritis is often premature: 10 years after disease onset, more than 50% of people with RA and 30% of people with OA were found to be no longer working (28). Although changes in activity level at this stage of development may be quite normal, decisions that are made by the patients, based on their own wisdom and understanding of themselves, will contribute most effectively to coherence and integrity in the later stages of life.

Research has shown that as individuals age, a wide variety of limitations and personal failings are attributed to old age. The older a patient is, the more likely he or she and others will attribute even mild short-term symptoms to aging; this attribution is associated with the utilization of passive rather than active coping strategies (29,30). This kind of explanation carries with it the message that there is nothing that can be done about the older person's failings.

Because age cannot be changed, an explanation that says "I can't go out with my friends because I'm old and have arthritis" suggests there is nothing one can do but accept the situation. On the other hand, an explanation that says "I can't go out with my friends because I get tired easily" allows for the possibility of alternative plans and suggests that things are not hopeless. Health professionals may fall prey to these kinds of ageist conclusions as well. Younger patients tend to be evaluated more positively in the clinic setting and older patients are seen less positively, exacerbating the likelihood that the older patient will revert to a passive patient role (31). Just when rheumatic disease might finally feel normal, the need to confront and challenge these assumptions is most compelling.

GUIDELINES FOR THE HEALTH CARE PROVIDER

Factors to Consider

The theoretical models on which this chapter is based suggest some factors to be considered in the individual with rheumatic disease.

Age-related Processes. Age is merely a marker for developmental changes that typically occur in a certain order; great individual variability exists with respect to when and if specific events will occur. Motor skills develop at different rates in children, adolescents pursue their efforts to separate from parents at their own pace, not all adults marry and/or have children, and older adults vary greatly in their desire to remain active and involved in the world. Recognizing the variability in patients' lives will help prevent the professional from communicating to them a lack of "normalcy" if their course is somewhat different from the typical. It also may protect the professional from concluding too quickly that variations from the norm are a result of the disease.

History-related Processes. For each generation, at each stage of life, the world offers different experiences. Many young women struggle to balance marriage, family, and profession in a way that was less common for the wives and mothers who preceded them. Similarly, a patient's mental image of a severely disabled grandparent and his/her own likelihood of becoming similarly disabled does not take into consideration advances in medical care. It may sometimes be necessary to uncover and then dispel preconceived notions that are no longer relevant but may block progress in treatment.

Developmental Contextualism. Developmental changes of an individual do not occur in a vacuum. At each step, the process of adjustment is influenced by characteristics of the individual, the individual's family, and the individual's social world (e.g., work, school, friends), as well as by larger socioeconomic factors, such as the latest rules governing health insurance and access to care. All of these factors are present in the office of the health care provider as he/she attempts to assist the patient in dealing with this latest developmental challenge.

Developing a Treatment Plan. The ability of patients to manage their arthritis will be, to an extent, a function of the social context in which they are embedded. The demands of family, school, and work must be considered in the development of a treatment plan. The efforts of the professional to implement a successful treatment plan should include recognition that the patient's understanding of his/her disease comes from the social context, and that treatment will, in turn, influence that context. Successful treatment efforts will ascertain the individual's current illness representations (32), providing clarification and facts as necessary but also acknowledging and respecting deeply held beliefs (see Chapter 12, Social and Cultural Assessment), which may be more or less at odds with traditional Western medicine. Both professional and patient must work together to resolve the disparity. Ignoring these cultural beliefs will likely doom the traditional treatment plan to failure.

The successful treatment plan will ascertain the individual's current life goals. Each individual brings strengths and weaknesses to the experience of rheumatic disease, as well as an identity made up of a variety of valued roles and abilities. A treatment plan that specifies no tennis may be fine for the marginally athletic patient, but may be a serious blow to the professional tennis coach. To design a treatment plan that respects the needs of the individual and maximizes the likelihood of success, it is essential to determine patient expectations regarding the management of this illness and its place in his/her life. Finally, the plan should develop treatment goals, in conjunction with the patient, that are based on the realities of the disease and the realities of the patient's life.

Human development is a complex and highly individual process. To serve patients well, rheumatology health professionals need to invest time and attention to learning the unique needs and goals of each individual. It is this willingness to listen and respond to the patient that is the hallmark of the rheumatology health care team.

The author of this chapter would like to acknowledge the contributions of Theresa J. Brady, PhD, who co-authored this chapter in the first edition and whose perspective continues to be reflected here.

REFERENCES

1. Erikson E. Childhood and society. New York: Norton; 1964.
2. Havighurst RJ. Developmental tasks and education. New York: Longmans, Green; 1953.
3. Seiffge-Krenke I. Chronic disease and perceived developmental progression in adolescence. Dev Psychol 1998;34:1073–84.
4. Baldwin AL. Theories of child development. New York: Wiley; 1967.
5. Simmeonsson RJ. Theories of child development. In: Walker CF, Roberts MC, editors. Handbook of clinical psychology. New York: Wiley-Interscience; 1992, pp. 26–46.
6. Harter S. Processes underlying the construct, maintenance, and enhancement of the self-concept in children. In: Suls J, Greenwald A, editors. Psychological perspectives on the self. Hillsdale, NJ: Erlbaum; 1986, Vol. 3, pp. 137–81.
7. Bornstein MH, Lamb ME. Developmental psychology: an advanced textbook. Hillsdale, NJ: Lawrence Erlbaum, 1992.
8. Lerner RM. Developmental contextualism and the life-span view of person-context interaction. In: Bornstein M, Bruner JS. Interaction in human development. Hillsdale, NJ: Lawrence Erlbaum; 1989.
9. Baltes PB, Reese HW, Lipsitt LP. Life-span developmental psychology. Annu Rev of Psychol 1980;31:65–110.
10. Cassidy JT, Petty RE. Textbook of pediatric rheumatology. 2nd ed. NY: Churchill Livingstone; 1990.
11. Varni JW, Bernstein BH. Evaluation and management of pain in children with rheumatic diseases. Rheum Dis Clin North Am 1991;17:985–1000.
12. Hagglund KJ, Schopp LM, Alberts KR, Cassidy JT, Frank RG. Predicting pain among children with juvenile rheumatoid arthritis. Arthritis Care Res 1995;8:36–42.
13. Varni JW, Wilcox KT, Hanson V. Mediating effects of family social support on child psychological adjustment in juvenile rheumatoid arthritis. Health Psychol 1988;7:421–31.
14. Bartholomew LK, Koenning G, Dahlquist L, Barron K. An educational needs assessment of children with juvenile rheumatoid arthritis. Arthritis Care Res 1994;7:136–43.
15. Frank RG, Thayer JF, Hagglund KJ, Vieth AZ, Schopp LH, Beck NC, et al. Trajectories of adaptation in pediatric chronic illness: the importance of the individual. J Consult Clin Psychol 1998;66:521–32.
16. Westbrook LE, Bauman LJ, Shinnar S. Applying stigma theory to epilepsy. A test of a conceptual model. J Pediatr Psychol 1992;17:633–49.
17. Varni JW, Walco GA, Katz ER. A cognitive-behavioral approach to pain associated with pediatric chronic disease. J Pain Symptom Manage 1989; 4:238–41.
18. Manaster GJ. Adolescent development: a psychological approach. Itasca, IL: FE Peacock Publishers, Inc; 1989.
19. Ungerer JA, Horgan B, Chaitow J, Champion GD. Psychosocial functioning in children and young adults with juvenile arthritis. Pediatrics 1988; 81:195–202.

20. Eiser C, Berrenberg JL. Assessing the impact of chronic disease on the relationship between parents and their adolescents. J Psychosom Res 1995;39:109–14.

21. Bradley LA. Psychological dimensions of rheumatoid arthritis. In: Wolfe F, Pincus T, editors. Rheumatoid arthritis: pathogenesis, assessments, outcomes, and treatment. New York: Marcel Dekker; 1994, pp. 273–95.

22. Revenson TA, Majerovitz SD. The effects of chronic illness on the spouse. Social resources as stress buffers. Arthritis Care Res 1991;4:63–72.

23. Turner Cobb JM, Steptoe A, Perry L, Axford J. Adjustment in patients with rheumatoid arthritis and their children. J Rheumatol 1998;25:565–71.

24. Kobasa SCO, Bochnak E, McKinley PS. Patient identity in women with SLE. Arthritis Care Res 1991;4:S22.

25. Reisine S, Fifield J. Family work demands, employment demands and depressive symptoms in women with rheumatoid arthritis. Women's Health 1995;22:25–45.

26. Reisine S, Fifield J. Expanding the definition of disability: implications for planning, policy, and research. Milbank Q 1992;70:491–508.

27. Smith CA, Dobbins CJ, Wallston KA. The mediational role of perceived competence in psychological adjustment to arthritis. J Appl Soc Psych 1991;15:1218–47.

28. Boutaugh M, Brady T, Callahan L, Gibofsky A, Haralson K, Lappin D, et al. Quality of life action plan. Atlanta: Arthritis Foundation; 1993.

29. Leventhal EA, Prohaska TR; Age, symptom interpretation, and health behavior. J Am Geriatr Soc 1986;34:185–91.

30. Erber JT, Szuchman LT, Rothberg ST. Age, gender, and individual differences in memory failure appraisal. Psychol Aging 1990;5:600–3.

31. Greene MG, Adelman R, Charon R, Hoffman S. Ageism in the medical encounter: an exploratory study of the doctor-elderly patient relationship. Language & Communication 1986;6:113–24.

32. Schiaffino KM, Cea CD. Assessing chronic illness representations: the Implicit Models of Illness Questionnaire. J Behav Med 1995;18:531–48.

SECTION B: DIAGNOSIS AND ASSESSMENT

History and Physical Assessment

LISA A. NICHOLS, MSN, RN, CCRA

Over the past few decades, our understanding of rheumatic diseases has increased greatly due to technologic advances in joint imaging and clinical immunology. However, an extensive history and complete physical examination remain the basis of a sound evaluation of the patient with musculoskeletal complaints. It is estimated that 1 of every 6 visits to a primary care provider is motivated by musculoskeletal problems, which range from straightforward sprains and strains to complicated systemic diseases, such as systemic lupus erythematosus (SLE) or rheumatoid arthritis (RA). The examiner must have a working knowledge of the rheumatic diseases to recognize the appropriate path to follow when first questioning and examining the patient (1–6).

THE RHEUMATIC HISTORY

The history should be obtained from the patient in a private setting, before the physical examination is conducted. When possible, the interviewer should face the patient with no barriers between. If the patient is in pain or has difficulty sitting without support, he or she can sit in a chair with arms and a back, or perhaps recline rather than sit on the examining table. Attending to the patient's comfort at the outset will help establish a positive patient–provider relationship. Providing a nonthreatening environment can aid in gaining the patient's trust and help allay fears. The interview should begin with a general open-ended question such as "What is it that brings you in to see me today?" This will help elicit the chief complaint. It is important to listen to the exact words the patient uses to describe the symptoms, as well as note any nonverbal clues. The clinician should resist the temptation to hurry the patient along by offering language to describe the problem. If the patient is reluctant to give information spontaneously, or has difficulty describing symptoms, more direct questioning by the interviewer may be needed. When assessing the pediatric patient, both the child and the child's parent or guardian should be questioned about current complaints and past examination findings (7).

Assessing the Chief Complaint

A systematic approach should be used when attempting to elicit information. Assessment of 7 particular symptom details can provide clues of diagnostic importance: location, character,

quantity, course, aggravating and alleviating factors, setting, and associated manifestations (7). The pain associated with rheumatic conditions most frequently causes patients to seek out a health care provider.

The precise *location* of the pain is essential to determine whether the pain is articular or nonarticular. Pain described as "deep" or difficult to pinpoint with one finger is likely to be articular, whereas pain described as "superficial" and/or easily pinpointed along tendons or to adjacent joint structures is likely to be extraarticular.

The *character* or quality of the pain may best be described by the patient in comparison to another type of pain, such as "like a toothache" or "similar to labor pains." The origin of the pain can often be inferred from the patient's description. Muscular pain or myalgia is usually described as "crampy" or "throbbing," whereas neurologic pain is described as "pins and needles" or "electric shocks."

The *quantity* or intensity of pain is sometimes difficult to assess, as patients have different pain thresholds. Some patients, because of a need to convince the provider of the severity of the pain, may actually inflate the pain intensity. Children may best express their perception of pain by use of a cartoon pain assessment scale with several faces ranging from smiling to crying. The child chooses the face that best represents how he or she feels (8).

The *course* of the pain, including date and type of onset (e.g., insidious or sudden), duration, and progression may be of diagnostic importance. For example, pain may be acute (less than 6 weeks duration) with conditions such as gout or infectious arthritis, or it may be chronic (greater than 6 weeks duration) in osteoarthritis (OA) or RA. Joint pain may be intermittent (as in gout), additive (RA or OA), or migratory. Migratory articular pain implies a rapidly changing pattern of joint involvement and should suggest either rheumatic fever or viral or gonococcal arthritis. Nocturnal pain in a child may suggest growing pains, osteoid osteoma, or an inflammatory condition.

Aggravating and alleviating factors, such as rest or activity, heat or cold, should be assessed. The setting in which pain occurs may provide clues to causality, such as pain related to the performance of repetitive physical movements on the job in a patient with wrist pain. Musculoskeletal pain in a child that occurs only during the school week may suggest a school-related stressor. Associated manifestations, whether local (bony enlargements), constitutional (weight loss), or emotional (depression), can help determine the nature of the underlying process.

Joint swelling is an important component to many rheumatic diseases. Swelling may be subjective (i.e., perceived by the patient) or objective. As with pain, patients should be questioned about the location, pattern of onset, and aggravating or alleviating factors related to the swelling. Location is important in determining whether the swelling is localized to a discrete structure, as in a bursa, or to a broader area, such as a dependent limb. The pattern of onset may give clues to the acuteness of the problem, such as a traumatic injury. Aggravating and alleviating factors may include activity, rest, and response to medications.

Limitation of motion is commonly described by the patient in terms of interruption in their activities of daily living. Questions about the patient's ability to bathe, toilet, feed, dress, ambulate at home, and perform normal work or play activities should be addressed. Length of time the limitation has persisted and how the patient has adapted are important. Assessment of the use of ambulatory aids, such as canes or crutches, and assistive devices such as jar openers and dressing aids is necessary. The pattern of onset may have diagnostic importance. Sudden limitation of motion may be related to a tendon rupture, whereas a gradual limitation, as in contracture formation, may be caused by a chronic inflammatory condition.

Stiffness is the feeling of discomfort or restriction of movement after a period of inactivity. Morning stiffness of greater than 1 hour is a hallmark symptom of inflammatory arthritis, such as RA, and is usually systemic. Stiffness that occurs after brief periods of inactivity and lasts less than 60 minutes may occur in noninflammatory conditions such as OA. This sensation is most often perceived close to the affected joints. Patients may have difficulty quantifying the amount of stiffness they experience. Many are unclear as to what the interviewer means by stiffness. Some patients liken stiffness to pain, soreness, weakness, or fatigue. A generally accepted method of questioning patients about the duration of morning stiffness is to ask if they feel stiff upon awakening in the morning and the time stiffness is first noted. This is followed by inquiries to determine when the patient is most limber. The duration of stiffness is the time elapsed. Because patients may feel more stiff on some days and less on others, it is best to have them give an average of morning stiffness for the past week, rather than just on the day of the interview.

Weakness is defined as a decrease in, or loss of, muscle strength. It may coexist with other constitutional symptoms, such as stiffness and fatigue; therefore, it is sometimes difficult for patients to separate weakness from other symptoms. Actual muscle weakness is seen only when muscles are being used, and it is frequently noted by an inability to carry out activities of daily living. Questions should focus on the patient's ability to perform the following functions: ambulating, gripping, chewing, swallowing, and toileting. The weakness manifested in inflammatory myopathies is usually present in proximal muscles, whereas neuropathies cause distal muscle weakness. Patients with true myopathies have little trouble distinguishing between muscle weakness and generalized fatigue.

Fatigue is one of the most common constitutional complaints associated with rheumatic disease (see Chapter 37, Fatigue). It is defined as a feeling of "weariness, exhaustion, or lassitude . . . frequently associated with a decreased capacity for work" (9). Fatigue is assessed by determining the time of onset, frequency, degree of severity, and impact on activities of daily living. Accompanying psychosocial stressors, diet, sleep patterns, and activity level should be determined. Fatigue is often prominent in inflammatory and noninflammatory conditions (e.g., RA and fibromyalgia, respectively).

Other Pertinent History

A history of any previous therapy for the current problem should be sought. If similar symptoms have occurred before, it is likely that other providers have been consulted. Previous use of prescription or nonprescription medications, physical therapies, natural or home remedies, and other nontraditional treatments should be elicited. Questions might encompass length of previous therapy, adherence, presence of side effects, acceptability of cost, and the patient's perception of success or failure of these modalities. In addition, all of the patient's current medications for seemingly unrelated illnesses should be reviewed to rule out potential drug interactions or the possibility of drug-induced rheumatic symptoms, such as drug-induced lupus.

Exploring the patient's past medical and sexual history can help determine previous serious illnesses and surgeries, as well as identify conditions pertinent to the current illness. For example, urethritis that predates the onset of heel pain may be a significant clue to a diagnosis of Reiter's syndrome. The family history may also reveal information of diagnostic importance. Some rheumatic diseases have a genetic basis. For example, the HLA-B27–associated spondylarthropathies (ankylosing spondylitis, Reiter's syndrome, psoriatic arthritis, and enteropathic arthritis) can occur in several family members, even children. A family history of lupus in a child with SLE is not unusual, although chronic rheumatic diseases of childhood are seldom familial. A negative family history should also be noted. Potential environmental triggers, occupational exposure, travel, or recent viral or bacterial infection should not be overlooked. Finally, a careful developmental history should be obtained.

Review of Systems

The final part of the history is the review of systems. Because many rheumatic diseases are systemic in nature, a complete review of all body systems is another opportunity to identify important diagnostic symptoms or comorbid conditions. Examples of positive findings in the review of systems relevant to rheumatic diseases are included in Table 1.

THE PHYSICAL EXAMINATION

As with the history, the physical examination should take place in a private setting. Often patients with rheumatic disease are unable to seat themselves on the examination table without assistance. Conventional tables may have too high a step for the patient with muscle weakness or lower extremity disease. If necessary, the majority of the physical examination can be performed with the patient seated in a chair. A motorized examination table that can be lowered to a height of approximately 24–36 inches is preferable.

Physical examination of the child is similar to an adult, with two notable exceptions. First, a developmental assessment of

Table 1. Positive findings in the review of systems relevant to rheumatic diseases.*

System	Symptoms/complaints	Diagnosis to consider
Integument	Nail pitting	Psoriatic arthritis
	Nodules	RA
	Tophi	Gout
	Photosensitivity	SLE, scleroderma
	Rashes	Vasculitis, dermatomyositis, Lyme disease, psoriatic arthritis
Head and neck	Alopecia	SLE, scleroderma
	Dysphagia	Scleroderma, polymyositis
	Dry eyes/mouth	Sjögren's syndrome
	Jaw claudication	Temporal arteritis
	Nasal ulceration	Wegener's granulomatosus, SLE
Chest	Cough	Interstitial pulmonary fibrosis
	Chest pain	Pericarditis, pleuritis, costochondritis
Abdomen	Abdominal pain	Mesenteric vasculitis, peptic ulcer
Genitourinary	Penile ulceration	Behçet's syndrome, Reiter's syndrome
	Penile/vaginal discharge	Reiter's syndrome
	Microscopic hematuria	Lupus nephritis
Neurologic	Paresthesias	Carpal tunnel syndrome
	Seizures	Lupus cerebritis
	Headache	Temporal arteritis
Other	Fever	Systemic juvenile arthritis, septic arthritis, vasculitis
	Fatigue	Fibromyalgia, RA, SLE
	Weakness	Polymyositis

* RA = rheumatoid arthritis; SLE = systemic lupus erythematosus.

the child should be made to determine whether the child is maturing at an age-appropriate pace. Second, it is wise to modify the order of the examination, saving potentially painful or distressing aspects of the examination until last. Most of the examination can be conducted with the child sitting on the parent or guardian's lap.

The General Physical Examination

Examination of the patient with rheumatic disease should not be limited to the musculoskeletal system. As with the history, particular attention should be paid to other organ systems that may be involved. Concomitant illnesses, such as peptic ulcer disease, may also affect treatment selections.

The examination should begin with vital signs, including temperature, respirations, pulse, blood pressure, and weight. Unintentional weight loss may be a feature of neoplasia, chronic infection, or inflammatory disorders. Weight loss may be insidious early in the disease course, and is often only noted through serial evaluation. The adult patient should change into a gown and remove the shoes and socks to allow for complete inspection and evaluation of skin, nails, and extremities. It may not be necessary to thoroughly undress the child. Exposing small areas as they are assessed helps keep the child warm and feeling more in control.

The skin, hair, scalp, and nails are usually examined first. Special attention should be paid to the presence of any nodules, tophi, rashes, ulcerations, telangiectasias, alopecia, or Raynaud's phenomenon. Thorough pulmonary and cardiac examinations are required and are of particular importance when systemic sclerosis, SLE, or vasculitis are suspected. Careful neurologic examination is necessary when assessing for SLE, vasculitis, or nerve entrapment syndromes.

The Musculoskeletal Examination

Examination of the musculoskeletal system is best undertaken in a systematic manner. Many examiners begin at the head and

move downward, while others begin with the upper extremities, move toward the trunk and then downward to the feet. The latter approach is less threatening to the patient, as the examination begins in a socially neutral location—the hands. Throughout the examination, the patient should be as comfortable as possible. Support should be provided above or below an inflamed joint when moving it through range of motion, rather than holding on to the joint itself. Movements should be slow and fluid, not sudden or forceful. A relaxed patient is better able to tolerate a thorough examination, thus allowing a more accurate assessment.

The basic maneuvers of a musculoskeletal examination include inspection, palpation, range of motion, and assessment of function. Inspection and palpation are usually performed simultaneously. Similarly, range of motion and function can often be assessed together. For example, while a patient is demonstrating active range of motion of the shoulder, the examiner can ask if the patient is able to style her hair.

Joint Findings

The most common joint abnormalities are swelling, tenderness, warmth, crepitus, limitation of motion, and sometimes deformity. Swelling can result from several causes, such as bony overgrowth, joint effusion, or synovial proliferation, and it may be assessed by inspection and direct palpation of the joint. Tenderness is assessed by gentle, yet firm, palpation over the joint. Using both hands, the examiner should palpate the joint in all planes, anterior to posterior and medial to lateral. Enough pressure is exerted when the nail beds of the examiner's fingers or thumbs blanch. Observing the patient's facial expressions, as well as listening to verbal cues, is often useful. Warmth of the joint is best confirmed by comparison with the opposite joint. Skin color changes may also be present.

Crepitus is the palpable or audible grating sensation produced by roughened articular or extraarticular surfaces rubbing against each other. Some crepitus is appreciated in normal joints, but severe cracking or grating is usually indicative of chronic degenerative processes. When assessing limitation of motion, it is helpful to understand the normal ranges of joint motion. Range of motion should be assessed actively as well as passively. The only exception is the cervical spine, which should never be passively moved. Limitation of motion can occur either actively or passively; however, because patients are limited by their own pain, passive range of motion is usually greater, and therefore is a more accurate measure. Deformity denotes malalignment of the joint, which may result from various causes, such as bony enlargement, joint subluxation, contracture, or destruction of ligamentous support.

Examination of Specific Joints

The Small Joints. The temporomandibular (TM), acromioclavicular (AC), sternoclavicular (SC), and sternomanubrial (SM) joints deserve inclusion in the examination. Despite their size, these joints can exhibit pain, swelling, and crepitus. The TM joint is located at the junction of the articular tubercle of the temporal bone and the condyle of the mandible. It is assessed for warmth, pain, and swelling by direct palpation over the joint just anterior to the tragus. Crepitus can be discerned by inserting the index fingers just inside the external ear canal and gently pulling forward while the patient opens and closes the mouth. Range of motion is adequate if the patient is able to insert the width of two fingers inside the mouth. The AC joint is located by tracing the clavicle laterally to the acromion process. The SC joint is medial, where the clavicle meets the sternum. These 2 joints are assessed for tenderness, swelling, and crepitus. Motion of the AC is assessed by firmly pulling down on the forearm. The SC joint has minimal motion, but can be assessed by having the patient shrug the shoulders. The SM joint is located where the manubrium articulates with the body of the sternum. This joint has no motion, but it may be tender or swollen.

Shoulder. The shoulder is a ball and socket joint formed by the head of the humerus and the glenoid fossa of the scapula. Knowledge of shoulder anatomy is essential to assess the origin of symptoms. Pathology can occur in the glenohumeral joint, the rotator cuff, the subacromial bursae, the bicipital tendon, or the axillae. The shoulder is best examined from the front, so that both shoulders can be compared. The shoulder is inspected and palpated for warmth, swelling, tenderness, muscle spasm, or atrophy. Range of motion is assessed by having the patient perform the following procedures: raise arms forward in a wide arc and touch palms together above the head; with elbows flexed and hands on head, move arms posteriorly; raise arms extended in a sideways arc and touch palms together above head; and rotate the arm internally behind the back and touch between the scapulae. Normal ranges of motion are forward flexion 90°, backward extension 45°, abduction 180°, adduction 45°, internal rotation 55°, and external rotation 40–45° (3).

Elbow. The elbow is a hinge joint formed by 3 bony articulations: the humero-ulnar, radiohumeral, and the proximal radio-ulnar. The elbow is surrounded by one large (the olecranon) and several small bursae. This joint should be inspected for subcutaneous nodules, tophi, and the presence of olecranon bursitis. Palpation is conducted with the elbow flexed to approximately 70°. Synovitis is best appreciated in the medial paraolecranon groove. Normal elbow extension is 0–5°, while flexion is 135° or greater. Synovitis can cause loss

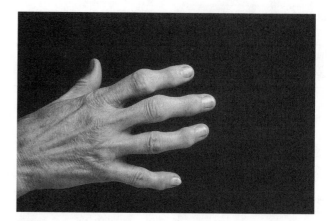

Figure 1. Bony enlargement of the distal interphalangeal joints (Heberden's nodes) and proximal interphalangeal joints (Bouchard's nodes) are common findings in osteoarthritis. These changes are more frequent in postmenopausal women and show some genetic predisposition. Reprinted from the Association of Rheumatology Health Professionals Teaching Slide Collection, 3rd edition.

of full extension, and if chronic, may result in flexion contracture (inability to fully extend to 0°).

Wrist and Hand. The wrist contains 8 carpal bones arranged in 2 rows; the proximal row articulates with the radius. The wrist normally has 60–70° of extension and 80–90° flexion. Ulnar to radius deviation at the wrist is 30° and 20°, respectively. The wrist is inspected and palpated for synovitis, warmth, thickened tendons, cystic swelling, and deformity. Mild synovitis may manifest as pain on movement. Dorsal/ventral instability with or without bogginess of the ulnar styloid is known as the *piano key sign.* Compression of the median nerve in the carpal tunnel is tested by placing the wrist in severe flexion (60°) for at least 1 minute. When numbness or paresthesias are noted along the distribution of the median nerve (first 3 digits and medial half of the fourth), it is known as a positive *Phalen's sign.* This maneuver may be difficult for the patient with acute synovitis. An alternative maneuver is to percuss repeatedly along the volar aspect of the wrist. A tingling or feeling of electric shock in the same median nerve distribution is known as *Tinel's sign.*

Another clinical sequelae of prolonged median nerve compression in the carpal tunnel is thenar muscle atrophy, noted on the palm at the base of the thumb. *Dupuytren's contracture* may be noted as thickening and contracture of the palmar aponeurosis, causing severe flexion of the fourth and fifth fingers. *DeQuervain's tenosynovitis* is a common cause of wrist pain due to inflammation and stenosing of the tendon sheaths at the base of the thumb near the radial styloid. It is assessed by having the patient flex the thumb into the palm, then grip the fingers over the thumb and move the hand downward (ulnar deviated). If tenosynovitis is present, this maneuver may produce exquisite tenderness on the radial side of the wrist.

The metacarpophalangeal (MCP), proximal interphalangeal (PIP), and distal interphalangeal (DIP) joints comprise the small joints of the hands. They are hinge joints held in place by tendons and ligaments. Range of motion of these joints is most easily assessed by having the patient slowly flex the fingers to form a fist. Loss of extension in any single digit is best expressed as the number of degrees lacking full extension. Hands should be inspected for swelling, deformity, and skin and nail changes. Rheumatoid arthritis predominantly affects the MCP and PIP joints. Common deformities include *swan neck deformity,* involving hyperextension of the PIP joint and flexion of the DIP joint, and *boutonniere deformity*, or flexion contracture of the PIP joint with hyperextension of the DIP joint. Osteoarthritis predominantly affects the first carpometacarpal joint and the DIP joints. Osteophytic nodules that form on the PIP and DIP joints are known as *Bouchard's nodes* and *Heberden's nodes*, respectively (Figure 1). Scleroderma can cause the skin over the fingers to have a tight, shiny, atrophic appearance *(sclerodactyly)*. Pitting of the nails and dystrophic changes *(onycholysis)* may be seen in psoriatic arthritis.

Hip. The hip is a major weight-bearing ball and socket joint, formed by the head of the femur and the pelvic acetabulum. It is surrounded by strong ligaments and bursae. Inspection of the hip begins with gait assessment. Before palpating the hip, instruct the patient to indicate where pain is located. Often patients will point to the lateral side and describe the pain as being in the "hip joint," when in reality they are pointing over the trochanteric bursa. True hip pain is manifested anteriorly in the groin fold. The hip has a wide range of motions. Extension (normal 30°) can be measured several ways, including having the patient drop the leg off the table; or from a standing position moving one leg backward; or lifting the leg off the table while lying supine. Flexion (normal 120°) is asssessed with the patient supine and drawing one knee up to the chest without bending the back. While in this position, the opposite hip can be checked for a flexion contracture. Abduction (normal 45°) is moving the leg away from the midline. Adduction (normal 20° to 30°) is moving the leg across the midline. Internal and external rotation are performed with the knee and hip flexed to 90°. Rotating the heel medially causes external rotation (normal 45°) and outwardly causes internal rotation (normal 35°). Hip movement can be quickly measured by placing the heel medially to the opposite knee and slowly lowering the flexed knee toward the table.

Knee. The knee is a large diarthrodial joint supported by a series of ligaments and surrounded by several bursae. Normal knee extension is 0°; normal flexion is 135°. The knee is inspected for swelling, deformity such as *genu varum* (bow legs) or *genu valgum* (knock knees), flexion contracture, locking or buckling, Baker's or popliteal cysts, and skin changes. The knee is palpated with the patient supine and in full extension. The patella should move easily medially and laterally, and may ballot if a large effusion is present. Minor knee effusions are best palpated after milking the fluid away from the medial side and then tapping the lateral aspect of the knee with the other hand. If an effusion is present, a small wave or bulge of fluid will reappear on the medial aspect *(bulge sign).*

Stability of the collateral ligaments is tested by placing the patient supine with the knee at full extension. One hand stabilizes the femur on either side of the knee and acts as a fulcrum, while the other hand grasps the ankle and moves the lower extremity in the direction of the braced hand to assess the contralateral collateral ligament. Excess movement may indicate collateral ligament laxity or damage. The cruciate ligaments are tested by having the patient flex the hip to 45° and the knee to 90°. The examiner fixes the foot position. The fingers are then placed posteriorly in the popliteal space behind the knee, with the thumbs anteriorly over the joint line. The lower extremity is pulled forward or pushed backward to assess the cruciate ligaments. Increased forward motion denotes pathology with the anterior cruciate ligament. Increased posterior

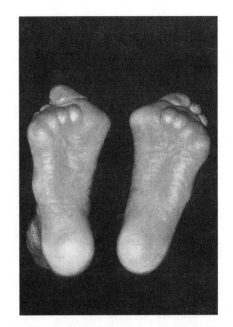

Figure 2. Chronic inflammation at the metatarsophalangeal (MTP) joints causes damage resulting in subluxation of the toes upwards. With the MTP joints displaced, weight bearing is not shared through the toes, but falls directly on the prominent metatarsal heads. This results in pain on weight bearing and difficulty in walking, and can cause the metatarsal heads to erode through the skin on the sole of the foot. Reprinted from the Association of Rheumatology Health Professionals Teaching Slide Collection, 3rd edition.

motion may indicate posterior cruciate damage. A positive finding is known as a *drawer sign.* Other findings related to knee pathology are quadriceps atrophy, crepitation on movement secondary to cartilage degeneration, and tenderness over the anserine bursa, on the anteromedial tibial plateau below the knee.

Ankle and Foot. The ankle is a hinge joint formed by the distal ends of the tibia and fibula and the proximal talus. This joint is limited in motion to plantar flexion (50°) and dorsiflexion (20°). The subtalar joint (articulation of the talus and the calcaneus) is responsible for inversion and eversion (5° each direction). The foot includes the intertarsal joints (midfoot), and the metatarsophalangeal (MTP) and interphalangeal (IP) joints of the toes. The metatarsal heads and the calcaneus are the weight-bearing portions of the foot. Midfoot range of motion is assessed by stabilizing the calcaneus and inverting and everting the forefoot (MTP and IP joints). Forefoot range of motion can be checked by having the patient flex and extend the toes.

The foot and ankle should be inspected in weight-bearing and non-weight-bearing positions, both with and without footwear. Assessment should include swelling, deformity, nodules, tophi, nail changes, and calluses. Swelling of the ankle joint is sometimes difficult to differentiate from generalized edema. True ankle joint effusions are noted as a non-pitting fullness anteriorly and/or posteriorly around the malleoli. Ankle synovitis causes tenderness on movement. The feet and toes are commonly affected in RA, OA, and gout; deformities may include lateral deviation of the great toe *(hallux valgus)*, hyperextension of the MTP joint *(hammer toe)*, and dorsal subluxation of the MTP joint *(cockup deformity)* (Figure 2). Calluses and abnormal patterns of shoe wear can be important clues in assessing foot problems.

Spine. The spine supports the upright posture of the body and provides protection for the spinal column. Spinal range of motion provides flexibility for the trunk. The vertebral column as a whole produces 90° of flexion. The trunk (minus the cervical spine) extends to 30° posteriorly, and 50° laterally in either direction. The cervical spine provides 45° of flexion, 50–60° of extension, 60–80° of rotation, and 40° of lateral bending. In the RA patient, cervical range of motion is always done actively, as there is a possibility for subluxation of C1 and C2. The spine should be inspected first as a whole and then by section. A thorough examination requires the patient to be standing, with the entire back, shoulders, hips, legs, and feet visible. The spine is inspected for symmetry, abnormal curvature (scoliosis, kyphosis, lordosis), and paravertebral spasm. Palpation is performed systematically from the top down and from side to side. Ankylosing spondylitis commonly affects the thoracic and lumbar spine, causing forward protrusion of the head, decreased chest expansion, thoracic kyphosis, and loss of lumbar lordosis. The *Wright–Schöber test* measures forward flexion of the lumbar spine. A line is drawn at the level of the posterior-superior iliac crests, with a second line 10 cm above the first. The distance between the two marks increases 5 cm or more with normal lumbar mobility and less than 4 cm in the case of decreased lumbar mobility.

The sacrum is a triangular bone formed by the union of 5 sacral vertebrae. The lateral aspect of the sacrum has a large auricular surface for articulating with the ileum of the hip. These sacroiliac joints are assessed with the patient lying on his or her side. The examiner exerts steady downward pressure over the upper iliac crest. Localization of pain to the sacroiliac area is a positive sign of sacroiliitis, a common feature of ankylosing spondylitis. The *straight-leg raising test* is a screening tool for neurologic or muscular low back pain. This is done with the patient supine and one knee in full extension. The leg is gradually raised until symptoms occur, usually within 30–80° of flexion. Pain is aggravated by forced dorsiflexion of the foot and relieved with flexion of the knee.

SUMMARY

A thorough history and physical examination of the musculoskeletal and selected other systems are the most important components of the evaluation of rheumatic complaints. Too much reliance on or inappropriate interpretation of laboratory testing and radiologic procedures may cloud the diagnostic picture, rather than guide the evaluation and plan of care. Early assessment and intervention can positively impact the morbidity and mortality of patients with rheumatic diseases. A careful history and physical examination can also yield the economic benefits of better utilization of clinician time and resources and decreased costs to patients.

REFERENCES

1. Cush JJ, Kavanaugh AF, Olsen NJ, Stein CM, Kazi S, Saag KG. Rheumatology diagnosis and therapeutics. Baltimore: Williams & Wilkins; 1999.
2. Cush JJ, Lipsky PE. Approach to articular and musculoskeletal disorders. In Fauci AS, Braunwald E, Isselbacher KJ, Wilson JD, Martin JB, Kasper DL, Hauser SL, Longo DL, editors. Harrison's principles of internal medicine, 14th ed. New York: McGraw Hill; 1998.
3. Moder KG, Hunder GG. Examination of the joints. In Ruddy S, Harris ED, Sledge CB, editors. Kelley's textbook of rheumatology, 6th ed. Philadelphia: WB Saunders; 2000.
4. Polly HF, Hunder GG. Rheumatologic interviewing and physical examination of the joints, 2nd ed. Philadelphia: WB Saunders; 1978. Hoppenfeld S. Physical examination of the spine and extremities. New York: Appleton-Century-Crofts; 1976.
6. American College of Rheumatology Ad Hoc Committee on Clinical Guidelines. Guidelines for the initial evaluation of the adult patient with acute musculoskeletal symptoms. Arthritis Rheum 1996;39:1–8.
7. Bickley LS, Hoekelman RA. Bates' guide to physical examination and history taking, 7th ed. Philadelphia: Lippincott Williams & Wilkins; 1999.
8. Cassidy JT, Petty RE. Textbook of pediatric rheumatology, 4th ed. Philadelphia: WB Saunders; 2000.
9. American Rheumatism Association Glossary Committee. Dictionary of the rheumatic diseases. Volume 1: signs and symptoms. New York: Contact Associates International, Ltd; 1982.

Audiovisual Resources

Title: The Joint Exam and You
Copyright: The University of Texas Southwestern Medical Center, 1991
Write to: The University of Texas Southwestern Medical Center
            Rheumatic Diseases Division
            Dallas, Texas, 75235-8577
            214-648-3466
Title: Physical Examination of the Musculoskeletal System, 3rd ed.
Copyright: JB Lippincott Company, 1995
Write to: 227 East Washington Square
            Philadelphia, PA 19106-3780
            800-523-2945
            ISBN: 0397-55225-4

Diagnostic Laboratory Tests and Imaging

MARK H. WENER, MD, FACR

Diagnostic tests and radiographic imaging have great importance in diagnosis and assessment of rheumatic diseases. They are an integral part of the American College of Rheumatology (ACR) classification criteria for many of the common rheumatic diseases, including rheumatoid arthritis (RA), systemic lupus erythematosus (SLE), and degenerative joint disease, and are widely used in routine clinical diagnosis. Sometimes negative results of tests are useful, as in the diagnosis of fibromyalgia and exclusion of inflammatory joint disease. Despite the usefulness of diagnostic tests, it is important to remember that no rheumatic disease is established by tests alone. The careful integration of history, physical examination, laboratory tests, and imaging is necessary to establish a diagnosis.

Laboratory tests assist in disease management in several ways: 1) establishing a diagnosis; 2) determining prognosis; 3) monitoring disease activity, progression, or damage; 4) monitoring drug or therapeutic toxicities; 5) establishing complications of the underlying disease process; and 6) excluding alternative diagnoses or complications. The optimal diagnostic test should be *sensitive* (able to identify a disease when present) and *specific* (able to identify that the disease is not present). An evaluative or monitoring test should be sensitive to change in the disease state over time. Ideally, tests should be inexpensive, standardized, easily performed, and readily available. Diagnostic testing is of great importance in establishing treatment modalities, whether these are medicines, exercises, or lifestyle adjustments.

GENERAL LABORATORY TESTING

Rheumatic disorders and treatments can affect major body systems. General laboratory testing reveals multi-system organ involvement and specific organ function. It is important to test the patient at baseline and periodically during the course of treatment to detect disease improvement, progression, and medication toxicity. A flow sheet for laboratory data is a valuable tool for the health care provider to assess the overall disease state and toxicity.

Hematology

A complete blood count including hemoglobin, hematocrit, white blood cell count with differential, and platelet count is one of the most common baseline tests in systemic rheumatic diseases. It is used not only for rheumatic disease diagnosis and monitoring, but also for detection of anemia or other blood disorders.

Understanding the cause or mechanism of anemia is important for characterizing the disease and for selecting and monitoring treatment. For example, anemia due to accelerated hemolysis is caused by autoantibodies directed against red cells in many patients with SLE. Similarly, leukopenia and thrombocytopenia caused by autoimmunity are common in SLE and may occasionally be seen as part of the underlying disease process in RA. Many rheumatic diseases such as RA, SLE, and systemic sclerosis are associated with an anemia termed *anemia of chronic disease.* In this type of anemia, the red cells typically have normal shape and hemoglobin content (normocytic and normochromic). The anemia does not respond to administration of iron; in fact, the problem is caused by the inflammation, which alters the availability of iron for the developing red blood cell in the bone marrow. This is in contrast to the iron-deficiency anemia that develops as a consequence of gastrointestinal bleeding from nonsteroidal anti-inflammatory drugs, in which the cells are small and the hemoglobin content low, and which typically responds to iron therapy. Therapy with drugs such as methotrexate may result in a macrocytic anemia, where red cells are large. Modest anemia (hemoglobin levels as low as 10 g/dl) is commonly seen in rheumatic diseases and is ascribed to anemia of chronic disease when normocytic and normochromic. More severe anemia should always be investigated to determine whether it is related to drug toxicity or serious complications of the underlying rheumatic disease.

Knowledge of hematologic abnormalities is important in designing exercise programs, education, activities of daily living, and medical treatment. For example, the provider needs to be aware when prescribing medications that bleeding may occur when platelet counts are low, or infections may occur when white cell counts are low. When the patient has anemia, he or she may experience general loss of energy and endurance.

Urinalysis

Urinalysis is one of the most informative, easy to perform, and cost-effective laboratory tests. Analysis for protein and microscopic presence of cells is important as a diagnostic aid in SLE, which has a high incidence of nephritis. Proteinuria is one of the ACR classification criteria for SLE. Nephritis can be reflected as increased urinary protein, white or red cells, and the presence of casts on microscopic analysis. When present, proteinuria should be quantitated by a timed collection (typically 24 hours).

Urinalysis is used to monitor for toxicities related to gold or penicillamine treatment of RA because of the associated renal toxicity manifested by proteinuria (both drugs) and hematuria (gold). Trace and modest proteinuria frequently can be managed by reducing the dosage of medications. Large amounts of proteinuria may require cessation of drugs. There are multiple potential causes of nephritis, and renal biopsy may be performed to determine the renal histopathology that is resulting in the protein loss.

Chemical Analysis of Blood

Routine blood chemistries are commonly measured as a panel of tests. Serum electrolytes, renal function tests (blood urea nitrogen and creatinine), liver damage and function tests, and mineral metabolism tests are often included. Most medications are metabolized by the liver and excreted by the kidneys, and the possibility of drug toxicity may be monitored with such tests. Toxicity may be reflected as a decrease in serum albumin, a rise in liver damage indicators such as alanine aminotransferase (ALT) and aspartate aminotransferase (AST), or an increase in blood urea nitrogen or creatinine (renal function). For example, an increase in ALT and/or AST in a patient taking methotrexate or other drugs for RA is an indication of potentially significant liver toxicity, which may require reduction or cessation of the drug.

Elevated serum uric acid is useful in the diagnosis of gout, although the diagnosis can be established with certainty only if sodium urate crystals are seen in tissue or synovial fluid. The higher the level of serum uric acid above the normal range (2.5 to 8 mg/dl), the greater the risk of development of gout. Nevertheless, there are limitations to using serum uric acid as a diagnostic test. Transient and persistent hyperuricemia is common, and not all hyperuricemic patients develop gout. Furthermore, a normal uric acid may be seen in patients at the time of their acute gout attacks. Once a diagnosis of gout is established, monitoring the serum uric acid is helpful to determine the appropriate dosing of the medications.

Serum measures of muscle damage, including creatine kinase (CK, previously known as creatine phosphokinase or CPK), myoglobin, and aldolase, are used to diagnose and monitor patients with polymyositis and dermatomyositis. The highest and most persistent levels of these muscle damage markers are seen in the inflammatory myopathies and can be used as a therapeutic indicator, because they will decrease with disease improvement. These measures can be elevated in conditions involving muscle breakdown or necrosis, such as intramuscular injections, extreme exercise, or myocardial infarction. Lactate dehydrogenase and AST may be elevated in muscle disease and mistaken for abnormalities of liver function. A serum CK-MB, while appropriate as a sensitive measurement of heart damage, is not a sensitive measure of skeletal muscle damage such as occurs in patients with myositis.

Viral Screening Tests

Many of the drugs used to treat rheumatic diseases can cause liver damage; it is thus common to screen for preexisting liver disease before starting these drugs. In addition, various forms of vasculitis and other rheumatic conditions are associated with hepatitis infections. Tests for hepatitis B commonly include measurement of hepatitis B surface antibody (HBsAb) and surface antigen (HBsAg). A positive test result for HBsAb indicates that the patient is protected from hepatitis B, either because of previous infection or previous immunization. A positive test result for HBsAg indicates that the patient is infected with hepatitis B, and follow-up tests are indicated.

Hepatitis C infection is relatively common, affecting about 1% of the U.S. population. The screening test for hepatitis C virus is performed by testing for antibodies to hepatitis C. If the antibody test result is positive, followup testing is performed to detect circulating hepatitis C RNA, which confirms active infection. In patients with positive antibody test results but negative RNA test results, the infection could be cured or the virus may still be present in the liver. Sometimes, repeat testing for hepatitis C RNA is performed to determine if a negative test result becomes positive, or to quantify the concentration of virus in patients known to be infected.

COMMON SEROLOGIC TESTS

Autoantibodies

An autoantibody is an immunoglobulin that is directed against a normally occurring protein or cellular component (see Chapter 3, Immunology, Inflammation, and Genetics). Autoantibodies may react with soluble serum proteins, such as antibodies directed against immune globulin (rheumatoid factor), or they may be directed against cell components such as cytoplasmic or nuclear antigens (antinuclear antibody). Autoantibodies are common in RA, SLE, and diffuse connective tissue diseases. Tests for autoantibodies are commonly performed in patients with musculoskeletal complaints.

Rheumatoid Factor

The commonly observed rheumatoid factor (RF) in RA is an IgM antibody that is directed against the constant portion of IgG. In some laboratories, it is detected by an agglutination test using latex particles or sheep red blood cells. In this test, the latex particles or sheep cells are coated with IgG and reacted with the patient's serum. If IgM rheumatoid factor is present, the latex particles or sheep cells clump or agglutinate. The test is quantified by serial 2-fold dilution of the serum, and the titer (the highest serum dilution at which visible agglutination occurs) is determined. A typical significant positive result of this test would be 1:160, indicating that the serum test had visible agglutination at a 1:160 dilution of serum, but no agglutination at the next dilution (i.e., 1:320). In larger laboratories, rheumatoid factor is more commonly measured on an instrument called a nephelometer, which measures the amount of light scattering that is caused to a beam of light passing through a solution. Nephelometric techniques provide better quantification and may be automated. Results are typically reported in international units per ml, where a typical significant positive result might be 50 IU/ml.

No matter how it is measured, rheumatoid factor is not diagnostic of RA. In early or mild RA, many patients will test negative for rheumatoid factor. However, 70–80% of patients with RA will become rheumatoid factor positive (1). The test cannot be used alone to diagnose RA, but it is one of the ACR classification criteria. A positive rheumatoid factor is also a prognostic test, since high titers of RF are associated with increased disease severity, the development of erosions, extra-articular manifestations, and greater disability (2). Rheumatoid factor does not change rapidly with treatment, so there is little

Table 1. Conditions associated with positive tests for rheumatoid factor.

Rheumatic diseases
   Rheumatoid arthritis (~70%)
   Sjögren's syndrome (~90%)
   Systemic lupus erythematosus (~20%)
   Cryoglobulinemia syndrome (90%)
Lung diseases
   Interstitial fibrosis
   Silicosis
Infections
   Hepatitis C virus infection
   Acute viral infections
   Endocarditis
   Tuberculosis
Miscellaneous
   Sarcoidosis
   Malignancies
   Aging

reason to repeat this test once a high-positive result is found. Rheumatoid factors are also found in some patients with SLE and in a form of vasculitis known as the mixed cryoglobuline-mia syndrome.

False-positive results for rheumatoid factor also limit the diagnostic specificity of this test. The incidence and titer of rheumatoid factor increase somewhat with age until patients reach the age of 70 or 80 years (3). Many other rheumatic diseases, as well bacterial endocarditis, tuberculosis, osteomy-elitis, and chronic viral and parasitic infections may be asso-ciated with positive test results for rheumatoid factor (Table 1). Recent attention has been paid to the fact that positive RF test results are also seen in many patients with chronic hepatitis C infection.

Antinuclear Antibodies

Antinuclear antibodies (ANA) are commonly seen in autoim-mune rheumatic diseases. A positive ANA test is not diagnos-tic of connective tissue disease, but ANA are seen with a high frequency in SLE, systemic sclerosis, Sjögren's syndrome, polymyositis, and RA. Approximately 95–99% of patients with SLE will be ANA positive over the course of their disease (4).

The ANA test is usually performed as an indirect immuno-fluorescence test using the patient's serum overlaid onto a cell substrate. The human cell line HEp-2 (an immortalized cancer) is commonly used as the substrate. After the serum is allowed to react with the substrate cells, the extra serum is washed off. Next, a fluorescent labeled antibody to normal human IgG is allowed to react with the substrate. The fluorescent labeled antibody binds to the serum antibody, which has bound to the substrate. This can be detected by a technologist looking at the reacted substrate with a fluorescence microscope.

The ANA test is a screening test with a high degree of sensitivity for the diagnosis of SLE. Unfortunately, it is also associated with many false-positive test results, particularly when the ANA is present at low titer. In general, ANA titers of less than 1/80 have less clinical significance than do those of higher titer. However, positive test results must always be interpreted in light of the history, physical examination, and other laboratory tests to establish a diagnosis of SLE or related rheumatic diseases.

The ANA patterns as seen under the fluorescence micro-scope have some importance, but are rarely diagnostically specific. The pattern with the greatest diagnostic significance is the anti-centromere pattern, which is typically associated with systemic sclerosis, and most often with limited cutaneous systemic sclerosis. The nucleolar pattern is also associated with systemic sclerosis. The diffuse and speckled patterns have little direct diagnostic significance, since they are seen in patients with SLE or a variety of other conditions. When present in low titer, the diffuse and the speckled patterns are most commonly seen in patients without an underlying rheumatic disorder.

If ANA are present and the patient has clinical features that suggest an autoimmune rheumatic syndrome, more specific testing is indicated (5) (Table 2). The antibody against double-stranded or native DNA (anti-dsDNA) is most closely associ-ated with the peripheral or diffuse ANA pattern and has high specificity for the diagnosis of SLE. About 80% of patients with SLE will develop anti-dsDNA at some time in their disease course. When present in large amounts, anti-dsDNA is typically associated with diffuse proliferative lupus nephritis and a risk for more severe SLE. Measurements of anti-dsDNA tend to change with disease activity, so this measure is often repeated to help monitor disease activity.

Another antibody, anti-Sm (named for a lupus patient, Mrs. Smith, from whom the antibody was originally obtained) also has high specificity for SLE, but it is present in only about 20–40% of SLE patients. Anti-Sm leads to a speckled ANA

Table 2. Antinuclear antibodies and related autoantibodies in various diseases.*

Antibody	Frequency of positive test result								
	Nl	SLE	Drug LE	MCTD	Sjögren	SSc	CREST	DM/PM	RA
ANA	**1–30**	**95–99**	**100**	**95**	**70–90**	**80**	**80**	**80**	**50**
dsDNA	1–2	**60–80**			30				
Histones		60	**90**						
RNP		40		**90**		15	10	15	
Sm		**30**							
Ro (SSA)	1–5	**40**			**50–90**				5
La (SSB)		**15**			**60**				
Scl-70						**30**	10		
Centromere						30	**85**		
Jo-1								**30**	

* Numbers show the percentage of patients with a given diagnosis that have the corresponding serum autoantibody. The most important associations are highlighted in **bold**. ANA = immunofluorescence ANA; Nl = normal; SLE = systemic lupus erythematosus; Drug LE = drug-induced lupus; MCTD = mixed connective-tissue disease; Sjögren = primary Sjögren's syndrome; SSc = systemic sclerosis (scleroderma); CREST = CREST syndrome variant of systemic sclerosis, i.e., limited cutaneous systemic sclerosis; DM/PM = dermatomyositis/polymyositis; RA = rheumatoid arthritis.

pattern. Another important antibody with a speckled ANA pattern is the RNP antibody, seen in sera of patients with SLE or an overlap disease known as mixed connective tissue disease. Other diagnostically useful autoantibodies associated with positive ANA tests include antihistone antibodies, associated with drug-induced lupus and spontaneous SLE, and anti-Scl70 (anti-topoisomerase I), associated with diffuse cutaneous systemic sclerosis (or scleroderma). Antibodies to SSA (anti-Ro) and anti-SSB (anti-La) are associated with primary Sjögren's syndrome and with SLE, particularly forms of SLE with prominent skin involvement but without prominent renal disease.

Antineutrophil Cytoplasmic Antibodies

Recently, the diagnostic value of antibodies directed against neutrophilic polymorphonuclear leukocyte (neutrophil) cytoplasmic antigens has been appreciated. Antibodies to neutrophil cytoplasmic antigens (ANCA) occur in 2 immunofluorescent patterns: a "classic" diffuse cytoplasmic (cANCA) distribution, and a perinuclear (pANCA) pattern. The cANCA pattern is associated strongly with the form of vasculitis known as Wegener's granulomatosis, and it may be seen in related forms of vasculitis. In general, the greater the severity and extent of clinical involvement, the higher the titer of cANCA. About 95% of patients with active generalized Wegener's have a positive ANCA, versus about 60% of patients with inactive generalized Wegener's and 60% of active limited (localized) Wegener's. Also, antibody titers generally fall in response to treatment and rise in association with clinical deterioration. The cANCA pattern is highly specific for these clinical entities, although there are a few cases of cANCAs reported in patients with other diagnoses. The cANCA immunofluorescence pattern is almost always caused by antibodies to a neutrophil granule enzyme known as proteinase-3; these antibodies can be identified by an ELISA test for anti-proteinase-3. The pANCA pattern has been observed in association with a variety of diseases, including various forms of vasculitis, inflammatory bowel disease, SLE, RA, and juvenile rheumatoid arthritis. Several different antigens are recognized by pANCA; however, antibodies directed against the neutrophil myeloperoxidase enzyme are those most closely linked to vasculitis.

Antiphospholipid (APL) Antibodies

Antibodies directed against phospholipids have received considerable attention in the last few years because of new appreciation of clinical associations and development of newer techniques for their measurement. The VDRL test and other serologic tests for syphilis employ reagents containing the phospholipid cardiolipin in the antigen mixture, and for decades, patients with SLE have been known to have false-positive test results for syphilis. Use of more specific assays led to the recognition that approximately 40% of patients with SLE have antibodies to cardiolipin. Another phenomenon seen in some patients with SLE is the lupus inhibitor or lupus anticoagulant, which is a type of autoantibody causing a prolonged activated partial thromboplastin time (PTT, clotting test). Studies have demonstrated that the lupus inhibitor is also an antibody directed against phospholipids and phospholipid-binding proteins. In those laboratory tests, lupus inhibitors led

to a prolonged PTT, and therefore might be predicted to lead to bleeding. In contrast, patients with these autoantibodies have an enhanced risk of thrombosis, including arterial and venous thromboses. In recognition of the increasing importance of the antiphospholipid syndrome in patients with lupus, the American College of Rheumatology classification criteria for SLE were modified to include the presence of antiphospholipid antibodies as part of the epidemiologic classification criteria (6).

In considering a patient with possible antiphospholipid syndrome, measurement of both the lupus inhibitor and anticardiolipin antibodies, and possibly a serologic test for syphilis, is appropriate, since the presence of one APL does not correlate well with the presence of another. In general, IgG anticardiolipin has a higher predictive value than IgM or IgA anticardiolipin, and the higher the elevation, the greater the positive predictive value for an association with antiphospholipid syndrome. It has been suggested that at least part of the anticardiolipin activity may be caused by antibodies to one or more protein cofactors that bind to cardiolipin or other phospholipids. The most important of these protein cofactors appears to be a phospholipid-binding protein known as beta-2-glycoprotein I (β2GPI). Because of both biologic and technical variation in APL assays, the presence of antibodies in high titer and detection of more than one antibody (e.g., anticardiolipin and anti-β2GPI) gives greater credence to the clinical significance of these antibodies in a given patient.

COMPLEMENT

The complement system is a series of proteins that play an important role in fighting infection and enhancing the inflammatory process (7). Complement is thought to be involved in disorders that involve immune complexes such as SLE or certain forms of vasculitis. When immune complexes are formed and cleared from the body, the complement level is decreased.

There are 3 common measurements for serum complement: the protein components C3 and C4, and CH_{50} (total hemolytic complement), which is a biologic measure of the entire complement pathway. In the rheumatic diseases, low levels of CH_{50}, C3, and C4 are usually related to consumption of complement by immune complex activation of the classical pathway (7). Rarely, reductions are related to an absence of one of the complement proteins. Complement measurement is particularly useful in SLE, due to its association with active disease. A decrease in complement level may precede the development of disease flares, particularly renal disease. Serial measurement of complement levels is frequently performed to assess disease activity in patients with SLE.

HLA ANTIGENS

Human leukocyte antigens (HLA) are present on the surface of nucleated cells, and play a central role in determining the genetic predisposition to a variety of immune-mediated processes, including autoimmune diseases. Currently, only HLA-B27 is commonly measured in the diagnosis of rheumatic diseases. This antigen is found in 5% to 10% of the U.S. population, but it is present in 95% of patients with ankylosing

Table 3. Synovial fluid analysis in rheumatic disease.*

	GROUP			
	I	II	III	IV
Clarity	Clear	Translucent	Opaque	Bloody
Type	Noninflammatory	Inflammatory	Infectious	Traumatic
Cell count/type	<2000/mono	2K–20K/mono, PMN	20K–200K/PMN	RBC
Disorder	DJD, ONB	RA, SLE, crystalline arthritis	Infectious, crystalline arthritis	Trauma, bleeding disorders

* PMN = polymorphonuclear, mono = mononuclear, ONB = osteonecrosis of bone, SLE = systemic lupus erythematosus, RA = rheumatoid arthritis, DJD = degenerative joint disease.

spondylitis, 80% of patients with Reiter's syndrome, and a high percentage of patients with other spondylarthropathies and acute anterior uveitis (8). The presence of HLA-B27 is not diagnostic for ankylosing spondylitis, but it may provide helpful clinical information in early disease when x-ray changes have not yet occurred. Testing for HLA-B27 may be misleading, because the antigen is also seen in patients without disease. In the future, HLA typing of patients with other disorders may be useful to establish the diagnosis or prognosis and to help select specific therapies.

SYNOVIAL FLUID ANALYSIS

Aspiration and examination of synovial fluid can be important in the diagnosis of joint swelling. Synovial fluid is usually clear, acellular, viscous, and low in volume. Alterations in the appearance, volume, and cellular content of synovial fluid are useful in diagnosis.

Based on a visual inspection of clarity and color, the synovial fluid is classified into 1 of 4 groups (9). Group I fluids are noninflammatory, with a low white blood cell count (<1,000/μl), and are usually associated with conditions such as osteoarthritis. Group II fluids are inflammatory, with an intermediate white blood count (in the range of 10,000/μl), and are associated with diseases such as RA. Group III fluids are purulent, with high white blood cell counts (in the range of 100,000/μl), and are typically associated with infections. Group IV fluids are hemorrhagic, with blood typically arising from trauma or bleeding disorders (Table 3). This grouping is a continuum. Depending on the severity of the disorder and the timing of the aspiration, a patient with a given diagnosis may have fluids in different groups. For example, during a quiescent period in a patient with gout, the synovial fluid could be in Group I; at the beginning of a flare, the patient could have a Group II fluid; and with severe gout attacks, the same patient could have synovial fluid which is opaque due to cell counts as high as 100,000/mm^3 (Group III).

The microscopic examination and culture of synovial fluid is extremely important. All synovial fluids in Groups II, III, and IV should be cultured when the diagnosis is unknown and infection is suspected. The culturing of organisms from synovial fluid establishes a diagnosis of infectious arthritis and allows treatment (specific antibiotics), which can result in cure.

In addition to cell counts and differentials, synovial fluid should be examined for crystals. Gout and calcium pyrophosphate dihydrate (CPPD) crystal deposition disease, two naturally occurring crystalline arthropathies, are diagnosed by the demonstration of birefringent crystals, using polarized light microscopy. In each of these conditions, the crystals may be ingested by a polymorphonuclear leukocyte. The CPPD crystal will have a rhomboid or rectangular shape and be weakly birefringent. If a first-order red compensator is used, CPPD crystals will show positive birefringence, demonstrating blue color when the long axis of the crystal is parallel to the "slow" direction noted on the housing of the compensator. Gouty crystals (monosodium urate) are needle-shaped and show strong negative birefringence, having a bright yellow appearance when the needle is parallel to the "slow" direction of the red compensator.

ACUTE PHASE REACTANTS

Among the body's internal responses to inflammation, infection, or other major injuries is a signal to change the production of proteins in the liver and other protein-synthesizing tissues. Proteins whose serum concentrations change in response to inflammation are called *acute phase reactants* (10,11). Many acute phase reactants demonstrate increased synthesis by the liver, including fibrinogen, prothrombin, haptoglobin, C-reactive protein (CRP), serum amyloid A protein, and others. The concentration of some of the acute phase proteins (e.g., fibrinogen) may increase modestly. Others (e.g., CRP) may increase by factors of up to 100 or more in concentration. Acute phase reactants are a common component of acute inflammation, but they also accompany chronic inflammation seen in the rheumatic diseases. These reactants can be measured directly, through measurement of CRP, and indirectly, through measurement of the erythrocyte sedimentation rate (ESR).

The ESR is the most common measurement of acute phase proteins in the rheumatic diseases. This simple test can be performed in the office with minimal equipment and requires only 1 hour for the red cells to sediment in a measured tube. The Westergren ESR uses a 100-mm tube to measure the sedimentation rate of cells over the 1-hour period. Sedimentation of the red cells is directly related to the quantity of acute phase proteins that are synthesized by the liver, particularly those with an asymmetric shape such as fibrinogen. However, this test is nonspecific, and positive findings may be seen in people who have no illness or who have illnesses such as anemia, which are not related to development of acute phase proteins. In addition, incorrect storage of the blood for more than a few hours may lead to errors in measurement.

Another measure of the acute phase response is the quantitation of serum CRP. The concentration of CRP rises more rapidly and returns to normal more quickly than the changes in ESR. Unlike the ESR, the CRP is not affected by anemia, nor is it very susceptible to incorrect results caused by specimen handling.

The measurement of acute phase reactants is important in rheumatic diseases, because elevations are generally consistent

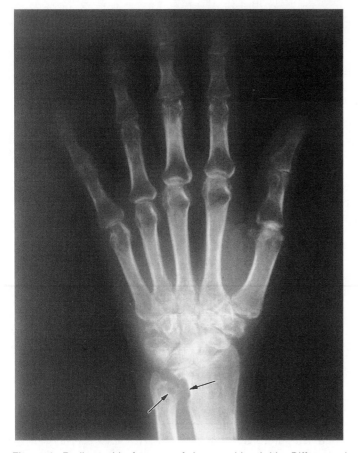

Figure 1. Radiographic features of rheumatoid arthritis. Diffuse and periarticular osteopenia, symmetric joint space loss, and multiple erosions are present in this advanced case. Large erosions are seen at the distal radial-ulnar articulation (arrows).

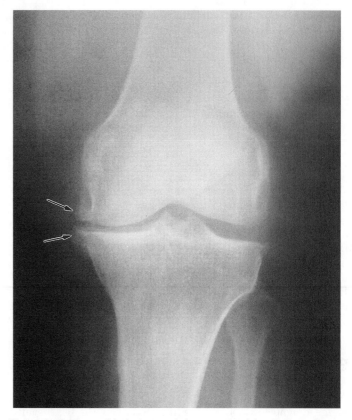

Figure 2. Radiographic features of degenerative joint disease. Osteophytes (arrows) and asymmetric medial cartilage loss are present in this knee x-ray.

with the presence of an inflammatory process, and normal values suggest that an inflammatory process is not present. Serial measurement of acute phase reactants may be used to monitor the disease course, particularly for patients with RA, polymyalgia rheumatica, and giant cell arteritis.

The upper limit of the reference normal range for both the ESR and CRP are influenced by age and gender. Patients above the upper limit of normal for young adults but below the upper limit of normal for their age range may have an inflammatory process, or may have mildly elevated acute phase reactants based on age and sex alone. Simple bedside formulae for the upper limit of normal for the ESR are, for women, (age + 10)/2; and for men, age/2 (12). For CRP, the upper limit of the reference range is age/50 for males, and age/50 + 0.6 for females, in units of mg/dL (13).

IMAGING TECHNIQUES

Radiography

The routinely performed radiograph, or x-ray, is the basic imaging technique for diagnosis and staging of all rheumatic diseases. Radiographs form a basis for monitoring disease progression. Plain x-rays are a component of the ACR classification criteria for RA and degenerative joint disease, and are integral components of the diagnosis of ankylosing

spondylitis, diffuse idiopathic skeletal hyperostosis, and the spondylarthropathies. Radiographs have the advantage of ready availability, relatively low cost, and the absence of a need for specialized equipment or diagnosticians.

Radiographic changes in the rheumatic diseases are best exemplified by inflammatory arthritis and degenerative joint disease. The classic example of inflammatory arthritis is RA, in which there is symmetric joint disease with soft-tissue swelling, the development of periarticular osteopenia, marginal erosions, and loss of articular cartilage (Figure 1), coupled with the development of joint malalignment and characteristic deformities.

Degenerative joint disease (Figure 2) also has articular loss; unlike RA however, loss occurs in an asymmetric pattern. There is increased subchondral bone density or sclerosis and the development of marginal osteophytes, or local areas of new bone formation. Involvement of weight-bearing joints is common; however, some forms of degenerative joint disease may occur in non-weight-bearing joints, as exemplified by the degenerative changes in the distal interphalangeal joints of the hands (Heberden's nodes).

Plain x-ray technique may be enhanced by the use of arthrography, in which radiocontrast dye (usually an iodinated water-soluble material) is injected into a joint. Arthrography is useful in diagnosing cysts and other herniations from joints (Figure 3A). As less invasive imaging techniques such as ultrasound and magnetic resonance imaging have become more common, arthrography is employed with less frequency.

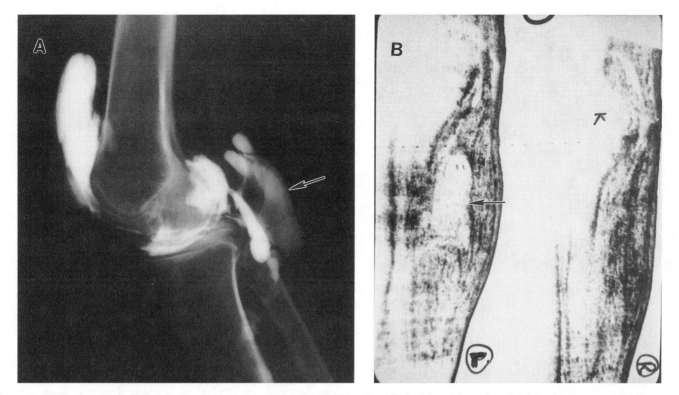

Figure 3. Popliteal cysts. **A,** Arthrography clearly demonstrates the small popliteal (Baker's) cyst (arrow) on this lateral knee x-ray. **B,** Ultrasonography in a dissecting Baker's cyst shows an echogenic-free mass in the mid-calf (arrow). L = left leg; R = right; K = knee.

Ultrasonography and Radionuclide Imaging

The use of ultrasound in the diagnosis of musculoskeletal disorders has the advantage of being inexpensive and readily available. It is most valuable in assessment of soft tissues and in superficial parts of the body. A common use of ultrasound is in the diagnosis of cysts at the knee (Figure 3B) or in cardiac examination in SLE or RA, where pericardial effusions may be seen. Ultrasound is increasingly being used to diagnose rotator cuff tendinitis and tears.

Radionuclide imaging or scintigraphy is used in the rheumatic diseases, primarily with the radionuclide Technetium[99], which is used for bone scans, indicating the presence of inflammation in and around bone. In a 3-phase bone scan, the early phase is an indicator of blood flow and transudation of fluid from vascular areas. Later in the test, the radionuclide is deposited in bone. The late phase indicates clearance of the tracer from bone. Early-phase studies are of value in the assessment of inflammation because increased radionuclide uptake occurs in areas of inflammation related to the rheumatic diseases. The 3-phase scan can be helpful in the diagnosis of reflex sympathetic dystrophy (also known as complex regional pain syndrome), which can be a perplexing diagnostic problem.

Radionuclide scanning is a very sensitive technique for detecting inflammation (including inflammation due to infection and nondisplaced fractures) in structures that are not readily accessible to physical examination or arthrocentesis, such as the spine, sacroiliac joints, and other deeper structures. The disadvantages of radionuclide scans are high cost, prolonged examination time, and the need for special facilities. Furthermore, the relatively poor resolution is a limitation. Radionuclide scanning has been combined with computer-aided reconstruction techniques to improve resolution, a process known as SPECT (single positron emission computed tomography) scanning. However, the high resolution and sensitivity provided by computed tomography and magnetic resonance imaging generally make those techniques preferable to radionuclide scanning.

Computed Tomography and Magnetic Resonance Imaging

The development of computed tomography (CT) and magnetic resonance imaging (MRI) has greatly enhanced the diagnostic potential of imaging techniques in the rheumatic diseases. These techniques better visualize soft tissues and deep structures within the body, such as the spine and pelvis. In CT, computer reconstruction permits greater resolution between bone and soft tissue and detection of disorders that are in a small area within a larger organ or tissue. Thus, more precise anatomic diagnoses can be made (Figure 4). Spinal inflammatory and degenerative disease, osteonecrosis of bone, and cysts within deep joints such as the hip, which are not easily seen on plain x-rays, are easily diagnosed with CT.

MRI has the advantages of showing greater soft-tissue contrast and being free of radiation. Because of its greater soft-tissue resolution, it is of particular value for osteonecrosis of bone and soft-tissue lesions, such as inflammatory synovitis in deep structures of the body like the spine and pelvis. It is also of great value in such soft-tissue pathology as rotator cuff tears, tears of the meniscus in the knees, spinal disk disease with or without nerve root or spinal cord impingement (Figure 5), and other ligamentous and tendon pathology. Because of the high soft-tissue contrast, MRI is

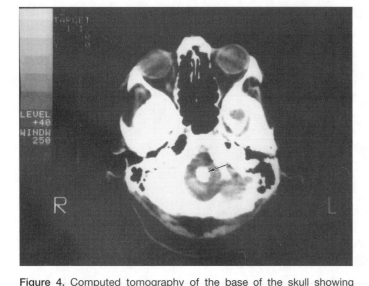

Figure 4. Computed tomography of the base of the skull showing migration of the dens of C2 (arrow) into the foramen magnum in a patient with rheumatoid arthritis.

supplanting arthrography and myelography in the rheumatic diseases. However, its high cost and need for special facilities are disadvantages.

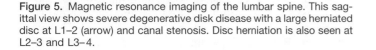

Figure 5. Magnetic resonance imaging of the lumbar spine. This sagittal view shows severe degenerative disk disease with a large herniated disc at L1–2 (arrow) and canal stenosis. Disc herniation is also seen at L2–3 and L3–4.

Dual Energy X-ray Absorptiometry

Osteoporosis is an extremely common problem in the rheumatology practice. It may be idiopathic, related to rheumatic disease, age-related, related to menopause, or iatrogenic from drugs such as corticosteroids. A measurement of the bone mineral content or bone mineral density (BMD) is imperative to monitor treatment of these patients, because studies show that fracture rate is directly related to bone mineral density.

Dual-energy x-ray absorptiometry (DEXA) allows precise and rapid quantification of the amount of bone with minimal radiation exposure. The BMD in a patient is expressed as a T score (the difference in standard deviation compared with peak bone mass in a young adult of the same sex and race) or a Z score (the difference in SD compared with healthy age-matched controls of the same sex and race). Persons with a BMD less than 1 SD below the mean in young adults (i.e., T score less than −1) are considered to have low BMD or osteopenia, while those with a BMD less than 2.5 SD below the mean in young adults (T score less than −2.5) are considered to have osteoporosis, according to the consensus criteria established by the World Health Organization.

The earliest changes of corticosteroid-induced bone loss can be detected in the lumbar spine using the techniques of quantitative computed tomography (QCT) or DEXA scanning. QCT provides information only on trabecular bone, while DEXA measures a combination of both cortical and trabecular bone. Because most medical practices do not have access to QCT, and because QCT requires a larger radiation exposure, DEXA measurement of both the lumbar spine and femoral neck is generally considered the imaging technique of choice. If only one site can be obtained, the lumbar spine should be imaged in men and women below age 60 and the femoral neck in men and women age 60 and above. Measurements of the lumbar spine in the elderly may be unreliable due to osteophyte formation at the vertebral bodies and facet joints.

Ideally, baseline bone mineral densitometry should be performed before long-term corticosteroid therapy is initiated, or very soon thereafter. BMD is the single most effective measure of future fracture risk and for establishing a diagnosis of osteoporosis. DEXA is useful for long-term monitoring of treatment effects; yearly repeat DEXA scanning can demonstrate stabilization or improvement in BMD after starting potent therapy for osteoporosis.

The author of this chapter would like to acknowledge the contributions of Thomas D. Beardmore, MD, who wrote this chapter in the first edition and whose perspective continues to be reflected here.

REFERENCES

1. Arnett FC, Edworthy SM, Bloch DA, McShane DJ, Fries JF, Cooper NS, et al. The American Rheumatism Association 1987 revised criteria for the classification of rheumatoid arthritis. Arthritis Rheum 1988;31:315–324.
2. Harris ED Jr. Clinical features of rheumatoid arthritis. In: Ruddy S, Harris ED Jr, Sledge CB, editors. Kelley's textbook of rheumatology. 6th ed. Philadelphia: WB Saunders; 2000. p. 967–1000.
3. Tighe H, Carson DA. Rheumatoid factors. In: Ruddy S, Harris ED Jr, Sledge CB, editors. Kelley's textbook of rheumatology. 6th ed. Philadelphia: WB Saunders; 2000. p. 151–60.
4. Tan EM, Cohen AS, Fries JF, Masi AT, McShane DJ, Rothfield NF, et al.

The 1982 revised criteria for the classification of systemic lupus erythematosus. Arthritis Rheum 1982;25:1271–1277.

5. Von Muhlen CA, Tan EM. Autoantibodies in the diagnosis of systemic rheumatic diseases. Semin Arthritis Rheum 1995;24:323–358.

6. Hochberg MC. Updating the American College of Rheumatology revised criteria for the classification of systemic lupus erythematosus (letter). Arthritis Rheum 1997;40:1725.

7. Piessens W. Immune complexes. In: Ruddy S, Harris ED Jr, Sledge CB, editors. Kelley's textbook of rheumatology. 6th ed. Philadelphia: WB Saunders; 2000. p. 175–183.

8. Arnett FC. Histocompatibility typing in the rheumatic diseases. Diagnostic and prognostic implications. Rheum Dis Clin North Am 1994;20:371–390.

9. McCarty D. Synovial fluid. In: Koopman WJ. Arthritis and allied conditions. 14th ed. Baltimore: Williams and Wilkins; 2001. p. 83–104.

10. Gabay C, Kushner I. Acute-phase proteins and other systemic responses to inflammation. N Engl J Med. 1999;340:448–454.

11. Volanakis J. Acute phase proteins in rheumatic disease. In: Koopman WJ, editor. Arthritis and allied conditions. 14th ed. Baltimore: Williams and Wilkins; 2001. p. 504–11.

12. Miller A, Green M, Robinson D. Simple rule for calculating normal erythrocyte sedimentation rate. Br Med J (Clin Res Ed). 1983;286:266.

13. Wener MH, Daum PR, McQuillan GM. The influence of age, sex, and race on the upper reference limit of serum C-reactive protein concentration. J Rheumatol 2000;27:2351–2359.

The Patient's Perspective

KATHLEEN S. LEWIS, RN, CMP, LPC

I arrived at work early to get some paperwork and patient assignments done before a staff meeting. As I rushed about making phone calls and talking to other team members, I began having chest pains that I just could not shake. They were a lot like the pains I'd experienced 3 months before when I threw an unexplained clot to my lung, spent a week in the hospital, and a month off from work.

Reluctantly, I called my supervisor to one side and told her about my pain. She checked me out and had me call my doctor. It was arranged that another nurse would drive me to the doctor's office after the staff meeting. I tried not to panic and to get as much work done as possible. I left work never to return.

THE DIAGNOSIS

A perfusion lung scan showed a clot at the same place in my left lung where a clot had formed 3 months earlier. Everyone was perplexed because I was on coumadin. They couldn't explain what was going on, and I felt scared and confused. The next few days were filled with tests and hubbub. The end result was that the doctors questioned if it was a clot at all and changed the diagnosis to exertional asthma. That diagnosis did not explain to me everything that was going on in my body. Along with shortness of breath and chest pain, I was experiencing fatigue, fever, joint pain, hair loss, and other unexplained symptoms. In the next few weeks while preparing to go to Hawaii with my husband, I got a sun lamp to start getting a tan. Strangely enough, I started getting a rash and spots on my chest. I headed back to the doctor to see what this was all about.

My doctor took a lot of blood and ran all sorts of tests but did not explain what he was looking for or suspecting. I left the office with more questions and fears than answers. My life was definitely changing at a fast pace in ways that I did not want. I had enough energy to be up for only short periods of time. It was difficult to function and carry out my activities of daily living, much less my roles as mother and wife. I was getting more and more frightened. At the same time, we were getting ready to leave on our trip to Hawaii.

Two days before we were to leave for Hawaii, I called Dr. Black's office to find out the results of my lab tests. After waiting for a period of time, the doctor came on the phone. "Kathleen, from all the labs it looks like you have systemic lupus. You need to see the rheumatologist when you come back from Hawaii. Be sure to wear a lot of sunscreen when you are out in the sun on your trip," Dr. Black's voice came across the phone like a cannon exploding in my ears. I kept hearing it as I drove to pick up the boys at soccer practice. At age 34 with 2 young sons and a husband, I felt my life would never be the same. I had gone from the ranks of the employed to the disabled.

As a visiting nurse, I usually saw patients only when they were in acute or terminal phases of their illnesses. I had no idea what it was like to live with a chronic illness like a rheumatic disease. Only after becoming a patient with chronic diseases (osteoarthritis, fibromyalgia, Sjögren's syndrome, osteoporosis, carpal tunnel, etc.) have I learned what it really is like to live with illness on a daily basis. In working and living with chronic illness for 23 years, I have become aware that there are differences in the challenges of living with acute, terminal, and chronic illness. Acute illness rapidly reaches crisis and resolution resulting in death or cure. Terminal illness is considered fatal, with death occurring in 2 to 3 months. I was only familiar with illness where you get sick, get better, and are well, or illness where you get sick, get worse, and die. With chronic illness I would neither die nor get well, but live with ongoing illness for the rest of a lifetime.

It seemed to me that people around me felt I was a failure, neurotic, a malingerer, different, or weird. I began to recognize the stigma associated with my illness and disability status. People seemed to say that maybe I was not doing something right, was being punished, or I just didn't have enough faith. It is hard to believe in this day and age of modern medicine that there is not a cure or pill for every ache or pain. Television commercials make it appear that there is a pill to take care of any medical problem that you might have—from hair loss to impotence.

CHALLENGES OF LIVING WITH CHRONIC ILLNESS

Victor Frankl says that living with a chronic illness is similar to the experience of being a prisoner of war: "Where there's an end of certainty . . . there's uncertainty of an end," (1). With acute and terminal illness, time will be short. An end is in sight. Chronic illness will last a lifetime. It is open-ended and ongoing with unpredictable fluctuations. Significant support people (health care professionals, family, friends, work associates) have come and gone through the years. I have experienced shifting of whole support systems over time.

The Physician−Patient Relationship

The physician−patient relationship, stretched over the years, becomes something of a marriage (2). It has been one of the most important bonds for me, accompanied by give and take, agreements and disagreements. I have found that it is a relationship best maintained with honesty, concern, and respect from both parties. A balanced working relationship is essential. Normal emotions have been and will be played out in this relationship. For me, anger, anxiety, and frustration were a part of the relationship. At times, a power struggle would develop to determine who was in control. The physicians and I might displace our feelings on each other. I could be upset about something else but blow up at the doctor, and vice versa.

It took time for me to build a sound physician–patient relationship. In this long-term relationship, the physician's opinions and judgments reached into many areas and decisions in my life. I have been frightened and at my lowest both physically and emotionally when trying to initiate these relationships. I have had as many as 8 doctors to deal with at a time. It can be crazy to try to relate to so many doctors at one time, especially when they may not agree with, or even talk to, one another.

At times my physicians have seemed God-like and felt like my lifeline. But I've realized that no physician can keep me in good health. The physician can only tell me what I need to do (3). He or she can help me learn to listen to my body and try to interpret what it is saying. Understanding this point has taken a lot of time and patience for me and for my physicians.

A physician's training is focused on relieving pain and suffering rather than helping patients learn how to live with it. Sometimes, when I have not responded to their treatments, physicians seem to feel they have been a failure. Over time, my chronic distress has presented my physicians with personal distress (4). Many times they have had to admit that they just did not know what to do. Physicians and patients each have their special needs. How these needs blend and collide has a bearing on the quality of health care (5).

In the managed care setting I have been forced to give up trusted, familiar health care professionals over and over as insurance plans merged, changed, and physicians jumped from one plan to another. In the 23 years that I have lived with rheumatic diseases, I have had to create completely new health care teams several times while simultaneously juggling serious health problems.

It has been frightening, devastating, and extremely difficult to have to start all over with a new health care team. Physicians need patients, just as patients need physicians. The relationship is intimate. They are both involved in different ways with the illness itself (5). I have found that I cannot replicate my medical history in spoken or written words that can fully convey what a medical team has lived through with me.

It can take a year or more to create that open, trusting working relationship needed to provide good medical care. New physicians have even questioned a diagnosis and treatment that I have lived with for years. Changing physicians or seeing yet another specialist is very upsetting and overwhelming.

Educating myself about my illness and test results has been essential so I can relate my history and medical condition as clearly and cogently as possible when I go to another physician. Getting copies of all of my labs and diagnostic tests over the years has proved invaluable, as vital information has been inadvertently lost. At one point a physician lost 12 years of my medical records.

Support Network

The duration of my illness has also presented a challenge to my support community. Significant others have tired, worn out, and become impatient over the years. Research has shown that spouses of patients experiencing chronic pain have higher levels of depression than the normal population. Treatment should include the whole family, not just the patient. The patient may live but the family may die (6).

Significant support people, like my husband, had their own needs and often inadequate resources to handle them. There were times when he needed a break and doubted his ability to go the distance. He seemed to become numb to my constant and ongoing needs and to lose the ability to tell what was and was not important because so much was happening all the time. After living with my health problems for 6 years, he left and filed for divorce.

We needed a broad base of support to balance the demands my illness put on us. This broad base of support might include the medical community, support groups, chat rooms, counseling, church affiliation, nuclear and extended family, friends, and neighbors. With a network of support, the burden could have been spread around and shifted so that everybody had a better chance of being able to go the distance.

When I was finally diagnosed with my chronic illness, my response was that I would rather die than live for a lifetime with how I was feeling. My husband felt we could handle anything as long as I did not die. We switched stances over the years.

We got caught up in the fear of what might happen in the days and years ahead, as well as in waiting and longing for that possible remission. The course of a rheumatic disease can be very uncertain, with remissions and flares coming and going unpredictably. Both flares and remissions presented adjustment challenges. I found out that it was very important to keep as much structure and schedule in my life as possible. I needed to deal with my illness one day at a time and not get stuck in the past or the future.

Credibility Gap

Many times I look great and the lab work appears normal, but I feel horrible. Other times I feel great but my labs are abnormal. I begin to feel crazy when my external and internal reality do not jibe. This dynamic sets up a credibility gap between me and my family, friends, and health care providers. Doubt, uncertainty, and confusion exists over what is real and what is in my head for all concerned.

At times I feel isolated, alone, and convinced that no one understands. I have been defensive, argumentative, and combative trying to prove my complaints. At other times I smile in denial and say everything is fine, only to crash later. Then, too, there are periods when I withdraw into myself and become bitter, angry, confused, and lonely.

Strangely, when you are ill, people seem compelled to tell you how good you look. When I became ill, you would have thought that I had become a beauty contestant rather than a patient living with pain, fatigue, and myriad other symptoms. I felt caught in the dilemma of whether or not to dress to cover up my illness so that I could "pass" as normal or to display my illness to appear credible. I found I became healthy when the illness became only a part of me and I began to dress to accentuate all of who I was.

I learned how to dress up a neck brace with scarves and turtlenecks so that people didn't even realize I was wearing it. Wearing skirts and pants with pleats and belts helped conceal a lumbar support and keep it in place. I found colorful wrist splints, and attractive silver ring splints to support finger joints.

Hats, sunscreens, and opaque makeup protected me from UV rays. Hats also covered my scant hair, and eventually became my trademark. I found it healthy to do these things, *if* my adaptive efforts were not intended to cover up my illness but to be an expression of all of me . . . style and illness. Trying to forget something is the best way to remember it.

Many times I am asked by patients and patient groups to "make" their family or support community understand what they are going through. I cannot make anyone understand my situation or theirs. I get caught in a power/control struggle when I try. When I can begin to accept my situation and establish realistic expectations for myself and my life, I am more at ease with myself and others. I am then able to identify key significant people who can listen and support me. I can let those who cannot realistically support me go their way understanding that it may have more to do with them than me.

Health care providers must learn to see the patient as an individual and listen to them. Patient education for everyone involved is essential to help them understand what complaints can be realistically treated and what ones cannot be treated without diminishing the reality of their complaints or credibility.

It has taken me a long time to learn what my individual disease patterns are—my symptoms and what makes me worse and what makes me better—and that not everything can be treated. Even though there may be no additional treatment, and laboratory tests may not validate how I feel, I can accept where I am and feel credible.

Keeping a Record

Learning to keep a journal or record of my health fluctuations helped me begin to see my disease patterns and report them to my health care professionals in an organized fashion. With documentation in hand, I possibly appear more credible and help the provider see what is really happening. A monthly calendar with symptoms and schedule briefly jotted down can be an efficient way to keep up with disease activity. There are health journals available for patients to keep these records.

I used to become frustrated with physician's visits because there would be so much to discuss with the physician and not enough time. Finally, I discovered that compiling an update of everything that has gone on since the last visit, including personal and financial factors, helped me make the best use of time. My update is as brief and succinct as possible. I keep a copy and give one to my physician.

Some clinicians fear that having the patient keep these records will cause them to focus more on their symptoms and encourage hypochondriac tendencies. But for me, keeping records helps me become more scientific about my illness and gives me a sense of control. By writing symptoms down I am able to forget about them and leave them documented on the paper. During this process, I began to see that there were times when I felt better, rather than having everything become blurred together. The health care provider can also help the patient focus on what is important to keep updated and allow us to have more of a role in our medical care (7).

Pacing

With acute and terminal illness there are sprints, frantic activity, rush orders, heroic efforts, heightened attention, and vigilance to bring about a cure or prepare for the inevitability of death. Enduring a chronic illness like rheumatic disease is more like running a marathon, which requires pacing, endurance, commitment, and flexibility.

I usually experience no rush orders and a lack of empathy or attention. It may take several months to find out the results of tests unless I ask the doctor to send me a copy of them. Only my symptoms are treated, not the illness itself. I must endure the illness, as well as the side effects of the medication or treatments, without a lot of frantic activity, empathy, or support. For me, illness-related activities simply become a way of life.

Tests are repeated over and over and expensive medications need to be taken on a routine basis, with no real expectation of getting back to "normal" or feeling better. Sometimes I become impatient, frustrated, or discouraged with how slowly things move. Patient education has helped my family and me understand the need for ongoing lab results, what they mean, and how medications are geared to balance gains against the risk of side effects. It has taken months, even years, to go through this trial-and-error process to find the medication that works best for me.

Interspersed with the slow pace of the chronic illness are acute and potentially life-threatening episodes. At these times the pace speeds up, and labs and diagnostic tests are done quickly, often accompanied by a lot of attention and empathy. When I initially began having kidney failure there was a lot of hubbub, concern, and activity around the kidney biopsy and outcome. However, once the disease activity leveled off, all concerned parties switched gears from the frantic sprint back to the marathon methodical pace once again. I am still in kidney failure, but that is no longer a major focus or concern. It has become a part of who I am, my normal abnormal, and to me no big deal at all.

Switching back and forth from a marathon to sprints can be difficult. The sprints break up the rhythm of my pace and drain energy needed to go the distance. All those concerned for me can become sick and tired of my being sick and tired. After an acute episode, I may not be able to return to the level of activity that I maintained before. It takes time, flexibility, patience, and communication for all involved to find a new pace and way of living with so many changes and shifts.

In a marathon, runners say that the twenty-first mile can feel like a "wall" where they do not think they can make it and want to give up. Their lungs burn and their legs feel like lead. All involved with chronic illness may hit a similar physical and emotional wall from time to time as the years stretch out. Patients may think of suicide when they hit the wall. Indeed, the chronically ill are more likely to commit suicide than the terminally ill (8). Health care providers should be acutely aware of this fact during times of increased stress, a sudden flare after a time of feeling better, a failed treatment, or long periods of no improvement. I have considered suicide at times, but have fought my way through to a better place.

Stress

With acute and terminal illness, stress may be intense and short-lived. Long-term stress associated with chronic illness requires long-term coping skills. My own thoughts can be one of my greatest stressors. My body responds to every thought, creating a mind/body feedback loop, changing my hormone release, heart and respiration rates, muscle tension, and immune functions. All of these bodily functions are affected by the thoughts related to my chronic illnesses.

McWilliams (9) states that "positive thoughts (joy, happiness, fulfillment, achievement, worthiness) have positive results (enthusiasm, calm, well-being, ease, energy, love). Negative thoughts (judgment, unworthiness, mistrust, resentment, fear) produce negative results (fear, anxiety, alienation, anger, fatigue)." To be healthy and realistic, I try to balance my positive and negative thoughts. I cannot constantly maintain positive thoughts. I need my negative thoughts as a part of my wisdom. Health care professionals can help patients balance their thoughts with realistic expectations through patient education, listening, and not discounting their fears and concerns.

My family and I needed help in becoming familiar and comfortable with my illness. Discussing the illness and handling the associated feelings with my health care provider created a type of systematic desensitization that helped reduce the fear and symptoms, and encouraged learning about my disease patterns. Instead of feeling phobic about chest pain, we learned to tell the difference between pain caused by pleurisy, pericarditis, or costochondritis. I figured out how much activity it took to trigger disease activity, how to slow down so it did not get worse, and what it took for me to get better.

Family members may experience the greatest stress when the patient reaches a plateau and all involved realize that this is as good as it gets. I distinctly remember the day my husband realized that my limited ability to engage in activity was not going to improve. The hope of complete remission faded. The dream that I might get back to "normal" was vanquished. Little did I know that was probably a major turning point in our marriage.

Stress comes not only from a diagnosed chronic illness, but also from associated daily events. The major life event of the diagnosis may translate into myriad daily life hassles, such as a poor night's sleep, remembering when and what medications to take, side effects of medications, fatigue, pain, dealing with the health care system, changing roles in the family, and loss of substantial gainful employment.

Richard Lazarus at the University of California, Berkeley suggests that you can balance the stress effects of every hassle you experience if you have 2 uplifting experiences, ranging from a pleasant time with your family to getting enough sleep (10). Dealing with the health care system can be a major hassle or stress for me, starting with the receptionist and continuing through the entire experience to the rescheduling clerk. Even after leaving the office there may be a long battle to get services reimbursed.

Every person in the physician's office can present me either with a hassle or an uplift. No matter how good the physician may be, the rest of the staff can neutralize the beneficial effects of an office visit. When already dealing with a rheumatic disease, I desperately need my encounter with the physician and his or her staff to be as uplifting and supportive as possible.

When your perceived demands are equal to your perceived resources, you are balanced. When your perceived resources do not equal your perceived resources, you are in distress (11). When I perceive my health care team as a resource rather than a demand, it makes a great difference in my outcome.

Since my diagnosis with a chronic rheumatic disease, the demands on me and on my family have increased, and the resources to deal with those demands have decreased. I've learned to increase my resources by attending support groups and self-help classes, engaging in exercise at my level of physical fitness, practicing meditation and relaxation techniques, educating myself about my illness and my treatments, getting counseling, learning how to ask for what I need, and leaving a physician when he or she is not working for me.

As a patient these resources have helped me balance the load and make it through one challenge at a time. It took a lot for me to become ill, and it takes a lot to stay as healthy as possible. Medications are only a small part of getting better. For me, working on a mind/body/spirit level is essential to maintain as much health as possible. My "coping" resources help me balance out the demands of stress. They include self-disclosure, self-directness (assertiveness), confidence, acceptance, social support, financial freedom, physical health, physical fitness, stress monitoring, tension control, structuring, problem solving, cognitive restructuring, functional beliefs, and social ease (12).

THE GRIEF PROCESS

Being diagnosed with a chronic illness may initiate a lifelong grief process for the patient and those who love her or him. This grief process is different from the grief associated with acute and terminal illness.

With chronic illness I found myself grieving present losses as well as those losses yet to come. The losses were, or maybe were not, as evident to those around me. Things I lost that needed to be grieved included my former good health, a good night's sleep, independence, privacy, body image, sense of control, relationships as they had been, established roles inside and outside the family, former social status, the ability to find health or life insurance, a sense of self-confidence, dreams and plans for the future, gainful employment and thereby financial security, familiar daily routines, hobbies, getting a glorious suntan in a bikini, modes of expressing sexuality. The list could go on and on.

Grieving the losses that result from a chronic illness presents special difficulties. The grieved object is present for all to see and reminds everyone of what was lost. I needed to do my own grieving while also experiencing the grief of those around me. Every person grieves in his or her own manner and time frame.

It took a long time for all involved to assess my newly imposed and fluctuating limitations and losses due to the illness. Almost everything about me was changed or affected to some degree (13). Flares and the promise of remission with rheumatic disease made it difficult to determine which losses were permanent and which were temporary.

Important tasks and maintaining family roles interrupted and sometimes delayed my personal grieving process. Seeing others grieve made me feel guilty that I could not continue my old familiar roles. I felt compelled to keep up the morale of others. I found out that my delayed grief could manifest itself by an immediate reaction of coldness, inability to express feelings that burst forth uncontrollably at a later time, or illness that didn't respond to treatment (14).

Grieving a chronic illness involves losses that are ongoing and open-ended, complicating and extending the time needed to grieve. I have found the emotional reaction to a chronic illness can be more crippling and enduring than the physical aspects of the illness (15). As Simonton (16) pointed out, "Harmony—balance among the physical, mental, and spiritual aspects of being—is central to health."

The all-absorbing identity of a diagnosed illness and disability threatened my own individual and sexual identity that usually so penetrated the fabric of my being that I had no consciousness of its presence. I became lupus and disability. When I introduced myself, the most important thing for people to know about me was that I had lupus. It took years to shrink lupus and disability down to size so that they became only a part of who I am.

The perceived loss of sexual identity along with the loss of a secure way of relating to others initiated more grief. The grief process itself caused difficulty in relating to others. Significant attachments were threatened by this breakdown of the ability to relate, creating yet another loss. Purtillo (17) stated that of the things that might be lost, privacy, body image, and relationships are the most important. When a patient seems to be stuck in any of the stages of the grief process and not able to move on with treatment, a counseling referral may be necessary.

Without grieving my losses, I ran the risk of developing such dysfunctional behaviors as severe reactions to separation, unexplained somatic responses, specific medical diseases, and altered relationships with others (18). When losses due to my illness were not grieved, the lifestyle changes needed to accommodate my illness could not be made. The illness would continue to control my life.

As grieving is worked through, "one can get the past in perspective and find meaning in the present" (19). As I grieved my losses, I began to accept my limitations and see new potentials. I then began to wade back into life and find new creative ways to carry out my life, be productive, express my sexuality, and relate to those around me.

Labeling what I was going through as a grief process was very helpful to me and gave me permission to grieve and go on with my life. Grief can be reawakened by a failed treatment, intercurrent illness, significant family transitions, increased loss of function, exacerbation of disease after a period of remission, and changes in the health care team (7). When a health care provider is aware of the grief process, they may help patients anticipate and understand emotional challenges. I have come to believe that dying is the easy part. Living, not just suffering with a chronic illness, is where the real challenge lies.

THE SICK ROLE OR A HEALTHY ROLE?

The sick role expectation in medical sociology requires the patient to be dependent, submissive, passive, unhappy, sad, nondirective, childlike—in other words, give up responsibility and mostly look sick. The sick role sanctions and grants temporary relief from personal, social, and vocational responsibility. The sick role is allowed with an impairment or physical limitation due to an injury or incurable illness for a limited amount of time and is not permanent. The person is expected to function to the optimum degree of his or her condition (20).

When I claim to be ill without acting out the sick role, many people will insist that I am not really ill. However, I have learned to live with illness without claiming the sick role all the time. Living out the sick role all of the time can be demeaning, limiting, and crippling. To some degree I need to listen to my body as a guide to activity, but not let my body determine my mood or attitude.

I have not found any truly healthy role models of how to manage illness. Some patients may become dependent and clinging from fear of their illness, a sense of vulnerability, or because they are living out the expected sick role. Other patients may choose fierce independence that is lauded and encouraged by our society's "hero" mentality. They may choose rigid independence out of fear of always being on the receiving end, or of rejection, inferiority, or embarrassment. They may be afraid of being labeled a complainer, hypochondriac, or lazy. Too much dependence or independence can create codependency. Interdependence seems to be the healthier choice.

I am trying to accept my limitations and identify my need for assistance. Being able to ask for what I need and set boundaries in an assertive, kind, firm, clear, specific, and direct manner can help greatly. In this way, I learn to bargain my limitations in a matter-of-fact way without whining or demanding. This type of communication can happen as I learn to accept myself, develop realistic expectations, and transact the business of communicating my needs. However, it has taken counseling for me and the whole family to reach this point.

My two sons and I started family counseling as my ex-husband and I were separating. We tried to negotiate realistic expectations for each other. One time we went by the counselor's office on my way to the hospital for surgery. We discussed which people they preferred to bring food. We set boundaries on their behavior with the house sitter during my hospital stay. What could have been a nightmare turned out to be as pleasant as possible under the circumstances. I continue to see the same counselor for assistance and guidance when I lose my way or perspective.

Many times patients are seen as noncompliant, resistant, and a problem when they are independent, think for themselves, and want to be active participants in their health care. Patients today tend to be educated consumers about their illness and its treatment. Although it may take more time, energy, and effort, health care providers should educate patients or refer them to good sources of information that will allow them to make informed decisions about their lives and illness.

With rheumatic disease treatment options, I try to be active in determining the course of my treatment, as risks are weighed against benefits. Being able to participate in these choices often makes a difference in my following through with the treatment or not. Some rheumatic disease medications may not produce therapeutic changes for weeks or months. Without this information, I might be tempted to stop taking the medication or question the physician's competence.

A patient's power is decreased and the clinician's power is increased when there is uncertainty in the course of an illness, outcome of treatment, or future actions. In my experience the situation is improved when the health care provider allows patients to be equal partners, to take an active role in their treatment, and to assume responsibility for themselves (5).

NEW HOPES AND GOALS

In the first 2 years after my diagnosis I lived from the couch to the bed and was in the hospital 3 times. But soon I realized that I needed realistic hopes and goals for the future. I began writing anything from poems to articles to occupy my time. Much to my disbelief, I even wrote a definitive article on systemic lupus erythematosus that was published in the journal, *Nurse Practitioner*. Eventually I wrote several books on living with chronic illness. My writing gave me something to fill my time, a sense of purpose, and much needed structure. I now speak around the country to patient and professional groups.

I began to realize that grief accompanies any big transition in life. I started doing grief support with friends facing significant changes in their lives. After the first 2 years, I ventured out of the house to attend a chaplaincy program for ministers' wives. Although the program was only 2 mornings a week, it was very difficult for me to keep the schedule. I ended up in a 3-month flare and in the hospital for a week—but I eventually made it back to the program and finished.

From that experience, I tentatively investigated what credentials I needed for counseling the chronically ill. I found a Master's degree program in rehabilitation counseling that would fit the bill and accommodate my limitations. It took me 5 years to complete a year and a half of coursework. During that time I also had 7 surgeries, went through a divorce, placed my mother in a nursing home, became the single mother of 2 teenage sons, had my first book published, began a counseling ministry out of my home, and lived with chronic illness on a daily basis. In trying to fill up my time and provide structure for my life, I found a whole new involvement in life and talents I didn't know I had.

CONCLUSION

I must emphasize the importance of my time with my health care providers. While any appointment is only a moment in the time I spend fighting the battles related to living with a chronic illness on a daily basis, it may be a "holy moment." Often I have waited a long time for the visit and will play and replay the meeting in my mind. My anxiety levels may be elevated, and later I may not remember or comprehend what was said. Many questions may come to mind the minute I walk out of the office door.

Having my health care provider reinforce what is discussed during that moment may be a lifesaver for me. Checklists, pamphlets, or written information in any form is helpful for me and my family. A sense that my physician hears me and takes me seriously is invaluable. I can leave the office feeling I have a partner and an advocate rather than an adversary or foe.

Having gone through my process, I feel better prepared to live my life as a patient with rheumatic disease, but also as a person who lives her life successfully. I've learned a great deal about my disease and how to cope better in working partnerships with my health care provider, my family, my friends, and indeed the world. I know my future holds better treatment and management options and that my confidence in dealing with the stresses and challenges put to me will continue to grow. My family has changed, my activities have changed, and my life has changed – with negative as well as positive consequences. While I would prefer *not* to have experienced some of the changes, my involvement and focus on communication makes the challenge of living with a chronic rheumatic disease a part of my life, and not a burden to be borne.

If you, too, are a patient, take heart. In all likelihood, you will be able to make lemonade from the lemons presented to you. If you are a health care provider, please communicate and work with your patients and their families. Education and communication are key components to making your patients' disease less burdensome. If you are a researcher, remember that we are hoping for a cure, but are willing to accept medications with fewer side effects as a good start. If you are a family member or simply a concerned reader, please recognize that many rheumatic diseases are multifaceted and have tremendous positive as well as negative impacts on our lives.

REFERENCES

1. Frankl EV. 1962. Man's search for meaning. Boston: Beacon Press; 1962.
2. Lewis KS. Successful living with chronic illness. Celebrating the joys of life. Dubuque, IA: Kendall/Hunt; 1994.
3. Chyatte SB. On borrowed time. Living with hemodialysis. Oradell, NJ: Medical Economics; 1979.
4. Lewis KS. Celebrate life: new attitudes for living with chronic illness. Atlanta: Arthritis Foundation; 1999.
5. Benet G. Physicians and their patients. London: Ballaire Tindale; 1979.
6. Lewis KS. Chronic illness and marriage: endings and beginnings. Humane Medicine 1989;5:54–57.
7. Lewis KS. Emotional adjustment to chronic illness. Prim Care Practice 1998;2:38–51.
8. Ford RD. Health assessment handbook. Springhouse, PA: Springhouse Corporation; 1987.
9. McWillaims R. You can't afford the luxury of a negative thought. Los Angeles: Prelude Press; 1995.
10. Lazarus RS: Little hassles can be hazardous to your health. Psychology Today 1981:XX;58–62.
11. Matheny KB. Stress coping: a qualitative and quantitative synthesis with implications for treatment. Counsel Psychol 1986;14:499–549.
12. Matheny K. The coping resources inventory for stress: a measure of perceived resourcefulness. Clin Psychol 1993;49:815–30.
13. Werner-Beland JA. Grief responses to long-term illness and disability. Reston, VA: Reston Publishing; 1980.
14. Mezer RR. Dynamic psychiatry. New York: Springer Publishing Company; 1976.
15. LeMaistre J. Beyond rage: the emotional impact of a chronic physical illness. Oak Park, IL: Alpine Guild; 1985.
16. Simonton OC. The healing journey. New York: Bantam Books; 1992.
17. Purtillo R. Similarities in patient response to chronic and terminal illness. 1976;56:279–84.
18. Lindeman. Symptomology and management in grief. In: Crisis intervention: selected readings. New York: Family Service Assoc of Am; 1965.
19. Cox-Gedmark J. Coping with physical disabilty. Philadelphia: The Westminister Press; 1980.
20. Shontz CS. The psychological aspects of physical illness and disability. Reston, VA: Reston Publishing; 1975.

CHAPTER 9

Functional Ability, Health Status, and Quality of Life

DONNA J. HAWLEY, EdD, RN

Functional status, health status, health-related quality of life, and quality of life are terms used to summarize disease outcomes that go beyond the physiologic consequences of disease. They describe outcome as the consequences of disease from the perspective of the individual's daily functioning. These outcomes are intended to represent what is important from the viewpoint of the patient.

DEFINITIONS

Moving along the continuum from functional status to quality of life, the terms become more abstract, more difficult to measure, and probably more important to the individual. *Functional status* is the ability to do the usual self-care activities of daily living such as eating, dressing, grooming, and toileting.

Health status is broader than functional ability and encompasses total physical, mental, and social well-being (1). It includes important aspects of health such as emotions and mood, symptoms (e.g., pain, sleep, fatigue), cognitive abilities, and social activities and roles.

Quality of life is more comprehensive and abstract than either functional or health status. It is influenced by numerous factors unrelated to an individual's health or disease (e.g., safe water, adequate housing, crime, and educational opportunities). Further, the perception of one's quality of life has meanings, preferences, and priorities unique to the individual (2). The totality of quality of life is very difficult to define and measure. For these reasons, evaluating the effect of disease on a person's quality of life has become more narrowly focused on health-related quality of life (HRQOL), which refers to a combination of functional ability, disease symptoms, social roles and activities such as work or school, and emotions and mood. Thus HRQOL represents a perception of well-being. Although health-related quality of life is more comprehensive than health status, the terms are frequently used interchangeably. Both refer to the aggregate effects of disease on the individual's life (1). In this chapter, the term "health status" will be used to refer to both health-related quality of life and health status. "Functional status" will refer to the ability to perform activities of daily living.

ASSESSMENT OF FUNCTIONAL ABILITY AND HEALTH STATUS

Assessment of functional ability and health status supplements the information obtained through more traditional assessments of health history, physical examination, laboratory tests, and radiography. Traditional assessments provide data about disease status. Data such as the number of tender joints, current degree of inflammation, and number of erosions are documented by physical examination, laboratory tests, and x-rays, respectively. Health status assessments provide additional information about how the patient is managing the disease and the consequences of the disease on the individual's everyday life from the patient's viewpoint. Direct observation, physician estimation of functioning, and self-report questionnaires have been used to assess both functional ability and health status.

Direct Observation

There are several standardized observational methods that may be used to evaluate one or more aspects of functional status. Hand function (button test), hand and arm strength (grip strength), lower extremity movement (walk time and timed-stands test), and range of motion (Keitel index) are listed in Table 1. With the exception of the time to walk 50 feet test (3,4), these measures have been shown to be valid and sensitive to change in clinical studies. Each relies on the motivation and cooperation of the patient. The amount of time needed to complete the Keitel index (>10 minutes using a health professional's time) may limit its use in routine clinical practice. The specially designed equipment needed for the button test and the timed-stands test requires an initial expenditure. Grip strength can be assessed quickly in a busy clinic setting at minimal cost. It is a standard outcome measure for many clinical trials and is sensitive to improvement in inflammation as well as function for a person with rheumatoid arthritis (RA) (3).

Clinician Estimation

Two common methods for assessing function are physician global estimate of disease activity and the American College of Rheumatology (ACR) Revised Criteria for Classification of Functional Status in Rheumatoid Arthritis. Physician global assessment is based on the subjective interpretation of the patient's symptoms, apparent functioning, and laboratory tests (4). Assignment of scores from 0 (no disease activity) to 4 (very severe activity) is recommended by some authors (4). While this measure has been shown to be sensitive to short-term change during clinical trials (3), similar findings have not been reported in practice situations (5,6). Physicians may tend to overestimate physical limitations compared to patients' perceptions, especially at higher levels of impairment in persons with RA (5). If health care professionals plan to use professional judgment to evaluate functioning in routine clinical practice, validating one's judgment through discussion with the patient would be appropriate and wise. Functional status may

Table 1. Examples of standardized measures for evaluating physical functioning in chronic rheumatic disorders using direct observation.

	Purpose	Measurement method	Comments
Grip strength (4)	Measurement of hand, wrist, and forearm strength.	Patient squeezes the cuff of a sphygmomanometer inflated to 30 mm Hg as hard as possible. The highest level on the mercury column of 3 attempts is recorded. May also be measured with Martin Virgorimeter (50).	Motivation, handedness, pain threshold, and muscle weakness will modify scores as well as involvement of any joint from the elbow to the hand. Grip strength has been shown to be sensitive to change in clinical trials (3).
Thumb to index strength	Hand and finger function.	Measured with Martin Virgorimeter (50).	Same as grip strength measurement.
Time to walk 50 feet (4)	Measurement of lower extremity function.	Individual walks 50 feet on a flat surface using any aids or assistive devices. Time is recorded to the nearest 0.1 second.	Motivation is influential. Low reliability, insensitive to changes in disease (3).
6-minute walk time (35,51)	Field test of fitness.		Motivation is influential. Low correlation with standard laboratory tests of physical fitness. Sensitive to change in exercise clinical trial in fibromyalgia. Little information available for other disorders (35, 51).
Jepson Hand Function Test, Grip Ability Test, Grip Function Test, Arthritis Hand Function Test	Various measures of hand function tested in persons with arthritis. Activities tested are based on activities of daily living.	Specific tasks (e.g., picking up cards, pouring water from a jug, writing) are performed in presence of evaluator.	May be used in clinical trials of specific hand treatments, following hand surgery, and in long-term outcome studies. Some tests require special equipment (3,52,53).
Button test (3,54)	Measurement of hand function, can be used in clinical practice.	Standard board with 5 buttons. Patients are timed while they unbutton and button using both right and left hands separately. Two scores are averaged.	Motivation is an important factor. Useful in disorders with direct effect on hand function (e.g., rheumatoid arthritis).
Timed-stands test (3,55)	Measurement of lower extremity function.	Number of seconds used in standing up and sitting down 10 times from a chair using only the lower extremities.	Motivation, age, and non-musculoskeletal comorbid conditions may affect scores. Sensitivity to change has not been determined (3,55).
Keitel index (4,56)	Upper and lower extremity function with emphasis on range of motion.	Measures 24 standard tasks of peripheral and axial joint motion performed by patients. Evaluation is by trained observer. Completion time 10–15 minutes (4).	Motivation may be a factor. Time and personnel to observe and score tasks are a factor in its use. Scale is sensitive to short-term change (3,57).

be classified using the ACR Revised Criteria for Classification of Functional Status in Rheumatoid Arthritis. These criteria, as listed in Table 2, may be used for the "rapid, global assessment of functional status by health professionals" (7). They are helpful in classifying groups of RA patients at one specific point in time; however, using these criteria to monitor change over time for individual patients is not recommended (7,8). More detailed assessments are needed to determine important clinical change over time.

Table 2. American College of Rheumatology revised criteria for classification of functional status in rheumatoid arthritis (ref. 7).*

Class	Description
Class I	Completely able to perform usual activities of daily living (self-care, vocational, and avocational)
Class II	Able to perform usual self-care and vocational activities, but limited in avocational activities
Class III	Able to perform usual self-care activities, but limited in vocational and avocational activities
Class IV	Limited ability to perform usual self-care, vocational, and avocational activities

* Usual self-care activities include dressing, feeding, bathing, grooming, and toileting. Avocational (recreational and/or leisure) and vocational (work, school, homemaking) activities are patient-desired and age- and sex-specific.

Self-Report Questionnaires

During the last 3 decades, numerous instruments and questionnaires have been developed to measure health status. These instruments vary in complexity from those measuring a single domain (such as ability to do activities of daily living or self-report pain levels) to more comprehensive instruments having several subscales that measure different aspects of health status. In addition to functional status, the multidimensional instruments contain measures of pain, mood, and emotional well-being; symptoms such as sleep disturbance, fatigue (energy level), gastrointestinal distress, and morning stiffness; social activities and role; cognitive ability; and work and work disability. Patients' global perceptions of health and disease and their satisfaction with their overall health are included in several instruments. Less commonly evaluated are perceived priority areas for health, attribution of health problems, indirect and direct costs of disease, and drug side effects.

Instruments are classified as generic or disease-specific. Generic instruments may be used to evaluate a variety of chronic conditions and to compare across diseases. Comparison with the general population or with "healthy" groups is also possible (9). Disease-specific instruments are more sensitive to particular problems or symptoms (10). For example, pain is more important to evaluate in the rheumatic diseases than it is for patients with hypertension. Lower extremity

Table 3. Domains of health status questionnaires, including major sections (X) and subsections (O) (modified from ref. 14, with permission).*

	Disease-specific instruments									Generic instruments		
	F-HAQ	HAQ	CLINHAQ	MHAQ	AIMS	AIMS2	WOMAC	FIQ	MACTAR	SF-36	SIP	NHP
Functional disability	X	X	X	X	X	X	X		X	X	X	X
Eating											O	
Body care											O	
Mobility					O	O					O	
Dexterity					O	O						
ADL/self-care					O	O						
Arm function						O						
Physical function					O	O						
Pain	X	X	X	X	X	X	X	X		X		X
Social activities and roles					X	X			X	X	X	X
Social roles/function						O				O		
Home management											O	
Social activities					O	O				O		
Recreation/pastime											O	
Social interaction/isolation											O	O
Social support						O						
Communication											O	
Work/work disability	X		X			X		X		X	X	
Symptoms												
Sleep/rest			X					X			X	X
Stiffness				X		X	X					
Fatigue/energy			X	X				X		X		X
Gastrointestinal problems			X	X								
Alertness/cognition											X	
Adverse drug reactions	X		X									
Global measures												
Global disease severity	X	X	X	X								
Global health/well-being			X	X				X		X		
Satisfaction			X	X		X						
Emotions/mood			X	X	X	X		X	X	X	X	X
Depression			O		O	O		O				
Anxiety			O		O	O		O				
Helplessness/attitude				O								
Financial aspects	X											
Indirect costs	O											
Direct costs	O											
Other areas												
Attribution of problems						X						
Priority areas: self-stated						X			X			

* F-HAQ = Full HAQ; HAQ = Health Assesment Questionnaire; CLINHAQ = clinical HAQ; MHAQ = Modified HAQ; AIMS = Arthritis Impact Measurement Scales, Original Version; AIMS2 = Arthritis Impact Measurement Scales, Version 2; WOMAC = Western Ontario and McMaster Universities Osteoarthritis Index; FIQ = Fibromyalgia Impact Questionnaire; MACTAR = McMaster Toronto Arthritis Preference Disability Questionnaire; SF-36 = Medical Outcomes Study 36-Item Short Form Health Survey; SIP = Sickness Impact Profile; NHP = Nottingham Health Profile.

function is especially important following hip or knee replacement for osteoarthritis (OA); however, limitations in activities related to hand functioning might be especially significant in early RA (11).

Disease-Specific Instruments

Health status instruments have been developed and validated for use across the rheumatic disorders and more specific instruments for use in a particular rheumatic disease. The Health Assessment Questionnaire (HAQ) and its modifications, the Arthritis Impact Measurement Scales (AIMS) and its revision, and the McMaster Toronto Arthritis Patient Preference Disability Questionnaire (MACTAR) are the more general of the disease-specific instruments. The Western Ontario and Mc-Master Universities Osteoarthritis Index (WOMAC) and the Fibromyalgia Impact Questionnaire (FIQ) are examples of instruments for use with OA of the hip and knee and fibromyalgia, respectively. Each of these instruments is briefly de-scribed below; the domains included in each instrument are listed in Table 3.

Health Assessment Questionnaire. There are 2 versions of the original HAQ: the functional disability scale and the full HAQ, both developed in the early 1980s. The full HAQ is over 20 pages long, changes periodically, and evaluates economic costs, medications and their side effects, use of health care services, comorbidity as well as functional disability, pain, and global disease severity. The second version, which is used extensively, is the short functional disability scale consisting of 24 questions. This instrument evaluates 8 activities of daily living including dressing, arising, eating, walking, hygiene, reach, grip, and general activities (e.g., running errands, getting in and out of a car) (12). Scores range from 0 (able to perform all activities without difficulty) to 3 (unable to do activities even with help). Visual analog scales measuring severity of pain during the last week and global disease severity are frequently included as part of the HAQ. In contrast to the full questionnaire, this instrument may be completed and scored in less than 5 minutes and is suitable for use in both research and clinical practice settings. The HAQ functional disability scale has been translated into several languages and is used throughout the world (13,14). The instrument is sensitive to change in clinical trials and in long-term outcome studies and it has been shown to predict mortality and future disabilities. It has been used in studies across the spectrum of rheumatic diseases (13,14).

Modified Health Assessment Questionnaire (MHAQ). The MHAQ includes a shortened version of the HAQ functional scale (8 items) plus items related to patient satisfaction with function and patient interpretation of his/her change in ability to perform routine activities (15). The MHAQ has been used extensively in clinical trials and long-term observational studies. Recent studies comparing the original HAQ functional ability scale to the MHAQ have indicated that the MHAQ does not describe the full range of disability (i.e., minimal impairment through inability to do the activities of daily living) as well as the HAQ (13,16).

Multi-Dimensional Modified HAQ (MDHAQ). The MDHAQ is a total assessment instrument that is appropriate for routine clinic practice. It includes the MHAQ plus items related to activity levels (walking, running, climbing stairs), pain, psychological distress, fatigue, global status, review of systems, and medications (17).

CLINHAQ. The CLINHAQ is a "derivative" instrument that integrates several scales and subscales from established instruments as well as including new ones (14). It contains the HAQ functional disability scale, 5 visual analog scales (i.e., pain, global disease severity, sleep disturbance, gastrointestinal distress, and fatigue), a pain diagram, and the anxiety and depression subscales from the original AIMS instrument. This instrument has been used for numerous reports of long-term outcome in the rheumatic diseases as well as in ongoing clinical practice (14,18).

Arthritis Impact Measurement Scales (AIMS). The AIMS, a comprehensive rheumatic disease health status instrument, has been published in 2 versions (20). Both instruments have been extensively validated and translated into several languages. The original AIMS examined the "impact" of arthritis in terms of both physical function (scales for mobility, physical activity, dexterity, and activities of daily living) and psychosocial aspects of chronic arthritis (subscales for social role, social activities, pain, depression, and anxiety) (19). AIMS2, published in early 1992, added new components that addressed issues of patient satisfaction, patient preference or priority areas for health status improvement, and attribution of symptoms/problems to arthritis. The instrument is the most comprehensive of all disease-specific health status instruments and was designed for use in clinical research. The length of both instruments (>20 minutes to complete) and the complexity of scoring have limited their use in routine clinical practice and clinical studies (21).

Recently a shortened version of the AIMS2, the AIMS-SF, has been developed (22). The new instrument retains the original 5-component structure (physical functions, symptoms, affect, social interaction, and role) of the AIMS2 but reduces the number of items by half. This shortened version may prove useful in large clinical studies and in practice, although additional demonstrations of its performance are needed (21,22).

McMaster Toronto Arthritis Patient Preference Disability Questionnaire. The MACTAR must be administered by an interviewer and is designed to elicit patient priorities or pref-erences. Patients are asked to describe limitation in activities including physical functioning (self-care), household, work, and leisure activities, social roles, and sexuality and then to rank the importance of doing these various activities without pain (23,24). The interviewer probes for answers using a detailed protocol. The instrument has been shown to be "valid and highly responsive" in clinical trials, but the cost of administration limits its applicability for clinical practice and long-term outcome studies (24).

Western Ontario and McMaster Universities Osteoarthritis Index. The WOMAC is a self-administered instrument designed to measure dimensions particularly relevant in osteoarthritis. It specifically measures pain, stiffness, and physical function activities associated with OA of the hip or knee (25). The instrument has been used in trials of nonsteroidal anti-inflammatory drugs and other pain medications (26–28), following hip and knee arthroplasty, for evaluation of lower extremity function in OA, RA, and in fibromyalgia (29–31). The WOMAC correlates strongly with pain, fatigue, and psychological distress, demonstrating that the instrument has a global outlook (31). Its brevity (<10 minutes to administer), availability in both questionnaire and visual analog formats, and responsiveness to change make it appropriate for use in clinical practice settings, particularly following knee arthroplasty. The instrument has been translated into several languages and validated.

Fibromyalgia Impact Questionnaire. The FIQ is a brief 10-item questionnaire designed specifically for the assessment of fibromyalgia. Items included are physical function, work status, depression, anxiety, sleep, pain, stiffness, fatigue, and well-being (32). The physical function component assesses ability to do common tasks such as shopping, making beds, walking several blocks, laundry, vacuuming, and yard work. Participants have the option of not responding to items they do not ordinarily do. Difficulties with such an approach have been noted. One study involving several groups of patients from different geographic areas found that the most difficult items were often omitted. This scoring approach leads to underestimation of functional difficulties and makes comparisons across groups problematic (33). The instrument has been used in studies evaluating interventions and in observational studies of fibromyalgia (32,34,35).

Generic Health Status Measures

Generic health status measures are not disease-specific; they examine the impact of a disease and its symptoms on a person's life. They are frequently used to assess health of the population; therefore, they may be used with both "healthy" subjects and those with illness and symptoms. These instruments are usually multidimensional and may include subscales that address different concepts such as pain, social isolation/interaction, and fulfillment of roles. They permit comparison across diseases and cultures and with "healthy" populations (9). Table 3 lists common generic health status instruments.

Nottingham Health Profile (NHP). The NHP was developed in England and has been translated and tested in several languages. It includes 38 dichotomous questions that evaluate physical abilities, pain, sleep, social isolation, emotional reactions, and energy level from the patient's viewpoint (36). The simple format and short completion time (10 minutes) are advantages, although the yes/no response format limits the scope of impact that can be expressed. Results are similar to the AIMS and HAQ on most equivalent scales, but are less sensitive to change (37,38).

Sickness Impact Profile (SIP). The SIP has been widely used in North America and Europe across numerous chronic diseases, including the rheumatic disorders. It contains 312 items within the dimensions of physical and psychosocial functioning. Specific sections include sleep and rest, eating, work, home management, recreation and pastimes, ambulating, mobility, body care and movement, social interaction, alertness behavior, emotional behavior, and communication (39). The SIP can be self-administered or administered by an interviewer and takes 20–30 minutes to complete. While the SIP is one of the most comprehensive generic multidimensional health status questionnaires, its lack of a pain scale limits its use in the rheumatic disorders (38).

The Medical Outcomes Study Short Form 36 (SF-36). The Medical Outcomes Study SF-36 is the most widely used generic instrument and is frequently paired with a disease-specific instrument in clinical drug trials, long-term observational studies, and other clinical investigations (9,40). It evaluates 8 areas of health status including limitation in physical activities because of health problems, limitation in social activities because of health problems, limitation of social activities because of physical or emotional problems, limitation in usual role because of health problems, bodily pain, general mental health (psychological distress and well-being), vitality (energy and fatigue), and general health perceptions. A physical component and mental component are 2 commonly reported summary measures. The instrument can be completed in 5–10 minutes, scored quickly, and may be used in clinical practice, research, health policy, and population surveys. The SF-36 has been tested in large populations, and normative information is available for the US and several European countries (38). Questions concerning the sensitivity of the pain scale and the functional ability scales in severely ill or impaired populations have been raised (38,39). The SF-36 is an important instrument due to its use as an outcome measure for US health policy research. Ongoing efforts to translate and validate the instrument in many countries further illustrate its significance.

HEALTH STATUS ASSESSMENT IN CHILDREN

Assessment of the health-related quality of life and health status in children is complex. Developmental roles and tasks at different ages, parents' versus the child's opinion, and normal variability in growth and behavior are issues that must be addressed (41,42). Health status instruments for children are being developed that complement the reliable and well-validated instruments for assessment of adults. While functional classification systems including the ACR Functional Class and the Chronic Activity Limitations Scale have been used to describe functional limitations in children with rheumatic diseases, they have failed to describe adequately the physical limitations of these children. With both instruments, over 85% of the disabilities of children with juvenile rheumatoid arthritis (JRA) have been categorized in classes indicating no or only minor disruptions in functional ability (43).

The Child HAQ (CHAQ), the most commonly used instrument for children, is adapted from the functional status scale of the HAQ. It assesses functional ability, pain, and global severity. Each activity of daily living area from the adult HAQ (e.g., dressing, eating, and arising) has an age-appropriate assessment item. For example, able to remove socks was added to the dressing and grooming area because a healthy 1-year-old can perform this activity but could not accomplish the other listed activities. The instrument may be completed by the child or by parents as appropriate (44).

The Juvenile Arthritis Quality of Life Questionnaire (45) and the Childhood Arthritis Health Profile (42,46) are more comprehensive instruments than the CHAQ. Each addresses the health quality of life domains beyond function such as pain, psychosocial functioning, symptoms, and areas of family, friends, and school. Both instruments are beginning to be used in clinical practice.

Other instruments developed for use in children include the Juvenile Arthritis Functional Assessment Scale (JAFAS) and the Juvenile Arthritis Functional Assessment Report (JAFAR). The JAFAS includes 10 activities of daily living (e.g., buttoning a shirt or blouse, cutting food, walking, and bending) that are observed and evaluated by a health professional. In children 7 years and older, this instrument has been shown to discriminate between healthy children and children with JRA and between different ability levels of the chronically ill children (47). The JAFAS and JAFAR, an adaptation of the JAFAS, include 23 items and are designed as self-report instruments. Separate versions for proxy reports by parents or self-administration by the child are available (48).

USE OF HEALTH STATUS MEASURES IN CLINICAL PRACTICE

A variety of health status instruments have been developed and validated in clinical studies. They have been used as outcome measures in clinical trials of medications, educational interventions, and joint replacement surgery. These measures predict health care costs, length of stay in rehabilitation facilities, and even mortality. Although their usefulness in rheumatology outpatient care has been demonstrated (49), widespread integration of health status measures into routine clinical practice remains an important goal.

In selecting an instrument for use in clinical care, the length of the instrument and appropriateness to the practice setting are the major concerns. For routine monitoring of outpatients in a rheumatology practice, the HAQ functional ability scale, the MHAQ, and the CLINHAQ are the instruments of choice. They measure the important aspects of health status such as functional ability, pain, psychological distress, fatigue, and satisfaction, yet responding to all items takes less than 5 minutes. Patients may complete the questionnaires while sitting in a waiting room, and disruption of clinical routine is minimal. Scoring can be accomplished quickly so that important information (depression level, pain severity, and functional ability) is available immediately for use during the clinic visit (17,49).

In rehabilitation settings and evaluations following orthopedic surgery, other instruments may be used to assess outcome of treatment. Perhaps the more comprehensive AIMS or AIMS2 would be helpful, especially if repeated administrations are not required. Time for completion is longer than for the HAQ, MHAQ or the CLINHAQ; however, more comprehensive information is obtained. If one is studying outcome in osteoarthritis following orthopedic surgery, the WOMAC might provide the most meaningful information. The trade-off between costs of administration and comprehensive information remains the issue in selecting an appropriate instrument.

In primary care clinics, where a variety of chronic health problems are seen in addition to rheumatic diseases, the SF-36 may be the best choice. The availability of normative data in both the US and Europe makes adoption of this instrument for a primary practice clinic appealing. As shown in Table 3, domains included in the SF-36 are similar to the AIMS1 and AIMS2 and to aspects of the HAQ, CLINHAQ, and MHAQ. Like the disease-specific HAQ, the CLINHAQ, and the MHAQ, patients can complete the SF-36 in a few minutes without assistance. Rapid scoring is feasible, providing the health professional with ready access to important information.

SUMMARY

Health status assessment is rapidly becoming integrated into the health professional's traditional assessment tools of history taking, physical examination, laboratory tests, and radiography. While physical functioning may be evaluated by direct observation of the patient performing specific tasks, this approach is time-consuming, expensive, and limited to the few tasks that are observable in a clinical setting. Reliable, well-validated self-report health status instruments have been developed for use in clinical research and practice. These instruments may be specific to the rheumatic diseases or may be multidimensional assessments of health-related quality of life. Some, such as the SF-36 or versions of the HAQ, are more appropriate for routine clinical care. Others, such as AIMS or SIP, are best used for clinical research or in comprehensive outcome studies where they are administered once or infrequently. Regardless of instrument used, the assessment of health status is essential to the comprehensive understanding of how a disease affects someone's life; therefore, such assessment is also essential to quality patient care.

REFERENCES

1. Liang MH. The historical and conceptual framework for functional assessment in rheumatic disease. J Rheumatol 1987;14 Suppl 15:2–5.
2. Gill TM, Feinstein AR. A critical appraisal of the quality of quality-of-life measurements. JAMA 1994;272:619–26.
3. Anderson JJ, Felson DT, Meenan RF, Williams HJ. Which traditional measures should be used in rheumatoid arthritis clinical trials? Arthritis Rheum 1989;32:1093–9.
4. Decker JL, McShane DJ, Esdaile JM, Hathaway DE, Levinson JE, Liang MH, et al. Dictionary of the rheumatic diseases. Volume 1. Signs and symptoms. New York: Contact Associates International; 1982.
5. Kwoh CK, O'Connor GT, Regansmith MG, Olmstead EM, Brown LA, Burnett JB, et al. Concordance between clinician and patient assessment of physical and mental health status. J Rheumatol 1992;19:1031–7.
6. Kivela SL. Measuring disability–do self-ratings and service provider ratings compare? J Chronic Dis 1984;37:115–23.
7. Hochberg MC, Chang RW, Dwosh I, Lindsey S, Pincus T, Wolfe F. The American College of Rheumatology 1991 revised criteria for the classification of global functional status in rheumatoid arthritis. Arthritis Rheum 1992;35:498–502.
8. Stucki G, Stoll T, Bruhlmann P, Michel BA. Construct validation of the

9. Stewart AL, Greenfield S, Hays RD, Wells K, Rogers WH, Berry SD, et al. Functional status and well-being of patients with chronic conditions: results from the Medical Outcomes Study. JAMA 1989;262:907–13.
10. Fowler FJ, Cleary PD, Magaziner J, Patrick DL, Benjamin KL. Methodological issues in measuring patient-reported outcomes: the agenda of the work group on outcomes assessment. Med Care 1994;32:JS65–76.
11. Stewart AL, Painter PL. Issues in measuring physical functioning and disability in arthritis patients. Arthritis Care Res 1997;10:395–405.
12. Fries JF, Spitz P, Kraines RG, Holman HR. Measurement of patient outcome in arthritis. Arthritis Rheum 1980;23:137–45.
13. Wolfe F. Which HAQ is best? A comparison of the HAQ, MHAQ and RA-HAQ, a difficult 8-item HAQ (DHAQ), and a rescored 20-item HAQ (HAQ20): analyses on 2,491 rheumatoid arthritis patients following leflunomide initiation. J Rheumatol 2001;28:982–9.
14. Wolfe F. Health status questionnaires. Rheum Dis Clin North Am 1995; 21:445–64.
15. Pincus T, Summey JA, Soraci SA Jr, Wallston KA, Hummon NP. Assessment of patient satisfaction in activities of daily living using a modified Stanford Health Assessment Questionnaire. Arthritis Rheum 1983; 26:1346–53.
16. Stucki G, Stucki S, Bruhlmann P, Michel BA. Ceiling effects of the Health Assessment Questionnaire and its modified version in some ambulatory rheumatoid arthritis patients. Ann Rheum Dis 1995;54:461–5.
17. Pincus T, Wolfe F. An infrastructure of patient questionnaires at each rheumatology visit: improving efficiency and documenting care. J Rheumatol 2000;27:2727–30.
18. Wolfe F. Data collection and utilization: a methodology for clinical practice and clinical research. In: Wolfe F, Pincus T, editors. Rheumatoid arthritis: pathogenesis, assessment, outcome, and treatment. New York: Marcel Dekker; 1994. p. 463–514.
19. Meenan RF, Gertman PM, Mason JH. Measuring health status in arthritis: the Arthritis Impact Measurement Scales. Arthritis Rheum 1980;23:146–52.
20. Meenan RF, Mason JH, Anderson JJ, Guccione AA, Kazis LE. AIMS2: the content and properties of a revised and expanded Arthritis Impact Measurement Scales health status questionnaire. Arthritis Rheum 1992; 35:1–10.
21. Haavardsholm EA, Kvien TK, Uhlig T, Smedstad LM, Guillemin F. Comparison of agreement and sensitivity to change between AIMS2 and a short form of AIMS2 (AIMS2-SF) in more than 1000 rheumatoid arthritis patients. J Rheumatol 2000;27:2810–6.
22. Guillemin F, Coste J, Pouchot J, Ghézail M, Bregeon C, Sany J, et al, The French Quality of Life in Rheumatology Group. The AIMS2-SF: a short form of the Arthritis Impact Measurement Scales 2. Arthritis Rheum 1997;40:1267–74.
23. Tugwell P, Bombardier C, Buchanan WW, Goldsmith CH, Grace E, Hanna B. The MACTAR patient preference disability questionnaire–an individualized functional priority approach for assessing improvement in physical disability in clinical trials in rheumatoid arthritis. J Rheumatol 1987;14:446–51.
24. Verhoeven AC, Boers M, van der Linden S. Validity of the MACTAR questionnaire as a functional index in a rheumatoid arthritis clinical trial. J Rheumatol 2000;27:2801–9.
25. Bellamy N, Buchanan WW, Goldsmith CH, Campbell J, Stitt LW. Validation study of WOMAC: a health status instrument for measuring clinically important patient relevant outcomes to antirheumatic drug therapy in patients with osteoarthritis of the hip or knee. J Rheumatol 1988;15:1833–40.
26. Bellamy N, Kean WF, Buchanan WW, Gerecz-Simon E, Campbell J. Double blind randomized controlled trial of sodium meclofenamate (Meclomen) and diclofenac sodium (Voltaren): post validation reapplication of the WOMAC Osteoarthritis Index. J Rheumatol 1992;19:153–9.
27. Grace D, Rogers J, Skeith K, Anderson K. Topical diclofenac versus placebo: a double blind, randomized clinical trial in patients with osteoarthritis of the knee. J Rheumatol 1999;26:2659–63.
28. Peloso PM, Bellamy N, Bensen W, Thomson GTD, Harsanyi Z, Babul N, et al. Double blind randomized placebo control trial of controlled release codeine in the treatment of osteoarthritis of the hip or knee. J Rheumatol 2000;27:764–71.
29. Bellamy N, Buchanan WW, Goldsmith CH, Campbell J, Stitt L. Validation study of the WOMAC: a health status instrument for measuring clinically-important patient relevant outcomes following total hip or knee arthroplasty in osteoarthritis. J Orthop Rheumatol 1988;1:95–108.
30. Brazier JE, Harper R, Munro J, Walters SJ, Snaith ML. Generic and

condition-specific outcome measures for people with osteoarthritis of the knee. Rheumatology (Oxford) 1999;38:870–7.

31. Wolfe F. Determinants of WOMAC function, pain and stiffness scores: evidence for the role of low back pain, symptom counts, fatigue and depression in osteoarthritis, rheumatoid arthritis and fibromyalgia. Rheumatology (Oxford) 1999;38:355–61.

32. Burckhardt CS, Clark SR, Bennett RM. The fibromyalgia impact questionnaire: development and validation. J Rheumatol 1991;18:728–33.

33. Wolfe F, Hawley DJ, Goldenberg DL, Russell IJ, Buskila D, Neumann L. The assessment of functional impairment in fibromyalgia (FM): Rasch analyses of 5 functional scales and the development of the FM Health Assessment Questionnaire. J Rheumatol 2000;27:1989–99.

34. Mannerkorpi K, Nyberg B, Ahlmen M, Ekdahl C. Pool exercise combined with an education program for patients with fibromyalgia syndrome: a prospective, randomized study. J Rheumatol 2000;27:2473–81.

35. King S, Wessel J, Bhambhani Y, Maikala R, Sholter D, Maksymowych W. Validity and reliability of the 6 minute walk in persons with fibromyalgia. J Rheumatol 1999;26:2233–7.

36. Hunt SM, McKenna SP, McEwen J, Backett EM, Williams J, Papp E. The Nottingham Health Profile: subjective health status and medical consultations. Soc Sci Med [A] 1981;15:221–9.

37. Fitzpatrick R, Ziebland S, Jenkinson C, Mowat A. A comparison of the sensitivity to change of several health status instruments in rheumatoid arthritis. J Rheumatol 1993;20:429–36.

38. Scott A, Garrod T. Quality of life measures: use and abuse. Baillieres Best Pract Res Clin Rheumatol 2000;14:663–87.

39. Anderson RT, Aaronson NK, Wilkin D. Critical review of the international assessments of health-related quality of life. Qual Life Res 1993; 2:369–95.

40. Ware JE, Sherbourne CD. The MOS 36-item short-form health survey (SF-36).1. Conceptual framework and item selection. Med Care 1992;30: 473–83.

41. Feldman BM, Grundland B, McCullough L, Wright V. Distinction of quality of life, health related quality of life, and health status in children referred for rheumatologic care. J Rheumatol 2000;27:226–33.

42. Tucker LB. Whose life is it anyway? Understanding quality of life in children with rheumatic diseases. J Rheumatol 2000;27:8–11.

43. Lovell DJ. Newer functional outcome measurements in juvenile rheumatoid arthritis: a progress report. J Rheumatol Suppl 1992;33:28–31.

44. Singh G, Athreya BH, Fries JF, Goldsmith DP. Measurement of health status in children with juvenile rheumatoid arthritis. Arthritis Rheum 1994;37:1761–9.

45. Duffy CM, Arsenault L, Duffy KNW, Paquin JD, Strawczynski H. The juvenile arthritis quality of life questionnaire development of a new responsive index for juvenile rheumatoid arthritis and juvenile spondyloarthritides. J Rheumatol 1997;24:738–46.

46. Tucker LB, DeNardo BA, Abetz LN, Landgraf JM, Schaller JG. The Childhood Arthritis Health Profile (CAHP): validity and reliability of the condition-specific scales [abstract]. Arthritis Rheum 1995;38 Suppl 9:S183.

47. Lovell DJ, Howe S, Shear E, Hartner S, McGirr G, Schulte M, et al. Development of a disability measurement tool for juvenile rheumatoid arthritis: the Juvenile Arthritis Functional Assessment Scale. Arthritis Rheum 1989;32:1390–5.

48. Howe S, Levinson J, Shear E, Hartner S, McGirr G, Schulte M, et al. Development of a disability measurement tool for juvenile rheumatoid arthritis: the Juvenile Arthritis Functional Assessment Report for children and their parents. Arthritis Rheum 1991;34:873–80.

49. Wolfe F, Pincus T. Data collection in the clinic. Rheum Dis Clin North Am 1995;21:321–58.

50. Jones E, Hanly JG, Mooney R, Rand LL, Spurway PM, Eastwood BJ, et al. Strength and function in the normal and rheumatoid hand. J Rheumatol 1991;18:1313–8.

51. Pankoff B, Overend T, Lucy D, White K. Validity and responsiveness of the 6 minute walk test for people with fibromyalgia. J Rheumatol 2000; 27:2666–70.

52. Dellhag B, Bjelle A. A five-year followup of hand function and activities of daily living in rheumatoid arthritis patients. Arthritis Care Res 1999; 12:33–41.

53. Dellhag B, Bjelle A. A grip ability test for use in rheumatology practice. J Rheumatol 1995;22:1559–65.

54. Pincus T, Callahan LF. Rheumatology function tests–grip strength, walking time, button test and questionnaires document and predict long term morbidity and mortality in rheumatoid arthritis. J Rheumatol 1992;19: 1051–7.

55. Newcomer KL, Krug HE, Mahowald ML. Validity and reliability of the timed-stands test for patients with rheumatoid arthritis and other chronic diseases. J Rheumatol 1993;20:21–7.

56. Sullivan M, Ahlmen M, Bjelle A, Karlsson J. Health status assessment in rheumatoid arthritis. II. Evaluation of a modified Shorter Sickness Impact Profile. J Rheumatol 1993;20:1500–7.

57. Kalla AA, Smith PR, Brown GMM, Meyers OL, Chalton D. Responsiveness of Keitel functional index compared with laboratory measures of disease activity in rheumatoid arthritis. Br J Rheumatol 1995;34:141–9.

Additional Recommended Reading

Lorig K, Stewart A, Ritter PL, Gonzalez V, Lynch J. Outcome measures for health education and other health care interventions. Thousand Oaks (CA): Sage; 1996.

McDowell I, Newell C. Measuring health: a guide to rating scales and questionnaires. 2nd ed. Oxford (UK): Oxford University Press; 1996.

McHorney CA. Health status assessment methods for adults: past accomplishments and future challenges. Annu Rev Public Health 1999;200:309–35.

Evidence-Based Medicine and Evaluation of Clinical Trials

CHRISTOPHER LORISH, PhD

Providers, payers, and consumers of health care services are affected by not only the quantity and quality of care that patients receive but also health professionals' practice standards and working conditions. Proponents of evidence-based medicine (EBM) have developed some simple tools for assisting clinicians in their efforts to find and apply the best scientific evidence to clinical diagnosis and treatment.

Why is it important to be evidence-based practitioners now? In the past, clinicians often relied on regional practice norms and experience. However, care of many diseases is different from even 5–10 years ago, due to dramatic progress in diagnostic technology and pharmacologic treatments (and their potential interactions). Many diseases are being diagnosed earlier in their course, resulting in different patient groups and perhaps different experiences with treatments from past clinical experience. For instance, consider how the treatment of rheumatoid arthritis (RA) changed radically with the acceptance of methotrexate. Unlike the traditional CME programs, which are episodic and usually disease- but not patient-specific, EBM encourages continuous learning through frequent review of the scientific literature in response to a patient's specific clinical problems. Finally, the tools to access and use the best clinical science in practice have developed rapidly and continue to evolve, making it easier to access information.

Evidence-based medicine depends on a clinical science literature of well-designed, internally valid studies of diagnostic and treatment procedures. In addition, this same literature can be used to inform legislative debate and administrative decisions and to counterbalance the marketplace inclination to maximize cost reductions and profit, possibly at the patient's expense. Unlike medicine, other health disciplines have not had the advantage of government and industry support for clinical studies, resulting in a much more limited clinical science base.

Arthritis health professionals need to be critical consumers of the research literature to maintain credibility with their patients and colleagues and to influence the scientific and, possibly, national debate on effective practice. Reading the scientific literature critically is a necessary but not sufficient condition. Other skills and techniques for applying the best clinical science to practice are being formalized in the EBM movement (1,2) and will be touched upon briefly in this chapter. Ironically, a commitment to applying the best clinical science to practice may put individuals and professional groups at odds with policymakers desirous of cutting health care costs. The most efficacious diagnostic or treatment procedure may not be the least expensive.

THE SCIENCE OF CLINICAL TRIALS

The shift in health care from a focus on process-oriented quality standards to outcomes has found its research analogue in studies testing comparative diagnostic and treatment effectiveness. Supported mostly by pharmaceutical companies and government agencies like the National Institutes of Health, the best diagnostic and treatment effectiveness studies use randomized, controlled clinical experiments to determine which of 2 or more diagnostic or treatment methods produces the most accurate assessment or greatest amount/most rapid return to health with the least harm (3). An everyday analogy to the randomized clinical trial is the professional automobile race in which a group of comparable automobiles that differ mostly on the basis of the driver's skills are all subjected to comparable racing conditions to determine the relative speed and time each driver took to complete the race. Although luck and mechanical durability play a role, differences in the drivers' skill is presumed to be the reason one auto crosses the line before another, because other influences on the final standings are more or less equal before and during the race.

In medicine, randomized, controlled studies are commonly conducted in which, for example, a new nonsteroidal anti-inflammatory drug (NSAID) is compared to aspirin or another NSAID in its relative ability to reduce pain, inflammation, and improve function using comparable patients and study conditions. In physical therapy, comparing manual therapy treatment to electrical stimulation to reduce pain and increase function in acute low back pain is another example. No one clinical trial can answer all the questions surrounding a treatment's efficacy— for example, which patient groups under what treatment conditions benefit the most for the longest period of time with the least side effects. Thus, multiple studies of a diagnostic or treatment procedure are needed.

The accumulation of results from well-designed and -conducted randomized clinical trials permits health professionals to use scientifically verified or evidence-based diagnostic and treatment procedures, rather than relying primarily on personal experience, expert opinion, or tradition. However, clinical trials are expensive and time consuming and lag behind the development of new diagnostic and treatment technology, suggesting a continued role for experience and expert opinion.

BECOMING A CRITICAL CONSUMER OF RESEARCH

Clinical trials comparing diagnostic or treatment procedures are presented regularly in scientific journals, and all health professionals are faced with the task of making judgments about the value of a diagnostic or treatment procedure based on one or more of these published reports (4). To critically evaluate clinical research, the reader should look for answers to the following questions: 1) What kind of research study is being reported—descriptive or experimental? 2) How credible is the causal relationship between the treatment and desired outcome (i.e., internal validity)? and 3) How clinically important are the results (i.e., the magnitude of effects)?

CLINICAL EXPERIMENTS VERSUS DESCRIPTIVE STUDIES

All research begins with questions. Human comparative clinical trials assessing diagnostic and treatment effectiveness attempt to answer questions about the diagnostic accuracy or the onset, duration, and degree of desired and harmful effects caused by 2 or more treatments (3–5). Treatment effects can be measured based on changes in tissues or organ-system dysfunctions (impairments), functional limitations, or social, emotional, and role dysfunctions. Note the implicit causal sequence, that is, impairments cause functional limitations that cause role or other health status changes. Inclusion of measures from each of these levels in treatment effectiveness studies greatly increases their value because of the understanding of how impairments influence function (6).

Before conducting a clinical trial, data that more completely describe the workings of a condition or even a treatment often need to be obtained. Clinical observation derived from daily experience needs to be supplemented by more systematic descriptive studies to identify characteristics of the condition, its untreated consequences, and the range of desired and harmful effects when a treatment is applied. Descriptive studies may include laboratory studies detailing the characteristics of normal and pathologic tissues, epidemiologic studies of the incidence and prevalence of the condition, or correlational studies that identify potentially important causal relationships in the etiology or sequelae of a condition. They may be case studies describing in detail the course of a disease or the effects of a treatment on an individual. Surveys that solicit patients' opinions or descriptions of a disease, its effects, and costs are another kind of descriptive study. Qualitative studies that emphasize participant observation and detailed description to provide insight into the meaning of a disease or treatment for patients have become more common (7).

These kinds of descriptive studies lay the groundwork for clinical trials by systematically and fully elaborating the characteristics of a condition, its untreated effects, and the likely costs and benefits of a diagnostic or treatment procedure. In addition, they often provide important insights into what variables should be included or controlled in clinical experiments. For example, research to improve our understanding of fibromyalgia consists of both descriptive and comparative treatment efficacy studies, specifically tissue pathology, incidence and prevalence of the condition, functional limitations, and psychological, social, and role consequences (8).

Another key distinction between descriptive studies and experimental ones is that the latter attempt to demonstrate a causal relation between the application of a treatment and one or more desired outcomes. For example, does a patient education program cause a decrease in pain and an improvement in patients' social and role functioning? The findings of descriptive studies may suggest a causal connection; however, because descriptive studies do not exert control over other causal explanations for an outcome of interest, they do not provide definitive evidence for a causal relationship. The goal of a comparative clinical trial is to set up a test between 2 or more competitors that unambiguously demonstrates the causal relationship between the treatment and effect (3). As in the car race analogy, this is accomplished by using methods that control unwanted causal influences.

A close reading of the study's Methods section enables the reader to judge whether the study has serious threats to demonstrating a causal relationship between the treatment and outcome, termed *internal validity*. If no apparent threats to the study's internal validity exist, the reader examines the Results section of the report to determine if any treatment produced an effect greater than chance variation (i.e., whether the P value was equal to or less than 0.05 for the experimental diagnostic or treatment procedure). Sometimes authors also report indicators of the magnitude of the effect of a treatment (effect size) that can then be compared directly with treatment effect sizes from other studies. This helps clinicians determine how important or powerful the effect is on an outcome. By comparing effect sizes between similar studies, a clinician can judge the robustness of the effect when a diagnostic or treatment procedure is tested under different conditions with different groups of patients.

JUDGING THE CREDIBILITY OF CLINICAL EXPERIMENTS

Laboratory and clinical experiments follow rules of methodologic procedure and evidence to narrow the number of potential causes of an effect to the one of interest (9). This is no simple task when dealing with real people living in natural settings and affected by a host of known and unknown causal forces. Experimental researchers attempt to control for the effects of unwanted causes by eliminating them or exerting procedural and statistical controls. This increases the likelihood that the observed effect, like reduced pain, is due to the treatment (the cause of interest) and not to some other cause, such as the patient's motivation or use of another remedy. The number and success of these control efforts determine a study's internal validity. Studies that successfully apply controls are judged to have higher internal validity and the results are more likely to be judged credible. Thus, to answer the question, "How credible is the causal relationship between the treatment and outcome?," the most important criterion is the amount of control exercised over other causes that threaten internal validity.

Because no study in humans is ever able to rule out all possible causal explanations for the effect of interest, the judgment of internal validity is one of degree. Additional studies are usually needed to overcome the uncontrolled causes of prior studies. The accumulation of similar findings from many published studies with high internal validity gives that causal relationship the highest credibility. Unfortunately, clinical trials are published that are seriously defective in design, execution, or both, resulting in little confidence in their demonstration of a causal relationship, even if one or more of the outcomes achieves statistical significance. Sometimes authors discuss the limitations of their studies in the Discussion section, but the reader must still make a careful analysis of the article's Methods and Results sections to judge the study's internal validity.

Recent articles have summarized the procedural characteristics a clinical trial should evidence to obtain high internal validity (10,11). Rating schemes that give a summary score of a study's internal validity exist and have been used to evaluate the experimental literature (10,12). Whether or not a rating scheme is used to assess a study's internal validity, the reader's examination should focus on the Methods section. This section should include details about the selection and randomization of subjects, the procedures applied to each group, measurements taken and the procedures used to obtain them, statistical procedures used to rule out chance variation, and the methods used to maintain consistency of the treatment applications and measures for the study's duration. The first area the reader should assess is patient selection.

Inclusion/Exclusion Criteria

To control other causes (sometimes called biases), researchers use a variety of control procedures to eliminate, minimize, or make them explicit in the statistical analysis. Clinical experiments consist of comparisons of 2 or more groups that receive differing treatment, diagnostic procedures, or other interventions; therefore, study subjects have to be selected, assigned to groups, and compared. Because people vary in many ways, some of which can affect the outcome of interest, the first control measure that should be reported is the specific subject inclusion and exclusion criteria used. The use of inclusion/exclusion criteria helps control unwanted biases by ensuring a more homogeneous pool of subjects. Persons with characteristics known to affect the outcome are usually excluded. For example, in a study on the efficacy of electrical stimulation versus NSAID therapy for controlling pain, persons who have gastric problems or an aversion to electricity would probably be excluded because of an increased likelihood that they would not comply with the treatment, thereby reducing the treatment's full effects.

By carefully examining the inclusion/exclusion criteria of a study, the reader can obtain an idea both of what causes were controlled through exclusion and what other causes may have affected the outcome because they were not excluded. Because a study only examines the effects of a procedure on a sample of patients whose characteristics are defined by the study's inclusion/exclusion criteria, the applicability of the findings to other patients (*external validity*) is determined, in part, by the characteristics of the patients studied. A well-controlled study with an extensive list of inclusion/exclusion criteria may not generalize to patients with other characteristics. If inclusion and exclusion criteria are not extensive or, worse still, are not stated, then the study may be flawed. Unfortunately, numerous other causal explanations are usually possible in a study that reports few or no inclusion/exclusion criteria.

Random Assignment to Groups

Even with selection criteria that attempt to produce a study pool of more homogenous subjects, there will likely be causally important differences. To address this problem, subjects are randomly assigned to groups. Random assignment equili-

brates groups at the study's outset. That is, the distribution and effects of other subject characteristics that can influence the outcome are more likely to be the same in all groups, especially when groups are large. Thus, the treatment effect must be large enough to be differentiated from this background causal "noise" that has been more equally distributed among the groups.

Note that randomization at the outset does not guarantee that groups will remain comparable throughout the study, even if no experimental procedure is applied. For example, unexpected events (historical artifacts or bias) occur in studies, especially those that continue over months or years. These events may affect one study group more than another, making a cause look more or less effective at the study's end. Something as innocent as an elevator being out of service for a week in a weeklong leg-strengthening exercise study can make a treatment look more powerful than it really is. If the members of only one group had to walk the steps to get to the area where the exercises were performed, their end-of-study strength measures would likely be greater. The best research reports will discuss how the study was monitored for historical changes or changes in the study's procedures. When procedures are applied over several months, the authors should discuss how the effects of historical or procedural changes may have added ambiguity to the causal connection between the treatment and outcome of interest.

Although randomization helps equilibrate subject-related causal influences, it does not guarantee total comparability. The number of study subjects affects the likelihood that the distribution of subject characteristics is similar in both groups, as illustrated by the distribution of heads and tails when a coin is flipped 500 times versus 10 times. The former is most likely to achieve a 50-50 split, while the latter most likely would deviate from the 50-50 split. Even with randomization, a reader cannot be assured that groups were equilibrated at the outset if the group sizes were small, say 10 or less for each. In a study with a small number of subjects in each group, authors should provide additional evidence of group equivalency on characteristics most likely to influence the outcome.

Statistical Control

Statistical control refers to the method used when measures of variables known to be associated with the outcome are included in the statistical design and analysis planned before the study. The importance of this prior planning is that the investigator is more likely to recruit enough subjects for valid, statistical subgroup comparisons. For example, a study may examine the effects of 2 treatments but also include subgroups within each treatment, such as males and females, because the investigator believes that sex differences may affect the outcome. The investigator may also plan for comparisons between groups of patients within each of the treatments based on their motivation or other potentially important causal influences. Statistical procedures like analysis of variance (ANOVA) or multiple regression can test differences between these subgroups. The results from these planned subgroup analyses often help clinicians tailor their diagnostic or treatment procedures to the subgroups of patients for which a study found them to be most effective.

Readers of comparative studies should be alert to reports in which randomization and/or inclusion/exclusion criteria were not used, but extensive use is made of statistical procedures to "rule out" other causes. While statistical analysis can do this to a degree, it fails as a substitute for the other control mechanisms because most investigators do not measure all the relevant causal variables. In such studies, it is usually not hard to identify one or more alternative influences not measured in the study that could also explain the results.

Statistical analysis helps rule out whether random variation is a possible explanation of the results. A study that obtains "*P* values" equal to or less than 0.05 is considered to have effects that have a 5% or less chance of being due to random variation. Thus, these 3 control procedures—inclusion/exclusion criteria, randomization, and statistical design and analysis—proactively reduce bias, but often things occur during a study that threaten internal validity and require further scrutiny by the reader.

The Missing Data Threat

Data not collected on subjects (missing data) or subjects who quit the study after its start (dropouts) pose a serious threat to the equality of groups obtained by randomization. At the end of a study that has dropouts, it can no longer be assumed that groups have the comparability they possessed at the start. For example, in a study of 2 strengthening regimens, random assignment is the best way to ensure that differences in pre-study strength and other influences, like exercise motivation, are equally distributed between the groups at the outset. Confidence in the relative superiority of one regimen is greatly diminished if there is a significant number of dropouts or data not collected in any or all of the groups. The distribution of pre-study strength or other causes that could influence the outcome may have changed, and the effects of these causes can no longer be assumed to be comparable between the groups. Look for discussion of the number of study dropouts and amount of missing data, as well as what the authors tried to do to identify its effects on the results. The results of a clinical experiment with dropouts or missing data that exceed 20% (15% is the FDA standard) should probably be viewed with skepticism (11).

The Variable Treatment Implementation Threat

Poor control of treatment implementation and measurement procedures can lead to ambiguous cause–effect relationships. The report should convince the reader that 1) treatments were clearly different and consistently applied and/or followed by subjects; 2) subjects were not exposed to other treatments, such as home remedies or other prescribed medications, outside of the study; and 3) measures were appropriate (*measurement validity*) and consistently applied (*reliability*). Treatments and measures haphazardly applied or frequently modified during the study result in a causal stew of unknown ingredients and effects.

This is especially problematic in studies in which patients must follow their treatment protocol without direct supervision from study personnel. Although patient logs, phone calls to patients, and more frequent visits to the clinic for taking measures are often used to encourage patients' adherence, the investigator or reader of the report cannot be as sure of subjects' adherence to the treatment protocol as when subjects come to a site where the treatment is applied. Even when

subjects come to a site for treatment, we usually do not know what subjects did at home or work that may have affected the outcomes.

Sometimes subjects, researchers, or data collectors knowingly or unknowingly alter their behavior because of their knowledge about the study. For example, a data collector might unknowingly encourage a treatment subject to try harder or respond differently. A person who administers a treatment might do more or less to a comparison group patient than the protocol calls for out of a "sense of fairness." Subjects may try to do more or less based on their interpretation of what they think is expected of them. Controlling these unwanted variations is best accomplished by trying to keep study subjects and all those that come in contact with subjects ignorant ("blinded") to their treatment group membership. Maintaining subjects' ignorance of the treatment received is especially important for minimizing bias in self-report measures.

The careful reader of a study should be aware of the steps taken to ensure the consistent implementation of the treatment and to keep subjects and study personnel blinded to the study group to which the subject belongs. For example, in a study comparing the efficacy of at-home exercise versus clinic-applied manual therapy techniques on low back pain, the report of a study with greater internal validity will include the following: 1) evidence that the subjects in the home exercise group did the same or at least similar exercises (within-group treatment homogeneity), and that each person did them correctly and regularly during the study period (treatment adherence); 2) evidence that subjects received no other treatments, such as acupuncture, chiropractic, or any others likely to affect the outcome measures during the study; 3) evidence that study personnel taking measures were blinded to a subject's group assignment and that the measures were taken consistently in the same way (intra- and inter-rater reliability). Indications that patients did less or more of the specified treatment or other treatments, that opportunities were missed to keep study personnel and subjects ignorant of a subject's group assignment, and low (<80%) intra- and inter-rater measurement reliability (self-report measures are often lower) are significant threats to internal validity and weaken the inference that one treatment was superior, even if one is statistically different from the other.

DETERMINING CLINICAL IMPORTANCE

Assume that an investigator has done a credible job of minimizing and identifying threats to internal validity and that the statistical analyses indicate that the differences between the groups were probably not due to chance variation. The reader of this study's report can more confidently believe that for the sample studied, one treatment was superior to another in producing a clinical effect. The reader must now ask whether applying the treatment to a patient would make an important difference to the patient's health or functioning. For example, a physical therapist may find 2 clinical experiments with high internal validity that reported significant differences between leg strength training regimens. In the first study, the statistically significant difference amounted to an advantage of 1 pound, and the other study found a statistically significant advantage of 50 pounds. How can both findings be statistically significant? A small difference between treatments can be

Table 1. Effect on pain classification of NSAID treatment versus placebo.*

	Better	Worse	Total
NSAID	25	10	35
Placebo	5	20	25
Total	30	30	60

Odds Ratio = (25/5)/(10/20) = 5/0.50 = 10
* NSAID = nonsteroidal antiinflammatory drug.

statistically different when a large sample and valid and reliable measurement are used. All things being equal, the training protocol that produced a 50-pound advantage is preferred because the magnitude of the effect is greater and because the 50-pound improvement is likely to have a greater effect on the patient's functioning.

Thus, to answer the question of a study's clinical importance, the reader needs a way to express the size of the effect if it is not given in the article, needs knowledge of other similar studies and the effect magnitudes that were found, and needs to make a judgment either on the basis of research or experience as to whether an effect is large enough to make a difference to a patient's health or functioning. Fortunately, there are some fairly simple computations, sometimes reported by a study's author, that allow a reader to express the study's effect size, which can then be compared to the effect sizes of other similar studies. Some are established, like the odds ratio (2) and effect size index (13). In addition, the evidence-based medicine movement has led to the development of a variety of newer clinical indicators of effect, such as the relative risk reduction, number needed to treat, absolute benefit increase, and others (1).

A recent development using these quantitative clinical and intervention indicators of effect is a methodology that synthesizes the effect sizes from multiple similar studies and reports an average effect size for a diagnostic or treatment procedure (14,15). These reports, called systematic reviews or meta-analyses, are published and available in such searchable databases as the Cochrane Collaboration, or Best Evidence (16). Familiarity with the effect sizes reported in a published systematic review can help a clinician decide whether an effect size found in a new study is comparatively important.

Odds Ratio

Some study outcomes are expressed as classifications or differences in kind, such as when a subject is classified at the end of a study as "recovered," "sick," or "deceased." The counts in these groups are then compared statistically by using the chi square test statistic or a variation. When 2 groups of subjects who receive differing treatments (such as treatment and placebo) are classified at the end of the study as either "improved" or "worse" on some outcome of interest, it is possible to express any relative advantage of the treatment group as an odds ratio, as shown in Table 1. In this example, the odds of having a pain rating of "better" is more than 10 times greater for those on the NSAID than for those receiving placebo. Odds ratios are easily computed and provide a convenient way of expressing comparative effect.

Treatment Effect Size

When study outcomes are expressed on a scale that differs by degree, such as amount of strength or pain, then it is possible to calculate a treatment's effect size index. Effect size can be calculated in different ways; one common way involves taking the difference between the end-of-study means of 2 interventions and dividing the result by the standard deviation of the mean of the control group. This yields a number that can be compared with effect size indices from other studies. If there are no prior studies, guidelines exist for classifying an effect as small, medium, or large (13).

Effect size index may also be used to calculate the number of subjects needed in a study to achieve a statistically significant result (13). In the research report, the author should indicate how the study's sample size was determined, preferably using an effect size estimate obtained from the most recent, similar study published. If no published study exists, the author may cite a pilot study effect size. This planning step avoids the unfortunate situation of reading a research report in which the internal validity was high, but there were not enough subjects to demonstrate statistical significance.

Meta-analysis

Another approach to determining a study's clinical significance is to place the obtained effect size in the context of similar studies. *Meta-analysis*, a quantitative study of studies, aggregates the effect sizes of other similar studies to produce an average effect size for a treatment (17). This quantitative approach to synthesizing findings from numerous studies on similar treatments and outcomes provides a quantitative accounting of our knowledge. For example, a meta-analytic study of the effect of NSAID therapy in similar patients would produce an average effect size that could be directly compared with splinting to reduce inflammation. Analyses of the average effects of a treatment and comparisons of effect sizes with other treatments for the same condition will help answer the question of which treatments are most efficacious and should be considered first-line therapy. Extant meta-analyses of interest to arthritis health professionals include patient education and psychoeducation interventions (18), multidisciplinary pain treatment (19), aerobic fitness (20), nursing interventions (21), and psychosocial treatments of depression (22). This approach to integrating findings is relatively new and requires a number of comparative trials before it can be completed. Because of the relative youth of the allied health disciplines, there may not be enough comparative experiments to conduct a meta-analysis on a specific treatment, leaving the therapist to gauge the clinical importance and relevance to practice on a study-by-study basis.

EVIDENCE-BASED PRACTICE

Sackett et al noted, "Evidence-based medicine is the conscientious, explicit, and judicious use of current best evidence in making decisions about the care of individual patients" (23). In the past, physicians and health professionals attended school to learn, among other things, the diagnostic and practice routines of the master clinicians. Out of school, the practitioner's diagnostic and treatment routines may change as a result of the

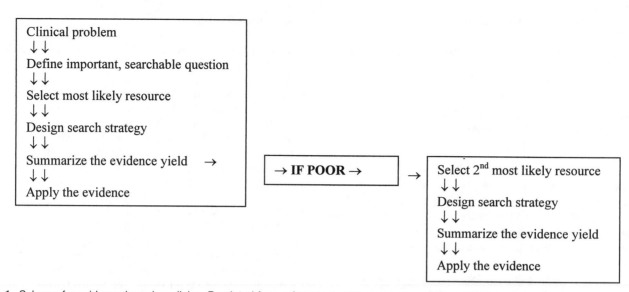

Figure 1. Schema for evidence-based medicine. Reprinted from reference 1, with permission of Churchill Livingstone.

accumulated wisdom of personal experience, regional or national diagnostic and treatment guidelines, or other influences such as patient demand, CME programs, or industry sales representatives. What was often missing in the past was an emphasis on finding the best clinical science and using that clinical science to address the needs of patients. In part to counter the influence of unscientific or special interest groups on medical practice, evidence-based medicine developed as both a commitment and methodology for clinicians to combine with their practice wisdom to provide the most effective care to patients.

Sackett et al (1) suggest using the evidence-based medicine schema shown in Figure 1 as a way of identifying and applying the best clinical evidence to a diagnostic or treatment decision. As the schema suggests, the method starts with a clinician asking a disease-specific diagnostic or treatment question such as: "What is the specificity and sensitivity of the straight leg raise for diagnosing lumbar disc deformity as the cause of low back pain compared with spinal column palpation?" Once the question is phrased, the most recent, relevant, internally valid, randomized clinical trials are sought. Fortunately, this literature is available in electronic databases and often in full text online from local medical libraries or the National Library of Medicine (NLM). By clicking on the Clinical Queries section of the NLM site (http://www.ncbi.nlm.nih.gov/entrez), it is possible to search for and retrieve only randomized trials on a diagnostic or treatment issue, thereby minimizing the time spent examining non-randomized trials. Most major medical school libraries now provide online access to the Cochrane Collaboration database, which reflects best evidence summaries of the clinical science literature on specific diagnostic and treatment topics. Additional search tools and databases summarizing the clinical literature can be accessed by clicking on the Search icon at http://www.shef.ac.uk/~scharr/ir/netting.

Once appropriate articles are identified, each must be evaluated using the internal validity concepts presented in this chapter. A good clinician should balance skepticism of reported results with respect for the strengths of a well-conducted study. In addition to assessing a study's credibility, questions of its applicability to a specific patient must be addressed. It is helpful to consider the following questions: 1) Who was studied and are they similar to my patients (age groups, sex, ethnic/racial groups, patient groups)? 2) Are this study's findings clinically relevant to my patient(s)? 3) Could I replicate these findings in my patients under similar circumstances? 4) Do the findings conflict with my clinical experience? 5) Were the subjects representative of patients who would actually use the treatment? 6) Was the comparison group clinically meaningful? 7) Were the findings strong enough to have clinical relevance (the effect size issue)? 8) Were the effects and side effects reliably measured?

Answering these questions fully and completely requires knowledge and skills beyond the scope of this chapter. However, there are resources that can guide clinicians' efforts to determine the value of a study. In addition to the Sackett et al (1) resource that helps clinicians develop the tools needed to answer these questions, clinicians can also access the *Journal of the American Medical Association*'s online Users Guide to the Medical Literature series that addresses most of these questions (http://www.cche.net/principles/content_all.asp).

REFERENCES

1. Sackett DL, Straus S, Richardson S, Rosenberg W, Haynes RB. Evidence-based medicine. How to practice and teach EBM. 2nd ed. Philadelphia: Churchill Livingstone; 2000.
2. Sackett DL, Haynes RB, Guyatt GH, Tugwell P. Clinical epidemiology. A basic science for clinical medicine. 2nd ed. Philadelphia: Lippincott, Williams & Wilkins; 1991.
3. Friedman L, Demets D. Fundamentals of clinial trials. St Louis: Mosby; 1996.
4. Robertson VJ. A quantitative analysis of research in physical therapy. Phys Ther 1995;75:313–22.
5. Liang MH, Andersson G, Bombardier C, Cherkin DC, Deyo RA, Keller RB, et al. Strategies for outcome research in spinal disorders. An introduction. Spine 1994;19(18Suppl):2037S–40S.
6. Gall E, Gibofsky A. Rheumatoid arthritis: clinical tools for outcome assessment. Atlanta: Arthritis Foundation; 1994.
7. DePoy E, Gitlin LN. Introduction to research. Understanding and applying multiple strategies. 2nd ed. St. Louis: Mosby; 1998.
8. Freundlich B, Leventhal L. The fibromyalgia syndrome. In: Schumacher HR, Klippel JH, Koopman WM, editors. Primer on the rheumatic diseases. 10th ed. Atlanta: Arthritis Foundation; 1997, pp. 247.

9. Spilker B. Guide to clinical trials. New York: Raven Press; 1991.

10. Guyatt GH, Sackett DL, Cook DJ. Users' guide to the medical literature. II. How to use an article about therapy or prevention. A. Are the results of the study valid? Evidence-Based Medicine Working Group. JAMA 1993; 270:2598–601.

11. Shekelle PG, Andersson G, Bombardier C, Cherkin D, Deyo R, Keller R, et al. A brief introduction to the critical reading of the clinical literature. Spine 1994;19(18 Suppl):2028S–31S.

12. Barr JT. Critical literature review: clinical effectiveness in allied health practices. Rockville, Md. Agency for Health Care Policy and Research, Pub #-940029; 1995.

13. Cohen J. Statistical power analysis for the behavioral sciences. 2nd edition. New York: Academic Press; 1988.

14. Cook D, Mulrow CD, Haynes RB. Systematic reviews: synthesis of best evidence for clinical decisions. Ann Intern Med 1997;126:376–80.

15. Lau J, Ioannidis JP, Schmid CH. Quantitative synthesis in systematic reviews. Ann Intern Med 1997;127:820–6.

16. Hunt DL, McKibbon KA. Locating and appraising systematic reviews. Ann Intern Med 1997;126:532–8.

17. Mulrow C, Cook D. Systematic reviews. Synthesis of best evidence for health care decisions. Philadelphia: American College of Physcians; 1998.

18. Mullen PD, Laville EA, Biddle AK, Lorig K. Efficacy of psychoeducational interventions on pain, depression, and disability in people with arthritis: a meta-analysis. J Rheumatol 1987;14(15 Suppl):33–9.

19. Flor H, Fydrich T, Turk DC. Efficacy of multidisciplinary pain treatment centers: a meta-analytic review. Pain 1992;49:221–30.

20. Crews DJ, Landers DM. A meta-analytic review of aerobic fitness and reactivity to psychosocial stressors. Med Sci Sports Exerc 1987;19(5 Suppl):S114–20.

21. Heater BS, Becker AM, Olson RK. Nursing interventions and patient outcomes: a meta-analysis of studies. Nurs Res 1988;37:303–7.

22. Scogin F, McElreath L. Efficacy of psychosocial treatments for geriatric depression: a quantitative review. J Consult Clin Psychol 1994;62:69–74.

23. Sackett DL, Rosenberg WM, Gray JA, Haynes RB, Richardson WS. Evidence based medicine: what it is and what it isn't. BMJ 1996;312: 71–2.

Additional Recommended Reading

Reading the Literature. Links to two readable series of articles for practitioners: *How to Read a Paper* (British Medical Journal) and Basic Statistics for Clinicians (Canadian Medical Association Journal) are available online at http://www.shef.ac.uk/~scharr/ir/netting. Click on Library icon to find the articles. Accessed 06/25/01.

Systematic Reviews and Journals. Links to two series of articles on systematic reviews are available online. The Annals of Internal Medicine series on systematic reviews and the British Medical Journal articles on meta-analysis are available at http://www.shef.ac.uk/~scharr/ir/netting. Click on the Library icon to find the articles. Accessed 06/25/01.

Implementing Evidence-Based Medicine. Links to a variety of online resources devoted to informing clinicians on how to use evidence-based medicine in practice are available at http://www.shef.ac.uk/~scharr/ir/netting. Click on the Implementing icon to find the resources. Accessed 06/25/01.

Psychological Assessment

JERRY C. PARKER, PhD; GAIL E. WRIGHT, PhD; and KAREN L. SMARR, MA

Characterizing the psychological aspects of the rheumatic diseases is difficult due to the diversity of diagnostic categories. Arthritis almost always results in pain and restricted movement, but some acute conditions, such as gout and septic arthritis, respond quickly to treatment and have minimal long-term psychological impact. However, in chronic conditions such rheumatoid arthritis (RA) and systemic lupus erythematosus (SLE), years of pain, functional losses, and deteriorated health are major challenges to the coping process. Many persons with chronic, debilitating arthritis manage to cope successfully. In some cases, however, either the disease-related stressors are too severe or the environmental resources are not sufficient to sustain a successful coping effort. Consequently, some persons with arthritis display psychological symptoms secondary to disease. In other cases, persons with arthritis present with pre-existing psychological problems.

The prevalence of psychological distress is difficult to estimate across a diversity of arthritic conditions and socioeconomic settings. Useful data, though, can be obtained from the primary care literature, where the prevalence of psychological problems has been shown to be relatively high. One study found that 26% of patients met criteria for a psychiatric disorder using the Diagnostic and Statistical Manual of Mental Disorders, 3rd Edition, Revised (DSM-III-R) (1,2). A survey of urban, low-income patients found that 18.9% screened positive for depression (3). Another study found that 15–40% of primary care patients met the criteria for a diagnosable mental disorder (4). There is little doubt that primary care settings are confronted with a high prevalence of mental, emotional, and behavioral problems.

In most rheumatology settings, psychological problems appear to be similarly prevalent. Estimates suggest that approximately 20% of persons with RA present with major depression (5). In a study of persons with SLE, 20.5% were found to have a concomitant psychiatric disorder (6). Approximately one-half of persons with either RA or osteoarthritis (OA) may experience loss in social relationships (7), which is a risk factor for depression. Several risk factors for depression have been identified in people with RA; these include high stress levels, low confidence in coping abilities, and high levels of physical disability (8). Although such psychological problems are far from universal, the literature convincingly shows that a substantial number of people with arthritis encounter psychological distress at some point in their lives. Those providing care to arthritis patients should be both vigilant regarding psychological problems and familiar with the process of psychological assessment.

IMPORTANCE OF PSYCHOLOGICAL PERSPECTIVE

Beyond recognizing the relatively high prevalence of psychological problems in medical settings, arthritis health profes-

sionals also need a keen appreciation of psychological concepts to provide optimal care for patients. Three broad psychological perspectives are important in the management of rheumatic disease: 1) the biopsychosocial model of illness; 2) the Institute of Medicine enablement model of disability; and 3) the empirical foundations for psychological interventions.

Biopsychosocial Model

For the past 400 years, the conceptualization of physical illness has been dominated by a biomedical framework. Illness has been viewed as a physiochemical abnormality requiring biologic management. The biomedical model is highly valid under many circumstances, and it has led to impressive therapeutic breakthroughs in such acute illnesses as infectious disease. Increasingly, though, the inadequacy of the biomedical model has been recognized, especially in chronic diseases such as arthritis. In these conditions, there is an intermingling of biologic, psychological, and sociologic determinants with regard to the onset, course, and outcomes of illness. Engel (9) coined the term, biopsychosocial model, to convey the multiple determinants of physical illness. For optimal health care, the psychological and social aspects of rheumatic disease must be thoroughly assessed and treated.

Institute of Medicine Enablement Model of Disability

Another psychological concept derives from the Institute of Medicine "enabling–disabling process" model of disability (10). Traditionally, tissue abnormalities and/or physiologic imbalances have been viewed as the primary determinants of disability. However, many persons with abnormalities at the cellular level never develop a failure of an entire organ system. Even persons who experience organ system failure do not necessarily develop functional disability. The enablement model views the individual's environment as either enabling or disabling. Enabling factors such as personal resilience (e.g., effective coping), access to appropriate care, and/or assistive devices allow for independence and enhanced functioning. Disability can occur when barriers exist and these factors are lacking. Therefore, disability is not a purely biologic phenomenon, but is also determined to a great extent by behavioral factors and the psychological processes of coping and adaptation. Consequently, from the disability perspective, the psychological symptomatology of persons with arthritis should be carefully assessed.

Psychological Interventions

The effectiveness of psychological interventions should also be considered by health care professionals. In general, psychological treatments work reasonably well. A meta-analysis of the effectiveness of cognitive therapy for depression found that the average therapy patient did better than 98% of the control subjects (overall effect size = 0.99) (11,12). These data, along with some additional studies, were reanalyzed with similar conclusions (13). Another study supported those results and indicated that cognitive therapy was superior to pharmacological treatment to prevent relapse in depression (14). In comparison, the average effect size for drug treatment in arthritis ranges from only 0.45 to 0.77 (15). Even in severe psychiatric disorders such as major depression, behavioral treatments are effective in approximately 55% of cases (16).

Regarding arthritis, a literature review on cognitive–behavioral or self-management interventions for RA or OA found reported benefits in pain, depressive symptoms, coping abilities, self-efficacy, and self-management behaviors (17). In addition, a stress management program for persons with RA has been shown to decrease helplessness, improve confidence in coping ability, and reduce pain, with benefits lasting up to 15 months (18). Evidence for the effectiveness of psychological interventions for persons with arthritis is impressive. Thus, psychological assessment can be viewed as an important prelude to beneficial psychological treatments.

APPROACHES TO PSYCHOLOGICAL ASSESSMENT

Psychological assessment is not a uniform procedure; it is a variety of approaches to the characterization of psychological/behavioral processes. There are 3 general approaches to psychological assessment: 1) diagnostic criteria; 2) unstructured clinical interviews; and 3) psychometric assessment. These approaches are not mutually exclusive. In fact, they often can be used in combination.

Diagnostic Criteria

A common approach to the assessment of psychological/psychiatric difficulties is the use of specific diagnostic criteria. In this approach, the symptoms characteristic of a given syndrome are systematically elaborated. The most common example is the Diagnostic and Statistical Manual-IV of the American Psychiatric Association (19), in which a classification of psychological/psychiatric states has been developed. The person conducting an assessment can search for the constellation of symptoms that characterize a particular diagnosis.

Diagnostic criteria have several advantages. The assessment process takes place in the context of a broad diagnostic classification system. Structured interviews guide the data-gathering process and minimize errors of omission. Also, when a psychological/psychiatric diagnosis is formulated, the associated clinical characteristics of the syndrome, such as natural history and prognosis, can usually be inferred. However, there are disadvantages to this approach. Many psychological manifestations do not conveniently fit into a structured diagnostic framework. Especially in the case of subclinical conditions, standard diagnostic frameworks simply may not apply. Diagnostic criteria are most useful in cases of moderate to severe conditions.

Clinical Interviews

Psychological assessment also can be approached through the use of unstructured clinical interviews. The examiner seeks to create a comfortable environment in which the examinee will feel free to discuss any psychological problems. The client-centered concepts of Raskin and Rogers provide the theoretical foundation for this approach (20). The interviewer asks open-ended questions and then listens in an accepting, nonjudgmental way. Subsequently, most examinees will articulate their individual, psychological concerns. The interviewer is thus able to gain an in-depth understanding of the patient's unique circumstances.

The unstructured interview provides an opportunity to access highly personal information that might otherwise be overlooked in a structured search for signs and symptoms. Another advantage is the rapport-building that usually occurs during a client-centered assessment; an excellent foundation may be established for future provider-patient interactions. The primary disadvantage of the client-centered approach is the lack of standardization of the data-gathering process. Determining the severity of a patient's psychological problems in comparison to other people may be difficult. Additionally, some patients are unable to articulate their personal problems, because they do not fully recognize and/or understand them. Therefore, unstructured clinical interviews are most valuable when augmented by other structured approaches.

Psychometric Assessment

Psychometric assessment refers to the examination of psychological characteristics and/or related behaviors through the use of psychological tests. A psychological test is defined as an "objective and standardized measure of a sample of behavior" (21). The behavioral characteristic to be examined must be objective and must be observable by others. Collection of test data must be standardized so that the stimuli and demands of the test can be reproduced. A psychological test is typically restricted to a sample of behavior, because the full range of an examinee's responses is not accessible. In short, psychological testing is simply a rigorous way of observing behavior.

There are several advantages to this approach. The quantification inherent in psychological testing permits an assessment of how much of a specific psychological or behavioral characteristic exists. Thus, the establishment of norm groups is possible. A second advantage is that the error inherent in psychological tests can be estimated, which permits a confidence interval to be established for a test score. Third, the psychometric approach is rigorous in terms of statistical and quantitative methodology; however, only a narrow range of behaviors is sampled. Thus, a psychological test may not adequately focus on a person's primary psychological concerns. The effectiveness of psychological tests may vary across populations due to ceiling or floor effects (i.e., scores primarily at the top or bottom of the scale). In general, such tests are most useful when complemented by other types of clinical data.

PREREQUISITES FOR PSYCHOMETRIC ASSESSMENT

In general, diagnostic criteria and clinical interviews can be used by anyone who learns the specific procedures. Psychometric assessment, however, requires more specialized training and is usually performed by psychologists or others with knowledge of psychometric theory. There are several prerequisites for accurate psychological assessment. First, there is the issue of *reliability*, or the assurance that a test yields similar results on successive administrations. Second, psychological tests must be *valid* in the sense of measuring what they purport to measure. Third, psychological tests should have a *small standard error*. Multiple administrations of the test should cluster tightly around the "true" score. Next, psychological tests must be interpreted in the context of *appropriate norm groups*. Fifth, psychological tests must be *standardized*, with procedures, stimuli, and task demands that are consistently reproducible. Finally, psychological tests must be used ethically with careful attention to confidentiality and rights to privacy. When these prerequisites are met, examiners skilled in psychometric theory can obtain valuable clinical data.

Types of Psychometric Assessment

There are literally hundreds of well-validated psychological tests that could be used in a rheumatology setting. However, the psychological domains most applicable for persons with arthritis include helplessness, depression, self-efficacy, coping/adaptation, social support, marital/family functioning, life stress, vocational preference, personality, and cognitive functioning. Each of these assessment domains warrants brief discussion. Some of the specific tests are referenced in more detail in Parker and Wright (22).

Helplessness. The concept of helplessness is particularly relevant to the care of persons with arthritis and is related to health outcomes (23). For many forms of arthritis, symptoms wax and wane; flares are generally unpredictable. Similarly, treatments for many forms of arthritis are only palliative. Therefore, persons with arthritis may perceive themselves as helpless and as having minimal control over their disease. Helplessness can be measured with the Arthritis Helplessness Index and the Rheumatology Attitudes Index (24).

Depression. Although not universal, depression is a significant clinical problem for some persons with arthritis. Persons with chronic diseases have a higher probability of developing depression than do persons who are healthy (25). Social isolation and economic distress have been identified as factors that can contribute to depression (26). Several measures have been developed to assess depression. Some, such as the Center for Epidemiological Studies-Depression Scale (27) and the Beck Depression Inventory (28), assess depressive symptoms using self-report instruments; others, such as the Hamilton Rating Scale for Depression (29), use a structured clinical interview format. Diagnostic tools that assess depression include the Primary Care Evaluation of Mental Disorders (PRIME-MD) (2).

Self-efficacy. Self-efficacy refers to a person's belief in his or her ability to accomplish a task or cope with a stressor (30). Self-efficacy for function, for pain, and for other symptoms have all been found to be related to important clinical outcomes, such as functional capacity and health status. In addition, it is an important factor in the success of patient education interventions (31). Self-efficacy can be measured with the Arthritis Self-Efficacy Scale.

Life Stress. *Stress* is a common but potentially confusing term. Sometimes it can refer to environmental stimuli that are judged to be taxing by the individual. At other times, stress may refer to a person's biologic response to taxing stimuli. It can also refer to an interaction between a person and environment that is dependent on the person's perception of his or her situation, rather than on the situation itself. Despite this diversity of definitions, stress is a common problem for many persons with arthritis. Disease-related problems such as chronic pain, functional losses, employment difficulties, and economic worries contribute to life stress. Paper-and-pencil measures of stress include the Social Readjustment Rating Scale, the Life Experiences Survey, the Hassles Scale, the Daily Stress Inventory, the Daily Life Experience Checklist (32), and the Perceived Stress Scale (33).

Coping and Adaptation. In the face of numerous stressors, persons with arthritis must adapt to rapidly changing circumstances. The coping process usually involves a primary appraisal or judgment as to whether a stressor poses a risk of threat or harm. If a threat or harm is perceived, a secondary appraisal typically occurs, including a judgment as to whether sufficient resources exist to cope with the stressor. If persons perceive that they do not possess sufficient coping resources, then the stressfulness of the situation dramatically intensifies. Thus, assessment of the coping/adaptation process is important in the care of persons with arthritis. Measures of the coping process that use questionnaire and interview formats include the Ways of Coping Scale, the Coping Strategies Questionnaire, and the Vanderbilt Multidimensional Pain Coping Inventory. Coping assessments that utilize daily diary methods include the Daily Coping Inventory (34), which has been adapted for chronic pain coping; daily spiritual and religious coping can be assessed using the Brief Multidimensional Measure of Religiousness/Spirituality (35).

Social Support. Social support refers to interpersonal relationships that are beneficial to a person's well-being. At best, social relationships offer support and understanding. At worst, they may offer criticism and blame. High levels of social support are generally associated with better adherence to medical regimens and more effective coping (36), although such findings are not universal (37). Social support can be measured with the Social Support Questionnaire, the Social Relationship Questionnaire, the Interview Schedule for Social Interaction (38), and the Interpersonal Support Evaluation List (39).

Marital and Family Functioning. In chronic illness, marital and family functioning is often severely challenged. When health status changes for one family member, other family members are required to adapt as well. In arthritis, changes in work capacity or the ability to perform social roles can contribute to marital/family distress. Therefore, assessment of marriage and family functioning is important and can be accomplished with measures such as the Locke–Wallace Marital Adjustment Test and the Spanier Dyadic Adjustment Scale.

Vocational Assessments. One of the greatest challenges in the care of persons with arthritis is maintaining gainful employment. Work-related difficulties and economic losses are common occurrences in the context of such rheumatic diseases as RA (40). Vocational rehabilitation can lead to dramatically improved quality of life. Vocational measures, such as the

Strong–Campbell Interest Inventory and the Holland Self-Directed Search, can be useful. In addition, vocational assessments can elucidate aptitudes and functional work capacities.

Personality Testing. Personality testing refers to the examination of enduring psychological or behavioral traits of an individual. In rheumatology settings, personality testing is typically reserved for situations in which serious psychological problems appear to be developing or when mental health difficulties precede rheumatic disease. The most common measure of personality is the Minnesota Multiphasic Personality Inventory II (MMPI-II). This lengthy questionnaire yields 10 clinical scales and 3 validity scales used to assess overall psychological status. For persons with arthritis, the MMPI-II has distinct disadvantages, because some items overlap with the signs and symptoms of rheumatic disease (41). For example, symptoms such as "tiring easily" or "having aches and pains" are associated with rheumatic disease, so they do not necessarily reflect mental health problems. Alternative measures of global psychological functioning include the Symptom Checklist-90-Revised, the Brief Symptom Inventory (42,43), and the Millon Clinical Multiaxial Inventory-II.

Cognitive Functioning. Rheumatic diseases do not typically involve cognitive dysfunction. The most notable exception is SLE, in which cognitive functioning and psychiatric symptoms may become prominent. Cognitive dysfunction also may occur in patients taking high-dose corticosteroids or certain other medications. In addition, arthritis patients may present with comorbidities that affect cognitive status, such as strokes, head injuries, or dementias. In these situations, neuropsychological testing can be helpful. Global intellectual functioning can be assessed with the Wechsler Adult Intelligence Scale-Third Edition (44) and the Kaufman Adult Intelligence Test-Revised. Memory can be assessed with the Wechsler Memory Scale-Revised and the Rey Auditory Memory Scale. Comprehensive neuropsychological examination can be accomplished with the Halstead-Reitan Neuropsychological Test Battery, which samples a wide range of cognitive, motor, and sensory capacities.

INDICATIONS FOR CONSULTATION

Beyond an awareness of specific psychological tests, health care providers also need to know when and how to request psychological/mental health consultations. An initial step in the process is to carefully explain to the patient the rationale for psychological referral. Understandably, persons with arthritis view their health-related problems as primarily medical, so a psychological referral may seem dissonant if not carefully explained. Conversely, a majority of persons with arthritis recognize that their chronic disease constitutes a major challenge to their coping capacities. When psychological referral is presented as being secondary to their arthritis, most patients easily accept, or even welcome, the opportunity to receive help. There are 5 key situations for which psychological/mental health consultation may be helpful: 1) psychiatric diagnosis; 2) psychotropic medications; 3) chronic psychological distress; 4) acute adjustment reactions; and 5) psychoeducational treatments.

Psychiatric Diagnosis. In the management of rheumatic disease, a well-formulated psychiatric diagnosis is sometimes critical. For example, treatments for depression vary widely depending on the specific diagnosis. For major depression, pharmacologic treatment is usually indicated. Conversely, for adjustment reaction with depressed mood, supportive counseling is typically the treatment of choice. Cognitive dysfunction may be secondary to such diverse etiologies as adverse effects of medication, major depression, or dementia; treatment varies depending on the specific etiology. Therefore, psychological assessment should be obtained in situations where psychological/psychiatric diagnoses may affect treatment strategies.

Psychotropic Medications. A related situation in which mental health assessment/consultation is indicated involves psychotropic medication. Many rheumatology health professionals do not possess extensive familiarity with either mental illness or psychotropic medications. A referral for psychological assessment or mental health consultation can result in more effective psychopharmacologic intervention for arthritis patients with concomitant psychiatric problems.

Chronic Psychological Distress. Persons with arthritis can present with an extensive history of psychological distress, even though they do not show evidence of full-blown psychiatric disturbance. For some patients, the burden of living with a chronic disease eventually overpowers their coping capacities. Patients who show signs of chronic psychological distress should not be overlooked; referral for psychological assessment and subsequent intervention can lead to improved quality of life.

Acute Adjustment Reactions. Acute adjustment reactions sometimes occur in persons with rheumatic disease, just as they do in the physically healthy population. Acute marital conflicts or family disturbances may develop. Concerns regarding employment, finances, or social circumstances may arise. Although acute life stressors are unavoidable, they are often particularly severe in the context of a chronic disease. Careful psychological assessment can lead to effective interventions.

Psychoeducational Treatments. There are numerous reports regarding the effectiveness of psychoeducational interventions. For example, the Arthritis Self-Management Program has been shown to be beneficial for persons with arthritis (45), and rheumatology teams are increasingly using the services of psychologists, counselors, and educators. Psychological assessment can be helpful prior to implementing a psychoeducational intervention. For some arthritis patients, group treatments that enhance opportunities for socialization are indicated. For others, an individual treatment approach may be more viable. When there is uncertainty about the best psychoeducational strategy, psychological assessment should be considered.

COLLABORATIVE CARE

There are 2 ways in which rheumatologists and mental health professionals can work together. First, psychologists and other mental health professionals can be treated as consultants; arthritis patients with concomitant psychological problems can simply be referred to mental health professionals working outside the arthritis team. The consultant model is easy to establish, but the mental health consultants may have little understanding of the unique needs of arthritis patients. In addition, some arthritis patients may not be comfortable receiving care in a mental health environment.

The second strategy for collaboration involves the direct participation of mental health professionals as members of the arthritis rehabilitation team. In this model, mental health professionals gain the opportunity to develop a deeper understanding of the needs of arthritis patients, and they can deliver their interventions within the overall context of the rheumatology setting.

REFERENCES

1. American Psychiatric Association. Diagnostic and statistical manual of mental disorders, 3rd edition. Washington, DC: American Psychiatric Association; 1987.
2. Spitzer RL, Williams JBW, Kroenke K, Linzer M, deGruy FV, Hahn SR, et al. Utility of a new procedure for diagnosing mental disorders in primary care: The PRIME-MD 1000 study. JAMA 1994;272:1749–56.
3. Olfson M, Shea S, Feder A, Fuentes M, Nomura Y, Gameroff M, et al. Prevalence of anxiety, depression, and substance use disorders in an urban general medicine practice. Arch Fam Med 2000;9:876–83.
4. Jencks SF. Recognition of mental distress and diagnosis of mental disorders in primary care. JAMA 1985;253:1903–7.
5. Creed F, Ash G. Depression in rheumatoid arthritis: aetiology and treatment. International Review of Psychiatry 1992;4:23–34.
6. Hay EM, Black D, Huddy A, Creed F, Tomenson B, Bernstein RM, et al. Psychiatric disorder and cognitive impairment in systemic lupus erythematosus. Arthritis Rheum 1992;35:411–6.
7. Wright GE, Parker JC, Smarr KL, Schoenfeld-Smith K, Slaughter JR, Buckelew SP, et al. Risk factors for depression in rheumatoid arthritis. Arthritis Care Res 1996;9:264–72.
8. Wright GE, Parker JC, Schoenfeld-Smith K, Smarr KL, Buckelew SP, Slaughter JR, et al. Risk factors for depression in rheumatoid arthritis. Arthritis Care Res 1996;9:264–72.
9. Engel GL. The need for a new medical model: a challenge for biomedicine. Science 1977;196:129–36.
10. Brandt EN Jr, Pope AM. Enabling America: assessing the role of rehabilitation science and engineering. Washington, DC: National Academy Press; 1997.
11. Dobson KS. A meta-analysis of the efficacy of cognitive therapy for depression. J Consult Clin Psychol 1989;57:414–9.
12. Gloaguen V, Cottraux J, Cucherat M, Blackburn IM. A meta-analysis of the effects of cognitive therapy in depressed patients. J Affective Disord 1998;49:59–72.
13. Gaffan EA, Tsaousis I, Kemp-Wheeler SM. Researcher allegiance and meta-analysis: the case of cognitive therapy for depression. J Consult Clin Psychol 1995;63:966–80.
14. Gloaguen V, Cottraux J, Cucherat M, Blackburn IM. A meta-analysis of the effects of cognitive therapy in depressed patients. J Affective Disord 1998;49:59–72.
15. Felson DT, Anderson JJ, Meenan RF. The comparative efficacy and toxicity of second line drugs in rheumatoid arthritis. Arthritis Rheum 1990;33:1449–61.
16. Depression Guideline Panel. Depression in primary care: volume 2. Treatment of major depression. Clinical practice guideline, number 5. Rockville, MD: U.S. Department of Health and Human Services, Public Health Service: 1993.
17. Hawley DJ. Psycho-educational interventions in the treatment of arthritis. Baillière's Clin Rheumatol 1995;9:803–23.
18. Parker JC, Smarr KL, Buckelew SP, Stucky-Ropp RC, Hewett JE, Johnson JC, et al. Effects of stress-management on clinical outcomes in rheumatoid arthritis. Arthritis Rheum 1995;38:1807–18.
19. American Psychiatric Association. Diagnostic and statistical manual of mental disorders, 4th edition. Washington, DC: American Psychiatric Association; 1994.
20. Raskin NJ, Rogers CR. Person-centered therapy. In: Corsini RJ, Wedding DFE. Current Psychotherapies. Itasca, IL: Peacock Publishers, Inc; 1989.
21. Anastasi A. Psychological testing. New York: Macmillan Publishing Company; 1988.
22. Parker JC, Wright G. Psychologic assessment in rheumatology. Rheum Dis Clin North Am 1995;21:465–80.
23. Callahan LF, Brooks RH, Pincus T. Further analysis of learned helplessness in rheumatoid arthritis using a "Rheumatology Attitudes Index". J Rheumatol 1988;15:418–26.
24. Nicassio PM, Wallston KA, Callahan LF, Herbert M, Pincus T. The measurement of helplessness in rheumatoid arthritis: the development of the Arthritis Helplessness Index. J Rheumatol 1985;12:462–7.
25. Rodin G, Craven J, and Littlefield C. Depression in the medically ill: an integrated approach. New York: Brunner/Mazel; 1991.
26. Hamilton M. Development of a rating scale for primary depressive illness. Br J Soc Clin Psychol 1967;6:278–96.
27. Radloff LS. The CES-D scale: a self-report depression scale for research in the general population. Applied Psychological Measurement 1977;1: 385–401.
28. Beck AT, Steer RA, Garbin MG. Psychometric properties of the Beck Depression Inventory: twenty-five years of evaluation. Clin Psychol Rev 1988;8:77–100.
29. Hamilton M. Development of a rating scale for primary depressive illness. Br J Soc Clin Psychol 1967;6:278–96.
30. Bandura A. Self-efficacy: toward a unifying theory of behavioral change. Psychol Rev 1977;84:191–215.
31. Fetzer Institute. Multidimensional measurement of religiousness/spirituality for use in health research: a report of the Fetzer Institute/National Institute on Aging Working Group. Kalamazoo, MI: John E. Fetzer Institute; 1999.
32. Stone AA, Neale JM. Development of a methodology for assessing daily experiences. In: Baum A, Singer J, eds. Advances in environmental psychology, environment, and health. Vol. IV. New York: J. Erlbaum; 1982.
33. Cohen S, Kamarck T, Mermelstein R. A global measure of perceived stress. J Health Soc Behav 1983;24:385–96.
34. Stone AA, Neale JM. Effects of severe daily events on mood. J Pers Soc Psychol 1984;46:137–44.
35. Fetzer Institute. Multidimensional Measurement of Religiousness/Spirituality for Use in Health Research: a Report of the Fetzer Institute/National Institute on Aging Working Group. John E. Fetzer Institute; 1999.
36. Wallston BS, Alagna SW, DeVellis BM, DeVellis RF. Social support and physical health. Health Psychol 1983;2:367–91.
37. Spanier GB. Measuring dyadic adjustment: new scales for assessing the quality of marriage and similar dyads. J Marriage Family 1976;1:15–28.
38. Fitzpatrick R, Newman S, Archer R, Shipley M. Social support, disability and depression: a longitudinal study of rheumatoid arthritis. Soc Sci Med 1991;33:605–11.
39. Cohen S, Mermelstein R, Kamarck T, Hoberman HM. Measuring the functional components of social support. In: Sarason IG, Sarason BR, eds. Social support: theory, research and applications. Dordrecht, Netherlands: Martinus Nijhoff Publishers; 1985.
40. Holland JL. Making vocational choices a theory of careers. New Jersey: Prentice-Hall; 1973.
41. Russell EW, Neuringer C, and Goldstein G. Assessment of brain damage: a neuropsychological key approach. New York: Wiley-Interscience; 1970.
42. Derogatis LR. Brief symptom inventory. Minneapolis: National Computer Systems; 1993.
43. Derogatis LR, Melisaratos N. The brief symptom inventory: an introductory report. Psychol Med 1983;13:595–605.
44. Wechsler D. Wechsler Adult Intelligence Scale-third edition: administration and scoring manual. San Antonio: The Psychological Corporation, Harcourt Brace & Company; 1997.
45. Lorig K, Lubeck D, Kraines RG, Seleznick M, Holman HR. Outcomes of self-help education for patients with arthritis. Arthritis Rheum 1985;28: 680–5.

Additional Recommended Reading

Blalock SJ, DeVellis RF, Brown GK, Wallston KA. Validity of the Center for Epidemiological Studies Depression Scale in arthritis populations. Arthritis Rheum 1989;32:991–7.

Parker JC, Bradley LA, DeVellis RM, Gerber LH, Holman HR, Keefe FJ, et al. Biopsychosocial contributions to the management of arthritis disability. Blueprints from an NIDRR-sponsored conference. Arthritis Rheum 1993; 36:885–9.

Pincus T, Callahan LF. Depression scales in rheumatoid arthritis: Criterion contamination in interpretation of patient responses. Patient Education and Counseling 1993;20:133–43.

Pincus T, Callahan LF, Bradley LA, Vaughn WK, Wolfe F. Elevated MMPI scores for hypochondriasis, depression, and hysteria in patients with rheumatoid arthritis reflect disease rather than psychological status. Arthritis Rheum 1986;29:1456–66.

Social and Cultural Assessment

LAURA ROBBINS, DSW, MSW

The field of rheumatology is changing rapidly due to the introduction of new diagnostic and pharmacologic agents; however, the cultural and ethnic composition of the patient population is changing as well. Clinicians today are challenged by the increasing number of patients from many cultures who speak different languages, who have varying levels of acculturation, and who come from varied socioeconomic backgrounds. These patients have unique ways of understanding illness and health, and they develop health care behaviors based on these beliefs. There has been a tendency to view patients of diverse cultures through the identification of specific, unifying characteristics that generalize cultural traits within groups (1). This unacceptable approach tends to stereotype patients. Instead, a systems approach that assesses culture as one aspect of the patient's experience is becoming more widely accepted (2–4). The patient-centered biopsychosocial model is the basis for this approach.

For any person living with a chronic illness, there are many emotional and physical challenges to everyday life activities and interpersonal relationships. These changes require a re-evaluation of goals and long-term commitments. Moreover, chronic diseases like rheumatoid arthritis (RA) and systemic lupus erythematosus (SLE) are often unpredictable, resulting in the need for emotional and social support from family members, friends, and ultimately the health care team. While social workers are trained to assess a patient's social and cultural background, it is not unusual for other health professionals to conduct similar assessments. The professional should possess the basic knowledge, skills, and training to evaluate a patient's coping patterns and level of social adjustment, as well as how that patient's culture determines medical understanding of the disease and its etiology. Clinicians should also have the tools to assess how patients may decide to take action to address their disease.

This chapter addresses the components of a comprehensive social and cultural assessment. Understanding the patient in the appropriate social and cultural context can enable you to make referrals to appropriate education and support programs that have been demonstrated to influence health outcomes (5).

THE ASSESSMENT METHOD

A comprehensive social and cultural assessment begins with evaluation of the patient's physical status, emotional state, and support system. This approach, grounded in the social work concept of "the person in the situation," focuses on the person, the situation, and the interaction between them (6). In the health care setting, the person is the patient, the situation may be medical crisis, and the interaction can be considered to be the process that evolves between the patient and his or her support system when attempting to cope with the medical condition. In chronic illness, the emphasis is on the *process* by which people learn to cope or function within their social network. The method also emphasizes communication skills and the patient's ability to articulate emotional, social, and physical needs to other people within their environment (7). The patient becomes an integral member of the medical team throughout the duration of the chronic illness.

The patient brings a unique history and understanding of the disease and contributes to the treatment process. Optimal health outcomes, particularly effective emotional and social functioning, are more likely to occur because the patient becomes a part of the evaluation and influences the treatment plan. The goal for the health care worker is to gain an understanding of the patient's emotional, social, and physical reaction to the medical situation in order to provide appropriate care. Through patient information and participation, the health professional and the patient should work together to assess the impact of the disease over the course of the illness.

The first step in this process is a complete social and cultural assessment. Depending on the individual's experiences, social supports, and level of physical activity, an assessment may take from one to several sessions. A written evaluation, completed at the end of the assessment, then becomes a part of the patient's medical record. Just as medications and treatments are reevaluated and adjusted periodically, the assessment should be reviewed and updated to reflect the ongoing disease. This continual review is particularly pertinent for patients with rheumatic diseases, because there may be episodes of increased disease activity. An assessment should be done during each hospitalization and updated during routine office visits.

THE SOCIAL ASSESSMENT

The Patient as Person

A social assessment begins with the person diagnosed with the rheumatic disease. The goal is to evaluate the person's life history and the impact of the diagnosis on the individual's current functioning. Unless fully unable to communicate, the patient is the best source of information about the impact of the illness. Scheduling the assessment interview with the patient alone is optimal. If this is not possible, asking family members for privacy is appropriate. It is not unusual, however, for an older person to have family members present during the assessment who will answer questions addressed to the patient. When this occurs, patients must be encouraged to answer the questions themselves in order to obtain pertinent information. Since disease is a family issue in some culturally diverse populations, it may be appropriate for the family to be present during the assessment. Assuring family members that their input is important can be useful and demonstrates that the family is vital to the patient as he or she learns to cope and adjust to the medical situation. It also allows the health care

Table 1. Social assessment sample questions.

Social impact questions
  Do you live close to the medical center?
  Who lives in your household with you?
  How do you get to and from the medical center?
  Are you presently working?
  What has changed about your current work schedule?
  Do you go to school?
  Who in your family is responsible for the cooking, shopping, child rearing, or the well-being of aging parents?
Emotional impact questions
  How has the relationship with your children changed since you learned that you have arthritis?
  How has your family reacted to the fact that you can no longer contribute to the household responsibilities?
  How do your friends react to you since you told them about your arthritis?
Interpersonal impact questions
  What did you and your partner enjoy that you can't enjoy now due to your arthritis?
  What do you discuss with your spouse about your arthritis?
  What are the kind of things that you and your spouse routinely discuss?
  How does your spouse feel about the changes in your relationship since you developed arthritis?
  Have your sexual relationships changed since being diagnosed?
Nonverbal assessment questions
  Does the patient ask questions during the interview?
  Does the patient indicate that he or she is listening by a head nod as I am talking?
  Does the patient appear distressed and perhaps too emotional to respond to questions?

professional to assess the family's adjustment to the changing physical and emotional situations caused by a chronic illness.

Most assessments begin with demographic details and information, including definitive or concrete questions related to age, marital status, parental status, level of education, sexual identity, work history, medical insurance, and religious affiliation. The assessment should also explore prior and current alcohol and drug use. Additional areas should address patient concerns related to housing arrangements, geographic location and proximity to health care services, and modes of transportation. As illustrated in Table 1, these questions should be phrased to elicit concrete responses. As questions begin to produce information, the responses are then used to evaluate the family constellation, support systems, belief systems, and the impact of arthritis on the patient's life.

Perhaps the most difficult part of evaluation involves assessing the significance of physical and emotional changes for the patient during interactions with people in their environment. Rapid, unplanned episodes of disease such as flares, increased pain, or medication side effects present unique challenges. To capture this process, it is helpful to begin by asking simple, direct questions aimed at evaluating changes that have occurred since the onset of the diagnosis. These change questions (Table 1), when directed to the patient, also address the person's interpersonal relationships with the significant people in the immediate social network. Similar questions should be asked about other relationships in the patient's extended environment and may include casual relationships with work colleagues, school peers, religious congregations, and recreational contacts. Generally, these questions begin with *"What is different about . . ."* or *"How has your life changed since. . . ."* Alterations in daily routines due to physical limitations can also shift social relationships and result in emotional distress. For example, the patient who has had to stop working due to

RA may lose not only contact with colleagues but also the supportive listening of available friends. Questions targeted towards change in the patient's life will provide information with which to assess disease impact.

Comparable questions about the nature of intimate personal relationships and recent changes since adjusting to a chronic illness also need to be explored. Questions about role shifts in family responsibilities between spouses and children are essential and should focus on the major daily responsibilities for the patient within the family system. Personal relationships and questions about sexual relationships must also be explored, although the clinician must be aware that not all cultures perceive sexual activity as something to be discussed outside the marital or adult relationship. A direct approach to questions is most effective, particularly when the information required is personal and private. With some culturally diverse populations, the clinician may need to first develop trust before asking personal questions. Knowledge about changes in sexual functioning as part of the assessment will assist in appropriate referral and in the treatment process.

Effective Communication

Good communication skills are fundamental in the patient and health professional relationship. Learning how to enhance discussions and increase the exchange of information will facilitate the ability to ask questions that are personal and confidential. This includes not only spoken verbal language but nonverbal interactions as well.

To enhance the patient–physician relationship, health professionals need specific tools for better communication. These include role modeling through demonstration of the following: the ability to ask for help, knowing how to verbalize questions and concerns, listening, and having the confidence to ask for clarification and additional information. Questions that begin with "how," "what," and "why" are effective because they tend to elicit answers that require explanations. Questions that lead to "yes" and "no" answers tend to hinder a free exchange of information. Direct questions might include *What do you discuss with your husband about your osteoarthritis?"* or *"How does your spouse feel about the changes in your relationship since you developed arthritis?"* Questions like these assess what has changed not only for the patient but for the family members as well.

Communication skills can be evaluated through observation as well as direct questions. You can observe whether someone is listening by asking yourself a series of questions (see Table 1). Awareness of how you, as the health professional, ask questions can greatly enhance the outcome of the assessment. Encourage patients to fully express their concerns about their medical situation. Urge them to ask all their questions regardless of how relevant they seem. Good communication allows a meaningful exchange of information during the assessment interviews.

The Social Environment

For people living with chronic illness, personal relationships are further broadened to include doctors, nurses, hospital personnel, and health insurance companies. In some cultural groups, this can include whole communities. Through this expanding social network, the patient is confronted with many new and unique situations that can be perceived as opportunities as well as obstacles. The way in which people cope with chronic illness depends largely on their experience with previous threats to their lives and lifestyles. Availability of food, shelter, transportation, medical care, employment, education, and recreational activities are examples of some resources necessary for basic survival.

However, patients also have psychosocial realities that are challenged when dealing with crisis (8). These realities are more obscure and include concepts such as role identity, self esteem, and perceived self worth. These qualities are expressed through interpersonal relationships. When chronic illness mandates changes in roles from full-time career woman, wife, and mother to full-time patient and part-time wife and mother, the patient's role status changes. This challenges the individual's identity and perceived self worth. Family structure and family members' perceptions of the patient's roles also change. Psychosocial challenges, although intangible, are as important as the concrete realities of food and shelter and can dramatically alter the former coping mechanisms of the person transformed to patient. While the individual exercises some control by choosing friends for social support, most social relationships with parents, siblings, and extended family members are inherited. The quality of these relationships can have a potent effect and create pressures over which the individual has no control (9). With chronic illness, there is an increased need for intermittent dependency, which can make a patient feel out of control and cause increased stress and anxiety. These feelings interfere with communication and normal interpersonal relationships.

Patients with rheumatic diseases often experience changes in physical mobility, financial status, role function, and emotional health. The goal of social assessment is to evaluate the extent to which changes have occurred in relationships between the patient and the social factors that make up his or her social environment. These factors are inextricably linked to culture and affect the patient's self worth and self esteem (10).

THE CULTURAL ASSESSMENT

Health Beliefs and Behaviors

A patient has certain beliefs, concerns, and perceptions about the medical diagnosis as well as the encounter with the health professional (11). These beliefs are determined by many factors including cultural influence. It would be artificial to separate the social experience from the cultural one, because a person's cultural group is made up of the family and social support network. Culture has a significant impact on the outcomes of treatment and health management. People acquire their own perceptions and beliefs about the origin of diseases and treatments that are sanctioned by their cultural group, learned in childhood, and expressed through behaviors. Through these shared cultural beliefs we come to value what is worthwhile, desirable, and important for our physical and emotional well-being. However, our cultural identity may differ from those of people we encounter in our daily contacts. Health professionals, for example, may not be of the same cultural background and often have a tendency to view their own cultural orientation as the standard against which other

Table 2. Cultural assessment sample questions.

Health professional self-assessment
What is my cultural heritage?
What was the culture of my parents and my grandparents?
With what cultural group do I identify?
What values, beliefs, opinions, and attitudes do I hold that are consistent with the dominant culture? Which are inconsistent? How did I learn these?
What unique abilities, aspirations, expectations, and limitations do I have that might influence my relations with culturally diverse individuals?
How do I communicate with my patients?
Do I change my communication styles to enhance discussion with my patients who come from different cultures than I do?

cultures are judged (12). Therefore, assessment of the person diagnosed with a chronic disease requires a culturally enlightened and culturally sensitive approach.

Culture is a filter through which we interpret experiences. Health beliefs, attitudes, and behaviors are defined within the cultural experience. In modern Western societies, explanations for illness are typically rooted in natural phenomena, such as infection with microorganisms or mechanical dysfunction. More recently stress has been identified as an explanation for illness. However, there are whole groups of people who attribute disease and illness to very different causes (13). How a person defines and copes with chronic disease and the health care experience can greatly modify the treatment plan and delivery of services.

There is no consensus on whether society should support cultural adaptation, cultural diversity, or a multicultural society, especially since the melting pot theory no longer shapes our society (14). Most health professionals do not have training in cultural diversity. Cultural sensitivity training exists, but often it is not required in academic programs. Although professionals may strive to be open-minded about different cultural groups, even the most well-intentioned professionals bring ethnocentric biases to the assessment of a person with different cultural attitudes and beliefs. Moreover, individuals who are not personally prejudiced or discriminatory may still distance culturally different groups if they avoid communication or fail to recognize how others interpret their behavior (15). There is a need for clinicians to recognize that their health beliefs and practices differ from those of other populations. In the Anglo-American culture, values of mastery over nature, individualism, competition, and directness vary significantly from values of harmony with nature, group welfare, cooperation, and indirectness characteristic of some ethnocultural groups (16). Recognizing and understanding the differences in these values will lead to understanding of culture-specific behaviors that influence health behaviors. Thus, the goal of the cultural assessment is to provide sensitive and effective health care to patients from differing cultures.

A cultural assessment should begin by self-assessment on the part of the health professional to evaluate his or her own cultural values and beliefs. This step is essential in order to assess personal biases. Recognizing one's own cultural identity and how it influences personal values, beliefs, and behaviors is a precursor to understanding and being able to assess a patient's cultural orientation. The self-assessment of cultural awareness is based on the premise that awareness of self is the first step to understanding others (17). As illustrated in Table 2, basic questions for self-assessment are designed to help health professionals recognize their own cultural identity through key

Table 3. Patient assessment.

Cultural identity
    To what ethnic group do you belong?
    What language do you speak most often with your family? With your friends?
    What religious group do you belong to? Do you attend services regularly? In what ways do you practice your religion?
Health beliefs
    How would you describe your arthritis symptoms?
    What does having arthritis mean to you?
    How do you believe that your arthritis can be treated?
    What do you believe caused your arthritis?
Health behaviors
    Who in the family makes the major decisions?
    Who do you go to in your community for advice about medical problems or treatment?
    When do you go for advice or treatment?
    Do you go to a healer or any other person for advice about your health (Chinese herbalist, spiritualist, minister)? What advice do you follow?
    What foods do you eat that you believe makes your arthritis better?
    What foods do you eat that you believe makes your arthritis worse?
    What other things do you do to deal with your arthritis?

questions focusing on one's own cultural orientation. In addition to creating self-awareness, such questions also assist the health professional in a general understanding of the influence of culture-specific beliefs and attitudes on health behaviors.

The cultural assessment must emphasize the patient's global beliefs, practices, and behaviors as well as health-specific ones. However, the goal is not only to understand beliefs, attitudes, and subsequent behaviors but to identify how they are important to the development of the individual's concept of self, the core for emotional and social functioning. Self-concept develops through socialization within the family unit, social networks, and community groups. Individuals develop a perception of self through interactions that are sanctioned and defined within their cultural group. Self-concept is formed by several factors including language, gender identity, and behaviors. Questions focused on the patient's attitudes and beliefs about health care reveal information about health behaviors practiced by the patient. Table 3 lists sample questions for obtaining cultural information about the patient that can be utilized in developing a treatment plan. These questions also help the health professional understand the way in which a person within a cultural group defines and treats diseases as well as the patient's perception of how they cope and function.

For example, in doing an assessment of a Latina woman newly diagnosed with RA, it would not be unusual for the patient to consult with family members about what and how much to discuss with the physician. Latino people frequently consult with other family members before following recommended medical treatment (18). When working with Latinos in the health care setting, culturally determined practices have to be recognized and respected in order to develop a patient–physician trust that can lead to positive health outcomes. As further illustration of the importance of culture, it is common for patients of some Asian cultures to be guarded about sharing emotional stress, and it is an uncommon health behavior to seek out mental health clinicians for assistance. However, in fact, little is known about the nature and distribution of mental disorders among Asian populations (19).

In the example of the Latina patient, it is probable that she may not follow the prescribed treatment plan if her husband or family was not consulted first. Although she has her own concept of self-identity, it is determined in relationship to

family roles. In general, there are many cultures in which it is expected that the husband, or dominant male figure, be consulted about important decisions, particularly if decisions will affect the family unit (20). Therefore, it is important to assess behaviors that are defined in relationship to other key family members or that may not overtly represent the patient's emotional state.

The Importance of Language

Language is another primary element that must be considered in any cultural assessment. While culture provides a sense of belonging and identification to a group of people and ascribes meaning and utilization to behaviors, it also provides meaning and function to language. Language shapes our world, defines our roles within society, and is the way in which we express our self-concept and identity (21,22). There can be severe handicaps to understanding the impact of chronic illness when language differences hinder communication.

Language complicates optimal health outcomes because it serves a vital role in social and survival functions. When doing cultural assessments, ask the patients what language they primarily speak, read, write, and think in when at home or with friends and family. Response to this question usually indicates which language the patient uses most often in familiar social situations. In the health care setting, patients who speak different languages often attempt to understand physician questions due to cultural values of respect for authority figures. Their marginal understanding of English can be conveyed by a nod of the head or by "yes" or "no" responses to questions. However, the patient usually does not fully understand the question or the instructions. When asking questions of someone who speaks English marginally, refrain from using questions that result in yes/no answers, and always ask the patient to repeat the information as an indicator of comprehension.

Whenever there is any indication that the patient does not comprehend your assessment questions, you should use an interpreter. There are concerns about the use of third-party information gathering, however. First, it is inappropriate to use family members to translate during an assessment. Due to time constraints in hospital and office settings, family members—particularly young children—and close friends are used for communication during interviews. This method of translation results in a breach of patient confidentiality, leads to inaccurate translation of questions and responses, and causes emotional distress for family members who themselves are coping with the patient's medical condition (23). When family members are not present, hospital and office staff may be asked to translate if they speak the same language. This practice is also inappropriate, because staff who have knowledge of the patient's condition will often paraphrase the questions asked during the assessment. Additionally, they will provide their own interpretation of the patient's medical situation in an earnest attempt to assist the patient. Important information can be misinterpreted and stripped of its significance, contributing to poor treatment outcomes.

However, translators can be effective if utilized appropriately. Models for the use of translators that include bilingual, bicultural people have been the most effective (18). Community-based agencies can provide professionally trained translators, and a growing number of agencies train translators to be available via phone to assist in the communication process.

Another effective model is the use of bilingual, bicultural patient advocates who are trained as translators for other patients from the same cultural group. While this model may appear to be labor intensive, the training and supervision of a cadre of patients is worth the initial investment to ensure the well-being of new patients. This model also allows for assessment of the patient's level of language and communication skills, as well as a determination of cultural health beliefs and practices.

In addition to language differences, specific cultures have clearly defined health beliefs and practices that differ from those of Western medicine. It would be unrealistic to expect that health professionals be knowledgeable about the plethora of cultures they may encounter. Cultural sensitivity is a place to start. To ensure ongoing cultural understanding, it may be necessary to engage a community leader as a key informant about the patient's culture to assist you in obtaining information (24). Community leaders often are identified within cultural groups as the informant for group-specific norms, beliefs, and attitudes. They also sanction culturally determined behaviors. There are large community health agencies serving Asian, Latino, African American, and Native American groups that specifically train their constituents to serve cultural groups in a variety of roles. Enlisting a cultural informant to assist in a social and cultural assessment greatly enhances the communication process between health provider and patient. Moreover, it ameliorates the mistrust, fear, and intimidation that some cultural groups feel towards Anglo-American institutions (25). A cultural informant does not replace the patient; rather, the informant collaboratively serves as a verbal translator and advocate for the patient. The patient's consent and permission should always be obtained prior to engaging a third party in the assessment process.

Acculturation

Culturally determined health beliefs and practices may vary within cultural groups due to the length of time the patient has lived in the United States. Socialization in the patient's native homeland or within a different culture also affects the health beliefs and practices of patients. Therefore, acculturation becomes a factor in doing an assessment, because people learn new behaviors when they are exposed to new cultures. If a patient from Russia has lived in the US for 15 years, the patient is probably more familiar with Anglo-American health beliefs and behaviors. It should be standard practice during an assessment to ask a brief question that addresses level of acculturation. A simple question, *"How long have you lived in . . . ,"* will provide a response that clarifies the patient's exposure to different cultural groups. The response to this question should then guide you when conducting the full cultural assessment.

THERAPEUTIC INTERVENTIONS

Once a social and cultural assessment is completed, it may be necessary to refer the patient for psychosocial treatment. Many therapeutic interventions are available; however, the type of referral depends upon the assessment. Casework is one of the most common treatments, which focuses on helping patients cope with their medical situation. In this model, the social worker uses counseling to assist the patient in making emo-

tional adjustments to chronic illness. Social workers can help the patient with concrete needs, such as financial evaluations and referrals for assistance. They also assist with problems relating to housing, medical insurance, disability, and transportation. Additionally, if it is determined that the patient is clinically depressed or has an existing personality disorder, a social worker can refer to a psychiatrist or psychologist as appropriate.

When the patient and family members assessment indicates interpersonal difficulties, family therapy may be needed. Referrals should be made to family social workers who can provide counseling and emotional support to the entire family. If more dysfunctional family problems are apparent, a family therapist with a psychology background is required. Consulting with a key informant, such as a clergy member, can be beneficial with some cultural groups in order to determine an appropriate referral.

For patients who are experiencing the normal adjustment in coping, such as mild depression, anger, or sadness due to the common adjustments of living with a chronic illness, a referral to a self-management or support group can be extremely beneficial. The Arthritis Foundation (www.arthritis.org) provides a list of such programs offered through its local chapters. Over time, participants in self-management programs report a decrease in depression, an increase in self-confidence, and an increase in self-management skills (26). Programs like these are excellent vehicles for empowering patients by providing educational information and social support.

Finally, traditional therapeutic interventions may not be relevant to some cultural groups. For many people, support and empathy originate from systems within the cultural group. For African Americans, religious affiliations often provide spiritual support and are a source of comfort during medical crises. In some Latino cultures, herbs and botanicals are obtained from within the community and are used to take control of the medical illness. And, in some Asian cultures, patients in emotional distress will keep their concerns within the family rather than seek outside assistance. When working with culturally diverse patients, the goal is to understand the client's emotional and social supports.

Utilizing a social and cultural assessment as a key component of evaluating the patient with rheumatic disease is a comprehensive model that ultimately enhances the treatment plan. This assessment is an important piece to the overall medical diagnosis, management, and treatment of the person who is challenged by a chronic disease.

REFERENCES

1. Carrillo JE, Green A, Betancourt J. Cross-cultural primary care: a patient-based approach. Ann Intern Med 1999;130:829–34.
2. Berlin EA, Fowkes WC Jr. A teaching framework for cross-cultural healthcare: application in family practice. West J Med 1983;139:934–8.
3. Scott CJ. Enhancing patient outcomes through an understanding of intercultural medicine: guidelines for the practitioner. Md Med J 1997;46:175–80.
4. Goldstein E, Bobo L, Womeodu R, Kaufman L, Nathan M, Palmer D, et al. Intercultural medicine. In: Jensen NM, van Kirk JA, editors. A curriculum for internal medicine residency: the University of Wisconsin program. Philadelphia: American College of Physicians; 1996.
5. Robbins L. Patient education and self-management. In: Klippel J, editor. Primer on the rheumatic diseases, 12th ed. Atlanta: Arthritis Foundation. In press.
6. Hollis F. Casework: a psychosocial therapy. 2nd ed. New York: Random House; 1972.

7. Turner F, editor. Social work treatment: interlocking theoretical approaches. New York: Free Press; 1979.
8. Perlman H. Social casework: a problem solving process. Chicago: University of Chicago Press; 1957.
9. Billingsley A. Black families in white America. Englewood Cliffs (NJ): Prentice-Hall; 1968.
10. Helman CG. Culture, health and illness: an introduction for health professionals. 3rd ed. Boston: Butterworth-Heinemann, 1994.
11. Eisenberg L. Disease and illness: distinctions between professional and popular ideas of sickness. Cult Med Psychiatry 1977;1:9–23.
12. Locke D. Increasing multicultural understanding: a comprehensive model. Newbury Park (CA): Sage; 1992.
13. Airhihenbuwa C. Health and culture: beyond the Western paradigm. Thousand Oaks (CA): Sage; 1995.
14. Marin G, Marin B. Research with Hispanic populations. Newbury Park (CA): Sage; 1991.
15. Kavanagh K, Kennedy P. Promoting cultural diversity: strategies for health care professionals. Thousand Oaks (CA): Sage; 1992.
16. Sigelman L, Welch S. Black Americans' views of racial inequity: the dream deferred. New York: Cambridge University Press; 1991.
17. Lum CK, Koreman SG. Cultural-sensitivity training in U. S. medical schools. Acad Med 1994;69:239–41.
18. A primer for cultural proficiency: towards quality health services for Hispanics. Washington (DC): The National Alliance for Hispanic Health, Estrella Press; 2001.
19. Sue S. Mental health. In: Zane N, Takeuchi D, Young K, editors. Confronting critical health issues of Asian and Pacific Islander Americans. Newbury Park (CA): Sage; 1994. p. 266–88.
20. Locke DC. Cross-cultural counseling issues. In: Pakmo AJ, Weikel WJ, editors. Foundations of mental health counseling. Springfield (IL): Charles C Thomas; 1986.
21. Sotomayor, M. Language, culture and ethnicity in developing self-concept. Soc Casework 1977;41:195–203.
22. Quillte J. Barriers to effective communication. In: Lipkin M Jr, Putnam SM, Lazare A, editors. The medical interview: clinical care, education and research. New York: Springer-Verlag; 1995. p. 110–21.
23. Putsch RW. Cross-cultural communication: the special case of interpreters in health care. JAMA 1985;254:3344–8.
24. Breckon D, Harvey J, Lancaster R. Community health education: settings, roles, and skills for the 21st century. Gaithersburg (MD): Aspen; 1994.
25. Robbins L, Allegrante JP, Paget S. Adapting the Systemic Lupus Erythematosus Self-Help (SLESH) course for Latino SLE patients. Arthritis Care Res 1993;6:97–103.
26. National Arthritis Foundation, 1314 Spring Street NW, Atlanta, Georgia, 30309.

Additional Recommended Reading

Braithwaite R, Taylor S, editors. Health issues in the black community. San Francisco: Jossey-Bass; 1992.
Journal of Multicultural Social Work. New York: The Haworth Press.
Carlson V. Social work and general systems theory. Berkeley: University of California, School of Social Welfare; 1957.
Molina C, Molina-Aguirre, M, editors. Latino health in the US: a growing challenge. Washington (DC): American Public Health Association; 1994.
National Alliance for Hispanic Health. A primer for cultural proficiency: towards quality health services for Hispanics. Washington (DC): Estrella Press; 2001.
Ponterotto J, Casas J, Suzuki L, Alexander C, editors. Handbook of multicultural counseling. Thousand Oaks (CA): Sage; 1995.
Rogler L. Implementing cultural sensitivity in mental health research: convergence and new directions. 3-part series in Psychline Inter-Transdisciplinary Journal of Mental Health 1999; Vol. 3, Nos. 1,2,3.

SECTION C: COMMON RHEUMATIC DISEASES

<table>
<tr><td>CHAPTER
13</td><td></td></tr>
</table>

CHAPTER
13

Pediatric Rheumatic Diseases

JANALEE TAYLOR, RN, MSN; and DIANE M. ERLANDSON, RN, MS, MPH

The rheumatic diseases of childhood comprise a wide variety of acute, but mostly chronic, illnesses occurring before the age of 16 and affecting connective tissues. They range from single organ to multisystem diseases. Although some are short-term or self-limiting, the majority are chronic and can result in lifelong functional limitations. The rheumatic diseases of childhood are classified into categories based on the nature of the disease or systems involved (1) (Table 1). These categories include inflammatory rheumatic diseases of childhood, noninflammatory disorders, skeletal dysplasias, heritable disorders of connective tissue, storage diseases, metabolic disorders, systemic diseases with musculoskeletal manifestations, and hyperostosis. This chapter will focus on select inflammatory diseases, juvenile rheumatoid arthritis (JRA), and the spondylarthropathies.

Most of the epidemiologic data on childhood rheumatic diseases have been generated from clinic-based populations, leading to wide variation in estimates of prevalence. The National Health Interview Survey (NHIS), a population-based cross-sectional study, estimates the prevalence of childhood rheumatic diseases to be 160,000–290,000 U.S. children (2). In 2000, the Maternal and Child Health Bureau and the National Center for Health Statistics initiated the first nationwide population-based study to determine the prevalence of children with special health care needs. This 3-year study will provide national- and state-based prevalence estimates of childhood chronic diseases, including rheumatic diseases.

The age of onset is disease specific. In general, rheumatic diseases of childhood are more common among girls, with the exceptions of systemic onset JRA, the seronegative spondylarthropathies, some of the vasculitides, and septic arthritis (3).

JUVENILE RHEUMATOID ARTHRITIS

Etiology and Classification

Although the etiology of JRA, a chronic inflammatory disease, is unknown, most theories take into account a genetic predisposition and environmental triggers. Research over the past decade has provided significant information on human leukocyte antigen (HLA) types and predisposition to JRA and other childhood rheumatic diseases. Evidence-based research on the HLA indicates a genetic underpinning to some of the childhood rheumatic diseases, especially JRA (4). Specific HLA genotypes have been associated with the type and course of JRA

(5). Laboratory research has also made strides in attempting to determine the pathogenesis of JRA. The interaction of T cells and cytokines, including tumor necrosis factor (6), on the synovium has led to the development of new treatments for JRA.

Criteria for classification and general nomenclature for JRA vary across continents. In the U.S. and Canada, physicians have adopted the American College of Rheumatology criteria for JRA (7), which describe 3 disease subtypes: pauciarticular, polyarticular, and systemic. This classification represents disease at onset, but may not accurately address the course and progression of disease. Other guidelines share similarities with the ACR criteria for JRA, but refer to the disease as juvenile chronic arthritis (European) and juvenile idiopathic arthritis (International League Against Rheumatism). In this chapter, the ACR criteria are used to describe JRA.

Diagnosis

Juvenile rheumatoid arthritis is a heterogeneous group of chronic arthritides characterized by exacerbations and remissions. The onset of arthritis must occur before 16 years of age and be present for at least 6 consecutive weeks to confirm the diagnosis. Exacerbations are an expression of the natural course of the disease, but frequently occur in response to trauma, infection, or treatment withdrawal. Similarly, remissions occur as part of the natural course of the disease or may be treatment-induced.

The diagnosis of JRA requires a thorough history and physical examination. The initial presentation of signs and symptoms depends on the type of JRA. In addition to arthritis, children may exhibit some or all of the following symptoms: fever, rash, fatigue, anemia, loss of appetite, stiffness, irritability, altered mobility, and change in or difficulty with activities of daily living, including play. Special attention should be given to joint signs and symptoms, pattern of arthritis and rash (if present), duration of signs and symptoms, extraarticular manifestations, antecedent illnesses or trauma, and response to treatment.

No single diagnostic laboratory or radiographic test will confirm the diagnosis of JRA. Instead, tests are used to support physical findings, identify risk factors, monitor therapy and response to treatment, and exclude other disease possibilities. Evaluation may include the following laboratory measures: complete blood count, liver and renal function tests, immuno-

Table 1. Classification of rheumatic diseases in childhood (RDC).*

Inflammatory RDC
  Chronic Arthropathies
    Juvenile rheumatoid arthritis
      Pauciarticular onset
      Polyarticular onset
      Systemic onset
    Spondylarthropathies
      Juvenile-onset ankylosing spondylitis
      Juvenile-onset psoriatic arthritides
      Arthritides with inflammatory bowel disease
      Reiter's syndrome
    Arthritis associated with infectious agents
      Infectious arthritis
        Bacterial
        Spirochetal (Lyme disease)
        Viral
        Other
      Reactive arthritis
        Acute rheumatic fever
        Post-enteric infection
        Post-genitourinary infection
        Other
  Connective Tissue Disorders
    Systemic lupus erythematosus
    Juvenile dermatomyositis
    The sclerodermas
      Systemic sclerosis
      Localized sclerodermas
      Mixed connective tissue disease
      Eosinophilic fasciitis
      Other
    Vasculitis
      Polyarteritis
        Polyarteritis nodosa
        Kawasaki disease
        Microscopic polyarteritis nodosa
        Other
      Leukocytoclastic vasculitis
        Henoch-Schönlein purpura
        Hypersensitivity vasculitis
        Other
      Granulomatous vasculitis
        Allergic granulomatosis
        Wegener's granulomatosis
        Other
      Giant cell arteritis
        Takayasu's arteritis
        Temporal arteritis
      Other
  Arthritis and Connective Tissue Diseases Associated with Immunodeficiencies
    Complement component deficiences
    Antibody deficiency syndromes
    Cell-mediated deficiencies

Noninflammatory Disorders
  Benign hypermobility syndromes
    Generalized
    Localized
  Pain amplification syndromes and related disorders
    Growing pains
    Primary fibromyalgia syndrome
    Reflex sympathetic dystropy
    Acute transient osteoporosis
    Erythromelalgia
  Overuse syndromes
    Chondromalacia patellae
    Plica syndromes
    Stress fractures
    Skin splints
    Tennis elbow, Little Leaguer's elbow, tenosynovitis

  Trama
    Osteochondritis dissecans
    Traumatic arthritis, noaccidental trauma
    Congenital indifference to pain
    Frostbite arthropathy
  Pain syndromes affecting back, chest, or neck
    Spondylolysis and spondylolisthesis
    Intervertebral disc herniation
    Slipping rib
    Costochondritis
    Torticollis
    Aneuralgic amyotrophy

Skeletal Dysplasias
  Osteochondrodysplasias
    Generalized
      Achondroplasia
      Diastrophic dwarfism
      Metatrophic dwarfism
    Epiphyseal dysplasias
      Spondyloepiphyseal dysplasias
      Multiple epiphyseal dysplasias
    Osteochondroses
      Legg-Calvé-Perthes disease
      Osgood-Schlatter disease
      Thiemann's disease, Köhler's disease
      Scheurmann's disease
      Freiberg's infraction

Heritable Disorders of Connective Tissue
  Osteogenesis imperfecta
  Ehler's Danlos syndromes
  Cutis laxa
  Pseudoxanthoma elasticum
  Marfan's syndrome

Storage Diseases
  Mucopolysaccharidoses
  Mucolipidoses
  Sphingolipidoses

Metabolic Disorders
  Osteoporosis
  Amyloidosis
  Rickets
  Scurvy
  Hypervitaminosis A
  Gout
  Ochronosis
  Kashin-Beck disease
  Mseleni disease
  Fluorosis

Systemic Diseases with Musculoskeletal Manifestations
  Hemoglobinopathies
  Hemophilia
  Diabetes mellitus
  Hyperlipoproteinemias
  Pseudohyperparathyroidism
  Secondary hypertropic osteoarthropathy
  Sarcoidosis

Hyperostosis
  Infantile cortical hyperostosis (Caffey's disease)
  Other

* Reprinted from reference 1, with permission of W.B. Saunders.

globulins, antinuclear antibody, and rheumatoid factor. The erythrocyte sedimentation rate is almost always elevated with systemic JRA and may be a helpful marker for monitoring disease. Active synovitis will yield an inflammatory synovial fluid; however, arthrocentesis is usually avoided in children because of its trauma. In early disease, radiographs may be of little diagnostic value, but should be considered to establish a baseline. Magnetic resonance imaging (MRI) plays a valuable role in determining early joint and tissue changes, as well as joint effusion, synovial hypertrophy, epiphyseal overgrowth, and the thinning or absence of articular cartilage even before joint space narrowing is visible on plain radiographs (8).

Types of JRA

The 3 subtypes of JRA are based on the presentation at onset and during the first 6 months of disease: pauciarticular (40–50%), polyarticular (~30%), and systemic onset (~20%). The prognostic indicators for JRA are subtype, rheumatoid factor (RF) status, the course of disease, and the response to and side effects of treatments.

Pauciarticular JRA. This subtype is characterized by synovitis in 4 or fewer joints. Arthritis is typically asymmetric with almost no systemic features. Rheumatoid factor is always negative, but ANA is positive in 60% of patients. Joints most commonly affected include the knee, ankle, and elbow.

An early onset subtype of pauciarticular JRA is most commonly seen in girls before the age of 5. Children with this subtype and a positive antinuclear antibody test are at high risk for developing uveitis, which is usually asymptomatic and detected only by a slit lamp examination performed by an ophthalmologist. If left untreated, the uveitis or its complications can result in visual impairment, including complete blindness.

Late onset pauciarticular JRA (age 10–12) is more common among boys and is often associated with the HLA-B27 class I gene. Weight-bearing large joints and entheses are commonly affected. Acute iritis may occur. These patients may later develop a spondylarthropathy. Children with pauciarticular JRA are frequently stiff but may not always complain of pain. However, the level of discomfort is usually manifested by other findings such as irritability or keeping the involved joint(s) in flexion or extension.

Polyarticular JRA. This subtype occurs more commonly in girls and is characterized by synovitis in 5 or more joints, occasional systemic features, and in some circumstances, positive rheumatoid factor test. The affected joints are usually symmetric and may include the small joints of the hands or feet, wrists, elbows, shoulders, cervical spine, temporomandibular joints, hips, knees, and ankles. Because the bursae and tendons are also lined with synovial tissue, bursitis and tendinitis are not uncommon.

Systemic features may include low grade fever, anemia, leukocytosis, mild hepatosplenomegaly, and lymphadenopathy. Pericarditis and uveitis are rare (9). Cervical spine disease, which can progress to fusion or subluxation, is common among children with polyarticular disease. When rheumatoid factor is positive (5–10%), subcutaneous nodules are often present, and aggressive joint disease often leads to more severe deformities. Total joint arthroplasty and other surgical interventions may be necessary during young adulthood.

Polyarticular JRA also affects normal growth and development. Fatigue, pain, stiffness, and depression all play a role in

limiting self-care, socialization, recreation, and participation in school and sports.

Systemic Onset JRA. This subtype occurs at any age with equal frequency in boys and girls. It is characterized by daily or twice-daily high spiking fevers, synovitis in one or more joints, and a classic rash (salmon pink, 2–5 mm in diameter, macular, erythematous perimeter) (9). The rash most often occurs with the fever and appears on the trunk and proximal extremities. Fevers typically occur in the afternoon or evening, rise to 39° C or higher, and return to baseline or below. Because fever can precede all other symptoms by months, these children are often initially evaluated for fever of unknown origin. Other commonly observed signs and symptoms of systemic onset JRA include malaise, irritability, severe anemia, leukocytosis, thrombocytosis, lymphadenopathy, hepatomegaly, splenomegaly, and serositis, including pericarditis, and/or pleuritis.

Systemic features of the disease, such as fever and fatigue, frequently impair function simply because the child feels too ill to do anything. Participation in recreational or school activities may depend on the timing of the fever spike. Other functional limitations relate to the degree of joint and organ involvement. Systemic features may resolve over the course of the disease. Growth retardation (<5th percentile) is common in systemic JRA. Almost half of the children with systemic onset JRA eventually develop a chronic polyarthritis that is usually erosive, especially in the hips. These children are more likely to develop long-term disabilities.

Impact of Disease

Physical Impact. Both localized and systemic growth disturbances can manifest themselves in JRA. Generalized growth disturbance is related to activity of disease, side effects of medications, and poor nutritional status. Growth retardation can worsen with prolonged disease activity and use of daily corticosteroids. The use of corticosteroids affects stature secondary to slow bone growth and vertebral compression fractures.

Locally, hyperemia surrounding the joint provides excess nourishment to the bones, leading to overgrowth. When this overgrowth occurs in an extremity or a phalange, a discrepancy in length and size becomes apparent. If the hyperemia subsides in a short period of time, the rate of growth normalizes and the "catch up growth phenomenon" allows the unaffected side to reduce or eliminate the discrepancy.

Localized growth disturbance in JRA can lead to significant or noticeable deformities. For example, retarded mandibular growth results in micrognathia, causing a recessed jaw, which becomes more apparent with accelerated skeletal growth, as well as such associated dental problems as crowding of teeth, abnormal bite, and abnormal location of tooth eruption (10). Cosmetically, this can be a devastating problem for a child or teen. Routine assessment of the temporomandibular joints allows early identification and treatment of problems. Referrals to experienced dentists or maxillofacial teams may be necessary for orthodontic and surgical management.

Other physical changes include joint abnormalities such as loss of motion, contractures, subluxation, and instability (11,12). Abnormalities usually occur when disease progression cannot be slowed or halted, or when physical or occupational therapy modalities fail. Ongoing synovitis can destroy not only the joint but the surrounding tendons and ligaments as well.

Sexual maturation also seems to be affected by JRA. Compared to their siblings, adolescent females with JRA (especially the polyarticular subtype) had menarche delayed by about 8 months (mean, 13.2 years) (13).

Protein calorie malnutrition and vitamin and mineral deficiencies have been linked to JRA in the last decade (14). Bone mineral density has also been reduced in about 30% of mild to moderately ill, prepubertal children with JRA. This poor mineralization is associated with more active and severe disease, as well as limitation in physical function (15).

The posture and gait of the child with JRA are altered because of insults to the lower extremities and spine. Pain, stiffness, fatigue, active synovitis, joint abnormalities, spinal aberrations, foot callosities, discrepancies in length of the long bones, muscle weakness, and atrophy all contribute to an abnormal gait. Whatever the reasons for the aberrations in posture or gait, they should be evaluated and corrected as soon as possible to avoid or minimize long-term repercussions.

Psychosocial Impact. The psychosocial impact of JRA is individual and requires initial and ongoing assessment by skilled professionals. Research often documents psychological difficulties in children with JRA (16); however, a recent study reported minimal social, emotional, and behavioral problems (17). Children with JRA were remarkably similar to case-control children on measures of social functioning, emotional well-being, and behavior.

The families of children with JRA often experience grief, not only at the time of diagnosis but also when exacerbations occur or when developmental milestones are delayed. The sense of loss of their "normal child" is overwhelming and recurrent. Not all family members go through the grieving cycle at the same time.

The child's or teen's perception of what is happening to his or her body, why it is happening, whether it will improve, and whether the disease will ever go away are all based on stage of cognitive development. This is best demonstrated at the age of 13 or 14, when a child is cognitively able to understand the concept of conservation. Only then can a child understand the concept of "chronic."

The ability to cope with the stress of a chronic disease is influenced by personal skills, strengths, experience with coping, presence of concurrent stresses, availability and access to support systems, and response to treatment (18). Problems that warrant further assessment and intervention include unexplained school absences, withdrawal from family and friends, depression, interpersonal and family discord, inappropriate (for age) dependency on parents, anxiety, and substance abuse. Additional psychological support should always be recommended to families as a part of their care plan. Children and families are usually much more receptive to psychological support if they are made to feel that referrals for such services are routine.

Function in the Developing Child

Because children are continuously growing and developing, assessing function should be age- and development-specific. Function in the home, at play, during recreation, at school, and out of doors should be assessed subjectively and, when possible, objectively. Pain, immobility, stiffness, weakness, and

malaise associated with JRA can impair the achievement of developmental tasks or cause a regression in development. Parents can also impede a child's progress when they start to do things for the child because he or she takes too much time or elicits sympathy. Competency at each stage of development provides the foundation for positive self-esteem, confidence in independent function, and an affirmation of identity.

Health care providers should not only perform a functional assessment, but provide the treatments and teaching needed to assure competency building. Parents should be actively involved in providing the necessary guidance, encouragement, and reinforcement. Because school provides a forum for learning new skills, school personnel should be involved in the process, when possible, to provide continuity.

Reliable measures of function in children with JRA include the Childhood Health Assessment Questionnaire, Juvenile Arthritis Functional Assessment Report, Juvenile Arthritis Functional Assessment Survey, Juvenile Arthritis Self-report Index, Juvenile Arthritis Quality of Life Questionnaire, Childhood Arthritis Health Profile, and the Child Behavior Checklist (19). Long-term outcomes are often determined in adulthood by measuring joint status, health status, function, quality of life, psychosocial status, educational level, and work capacity (see also Chapter 9, Functional Ability, Health Status, and Quality of Life).

Active disease has been reported in 31–55% of patients with JRA after 10 years of followup (20). Joint space narrowing and erosions are significantly correlated with poor functional outcome. In patients with polyarticular and systemic disease, radiographic changes occurred within 2.2–2.5 years after disease onset. Pauciarticular patients developed changes within 5.3 years (20). Prahalad and Passo (21) provide a review on outcomes in JRA.

In general, the long-term psychosocial outcome is favorable in most patients, but some differences may exist between subsets. Patients who have good social support systems appear to do best.

Treatment

The treatment program for a child with JRA is multifaceted and should involve more than just medication. All children with joint involvement should receive a physical and/or occupational therapy program and ongoing health teaching tailored to individual and family needs. Other essential components include regular ophthalmologic exams and psychological support. Some children may also benefit from the services of an orthopedic surgeon, physiatrist, podiatrist, dentist, or nutritionist.

The treatment program should provide the necessary direction for the overall plan of care. Even though goals should be child- and family-specific, the following goals should always be a part of the plan: 1) alleviate or eradicate the inflammation and pain; 2) prevent physical abnormalities, disability, and psychosocial problems; and 3) ensure achievement of developmental competencies. These goals are best achieved through the efforts of an interdisciplinary team of professionals experienced in rheumatic disease care, the child, and the family. Even though the child's pediatrician should be an integral part of the team, the pediatrician does not usually have long-term experience managing rheumatic diseases.

Given the restrictions on approvals for specialty services, it may become a challenge for interdisciplinary teams to provide long-term followup. Health professionals must provide convincing evidence to case managers as to the potential short- and long-term outcomes for the child if their services are not provided. Increased responsibility for daily disease management is placed on the family. Services that previously required hospitalization are now provided on an outpatient basis. Fortunately, there are some excellent self-help resources and books available to assist patients and families in meeting the needs of children with JRA.

Five aspects of care are considered essential for a comprehensive management program for a child with JRA: physical management, psychosocial care, nutrition, pharmacologic management, and non-rheumatologic care (22). All of these components are important and must be coordinated; however, pharmacologic management is the essential element.

Physical Management. Physical and occupational therapists play a central role in the management of a child with JRA. The goals of therapy are to improve motion and strength, preserve or enhance function, prevent disability, eliminate pain, and promote competency building consistent with the child's developmental stage. Assessment should include careful interviews with the child and parent, musculoskeletal examination, and subjective and objective functional evaluations. An effective treatment plan is developed in collaboration with the child and parent, because they know best how a therapy program will fit into their daily lives. The plan should, therefore, be incorporated into the usual family schedule.

All involved joints should be put through their full available range of motion on a daily basis; ideally, range of motion should be accomplished twice a day. Parents and children find daily exercise difficult to adhere to when results are not immediate and when the program becomes a source of conflict. When possible, the therapeutic program should be fun, interesting, and interactive. For children less than 6 years of age, exercise programs for 15–20 minutes twice daily are usually sufficient. Older children and adolescents will be less likely to perform exercise programs if they last longer than 30 minutes. When joints are actively inflamed, therapy continues but becomes passive or active assisted and is performed within the range of minimal discomfort. Therapists need to teach children and parents about the need to avoid forced or deep flexion in an inflamed joint. Prone lying is recommended for children with hip and knee contractures; this can be done with a pleasant distraction such as while listening to music, reading a book, or watching television.

Splinting may be used to maintain alignment, relieve inflammation, reduce flexion contractures, and provide support during functional activities. Careful serial casting in conjunction with physical therapy may also be useful management for flexion contractures. Cervical collars are used only with cervical subluxation to prevent forward flexion and stabilize the head. Properly fitted footwear can reduce lower extremity pain and improve both posture and gait. Such walking aids as crutches and walkers (with or without platforms) are used only when necessary to limit weight bearing. If upper extremity joints are involved, the use of these devices may precipitate further joint symptoms. Wheelchairs, scooters, and strollers are a last resort, as use of artificial mobility can lead to flexion contractures in the hips and the knees, cause muscle atrophy and osteopenia, and make the child more dependent.

Heat and cold therapies are commonly used to reduce pain and stiffness and relax muscles for treatment. These modalities must be used with discretion in children, because they may not be able to adequately verbalize discomforts. Heat modalities include warm water, hydrocollator packs, paraffin wax, heating pads, hot water bottles, whirlpools (with continuous professional supervision), electric blankets, and heat-retaining gloves. Moist heat is often the easiest and most readily available. Warm water may relax muscles and provide relief from pain, thus allowing an increase in the range of motion of affected joints. Pool therapy and aquatics are ideal forms of hydrotherapy for patients with arthritis. Children can do their exercises in the pool without the forces of gravity to add stress to the joints. Ultrasound is not commonly used in children, as it is contraindicated over growth plates. Cold modalities include ice or commercial chemical cold packs. Cold is usually applied until numbness occurs, or up to 10 minutes for the young child who cannot communicate numbness.

Joint protection and energy conservation take on a different meaning in children. When children feel well or when they are determined, they will do what they want regardless of the disease. Most pediatric rheumatology teams try not to limit the child. Pediatric occupational therapists are especially skilled in teaching children how to alter tasks so that the joints are protected without attracting notice. As a rule, children should be cautioned to avoid repetitive movements (jumping, running, playing interactive video games) and aggressive sports (contact sports, karate) that could affect involved joints. Children can and should be encouraged to participate in swimming, biking, and other activities that are less stressful to the involved joints.

Psychosocial Care. Normal psychosocial development may be compromised when a child has chronic disease. The interdisciplinary team must work to keep the child in school every day, ensure adequate skills and movement to play and participate in recreational activities, assist the child with peer relationships, and promote good child and family coping skills.

Many costs for families with children who have chronic illness are covered by public or private insurance plans. However, intangible and out-of-pocket expenses (missed work days, transportation, lodging, co-payments, dental care, orthotics) can have a significant impact on a family's financial resources. Often parents must utilize the Family Medical Leave Act to care for their children when ill or accompany them to appointments. The expertise and advice of the social worker is essential for identification of appropriate financial assistance, health coverage, and community resources.

Education is necessary for the family to live successfully with the disease and treatment, to improve overall outcomes, and to ensure informed decision-making. The staff nurse or advanced practice nurse is often the coordinator of the health team and is in a key position to explain the disease, the evaluation process, and management strategies to the family. Agencies such as the Arthritis Foundation and Arthritis Society have educational materials available to complement oral information. The Internet also offers a vast array of information about the disease and resources, all of which can be accessed at home or in the community. The Web sites of the Arthritis Foundation, American Juvenile Arthritis Organization, American Academy of Pediatrics, Family Voices, and the Maternal and Child Health Bureau all offer reliable and current information, links, and resources.

Nutrition. Diet has only recently received the attention it deserves in children with chronic diseases. Nutritional screening is now recommended for all children with JRA, especially in children with weight gain or loss that is not consistent with their predicted growth curve and when corticosteroids or cytotoxic drugs are prescribed. Because JRA impairs mobility, low energy expenditure in a child can cause rapid weight gain. Children and parents need the expert advice of a nutritionist to keep weight consistent with height and prevent excessive strain on weight-bearing joints. Because osteoporosis has been documented in JRA, it is important to evaluate bone mineralization. Dual-energy x-ray absorptiometry scans may be particularly important in children treated with corticosteroids or with a history of fractures.

Pharmocologic Management. Antiinflammatory and immunomodulator medications to alleviate inflammation are the mainstays of treatment for JRA. Recently, the standard approach to drug therapy for the child with JRA has been called into question. Numerous, well-documented studies suggest the need for more aggressive antiinflammatory treatment that suppresses disease activity early in the disease process to limit erosive disease and disability. The general approach to the pharmacologic management begins with nonsteroidal antiinflammatory drugs (NSAIDs). If the arthritis is not controlled by NSAIDs, a second-line medication such as methotrexate or sulfasalazine is added. Intraarticular corticosteroid injections are often used to treat limited joint disease. Newer medications such as etanercept (an anti-tumor necrosis factor) are also available. This medication can be used when methotrexate or sulfasalazine fail to produce a response or when intolerance occurs. If the disease is debilitating and recalcitrant, cytotoxic or experimental medications may be used.

NSAIDs can reduce the stiffness, pain, swelling, and sometimes the fevers associated with JRA; however, they do not alter the course of the disease. About 50% of children respond to these medications within 2 weeks and 25% take up to 3 months, with an average response time of 30 days (23). Dose levels, side effects, and cost vary among NSAIDs. Three NSAIDs have been approved for use in children in the U.S.: naproxen (10–20 mg/kg/day bid), tolmetin (20–30 mg/kg/day tid), and ibuprofen (30–50 mg/kg/day) (22). Almost half of the children who do not respond to the first NSAID may improve with another.

Most children tolerate NSAIDs well, but common side effects include abdominal pain, anorexia, or nausea. Effects on the central nervous system, mood alteration, and tinnitus have been reported. Additionally, pseudoporphyria may occur, especially in fair-skinned individuals (24). NSAIDs should always be administered with food to decrease gastric irritation. Gastrointestinal protective drugs such as antacids or H2 blockers may be added. Children on chronic NSAID therapy should be monitored for gastrointestinal, renal, and hepatic effects every 3–6 months as needed.

In some cases, acetaminophen may be used in conjunction with an NSAID to help control pain. Trials of cyclooxygenase-2 (COX-2) inhibitors, such as celecoxib and rofecoxib have not been conducted in JRA. Adult studies show that these drugs have fewer gastrointestinal effects than other NSAIDs.

Second-line agents are known as slow-acting antirheumatic drugs (SAARDs) or disease-modifying antirheumatic drugs (DMARDs). They include methotrexate, sulfasalazine, hydroxycloroquine, D-penicillamine, and gold. Methotrexate is now recommended early in the course of JRA because of its potential to reduce the pathologic impact of disease.

Methotrexate has also been employed as an additional treatment for uveitis. Methotrexate may be given orally (10–15 mg/m²/week) or parentally (up to 1 mg/kg/week). Initially, patients are often started with oral administration, but gastro-

Table 2. Frequency of ophthalmologic visits for children with juvenile rheumatoid arthritis (JRA) and without known iridocyclitis.*

JRA subtype at onset	Age of onset	
	< 7 years†	≥ 7 years‡
Pauciarticular		
ANA +	H§	M
ANA −	M	M
Polyarticular		
ANA +	H§	M
ANA −	M	M
Systemic	L	L

* High risk (H) indicates ophthalmologic exams every 3 to 4 months. Medium risk (M) indicates ophthalmologic examinations every 6 months. Low risk (L) indicates ophthalmologic examinations every 12 months. ANA = antinuclear antibodies. Reprinted from reference 28, with permission.
† All patients are considered at low risk 7 years after the onset of their arthritis and should have yearly ophthalmologic examinations indefinitely.
‡ All patients are considered at low risk 4 years after the onset of their arthritis and should have yearly ophthalmologic examinations indefinitely.
§ All high-risk patients are considered at medium risk 4 years after the onset of their arthritis.

intestinal absorption of the drug is highly variable. Subcutaneous injections of methotrexate may ultimately be more effective and better tolerated by the gastrointestinal tract in higher doses. Families are commonly trained to administer injections at home. The Pediatric Rheumatology Collaborative Study Group has established guidelines for the use of methotrexate in children (25), which should be closely followed. Adverse effects include oral ulcers (which can sometimes be decreased by giving folic acid at 1 mg/day), gastrointestinal irritation, hepatic injury, and bone marrow suppression. Risk factors for the development of liver fibrosis include hepatitis, diabetes mellitus, obesity, and alcohol use. Careful monitoring and avoidance of alcohol must be stressed with adolescents and young adults. The American College of Rheumatology has established guidelines for monitoring adults for liver toxicity that pediatric rheumatologists have adopted. Because of the potential teratogenic effects of methotrexate, age-appropriate counseling should be provided to adolescents and young adults regarding risk of pregnancy and use of contraception.

In general, oral corticosteroids are used infrequently in the treatment of JRA due to the significant long-term side effects and the difficulty of tapering the dose. However, they are often necessary in systemic JRA for life-threatening situations such as pericarditis, myocarditis, or macrophage activation syndrome. Corticosteroids may be administered as intravenous pulse therapy, orally, intraarticularly, or even topically. Side effects of greatest concern are growth cessation, weight gain, hypertension, Cushing's syndrome, osteoporosis, cataract formation, glaucoma, and decreased immune response. Doses below 0.2 mg/kg/day are not usually associated with significant cushingoid features and allow continued growth. Patients receiving long-term steroids should receive calcium and vitamin D supplementation. Additionally, patients on long-term steroids may require higher (stress) doses of corticosteroids at times of interim illnesses or surgical intervention. Deflazacort may eventually prove to be less hazardous than prednisone and prednisolone.

Topical steroids are commonly used to treat uveitis. When topical steroid eye treatment fails to reduce the inflammation, oral corticosteroids may be indicated. Localized therapy may also consist of intraarticular steroid injections for severely inflamed joints that are unresponsive to other treatment. These injections should only be employed after the possibility of infection has been eliminated.

Limited research has been conducted on the use of immune response modifiers in children. Etanercept, a TNF antagonist, is the first immune response modifier to be studied in children with polyarticular JRA (26). It appears to be as effective as methotrexate and has a good toxicity profile. When used in conjunction with methotrexate, there may be a synergistic effect (27). Etanercept appears to act relatively quickly, with clinical responses seen as early as a few weeks after the initiation of therapy. Most responses occur within the first 3 months. The most common side effects include a localized reaction at the injection site and upper respiratory infections and sinusitis. Serious infections have been reported in patients taking etanercept. It is advised that the medication be stopped if a patient develops a serious infection. Live virus vaccinations should not be administered with etanercept.

Nonrheumatologic Care. Nonrheumatologic care includes surgery, ophthalmologic care, and alternative therapies. The role of surgery in JRA is limited. Interventions that may be employed include soft tissue releases, arthroscopy, and arthroplasty. Three factors typically influence the decision to perform arthroplasty in children: 1) pain, 2) child's age with growth potential, and 3) the longevity of the possible prosthesis. Joint replacements are only advisable when the growth plates have closed. Children with polyarticular JRA, especially those who are rheumatoid factor positive and have unrelenting disease, may reach a time in the late teen or young adult years when pain and loss of function prompt the need for arthroplasty. Usually, a single joint, such as a hip or knee, is replaced. However, the need for multiple serial arthroplasties over many years is not uncommon. Prior to surgery, the appropriate therapists should evaluate the child or young adult and introduce the postoperative rehabilitation program.

Synovectomy was once popular, but the long-term outcomes of the procedure have not been significant. Tenosynovectomy may be indicated when hand function is deteriorating or to avoid tendon rupture or reduce nerve entrapment.

All children with JRA should have a baseline slit lamp examination by an ophthalmologist to determine if uveitis is present, as it is usually asymptomatic and can progress to blindness. Frequent examinations are also important for children taking corticosteroids and antimalarial drugs, as well as for children with cataracts or glaucoma. Ophthalmologic care and treatment for these children must be individualized to meet the child's needs. Table 2 provides a guideline for frequency of examination based on type of JRA at onset (28).

The use of alternative therapies is not uncommon in patients with chronic disease (See Chapter 33, Complementary and Alternative Treatments). As expected, many families choose remedies consistent with their culture. It is essential that health care providers encourage families to report what the child is using so that appropriate health education is provided.

As with all children who have a special health care need, the standard treatment program for a child with a rheumatic disease requires that care be family-centered, community-based, comprehensive, and culturally competent. In addition, all adolescents should have a transition in their care plan. For further discussion on these topics, visit the web sites of the American Academy of Pediatrics and the Maternal and Child Health Bureau.

SPONDYLARTHROPATHIES

The spondylarthropathies of childhood include juvenile ankylosing spondylitis, juvenile psoriatic arthritis, Reiter's syndrome (reactive arthritis), and inflammatory bowel disease (IBD) including ulcerative colitis and Crohn's disease. Even though these diseases may appear to be quite different from one another, there are several important similarities. Each can cause peripheral arthritis, acute iritis, enthesitis, sacroiliitis, and/or spondylitis; furthermore, each is always rheumatoid factor negative. All may present with the signs and symptoms of JRA (usually pauciarticular) at onset, sometimes long before other disease manifestations emerge to help finalize the diagnosis. Extra-articular manifestations, which may occur in the absence of joint involvement, include cutaneous diseases such as psoriasis, erythema nodosum, and pyoderma gangrenosum; bowel disease; acute uveitis; pulmonary disease; and genitourinary disease. Some bacterial infections such as salmonella, shigella, or campylobacter may play a role in triggering reactive arthritis.

Juvenile ankylosing spondylitis is considered the prototypical spondylarthropathy. Its etiology is unknown. There is a strong genetic predisposition with the class I HLA-B27 allele. HLA-B27 is present in approximately 90–95% of patients with juvenile ankylosing spondylitis. The disease is more common in males, with a mean age of onset greater than 10 years old. Initially, juvenile ankylosing spondylitis is commonly mistaken for JRA. Lower extremity joints are usually involved. Later in the disease, lumbar and sacroiliac disease becomes evident. Enthesitis is almost always present. Clinicians must carefully observe for enthesitis, psoriasis, nail changes (pitting or onycholysis), iritis, oral or anal lesions, urethritis, weight loss, fever, and hypoalbuminemia. Any of these symptoms should suggest a spondylarthropathy rather than JRA.

Initial pharmocologic management of the juvenile spondylarthropathies often consists of NSAIDs such as indomethacin, tolmetin, or naproxen. Second-line agents such as sulfasalazine or methotrexate are often utilized. Infliximab may also have a role in treatment, especially in patients with Crohn's disease. Apart from juvenile ankylosing spondylarthritis, the spondylarthropathies appear at times to have nothing to do with arthritis.

Physical therapy is a key part of any treatment program for a child with spondylitis and sacroiliitis, especially juvenile ankylosing spondylitis. It is imperative that the child exercise daily, preferably twice a day or more, to maintain back motion and posture. Lying prone, stretching, and swimming are important components of a physical therapy program. Children with peripheral arthritis require evaluation by a physical and/or occupational therapist, and often a therapeutic program similar to children with JRA. Special attention to axial flexibility, strengthening, chest expansion, and posture are central to physical management. A gastroenterologist and an experienced nutritionist should evaluate all children with inflammatory bowel disease during and after flares. Dermatologic consultation may be necessary for children with psoriasis.

The impact of disease on children with spondylarthropathies is very similar to that seen with JRA. In addition, children with Reiter's syndrome may be embarrassed or anxious about the urethritis and mucocutaneous lesions. For children with inflammatory bowel disease, abdominal cramping, flatulence, and diarrhea can be upsetting. The skin and nail lesions of psoriatic arthritis often have a significant impact on self-image. The lesions can be very difficult to hide, thus leaving the child open to ridicule. Psoriatic lesions on the scalp cause severe flaking and scaling, which other children and adults may perceive as the result of dirty hair. It is important to seek professional psychological screenings for these children and to make the necessary referrals for assessment and treatment when indicated.

THE SCHOOL SETTING

School participation is a child's work. The health care team should promote collaboration among the school staff, the parent, and the team, by providing education on juvenile arthritis to the school staff and input to the school program (Individual Educational Plan or 504 plan). When possible, therapy services can be provided during the school day, and school activities that are too difficult to accomplish or endure can be modified. Participation in physical education class should be encouraged; however, the program may need to be modified or adapted.

REFERENCES

1. Cassidy JT, Petty RE. Textbook of pediatric rheumatology. 4th ed. Philadelphia: W.B. Saunders; 2001.
2. Newacheck P, Taylor W. Childhood chronic illness: prevalence, severity, and impact. Am J Pub Health 1992;82:364–71.
3. Maddison PJ, Isenberg DA, Woo P, Glass DN. Oxford textbook of rheumatology. 2nd ed. New York: Oxford University Press; 1998.
4. Glass D, Giannini E. Juvenile rheumatoid arthritis as a complex genetic trait. Arthritis Rheum 1999;42:2261–68.
5. Van Kerckhove C, Luyrink L, Taylor J, Melin-Aldana H, Balakrishnan K, Maksymowych W, et al. HLA-DQA1*0101 haplotypes and disease outcome in early onset juvenile rheumatoid arthritis. J Rheumatol 1991;18:874–9.
6. Sakkas L, Platsoucas C. Immunopathogenesis of juvenile rheumatoid arthritis: role of T cells and MHC. Immunol Res 1995;14:218–36.
7. Klippel JH, Crofford LJ, Stone JH, Weyand CM. Appendix I. Criteria for the diagnosis of juvenile rheumatoid arthritis. In: Klippel JH, Crofford LJ, Stone JH, Weyand CM, editors. Primer on the rheumatic diseases. 12th ed. Atlanta: Arthritis Foundation; 2001, in press.
8. Graham T, Lovell D. Outcomes in pediatric rheumatic disease. Curr Opin Rheumatol 1997;9:434–9.
9. Jacobs J. Pediatric rheumatology for the practitioner. New York: Springer-Verlag; 1982.
10. Alepa R. Juvenile rheumatoid arthritis. In: Riggs G, Gall E, editors. Rheumatic diseases: rehabilitation and management. Boston: Butterworths; 1984.
11. Fraser PA, Hoch S, Erlandson D, Partridge R, Jackson J. The timing of menarche in juvenile rheumatoid arthritis. J Adolesc Health Care 1988;9:483–7.
12. Henderson C, Lovell D. Assessment of protein-energy malnutrition in children and adolescents with juvenile rheumatoid arthritis. Arthritis Care Res 1989;2:108–13.
13. Henderson C, Calkwell G, Specter B, Sierra R, Wilmott R, Campaigne B, et al. Predictors of total body bone mineral density in non-corticosteroid-treated prepubertal children with juvenile rheumatoid arthritis. Arthritis Rheum 1997;40:1967–75.
14. Erlandson D. Juvenile rheumatoid arthritis. In: Logigian M, Ward J, editors. Pediatric rehabilitation: a team approach for therapists. Boston: Little Brown Co; 1989.
15. Athreya B: The hand in juvenile rheumatoid arthritis. Arthritis Rheum 1977;20:573.
16. McAnarney ER, Pless IB, Satterwhite B, Friedman SB. Psychological problems of children with chronic juvenile arthritis. Pediatrics 1974;53:523–8.
17. Noll RB, Kozlowski K, Gerhard EC, Vannatta K, Taylor J, Passo M. Social, emotional, and behavioral functioning of children with juvenile rheumatoid arthritis. Arthritis Rheum 2000;43:1387–96.
18. Erlandson D: Helping the patient and family cope with systemic lupus erythematosus. In: Ahmed P, editor. Coping with arthritis. Springfield, IL: Charles C. Thomas Publisher; 1988.
19. Duffy C, Tucker L, Burgos-Vargas R. Update on functional assessment tools. J Rheumatol 2000;27(Suppl 58):11–4.
20. Levinson J, Wallace C. Dismantling the pyramid. J Rheumatol 1992;19:6–10.
21. Prahalad S, Passo M. Long-term outcomes among patients with juvenile rheumatoid arthritis. Frontiers Biosci 1998;3:13–22.
22. Giannini E, Petty R. Treatment of juvenile rheumatoid arthritis. In: Koopman WJ, editor. Arthritis & allied conditions: a textbook of rheumatology. 14th ed. New York: Lippincott, Williams & Wilkins; 2001, 1294–1310.
23. Lovell D, Giannini EH, Brewer EJ Jr. Time course of response to nonsteroidal antiinflammatory drugs in juvenile rheumatoid arthritis. Arthritis Rheum 1984;27:1433–7.
24. Lang B, Finlayson L. Naprosyn-induced pseudoporphyria in patients with JRA. J Pediatr 1994;124:639–42.
25. Pediatric Rheumatology Collaborative Study Group: FDA guidelines, drugs in children. Arthritis Rheum 1995;38:715–8.
26. Lovell DJ, Giannini EH, Reiff A, Cawkwell GD, Silverman ED, Nocton JJ, et al. Etanercept in children with polyarticular juvenile rheumatoid arthritis. Pediatric Rheumatology Collaborative Study Group. N Engl J Med 2000;342:763–9.
27. Weinblatt ME, Kremer JM, Bankhurst AD, Bulpitt KJ, Fleischmann RM, Rox RI, et al. A trial of etanercept, a recombinant tumor necrosis factor receptor:Fc fusion protein, in patients with rheumatoid arthritis receiving methotrexate. N Engl J Med 1999;340:253–9.
28. Section of Rheumatology and Section on Ophthalmology. Guidelines for ophthalmologic examinations in children with JRA. Pediatrics 1995;92:295–6.
29. Burgos-Vargas R, Pacheco-Tens C, Vazquez-Mellando J. Juvenile-onset spondyloarthropathies. Rheum Dis Clin North Am 1997;23:569–98.

Rheumatoid Arthritis

MARCIN GORNISIEWICZ, MD; and LARRY W. MORELAND, MD

Rheumatoid arthritis (RA) is a chronic, systemic inflammatory disorder of unknown etiology. It is frequently referred to as an autoimmune disease and is characterized by symmetric polyarticular pain and swelling, morning stiffness, malaise, and fatigue. RA has a variable course with remissions and exacerbations. Outcomes are variable as well, ranging from a remitting disease (rare) to a severe disease bringing disability and even premature death. The progression of joint damage in the majority of patients results in significant disability within 10 to 20 years.

EPIDEMIOLOGY

RA is a worldwide problem, with a prevalence of 0.5–1% of the adult population (1) and an annual incidence of 0.03% (2), although there is substantial variation across different studies and time periods. Overall, RA appears to be less common in Asia and Africa than in the United States and Europe (3), and it has been suggested that the incidence of RA decreases from northern to more southern European countries (4). The disease affects individuals at any age, including infants and the elderly; however, it is most common in women aged 40–50 years. RA is not very common in men under 45 years of age, but the incidence rises steeply with increasing age. In women, the incidence rises to age 45, plateaus until age 75, and then declines (5). Numerous studies have demonstrated increased mortality in patients with RA compared to the general population. There are reports of increased risk of death from gastrointestinal, cardiovascular, respiratory, hematologic, and infectious diseases (6–9).

ETIOLOGY AND PATHOGENESIS

The pathophysiology of RA has undergone intensive investigation over the last 10 to 20 years. It is well known that an individual's genetic background plays a critical role in the susceptibility to and severity of RA (10). Careful studies have revealed a 15% concordance in monozygotic twins, which is approximately 4 times greater than the rate in dizygotic twins and confirms a genetic component (11). The disease transmission is complex and likely involves many genes. The genes with the greatest impact lie in the class II major histocompatibility (MHC) locus. There is a strong association of the disease with a specific sequence on the beta chains of select HLA-DR haplotypes. This "shared epitope" contains amino acids 70 through 74 (glutamine-leucine-arginine-alanine-alanine) and is also known as QKRAA (12).

Although the search for a specific etiologic agent has been intense, the cause of RA has not been discovered. Its pathogenesis is likely multifactorial, with genetic background contributing to susceptibility, along with exposure to unknown environmental factors. Many theoretical and experimental arguments have supported infection as the triggering event in autoimmune disease, although no pathogens have yet been proven to initiate synovitis.

Infectious agents may invade the target organ directly, or infection outside the joint may trigger the arthritis through stimulation of autoimmunity, resulting in a sterile or "reactive" arthritis (13). This extraarticular infection possibly triggers disease through the mechanism known as molecular mimicry, which proposes that similarities in antigenic proteins between infecting agents and host tissues might result in the immune response against the pathogen being misdirected against the host tissue. Similar theories propose an autoimmune response directed at joint-specific antigens called "superantigens" that can activate multiple clones of T cells through a largely MHC-independent process. Examples of antigens that have been implicated are type II collagen, proteoglycans, heat shock proteins, cartilage protein gp39, and immunoglobulins (14,15). It is possible that RA may be multiple diseases, now defined by some common clinical manifestations, and there may not be a single predominant mechanism of initiation or perpetuation.

A current concept is that inflammation and tissue destruction in the rheumatoid synovium result from complex cell–cell interactions (Figure 1). The process may be initiated by an interaction between antigen-presenting cells (APC) and CD4$^+$ T cells. APC display complexes of class II MHC molecules and peptide antigens that bind to specific receptors on the T cells. This leads to clonal expansion of T cells, which stimulates synovial macrophages to secrete proinflammatory cytokines such as interleukin-1 (IL-1) and tumor necrosis factor alpha (TNF-α) (16).

Joint damage in RA results from proliferation of the synovial intimal layer to form a pannus that overgrows and invades adjacent cartilage and bone, evident on x-ray as loss of joint space and juxtaarticular bone erosion. Fibroblast-like synoviocytes and macrophages are the predominant cellular components of the invading pannus. Extracellular matrix damage resulting from synovial expansion is caused by several families of enzymes, including serine proteases and cathepsins. Matrix metalloproteinases (MMPs) produced mostly by synoviocytes in the intimal lining are probably the most important mediators of tissue destruction.

DIAGNOSIS AND CLINICAL HISTORY

Diagnosing a chronic illness such as RA, and separating it from other conditions that may be self-limited or have different outcomes, can be difficult. There are no early-onset, disease-specific features, and the characteristic hallmarks of the disease develop over time. There is no single diagnostic test that enables a diagnosis of RA to be made with certainty. Instead,

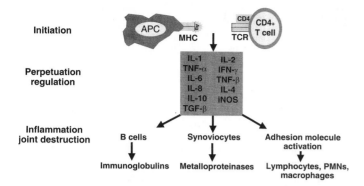

Initiation

Perpetuation regulation

Inflammation joint destruction

Figure 1. The immune-mediated inflammatory process of rheumatoid arthritis. APC = antigen-presenting cells; MHC = major histocompatibility complex; TCR = T-cell receptor; IL = interleukin; TNF = tumor necrosis factor; IFN = interferon; TGF = transforming growth factor; PMNs = polymorphonuclear cells. Adapted from Moreland LW, Heck LW Jr, Koopman WJ. Biologic agents for treating rheumatoid arthritis. Arthritis Rheum 1997;40:397–409.

diagnosis depends on the accumulation of characteristic symptoms, signs, laboratory data, and radiologic findings.

The clinical manifestations of RA are highly variable. The typical illness begins insidiously with slowly progressive development of symptoms over a period of weeks to months. Less often, the onset is acute, usually polyarticular. Symmetric arthritis affecting the metacarpophalangeal (MCP) joints and proximal interphalangeal (PIP) joints of both hands is the most characteristic early clinical feature. There is swelling with associated stiffness, warmth, tenderness, and pain. Edema of the synovium contributes to stiffness by mechanically interfering with joint motion.

The number of involved joints is highly variable, but the process is eventually polyarticular in most. Almost any joint may be affected but there is a predilection for peripheral joints with sparing of the axial skeletal. The joints involved most often are the PIP and MCP joints of the hands, wrists, elbows, ankles, metatarsophalangeal (MTP) joints, and temporomandibular joints. Involvement of shoulder, hip, sternoclavicular, and cricoarytenoid joints is less common (17).

Although RA is manifested primarily by joint involvement, it is a systemic inflammatory disease. Most patients experience such nonspecific systemic symptoms as fatigue, malaise, low-grade fever, and depression. These symptoms may precede other typical signs of disease by weeks or months. Because symptoms characteristically wax and wane, especially at the beginning of the illness, it is not unusual that the proper diagnosis is delayed for months.

Classification criteria for RA were drafted in 1956 by the American College of Rheumatology (ACR, formerly the American Rheumatism Association) and revised in 1987 (18) in an effort to provide guidelines for epidemiologic studies and clinical trials, not primarily intended for clinical diagnosis (Figure 2). The disease of patients who initially fulfill the diagnostic criteria may evolve into other connective tissue diseases.

PHYSICAL EXAMINATION

A complete physical examination is indicated in all patients with RA, not only to make the diagnosis but to establish a baseline

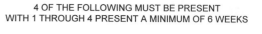

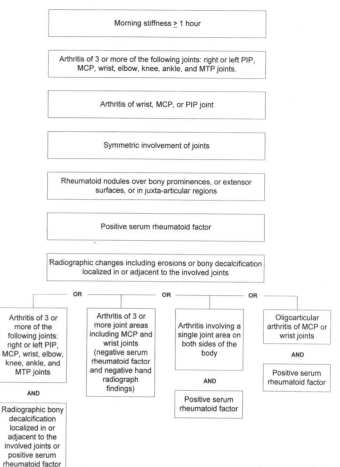

Figure 2. Classification criteria for the diagnosis of rheumatoid arthritis (18). PIP = proximal interphalangeal; MCP = metacarpophalangeal; MTP = metatarsophalangeal.

against which to assess disease progression. Pain and swelling are the key features that occur in joints affected by RA. Swelling may be due to synovial hypertrophy (detected by a "boggy" feel to a swollen joint) or effusion, demonstrated by fluctuation. This is most evident in the small joints of the hands and feet where the outline of the base of the proximal phalanx may become indistinct (Figure 3). In contrast to gout or septic arthritis, heat and redness are not prominent features of RA, although an involved joint is often warm on careful exam. When effusion contributes to swelling and is under increased pressure with joint flexion, a portion of the synovium may become trapped and separated from the rest of the joint, forming a cyst. The cyst may be seen in many peripheral joints but is most commonly recognized in the knee (Baker's cyst), which, when ruptured, may resemble acute thrombophlebitis. Tenderness and pain on passive motion are the most sensitive signs of inflammation, so it is important to apply gentle but firm pressure when examining a joint. A lateral squeeze of the MCP and MTP joint rows and assessment of grip strength are useful in detecting tenderness and restricted range of movement.

Subcutaneous nodules occur in about 30% of patients with RA, usually after the disease is established. They are not attached to underlying bone or overlying skin and are most commonly found over the extensor aspect of the proximal ulna,

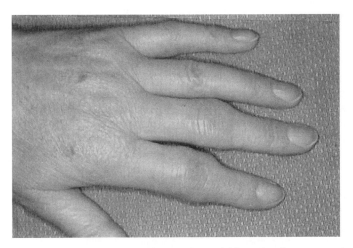

Figure 3. Swelling in the hand due to synovial hypertrophy.

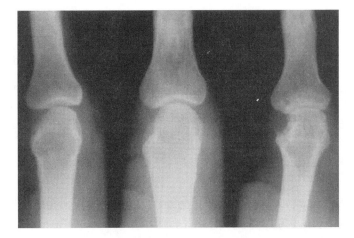

Figure 4. Erosive changes of a proximal interphalangeal joint.

although they also occur at other pressure locations. The characteristic joint deformities are late manifestations of disease that result from the physical stresses and local anatomy of involved joints. More than 10% of RA patients will develop deformity of the small joints of the hands within the first 2 years of disease, and at least one-third develop such deformities over time (19). Visible changes include hyperflexion or hyperextension of the joints of the fingers (boutonniere and swan-neck deformities), volar subluxation and ulnar deviation, hallux valgus (bunion), and "hammer toes." These changes occur in the majority of patients with disease lasting more than 10 years (20).

LABORATORY TESTS

No test is necessary to establish a diagnosis of RA, and all laboratory tests may be normal in certain patients. Routine tests are often not characteristic and lack specificity; however, certain data may contribute to the diagnosis and assessment of the severity of RA in an individual.

Rheumatoid factor (RF) was identified as an antibody (IgM, IgG or others) that binds to the Fc fragment of immunoglobulin G. It is detectable in the serum of 70–80% of patients with RA. It is unclear whether the production of RF is of pathologic relevance to RA, since RF production also frequently occurs in patients with systemic lupus erythematosus, Sjögren's syndrome, endocarditis, liver and chronic lung diseases, and other conditions (21). In addition, RF may be detected in the serum of apparently normal individuals, especially people over age 50 and smokers. In an individual patient, the titer does not correlate with the activity of disease, but it does appear that patients with very severe erosive arthritis or with extraarticular disease are likely to have relatively high titers. The presence of a positive serum RF does not establish a diagnosis of RA, but when combined with a typical clinical picture, it does help to confirm the clinical impression.

A mild anemia commonly occurs in RA. It is usually a normochromic, normocytic anemia of chronic disease; however, true iron deficiency anemia may also develop. The white blood cell count generally is normal, but occasionally may be elevated in patients with significant inflammatory disease; alternatively, it may be low in Felty's syndrome. Patients often have thrombocytosis, usually in association with active joint disease or extraarticular manifestations.

Acute phase reactants such as the erythrocyte sedimentation rate (ESR) and C-reactive protein (CRP), usually elevated in the presence of active inflammation, are much less specific than RF. They are useful in distinguishing RA from such noninflammatory conditions as osteoarthritis or fibromyalgia; however, a significant number of patients have normal values of these tests, despite clinical evidence of joint inflammation. Antinuclear antibodies (ANA) can be present in 20–40% of patients with RA, commonly those with extraarticular manifestations and with high titers of RF.

Synovial fluid analysis is usually not necessary when the diagnosis is already established, but arthrocentesis should be performed to rule out infection in patients who develop disproportionate discomfort and swelling of one joint.

RADIOLOGY

Radiologic findings vary depending on the duration and severity of the illness. A normal radiograph does not exclude a diagnosis of RA; in fact, early in the disease radiographs show nothing other than soft-tissue swelling. More than half of patients develop radiographic changes within the first 2 years of disease. The relationship between radiologic change and the consequences of RA for the patient has not yet been fully established. It is assumed, rather than proven, that the radiographic picture correlates with long-term disability.

Radiographic joint damage in RA has several features, including periarticular osteoporosis, joint space narrowing due to generalized cartilage loss, and juxtaarticular erosions, generally at the point of attachment of the joint capsule (Figure 4). In end-stage disease, large cystic erosions of bone may be seen together with bony proliferation and marked deformities. Erosions, typically in the MCP and PIP joints, are present in 15–30% of patients in the first year of the disease. In some patients, erosions occur first in the ulnar styloid or MTP joints. It is therefore important to evaluate both hands (including the wrists) and feet in all patients for whom a diagnosis of RA is suspected.

Cervical spine involvement is common. Joint destruction may lead to atlantoaxial (C1–C2) and subaxial malalignment (subluxation), vertebral endplate erosions, spondylodiscitis, and disc space narrowing without osteophytes. Anterior C1–C2 subluxation is the most frequent radiographic abnormality. The earliest and most common symptom is pain radiating toward the occiput; however, the correlation between the degree of subluxation and symptoms is poor. Plain radiographic views of the cervical spine (lateral, with the neck in flexion) should be considered for all RA patients scheduled for procedures requiring manipulation of the neck. Unrecognized C1–C2 disease may lead to cord compression, irreversible paralysis, even death.

SYSTEMIC AND NONARTICULAR MANIFESTATIONS

Extraarticular manifestations of RA usually occur in patients with relatively more severe disease, but rarely prior to the onset of arthritis. It is sometimes difficult to separate effects secondary to the disease itself from drug-induced side effects. In contrast to the predilection of classic RA for women, extraarticular manifestations of the disease are more common in men. This is especially true for pleural involvement, vasculitis, and pericarditis. Systemic involvement occurs more frequently in patients who are RF positive.

Cutaneous Manifestations

The most common cutaneous manifestations are *rheumatoid nodules*. They may arise within tendons or ligaments and can result in joint dysfunction and tendon rupture. Rarely, nodules may arise in visceral organs such as the lungs, heart valves, sclera, and vocal cords. Patients treated with methotrexate may occasionally have an increase in the size and number of rheumatoid nodules (22). The differential diagnosis should include gouty tophi, which may be found in similar locations. Very rarely biopsy of the nodule may be necessary if the diagnosis is uncertain.

About 10–15% of patients with RA develop *Sjögren's syndrome*, characterized by impaired secretion of saliva and tears, dry mouth (xerostomia), and dry eyes (keratoconjunctivitis). Cutaneous manifestations of Sjögren's syndrome include photosensitivity, Raynaud's phenomenon, annular erythema, and vasculitis. Patients are at increased risk of developing lymphomas, especially low-grade B-cell lymphoma.

Ocular Manifestations

Episcleritis, a self-limited process, and *scleritis*, a more serious problem that can lead to perforation of the globe and loss of vision, occur in less than 5% of RA patients. The distinction between episcleritis and scleritis is difficult, and all patients with suspected scleritis should be referred to an ophthalmologist.

Pulmonary Involvement

Pulmonary involvement in RA may present with several clinical scenarios. Pleurisy with or without effusion is the most common form of pulmonary disease, occurring in up to 70% of patients.

Most cases are asymptomatic, and a small pleural effusion may be discovered incidentally on a routine radiograph. The effusion is usually exudative, and the glucose concentration of the fluid is often very low. Interstitial lung disease is a common long-term manifestation of severe RA that usually follows the onset of joint symptoms by up to 5 years. It is more common in men, and smoking is a significant risk factor. Because of limited physical activity in patients with RA, it is often asymptomatic, but restrictive abnormalities on pulmonary function tests are common even in the absence of symptoms. The diagnosis should be suspected in any patient with RA with shortness of breath or dyspnea on exertion. Other rare pulmonary manifestations include bronchiolitis obliterans, pneumothorax, or rheumatoid pneumoconiosis (Caplan's syndrome).

Cardiac Involvement

Pericarditis and myocarditis are 2 major forms of cardiac involvement in RA. Up to 30% of patients have echocardiographic evidence of pericardial effusion, but symptomatic pericarditis is rare, usually developing during a generalized disease flare. Restrictive pericarditis with tamponade is unusual. Myocarditis and conduction abnormalities secondary to nodule formation in the heart have been reported rarely.

Renal Involvement

Renal involvement as an intrinsic part of the rheumatoid disease process is suggested but unproven. It is usually related to amyloidosis, vasculitis, or drug toxicity. Among drugs used in RA, those most commonly implicated in renal dysfunction include cyclosporine, gold, penicillamine, and nonsteroidal antiinflammatory drugs (NSAIDs).

Felty's Syndrome

This syndrome is characterized by the triad of neutropenia, splenomegaly, and deforming RA and may occur in about 1% of patients with RA. Patients are usually older than 50 years, have a high titer of RF, and often have a positive ANA and relatively severe arthritis with other extraarticular manifestations. When splenomegaly is not present, the diagnosis may be difficult. Recurrent bacterial infections, most commonly affecting the lungs and urinary tract, and chronic refractory leg ulcers are the major complications. Large granular lymphocyte syndrome (LGL) shares many clinical and laboratory features of Felty's syndrome, but is not exclusive to RA. In fact, LGL syndrome may represent a process that facilitates development of RA, rather than being a result of the disease itself. Up to 14% of patients with LGL syndrome may progress to leukemia, and exacerbation, rather than improvement, frequently follows splenectomy.

Vasculitis

Inflammation involving the blood vessels is found in as many as 25–30% of patients with RA on whom autopsies are performed. However, clinically evident disease is much less common. Classification of rheumatoid vasculitis is difficult because of the variability in both the size of the vessel involved and the histologic findings. Skin vasculitis is the most common manifestation, presenting as small digital infarcts along the nailbeds, palpable purpura, and petechiae. Neurovascular disease can lead to a mild distal sensory neuropathy or mononeuritis multiplex.

DIFFERENTIAL DIAGNOSIS

The diagnosis of RA, especially in its initial stages, can be difficult. The basic laboratory tests lack adequate sensitivity and specificity, and operator-dependent clinical assessment is subject to bias. Atypical early presentation with fluctuating symptoms, absence of rheumatoid factor, or single or asymmetric joint involvement, makes it more difficult to distinguish RA from other causes of acute or chronic polyarthritis.

The spondylarthropathies (Reiter's syndrome, reactive arthritis, inflammatory bowel disease) may appear similar to RA. Careful history and physical examination to look for heel pain and ocular or urethral symptoms are of greatest importance. The joint involvement in reactive arthritis is typically asymmetric oligoarthritis, usually of the weight-bearing joints with or without sacroiliac and spinal involvement. The characteristics of enthesopathy, such as inflammation at tendon insertion sites and "sausage" appearance of the fingers, may point to the diagnosis. Morning stiffness is unusual and RF is rare.

Inflammatory bowel disease (ulcerative colitis and Crohn's disease) may be associated with peripheral arthritis in up to 20% of patients. Not infrequently, arthritis is the first clinical symptom, and abdominal complaints may not be prominent. Lower extremity joints are involved predominantly, and large joint effusions are common. Involvement is usually asymmetric and erosions are not found.

Psoriatic arthritis may closely resemble RA, and joint symptoms may precede the onset of skin disease by many years. In a majority of patients, involvement of DIP joints, psoriatic skin lesions or family history of psoriasis, and characteristic nail changes (onychodystrophy, pitting), all point toward psoriatic arthritis. The presence of dactylitis and enthesitis, spinal involvement, and a characteristic radiographic picture with new bone formation or ankylosis clarify the diagnosis.

Osteoarthritis (OA) is most commonly confused with RA when it involves the hands, particularly the PIP joints. OA typically affects DIP joints with characteristic Heberden's nodes, and the carpometacarpal joint of the thumb. Stiffness is most bothersome after joint immobility, but in a small number of patients it may last for several hours. In general, OA is not associated with constitutional symptoms, RF, or abnormal levels of acute phase reactants. X-rays show narrowing of the joint space and osteophytes without erosions or cysts.

Gout, known as "the great masquerader," must always be considered before a diagnosis of RA is made. Features of gouty arthritis that mimic RA include polyarthritis, symmetric involvement, fusiform swelling of joints, and subcutaneous nodules. Radiographic findings may be similar, with overlapping appearance of the subcortical erosions of RA resembling small osseous tophi. Serologic tests may be misleading as well; often diagnosis of gout can be made only by arthrocentesis.

Polymyalgia rheumatica can usually be distinguished from RA by the absence of persistent small joint synovitis and by localization of symptoms in proximal muscles of the shoulders and pelvic girdle. Patients will have difficulty performing such activities as rising from a chair, climbing, or combing hair; whereas RA-associated difficulties include buttoning or opening jars.

Viral infections, such as rubella and parvovirus, can present as an acute polyarthritis, which differs from RA by the typically self-limited nature of symptoms. Furthermore, patients with viral arthritis may present with rash, low-grade fever, and a recent history of viral exposure.

Some typical findings in fibromyalgia may be seen in RA patients as well. These include morning stiffness, diffuse arthralgias and myalgias, subjective joint and soft tissue swelling, fatigue, and sleep disturbances. In fact, both of these conditions may be present simultaneously in a patient.

Other conditions that may simulate RA include systemic lupus erythematosus, systemic sclerosis, myositis, and less commonly, hypertrophic osteoarthropathy, hemochromatosis, hypothyroidism, bacterial endocarditis, hemoglobinopathies, sarcoidosis, and rheumatic fever.

TREATMENT

The ultimate goals of RA management are to reduce pain and discomfort, prevent deformities and loss of normal joint function, and maintain normal physical, social, and emotional function and capacity to work. Management begins with effective communication between physician and patient. It is very important to educate the patient and his or her family about the nature and course of the disease—the specific causes of the discomfort and the goals, problems, and expectations of treatment. Misunderstandings about the disease may lead to frustration, depression, and withdrawal.

Nonpharmacologic therapeutic options include reduction of joint stress, and physical and occupational therapy. Local rest of an inflamed joint can reduce joint stress, as can weight reduction, splinting, and use of walking aids and specially designed devices. Vigorous activity should be avoided during disease flares, although full range of motion of joints should be maintained by a graded exercise program to prevent contractures and muscular atrophy (see Chapter 26, Rest and Exercise).

Drug Therapy

The old approach to the treatment of RA was to begin with symptomatic treatment of inflammation using NSAIDs in addition to rest and corticosteroid injections. If the disease did not significantly improve, more potent disease-modifying antirheumatic drugs (DMARDs) were started. This is no longer the approach rheumatologists choose. Maintaining normal joint structure and anatomy can only be achieved by controlling the disease before any irreversible damage has occurred. Studies have revealed that DMARD therapy early in the course of RA slowed disease progression more effectively than did delayed use (23). This has led to a general agreement that the inflammation of RA should be controlled as completely as possible, as soon as possible, and that this control should be maintained for as long as possible. The currently available pharmacologic and biologic agents used to treat RA will be briefly reviewed.

Nonsteroidal Antiinflammatory Drugs. NSAIDs are probably the most frequently used drugs in treatment of RA, at least early in the disease process. The major effect of these agents is to reduce joint pain and swelling and improve joint function. There is no evidence that NSAIDs have any effect on the underlying disease process, and exacerbation of symptoms occurs quickly after metabolic elimination of the drugs. They are rarely, if ever, used alone for treatment of RA.

The major therapeutic effect of NSAIDs relates to their ability to suppress the synthesis of prostaglandins by inhibiting the enzyme cyclooxygenase, which exists in 2 isoforms: cyclooxygenase-1 and cyclooxygenase-2 (COX-1 and COX-2) (24). COX-1 is expressed in many tissues and is primarily responsible for the production of prostaglandins by endothelium and gastric mucosa, leading to homeostatic and cytoprotective effects. COX-2 is undetectable in most tissues; its expression increases during development and inflammation and can be induced by several proinflammatory stimuli. It is hypothesized that the antiinflammatory effects of NSAIDs are mainly the result of COX-2 inhibition and that inhibition of COX-1 is responsible for most of the gastrointestinal toxicity.

There are a large number of NSAIDs from which to choose, but their antiinflammatory potential is approximately equal. However, there is an unpredictable and varied individual response to different NSAIDs. If tolerated, maximum approved doses should be used, and if there is no clinical response after 2–3 weeks, another drug should be initiated.

The major side effects limiting the usefulness of currently available NSAIDs are gastrointestinal and renal toxicity. Gastrointestinal disturbance is secondary to direct damage to the gastric mucosa and suppression of gastroprotective prostaglandins. Ulcers, bleeding, and perforation occur in approximately 2–4% of patients who use NSAIDs for 1 year (25), therefore periodic assessment of hematocrit in patients taking NSAIDs for an extended duration is recommended. NSAIDs interfere with fluid and electrolyte homeostasis, resulting in fluid retention and hyperkalemia. Patients with pre-existing renal disease or diminished effective renal blood volume (CHF, cirrhosis, renal vascular disease) are at risk for effects of NSAIDs on glomerular perfusion; therefore, careful monitoring of creatinine and potassium levels is highly indicated.

Selective COX-2 inhibitors (celecoxib, rofecoxib, meloxicam) have been approved for use in RA. Their principal benefit is the lower risk of serious gastrointestinal adverse reactions compared to the nonselective NSAIDs (26–28). However, there is no evidence that highly selective COX-2 inhibitors have greater efficacy. Limited data are available concerning whether they are safer with regard to renal toxicity.

Corticosteroids. Corticosteroids have a long history in the treatment of many rheumatic diseases and they are still a key element in the management of RA. They produce rapid and potent suppression of inflammation with improvement in fatigue, joint pain, and swelling. One controlled study demonstrated a decrease in progression of joint erosion in patients treated with low-dose daily prednisolone (29). Prednisone is most frequently used for RA in a dose of 5–10 mg/day to minimize adrenal suppression. The therapy is often initiated in patients with significant functional decline and active disease while awaiting the full therapeutic effect of DMARDs. Once started, corticosteroid therapy is difficult to discontinue. Tapering should be gradual to avoid disease flares, e.g., 0.5–1.0 mg/day every few weeks to months.

A short course or even a single, high dose of corticosteroid can be administered in situations when rapid control of inflammation is desired. Occasionally, intraarticular injections may be used to control a local flare in joints with disproportionate involvement. The effects are sometimes dramatic but may be temporary.

All potential adverse effects should be fully discussed with the patient before initiating therapy. The immunosuppression and catabolic consequences associated with corticosteroids limit their long-term use in high doses and dictate the need for careful surveillance and preventive interventions to avoid undesired complications. Periodic assessment for steroid-induced osteoporosis has become a standard of care for patients on long-term corticosteroid therapy. Patients with and without osteoporosis risk factors should undergo bone densitometry to assess fracture risk. Hormone replacement therapy and bisphosphonates are recommended.

Disease-Modifying Antirheumatic Drugs. All patients with RA are candidates for DMARD therapy. DMARDs lack analgesic effect, and it may take weeks or months before any clinical benefit is recognized. They often only moderate the disease process, and some level of chronic inflammation usually persists. The disease generally recurs after the drug is discontinued. These agents may affect laboratory tests that measure acute-phase reactants and most have now been shown to slow the rate of progression of joint erosions and disability (30–32).

Antimalarial Drugs. Antimalarials (chloroquine and hydroxychloroquine) are commonly used drugs with a favorable toxicity/benefit profile. Chloroquine is more popular in Europe and appears to be more potent but more toxic than hydroxychloroquine (33), which is often used in early mild disease and as background therapy when another DMARD is started. There is no data to prove that hydroxychloroquine alone reduces or prevents radiographic damage from RA. Although very uncommon in the doses used in treating RA (200–400 mg daily), hydroxychloroquine may rarely cause ocular toxicity. Opinions differ with regard to the appropriate frequency of monitoring; nevertheless, patients should undergo ophthalmologic examination before starting therapy, and semiannually thereafter (34).

Methotrexate. As a result of its favorable efficacy and toxicity profile, low cost, and predictable benefit, methotrexate has become the most commonly used DMARD for RA. More than 50% of patients taking methotrexate continue the drug beyond 5 years, longer than any other DMARD (35). At lower doses, methotrexate has immunosuppressive and significant antiinflammatory effects. Initial dosage is 7.5–10 mg/week; this may be increased to 25 mg/week.

Mucositis, bone marrow suppression, and hepatocellular injury are the primary toxicities associated with use of methotrexate. Concomitant use of trimethoprim/sulfamethoxazole and administration during a superimposed infection may increase the risk for bone marrow suppression. Less common complications include interstitial pneumonitis and fibrosis, nephritis, and neurocognitive impairment. Opportunistic infections may rarely occur. Many gastrointestinal symptoms can be avoided by the concomitant use of folic acid, or changing to parenteral administration. Clinically significant liver disease is less frequent when patients with preexisting liver disease, alcohol abuse, or hepatic dysfunction are excluded from treatment. Use of methotrexate in patients with renal insufficiency or on dialysis should be avoided.

Guidelines for monitoring patients with RA while on methotrexate have been established. Baseline tests for all patients prior to initiation of therapy should include a complete blood count (CBC), serum creatinine, liver tests, and hepatitis B and C serologies. Recommendations for monitoring for hepatic safety have been published (36). Women of childbearing age must be warned to practice effective birth control, as methotrexate has potential for teratogenesis.

Sulfasalazine. Sulfasalazine is a combination of a salicylate and a sulfapyridine molecule. In addition to an antiinflammatory effect due to its salicylate component, sulfasalazine appears to have immunomodulatory effects similar to those of methotrexate. It is frequently used in combination with other DMARDs. The usual starting dose is 500 or 1000 mg/day, raised slowly to 2 or 3 g/day over 4–6 weeks. Gastrointestinal symptoms are the most common side effects, and are often resolved with dose attenuation. Hematologic consequences may include aplastic anemia, agranulocytosis, or hemolytic anemia. Regular monitoring of the CBC is recommended.

Leflunomide. Leflunomide is a prodrug; its active metabolite is an inhibitor of an enzyme mediating synthesis of pyrimidines. It has significant inhibitory effects on proliferation of lymphocytes and has demonstrated efficacy in the management of RA. The rate of progression of radiographic damage during a 12-month study in patients taking leflunomide was comparable to those taking methotrexate (37). It takes about 7–8 weeks for this drug to reach steady-state levels in the blood. To decrease this time, a loading dose of 100 mg/day for 3 days is recommended, followed by a maintenance dose of 10–20 mg/day.

Adverse events include reversible alopecia, skin rash, stomatitis, diarrhea, and elevation in liver enzymes. Routine monitoring of CBC and liver tests are required. Leflunomide is teratogenic. It may take up to 2 years after discontinuation for complete elimination, during which time pregnancy should be avoided. Excretion may be achieved more quickly by giving cholestyramine (8 g) 3 times a day for 10–11 days.

Gold Compounds. Due to their effectiveness in suppressing synovitis, gold compounds were the most popular remission-inducing agents in the 1970s and early 1980s. Preparations currently in use are aurothioglucose, administered parenterally, and auranofin, an oral preparation that is less effective and rarely used. The exact mechanism of action has not been established, but it is postulated that gold compounds act at many points in the sequence of inflammatory events. The administration of intramuscular gold requires regular office visits to monitor for toxicity and efficacy. If there is a favorable response, therapy can be maintained with 50 mg/month.

The most common adverse effects are mucocutaneous reactions including stomatitis, pruritis, and various forms of dermatitis. Proteinuria may occur; it is usually mild, and rarely in nephrotic range. Leukopenia, thrombocytopenia, and aplastic anemia are rare but potentially fatal consequences. Blood counts and urinalysis should be performed prior to each injection during the first year of treatment. Due to their toxicity and existence of many new alternatives, gold compounds are less often used in today's practice.

Cytotoxic Drugs. Cytotoxic drugs, including azathioprine, cyclophosphamide, and cyclosporine, are generally reserved for patients with refractory RA who have failed conventional therapy. Despite their efficacy profile, use of these drugs in RA is limited due to their toxicity and existence of new alternatives. They should be reserved only for patients with aggressive disease and life-threatening extraarticular manifestations.

Biologic Agents. Tumor necrosis factor (TNF) is known to play a central part in the pathogenesis of RA. This pro-inflammatory cytokine triggers several important events that lead to the synovitis and tissue destruction exhibited in RA. It stimulates production of other pro-inflammatory cytokines, induces production of metalloproteinases, regulates cell proliferation and apoptosis, and increases expression of adhesion molecules.

In the past few years, 2 biological response modifiers capable of neutralizing TNF have been developed, tested, and approved for patients with RA. The anti-TNF drugs etanercept and infliximab inhibit inflammation by sopping up TNF before it reaches its cell-bound receptor. Etanercept is a genetically engineered molecule containing 2 human soluble TNF receptors attached to the Fc portion of the human IgG. The clinical utility of etanercept in adults with RA has been assessed in clinical trials involving more than 500 patients (38–41). Etanercept produced significant improvements in all measures of disease activity, including the rate of progression of joint damage. The recommended dosage for adults is 25 mg by subcutaneous injection twice weekly.

Infliximab is a chimeric (part-mouse, part-human) monoclonal antibody to TNF administered by intravenous infusion. Infliximab reduces inflammatory activity and improves quality of life (42), and in combination with methotrexate inhibits radiographic progression over one year in up to 50% of patients (43,44). Administration of methotrexate with infliximab significantly reduces the formation of antibodies directed against the murine portion (45). Infliximab is currently recommended for use only with concomitant methotrexate therapy.

Initiation of therapy with a TNF inhibitor should be accompanied by a complete physical examination and careful evaluation to rule out underlying infections. There have been reports of patients receiving these agents who developed opportunistic infections, including sepsis and disseminated tuberculosis, some of which were fatal. To date, overall tolerance to these agents has been acceptable. In the published trials, there were no serious adverse effects for either anti-TNF agent. Post-marketing surveillance data has yielded rare reports of demyelination with TNF inhibitors, although a true association remains to be determined. Injection site reactions consisting of erythema, itching, pain, or swelling are the most common adverse effects during administration of etanercept. These generally occur during the first month and do not preclude continuation of therapy. It is mandatory to withhold therapy in the setting of acute bacterial infection, resuming treatment only after the infection has resolved. Patients should be reminded to call their physician immediately if they develop any signs or symptoms of infection. Anti-DNA and anticardiolipin antibodies have been seen in patients receiving both therapies, but the significance has not been fully defined. There is no clear answer as to what level of disease activity would be most appropriate to initiate or discontinue TNF-blocking therapy. Due to their cost and restrictions in insurance coverage, the biologic agents have been used primarily in patients with RA whose symptoms are resistant to DMARD treatment.

Combination Therapy. The use of combinations of DMARDs when a single agent fails to control clinical symptoms of RA is generally accepted (46), although the most effective way of providing combination therapy is under debate. Some propose initiating treatment in a "step-up" approach by adding new agents in patients whose disease has failed to respond to a single drug, while others recommend beginning with combination therapy early in the disease and using a "step-down" method once disease is under control. Clinical trials have showed promising results with increased efficacy and acceptable toxicity using a triple combination of methotrexate, sulfasalazine, and hydroxychloroquine (47,48). Combinations of biologic agents with methotrexate have been studied and found to be beneficial as well. Further studies will determine the optimal clinical use of combination therapy.

REFERENCES

1. Heath CW Jr, Fortin PR. Epidemiologic studies of rheumatoid arthritis: future directions. J Rheumatol. 1992;32(Suppl):74–7.

2. Lawrence RC. Rheumatoid arthritis: classification and epidemiology. In: Klippel JH, Dieppe PA, editors. Rheumatology. London: Mosby-Year Book; 1994.

3. Mijiyawa M. Epidemiology and semiology of rheumatoid arthritis in third world countries. Rev Rhum Engl Ed 1995;62:121–6.

4. Guillemin F, Briancon S, Klein JM, Sauleau E, Pourel J. Incidence of rheumatoid arthritis in France. Scand J Rheumatol 1994;23:264–8.

5. Symmons DP, Barrett EM, Bankhead CR, Scott DG, Silman AJ. The incidence of rheumatoid arthritis in the United Kingdom: results from the Norfolk arthritis register. Br J Rheumatol 1994;33:735–9.

6. Gabriel SE, Crowson CS, O'Fallon WM. Mortality in rheumatoid arthritis: have we made an impact in 4 decades? J Rheumatol 1999;26:2529–33.

7. Prior P, Symmons DP, Scott DL, Brown R, Hawkins CF. Cause of death in rheumatoid arthritis. Br J Rheumatol 1984;23:92–9.

8. Wallberg-Jonsson S, Ohman ML, Dahlqvist SR. Cardiovascular morbidity and mortality in patients with seropositive rheumatoid arthritis in northern Sweden. J Rheumatol 1997;24:445–51.

9. Gabriel SE, Crowson CS, O'Fallon WM. Comorbidity in arthritis. J Rheumatol 1999;26:2475–9.

10. Stastny P. Association of the B-cell alloantigen DRw4 with rheumatoid arthritis. N Engl J Med 1978;298:869–71.

11. Silman AJ, MacGregor AJ, Thomson W, Holligan S, Carthy D, Farhan A, et al. Twin concordance rates for rheumatoid arthritis: results from a nationwide study. Br J Rheumatol 1993;32:903–7.

12. Nepom GT, Byers P, Seyfried C, Healey LA, Wilske KR, Stage D, et al. HLA genes associated with rheumatoid arthritis. Identification of susceptibility alleles using specific oligonucleotide probes. Arthritis Rheum 1989;32:15–21.

13. Ebringer A, Wilson C, Tiwana H. Is rheumatoid arthritis a form of reactive arthritis? J Rheumatol 2000;27:559–63.

14. Albani S, Carson DA, Roudier J. Genetic and environmental factors in the immunopathogenesis of rheumatoid arthritis. Rheum Dis Clin N Am 1992;18:729–40.

15. Van Eden W: Heat shock proteins as immunogenic bacterial antigens with the potential to induce and regulate autoimmune arthritis. Immunol Rev 1991;121:5–28.

16. Arend WP, Dayer JM. Inhibition of the production and effects of interleukin-1 and tumor necrosis factor alpha in rheumatoid arthritis. Arthritis Rheum 1995;38:151–60.

17. Fleming A, Crown JM, Corbett M. Early rheumatoid disease. I. Onset. II. Patterns of joint involvement. Ann Rheum Dis 1976;35:357.

18. Arnett FC, Edworthy SM, Bloch DA, McShane DJ, Fries JF, Cooper NS, et al. The American Rheumatism Association 1987 revised criteria for the classification of rheumatoid arthritis. Arthritis Rheum 1988;31:315–24.

19. Fuchs HA, Sergent JS. Rheumatoid arthritis: the clinical picture. In: Koopman WJ, editor. Arthritis and allied conditions. Baltimore: Williams & Wilkins; 1997.

20. Komusi T, Munro T, Harth M. Radiologic review: the rheumatoid cervical spine. Semin Arthritis Rheum 1985;14:187–95.

21. Koopman WJ, Schrohenberg RE. Rheumatoid factor. In: Utsinger PD, Zvaifler NJ, Ehrlich GE, editors. Rheumatoid arthritis: etiology, diagnosis and therapy. Philadelphia: JB Lippincott; 1985.

22. Kerstens PJ, Boerbooms AM, Jeurissen ME, Fast JH, Assman KJ, van de Putte LB: Accelerated nodulosis during long term methotrexate therapy for rheumatoid arthritis: an analysis of 10 cases. J Rheumatol 1992;19:867–71.

23. Egsmose C, Lund B, Borg G, Pettersson H, Berg E, Brodin U, et al. Patients with rheumatoid arthritis benefit from early 2nd line therapy: five year followup of a prospective double blind placebo controlled study. J Rheumatol 1995;22:2208–13.

24. Masferrer JL, Zweifel BS, Seibert K, Needleman P. Selective regulation of cellular cyclooxygenase by dexamethasone and endotoxin in mice. J Clin Invest 1990;86:1375–9.

25. Borgini MJ, Paulus HE. Rheumatoid arthritis. In: Weisman MH, Weinblatt ME, Louie JS, editors. Treatment of rheumatoid arthritis, 2nd ed. Philadelphia: WB Saunders (in press).

26. Simon LS, Weaver AL, Graham DY, et al. Anti-inflammatory and upper gastrointestinal effects of celecoxib in rheumatoid arthritis: a randomized controlled trial. JAMA 1999;282:1921.

27. Emery P, Zeidler H, Kvien TK, et al. Celecoxib versus diclofenac in long-term management of rheumatoid arthritis: randomized double-blind comparison. Lancet 1999;354:2106.

28. Bombardier C, Laine L, Reicin A, Shapiro D, Burgos-Vargas R, Davis B, et al. Comparison of upper gastrointestinal toxicity of rofecoxib and naproxen in patients with rheumatoid arthritis. N Engl J Med 2000;343:1520–8.

29. Kirwan JR. The effect of glucocorticoids on joint destruction in rheumatoid arthritis. The arthritis and rheumatism council low-dose glucocorticoid study group. N Engl J Med 1995;333:142–6.

30. Iannuzzi L, Dawson N, Zein N, et al. Does drug therapy slow radiographic deterioration in rheumatoid arthritis? N Engl J Med 1983;309:1023.

31. Weinblatt ME, Polisson R, Blotner SD, et al. The effects of drug therapy on radiographic progression of rheumatoid arthritis: results of a 36-week randomized trial comparing methotrexate and auranofin. Arthritis Rheum 1993;36:613–19.

32. Smolen JS, Kalden JR, Scott DL, et al. Efficacy and safety of leflunomide compared with placebo and sulfasalazine in active rheumatoid arthritis: a double-blind, randomized, multicentre trial. Lancet 1999;353:259–66.

33. Felson DT, Anderson JJ, Meenan RF. The comparative efficacy and toxicity of second-line drugs in rheumatoid arthritis. Results of two metaanalyses. Arthritis Rheum 1990;33:1449–61.

34. Bernstein HN. Ophthalmologic considerations and testing in patients receiving long-term antimalarial therapy. Am J Med 1983;75:25.

35. Alarcon GS, Tracy IC, Blackburn WD Jr. Methotrexate in rheumatoid arthritis. Toxic effects as the major factor in limiting long-term treatment. Arthritis Rheum 1989;32:671–6.

36. Kremer JM, Alarcon GS, Lightfoot RW Jr, Willkens RF, Furst DE, Williams HJ, et al. Methotrexate for rheumatoid arthritis: suggested guidelines for monitoring liver toxicity. Arthritis Rheum 1994;37:316–28.

37. Sharp JT, Strand V, Leung H, Hurley F, Loew-Friedrich I. Treatment with leflunomide slows radiographic progression of rheumatoid arthritis: results from three randomized controlled trials of leflunomide in patients with active rheumatoid arthritis. Arthritis Rheum 2000;43:495–505.

38. Moreland LW, Baumgartner SW, Schiff MH, Tindall EA, Fleischmann RM, Weaver AL, et al. Treatment of rheumatoid arthritis with a recombinant human tumor necrosis factor receptor (P75)-Fc fusion protein. N Engl J Med 1997;337:141–7.

39. Moreland LW, Schiff MH, Baumgartner SW, Tindall EA, Fleischmann RM, Bulpitt KJ, et al. Etanercept therapy in rheumatoid arthritis. A randomized, controlled trial. Ann Intern Med 1999;130:478–86.

40. Weinblatt ME, Kremer JM, Bankhurst AD, Bulpitt KJ, Fleischmann RM, Fox RI, et al. A trial of etanercept, a recombinant tumor necrosis factor receptor:Fc fusion protein, in patients with rheumatoid arthritis receiving methotrexate. N Engl J Med 1999;340:253–9.

41. Bathon JM, Martin RW, Fleischmann RM, Tesser JR, Schiff MH, Keystone EC, et al. A comparison of etanercept and methotrexate in patients with early rheumatoid arthritis. N Engl J Med 2000;343:1586–93.

42. van der Heide A, Jacobs JW, Bijlsma JW, Heurkens AH, Booma-Frankfort C, van der Veen MJ, et al. The effectiveness of early treatment with second-line antirheumatic drugs. A randomized, controlled trial. Ann Intern Med 1996;124:699–707.

43. Lipsky PE, van der Heijde DM, St Clair EW, Furst DE, Breedveld FC, Kalden JR, et al. Infliximab and methotrexate in the treatment of rheumatoid arthritis. N Engl J Med 2000;343:1594–602.

44. Maini R, St Clair EW, Breedveld F, Furst D, Kalden J, Weisman M, et al. Infliximab (chimeric anti-tumor necrosis factor alpha monoclonal antibody) versus placebo in rheumatoid arthritis patients receiving concomitant methotrexate: a randomized phase III trial. ATTRACT study group. Lancet 1999;354(9194):1932–9.

45. Maini RN, Breedveld FC, Kalden JR, et al. Therapeutic efficacy of multiple intravenous infusions of anti-tumor necrosis factor a monoclonal antibody combined with low-dose weekly methotrexate in rheumatoid arthritis. Arthritis Rheum 1998;41:1552–63.

46. Pincus T, O'Dell JR, Kremer JM. Combination therapy with multiple disease-modifying anti-rheumatic drugs in rheumatoid arthritis: a preventive strategy. Ann Intern Med 1999;131:768–74.

47. O'Dell JR, Haire CE, Erikson N, Drymalski W, Palmer W, Eckhoff PJ, et al. Treatment of rheumatoid arthritis with methotrexate alone, sulfasalazine and hydroxychloroquine, or a combination of all three medications. N Engl J Med 1996;334:1287–91.

48. O'Dell J, Leff R, Paulsen G, Haire C, Mallek J, Eckhoff PJ, et al. Methotrexate(M)-Hydroxychloroquine(H)-Sulfasalazine(S) versus M-H or M-S for rheumatoid arthritis: results of a double-blind study. Arthritis Rheum 1999;42:S117.

Connective Tissue Diseases

ROSALIND RAMSEY-GOLDMAN, MD, DrPH

The term *connective tissue disease* describes a group of systemic rheumatic syndromes that share similar clinical and pathologic features of widespread inflammation. These diseases are associated with antinuclear antibodies and immune-mediated tissue damage. The connective tissue diseases share a defect of the immune system characterized by a loss of tolerance to self-antigens resulting in the development of antibodies that are directed at nucleic acids and other intracellular proteins. The connective tissue diseases are often referred to as autoimmune diseases. The basic cause of the defective immunity in these diseases is uncertain, but likely involves an interaction between genetic factors and presumed, as yet unidentified, environmental agents. The prevalence, sex, peak age distributions, and primary organ systems affected in the major connective tissue diseases are displayed in Table 1.

SYSTEMIC LUPUS ERYTHEMATOSUS

Systemic lupus erythematosus (SLE) is a chronic inflammatory autoimmune disease that occurs predominantly in women during their childbearing years. The disease course is marked by exacerbations and remissions. The clinical spectrum of SLE is wide and ranges from a benign, easily treated disease with rash, arthritis, and fatigue to a very severe and life-threatening illness with progressive nephritis leading to renal failure or irreversible central nervous system damage (Table 2) (1–3). Treatment is directed towards reversing inflammation, and if present, coagulopathies. The overall therapeutic goals are to prevent organ damage, relieve symptoms, and minimize long-term toxicity from medications.

Diagnosis

Diagnosis is not difficult when many typical symptoms and signs are present, but it may be problematic when the disease manifests as only a few complaints or when problems occur over time. The diagnosis is made largely on clinical grounds with the support of laboratory tests. Criteria have been developed for disease classification and were revised in 1997 (2). Although these criteria were established primarily for research purposes, they serve as useful reminders of those features that distinguish lupus from other connective tissue diseases. However, it is important to remember that the range of clinical manifestations in SLE is much greater than the 11 classification criteria and that disease severity may vary widely, even in patients with the same clinical criteria.

Clinical Features

Specific skin rashes seen in lupus include malar, discoid, and subacute lesions. Acute inflammatory rashes occur over the malar regions of the face, known as the "butterfly rash" (Figure 1, left); between the interphalangeal joints of the fingers; or on areas of the trunk or the upper extremities. Chronic, scarring rashes, termed *discoid lupus*, may develop and have a predilection for the face, scalp, ears, and upper extremities (Figure 1, right). Subacute lesions are typically symmetric and widespread in distribution, resembling psoriatic lesions, or the scaly

Table 1. Epidemiology of the connective tissue diseases.

	Prevalence* (female:male)	Peak ages (years)	Primary organs affected
Systemic lupus erythematosus	15–50 (10:1)	15–40	Skin, kidneys, joints, central nervous system
Scleroderma	10–20 (5:1)	30–50	Skin, lungs, kidneys, gastrointestinal tract
Inflammatory myopathy	5–10 (3:1)	5–15 and 30–50	Muscle, lungs, skin
Sjögren's syndrome	10–40 (9:1)	30–50	Exocrine glands

* Per 100,000 population.

Table 2. Clinical and laboratory findings in systemic lupus erythematosus.*

Constitutional signs	Musculoskeletal
Fever	**Arthritis**/arthralgia
Fatigue	Subcutaneous nodules
Anorexia	Myositis
Weight loss	Osteonecrosis
Myalgias	Deforming arthropathy (Jaccoud's)
	Osteoporosis
Mucocutaneous	**Cardiopulmonary**
Photosensitivity	**Pleuritis/pericarditis**
Malar rash	Endocarditis (Libman-Sacks)
Oral/nasal ulcers	Pneumonitis
Discoid rash	Raynaud's phenomenon
Alopecia	Thrombophlebitis
Xerostomia/xerophthalmia	Coronary artery disease
Renal	**Neurologic/psychiatric**
Active urine sediment (nephritis)	**Seizures**
Proteinuria (nephropathy)	Stroke syndromes
Renal vein thrombosis	Movement disorders
	Psychosis
	Cognitive dysfunction
Hematology	**Immunologic studies**
Lymphopenia or leukopenia	**Antinuclear antibody**
Anemia/**hemolytic anemia**	**Lupus anticoagulant**
Thrombocytopenia	**Anti-DNA and Anti-Sm**
False positive STS	**Antiphospholipid antibodies**
Increased PTT	Depressed serum complement levels

* Criteria for classification of systemic lupus erythematosus developed by the American College of Rheumatology are indicated in bold print (Arthritis Rheum 1982;25:1271–1277, and Arthritis Rheum 1997;40:1725). STS = serologic test for syphilis; PTT = partial thromboplastin time.

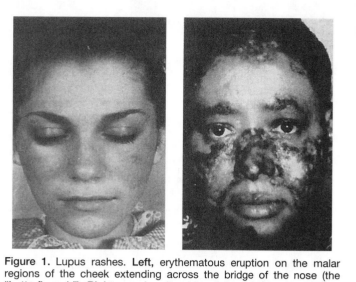

Figure 1. Lupus rashes. **Left,** erythematous eruption on the malar regions of the cheek extending across the bridge of the nose (the "butterfly rash"). **Right,** scarring discoid rash involving malar distribution. Reprinted from the Clinical Slide Collection on the Rheumatic Diseases, copyright 1995. Used by permission of the American College of Rheumatology.

papules may coalesce to form annular rings. Most specific lupus rashes are photosensitive. There are also many nonspecific cutaneous manifestations in lupus, including alopecia, oral ulcers, periungual erythema, livedo reticularis, urticaria, and panniculitis.

The most frequent pattern of arthritis seen in SLE is a symmetric polyarthritis that can resemble rheumatoid arthritis (RA). In contrast to RA, however, 10% of SLE patients develop a nonerosive, deforming arthropathy of the hands referred to as *Jaccoud's arthropathy*, which develops as a consequence of recurrent inflammation of tendons and other supporting structures of the joints. The deformities are easily reducible, and bone erosions are not evident on radiographs of the hands. Persistent monarthritis, particularly of the shoulders, hips, or knees, suggests osteonecrosis (avascular necrosis), or less commonly, septic arthritis (4). Tenosynovitis has been noted in up to 13% of patients (4). Both cortical and trabecular bone loss have been documented in lupus patients, putting them at risk for osteoporosis. Prevalence estimates of low bone mineral density range from 5–40%; in one study, self-reported symptomatic fractures in a lupus cohort occurred 5 times more often than expected when compared with population-based controls (5).

Hematologic manifestations of SLE include anemia, leukopenia, and thrombocytopenia. Most blood count abnormalities are mild and do not result in clinical problems. Such severe abnormalities as acute hemolytic anemia or aplastic anemia and severe thrombocytopenia with platelet counts <50,000/mm^3 are rare.

Cardiopulmonary manifestations include the common symptoms of pleurisy and pericarditis. Chronic interstitial inflammation can lead to pulmonary fibrosis. Valvular abnormalities have been noted in up to 25% of patients, but cause clinical complications infrequently. An increasing frequency of coronary artery disease has been noted as lupus patients live longer. The pathogenesis of accelerated atherosclerosis in these patients is likely to be multifactorial, relating to underlying vascular inflammation and arterial wall injury, adverse effects of corticosteroids, the high prevalence of renal disease and

hypertension, and an increased thrombosis risk in the setting of antiphospholipid antibodies (6).

Although many patients with lupus have some glomerular abnormality, clinically apparent nephritis develops in approximately 50% of patients (7). In most patients, the presence of lupus nephritis is first detected on routine screening studies with abnormal findings on urinalysis and/or elevations of the blood urea nitrogen (BUN) or serum creatinine. The extent of the evaluation required depends on the type and degree of abnormalities found. For example, the finding of low-grade proteinuria on dipstick (trace to 1+) and occasional red or white blood cells is generally a sign of mild renal disease that can be closely followed without the need for extensive evaluation or change in drug therapy. On the other hand, higher levels of proteinuria, greater numbers of cellular elements (particularly cellular casts) in the spun urinary sediment, or clinical signs of renal disease, such as peripheral edema or hypertension, clearly indicate the need for a thorough evaluation to determine appropriate drug treatment.

A renal biopsy is usually required to determine whether proliferative changes are mild (mesangial or focal proliferative nephritis) or severe (diffuse proliferative nephritis), or whether membranous nephropathy is present. From a prognostic standpoint, the biopsy is helpful in documenting glomerular sclerosis or tubulointerstitial disease, so-called chronicity features associated with an increased risk of end-stage renal failure (8).

The range of potential neuropsychiatric manifestations in patients with lupus is extensive (9). Clinical findings of central nervous system involvement include organic brain syndromes, psychoses, seizures, stroke syndromes, transverse myelitis, and headaches. Minor psychiatric disorders such as depression or disturbances of mental function are frequent, yet in many patients it may be difficult to determine if they are secondary to underlying SLE, treatment, or to the stresses associated with chronic illness. Peripheral nervous system syndromes include motor or sensory polyneuropathies, mononeuritis multiplex, and rarely, Guillain-Barré syndromes. The evaluation of patients with neurologic or psychiatric illnesses is complicated by the frequent failure to detect any abnormalities on routine testing with lumbar puncture, electroencephalograms, and magnetic resonance or computerized tomography scans.

Management

The foundation for managing SLE is lifelong monitoring to detect flares of disease early and to institute prompt, appropriate therapy. Because of the complexity and unpredictability of the disease process, all patients need education, counseling, and support. Patients should be seen regularly, and a complete blood count, platelet count, serum creatinine, and urinalysis should be routinely performed. In those with known renal disease, 24-hour urine collection for protein, serum creatinine, cholesterol, calcium phosphorus, alkaline phosphatase, sodium, and potassium levels should also be checked every 1–3 months, or more often if the patient is unstable. In many patients, it may be helpful to monitor serum complement levels and anti-dsDNA antibodies at regular intervals. Guidelines for referral and management of SLE in adults have been published by the American College of Rheumatology (10).

Patients should be advised to avoid intense sun exposure and to regularly use sunscreens. If rashes are present, topical applications of corticosteroid preparations are often helpful, and discoid lesions may be injected directly with long-acting corticosteroid suspensions. Antimalarial drugs, particularly hydroxychloroquine, are recommended in patients with generalized lupus rashes or rashes that fail to fully respond to topical corticosteroids. Options for drug therapy for patients with refractory rashes include antimalarial combinations (hydroxychloroquine, chloroquine, quinacrine), dapsone, retinoids, azathioprine, thalidomide, and low-dose oral corticosteroids. Monitoring for toxicity of medications is essential (10).

The arthritis of SLE responds well to nonsteroidal anti-inflammatory drug (NSAID) therapy, low-dose corticosteroids, or hydroxychloroquine. However, oral weekly methotrexate may be needed to control joint symptoms in patients with chronic arthritis. Early physical and occupational therapy is important in patients with Jaccoud's arthropathy to prevent progression of malalignments and minimize functional disabilities.

Options for the medical management of osteonecrosis are limited. Corticosteroid usage should be minimized when possible; a steroid-sparing medication may be added if needed to control underlying lupus symptoms. Patients should be referred to experienced physical and occupational therapists for recommendations to reduce forces across the joint surfaces. Decompression core biopsy should be considered in patients in the early stages of the disease, as detected by magnetic resonance imaging scans. Patients with advanced osteonecrosis are candidates for total joint replacement.

Prevention of osteoporosis, especially in the setting of chronic corticosteroid use, includes limiting the dose and duration of corticosteroids, lifestyle modification, measurement of bone mineral density at the lumbar spine and hip every 1–2 years, and use of anti-resorptive medications as appropriate. Lifestyle modifications include avoiding smoking, limiting alcohol intake, starting and maintaining exercise, and ensuring adequate daily intake of elemental calcium (1200–1500 mg) and vitamin D (400–600 IU).

Severe hematologic manifestations can lead to serious complications requiring aggressive treatment with high-dose corticosteroids combined with intravenous cyclophosphamide. Additional treatment options for patients with severe thrombocytopenia include danazol, intravenous immune globulin, and splenectomy.

Drug therapy for lupus nephritis/nephropathy is determined by factors related to the prognosis and severity of the renal disease. In all patients with nephropathy, it is extremely important to aggressively control hypertension, use diuretics for fluid overload states, and treat hyperlipidemia with diet or drug interventions. Corticosteroids, typically moderate-to-high dose oral prednisone given in the morning, are the mainstay of initial drug therapy. Bolus intravenous methylprednisolone is often given at the start of therapy to rapidly control kidney inflammation, particularly in patients who are massively nephrotic or who have an extremely active urinary sediment with red blood cell casts. The dose of oral prednisone is gradually tapered after 4–6 weeks; the rate of reduction varies depending on how well the patient has responded and whether residual symptoms of SLE are present. In patients with diffuse proliferative glomerulonephritis, studies have shown that bolus intravenous cyclophosphamide reduces the risk of end-stage renal failure. Patients who develop end-stage renal failure are treated with hemo- or peritoneal dialysis and become candidates for renal transplantation.

Management of neurologic and psychiatric manifestations is

Table 3. Comparison of diffuse and limited scleroderma.

	Diffuse (%)	Limited (%)
Skin findings		
Telangiectasias	30	90
Calcinosis	5	50
Raynaud's	90	99
Musculoskeletal		
Arthralgias/arthritis	95	95
Tendon friction rubs	70	5
Myopathy	40	10
Gastrointestinal		
Esophageal dysmotility	80	80
Pulmonary		
Pulmonary fibrosis	70	30
Pulmonary hypertension	5	10–15
Renal crisis	10–15	0
Antinuclear antibodies	95	95
Anticentromere antibody	5	40–70
Anti-topoisomerase I (Scl-70)	25–50	10
Cumulative survival		
5 year	70	90
10 year	50	75

complex, with few therapeutic studies to guide treatment. The benefits of counseling, particularly in SLE patients with psychological disorders, have been demonstrated (11). Attention to standard neurologic practices, including anticonvulsant therapy for patients with seizures, anticoagulants for transient ischemia episodes, and acute and chronic stroke care, is important. Aggressive drug management with high-dose corticosteroids or bolus intravenous cyclophosphamide as used in lupus nephritis is indicated in acute settings in which vasculitis is suspected. Thrombotic thrombocytopenic purpura is a rare but important cause of neurologic disease in lupus patients, and represents the only clear, unequivocal indication for plasmapheresis.

For the first time since the 1970s, clinical trials are being conducted involving new indications for drugs with established use or new, targeted therapies based on advances in the understanding of the pathogenesis of lupus. Dehydroepiandrosterone (DHEA) may have steroid-sparing effects (12). The safety of estrogens as oral contraceptives or hormone replacement in patients with SLE is currently being investigated in an NIH-funded multicenter trial. Other options that may be useful for treating severe disease in the future include lymphocyte-specific immunosuppressive strategies, toleragens, and biologic modifiers that interfere with B cell activation and autoantibody production.

SCLERODERMA

Systemic sclerosis, or scleroderma, is a chronic disease characterized by degenerative, inflammatory, and fibrotic changes in the skin, blood vessels, joints and tendons, skeletal muscle, and the following internal organs: gastrointestinal tract, lung, heart, and kidney. The 2 major subtypes are diffuse cutaneous and limited cutaneous, based on clinical and serologic features and prognosis, as shown in Table 3 (13). Several other forms have also been recognized, including localized cutaneous and overlaps with other connective tissue disorders. Treatment is directed towards controlling symptoms; no therapy has definitively arrested progression of the disease.

Diagnosis

Diagnosis is aided by the pattern, severity, and tempo of cutaneous, vascular, and visceral involvement. In patients with diffuse scleroderma, there is a rapidly progressive, generalized skin thickening affecting the distal and proximal extremities and trunk. There is also an early tendency to develop internal organ involvement, particularly the intestinal tract, lung, heart, and kidney. In those with limited disease, skin thickening is restricted to the distal extremities and face. Limited scleroderma is often referred to as the CREST syndrome, which stands for typical clinical findings that can develop over many years: calcinosis, Raynaud's phenomenon, esophageal dysmotility, sclerodactyly, and telangiectasias. Localized scleroderma can occur in patches (morphea) or can follow a linear distribution. Visceral involvement does not occur in the localized forms. In some patients, scleroderma features overlap with other connective tissue disease, such as SLE or polymyositis.

Clinical Features

All patients with scleroderma experience Raynaud's phenomenon (14). Skin changes are first noted in the fingers in most patients. The skin goes through phases of early edema in which the skin is swollen, shiny, and taut, followed by a slowly progressive hardening. Hypo- and hyperpigmentation of the skin may also be seen. Ulcerations on the tips of the fingers from minor trauma are a nagging problem in many patients. Joint contractures result from fibrotic changes within tendon sheaths. Calcific deposits frequently ulcerate, yielding a white, chalky drainage, and secondary infections can ensue.

Gastrointestinal problems are extremely common in patients with scleroderma. Dysphagia, gastroesophageal reflux, or strictures of the esophagus may develop. The obstruction from the latter complication can be severe enough to require periodic dilatation. Bloating caused by dysmotility of the stomach or small bowel may lead to malabsorption. Dysmotility of the large bowel can lead to obstipation, rectal prolapse, or incontinence.

Several different types of lung pathologies are seen in patients with scleroderma, including diffuse inflammatory alveolitis, interstitial fibrosis, and pulmonary hypertension. The limiting symptom is dyspnea on exertion. In addition, scleroderma patients are at increased risk for the development of lung cancer.

Renal crisis usually occurs in the setting of early, worsening disease, manifesting as malignant hypertension, microangiopathy, visual disturbances, headache, or pulmonary edema (15). Rapidly progressive renal failure is a serious, life-threatening complication of scleroderma. Although rare, progressive renal failure can occur in the absence of hypertension.

Management

Supportive measures and monitoring for organ involvement are the mainstay of management. Organ-based therapy can be extremely beneficial (16). Regular soaking of the ulcers in an antiseptic solution, topical application of antibiotic ointment, and use of occlusive dressing is helpful; however, it may take weeks before ulcers fully heal. D-penicillamine may be beneficial in reducing diffuse, progressive skin involvement.

Treatment options for subcutaneous calcium deposits that develop on the hands and in periarticular tissues along bony eminences are limited. Nonsteroidal antiinflammatory drugs or oral colchicine may help reduce inflammation around the deposits; diltiazem, warfarin, and diphosphonates have been used with occasional success in patients with severe, progressive calcinosis. When calcific deposits ulcerate they can become secondarily infected, typically with staphylococcal species, and require antibiotic treatment. Surgical excision and drainage of large deposits should be reserved for patients with massive accumulations because of problems with wound healing and the high likelihood of recurrence.

Joint contractures should be aggressively treated with physical therapy. Surgical management of contracted fingers may improve appearances and decrease the development of digital ulcers, but may not result in improved function.

Mild Raynaud's symptoms are easily controlled with attention to such practical measures as adjusting the thermostat upward, avoiding exposure to cold, dressing warmly, using insulated mittens or gloves, and covering the head and neck. Patients who smoke should be strongly encouraged to quit. Battery-operated or chemical hand and foot warmers sold in sporting goods stores may help some patients. Warming hands in tepid water is usually an effective way to abort an attack. Biofeedback training may be helpful in patients who fail to respond to traditional conservative measures (17). Drug therapy should be reserved for patients with severe symptoms. Calcium channel blocking agents are often effective; however, the doses needed to improve symptoms are often associated with intolerable vasodilatory side effects such as headaches, flushing, dizziness, palpitations, or fluid retention. Other drugs helpful for severe, recalcitrant Raynaud's include prazosin or nitroglycerine preparations, used either as a paste applied to the digits or as a transdermal patch.

Dysphagia and gastroesophageal reflux require attention to such simple practical measures as elevating the head of the bed, avoiding alcohol and caffeinated beverages, and eating smaller, more frequent meals. However, antacids, proton-pump inhibitors, H2-receptor antagonists, and sucralfate used as a thick slurry prior to meals and at bedtime may be needed. If esophageal strictures develop, periodic dilatation is needed. Reducing the fiber and fat content of the diet helps minimize abdominal symptoms caused by dysmotility of the small bowel. Advanced involvement of the bowel leads to malabsorption and the need for oral liquid supplements or, in severe instances, intravenous hyperalimentation. Bacterial overgrowth may contribute to abdominal symptoms, including malnutrition, and should be treated with short, rotating courses of broad-spectrum antibiotics.

General measures of pulmonary care are important and include prevention of aspiration through the use of anti-reflux regimens, use of bronchodilators in patients with wheezing, administration of pneumovax, yearly influenza vaccinations, early treatment of respiratory infections, and strong encouragement for smokers to quit. Some studies suggest that intravenous cyclophosphamide may prevent progressive loss of lung function in patients with interstitial pulmonary fibrosis (18). Supplemental oxygen should be used as needed, and patients with advanced, end-stage disease are candidates for lung or heart-lung transplantation.

When renal crisis occurs, prompt and aggressive treatment of the hypertension using angiotensin-converting enzyme (ACE) inhibitors is critical (13). There is no role for cortico-

Table 4. Differential diagnosis of inflammatory myopathies.

Drug- and toxin-induced	Corticosteroids, colchicine, cimetidine, zidovudine (AZT), lovastatin, D-penicillamine, chloroquine, alcohol, heroin, cocaine
Endocrinopathies	Hyper- and hypothyroidism, acromegaly, Cushing's syndrome, Addison's disease
Electrolyte disturbances	Hypokalemia, hypercalcemia, hypocalcemia, hypomagnesemia
Neurologic diseases	Myasthenia gravis, amyotrophic lateral sclerosis, muscular dystrophy, Guillain-Barré syndrome, periodic paralysis
Infections	Viruses (influenza, coxsackie, HIV, adenovirus, hepatitis B, rubella), toxoplasmosis, trichinella, Rickettsia, bacterial toxins (staphylococcal, streptococcal, clostridia)

steroids, plasmapheresis, or immunosuppressive drugs in scleroderma renal crisis. Intravenous enalapril or short-acting oral ACE inhibitors may be used to acutely titrate the blood pressure to normal levels. Minoxidil is indicated in patients who fail to respond to maximum dosage of ACE inhibitors. Patients who progress to end-stage renal failure should be treated with hemodialysis (or peritoneal dialysis). The experience with renal transplantation in these patients is promising.

INFLAMMATORY MYOPATHIES

Patients with inflammatory myopathies present with proximal muscle weakness and a spectrum of clinical features. Two major forms of inflammatory myopathy are recognized: polymyositis and dermatomyositis (19). The syndromes differ clinically on the basis of whether rashes are present or absent. Differences in pathophysiology of the 2 disorders are thought to exist, with *polymyositis* regarded as a cellular-mediated immune process against muscle myofibrils, and *dermatomyositis* as an antibody-mediated injury of muscle capillaries. A third variant, called *inclusion body myositis*, has slightly different clinical features and unique findings on electron microscopy of muscle biopsy sections showing microtubular or filamentous inclusions. The inflammatory myopathies may develop in patients with other connective diseases (overlap syndromes) or may be associated with malignancy, especially dermatomyositis. In addition, there is an extensive differential diagnosis that must be considered in patients with proximal muscle weakness and suspected inflammatory myopathies (Table 4). Treatment for inflammatory myopathies should seek to control inflammation and prevent long-term damage to muscles, joints, and internal organs.

Diagnosis

Routine studies helpful in the evaluation of patients with suspected inflammatory myopathies include measurement of levels of various enzymes in the serum, electromyography, and muscle biopsy. Levels of creatine kinase and aldolase are sensitive markers of muscle inflammation. In addition, many patients have elevations of lactate dehydrogenase, serum glutamic-oxaloacetic transaminase, and serum glutamic-pyruvic transaminase and often mistakenly undergo assessments for liver disease. An electromyogram is helpful in discriminating between pure neurologic and myopathic disorders. However, muscle biopsy remains the only

means to establish the diagnosis with certainty. Magnetic resonance imaging and P-31 MR spectroscopy are developing technologies that may have a role in the diagnosis and management of these myopathies (20).

Clinical Features

Patients with inflammatory muscle disorders often present with weakness of the proximal muscles of the upper and lower extremities. Although muscle weakness is usually painless, myalgia and muscle tenderness may occur early in some patients with dermatomyositis. Patients commonly experience difficulties in performing simple functions like rising from a chair, climbing stairs, dressing, or grooming. The weakness may be of abrupt or insidious onset. Other muscle groups commonly affected include the neck flexors (such that the patient is unable to lift the head against gravity), muscles of the oropharynx or esophagus causing dysphagia, and diaphragmatic and intercostal muscles leading to dyspnea. Involvement of distal muscles is a late finding; impairment of distal muscles early in the disease course suggests inclusion body myositis. Ocular and facial muscles are essentially never involved in the inflammatory myopathies.

Constitutional symptoms, such as fever, chills, malaise, and weight loss may occur. A nonerosive arthropathy has been described with antibodies to transfer-RNA synthetases; the most common antibody found is directed against histadyl t-RNA synthetase (Jo-1).

Several distinctive rashes occur in patients with dermatomyositis. Scaly patches (*Gottron's papules*) form over the extensor surfaces of joints, most commonly over the proximal interphalangeal and metacarpophalangeal joints, elbows, and knees. The radial surfaces and pads of the fingers become dry and cracked with black pigment changes (mechanic's hands). Erythematous, often photosensitive rashes occur on the neck, shoulder, and upper chest (V sign or shawl sign), and on the malar region of the face. The facial rash can easily be confused with the butterfly rash of SLE; crossing of the nasolabial fold is a helpful physical finding that occurs in dermatomyositis. The upper eyelids may become edematous and develop a purplish (heliotrope) hue. Subcutaneous calcifications develop within muscle planes, particularly in childhood-onset dermatomyositis, and these may ulcerate, drain, and become secondarily infected.

Dyspnea in patients with inflammatory muscle disease may result from several different causes. Myositis of the diaphragm or intercostal muscles directly interferes with the mechanics of respiration; dysfunction of the pharyngeal muscles may result in aspiration; and involvement of the myocardium or cardiac conduction system leads to congestive heart failure. Interstitial alveolitis and progressive pulmonary fibrosis occur in a subset of patients, and are another manifestation associated with antibodies to transfer-RNA synthetases.

Management

Physical and occupational therapy play an important role in the evaluation and treatment of inflammatory muscle disease. In addition to providing assessments of muscle strength and functional assessments to help guide and monitor the response to therapy, active rehabilitation programs are a critical component of clinical care (21).

In most forms of inflammatory myopathy, therapy is initiated with high-dose corticosteroids, typically oral prednisone in doses of 1 mg/kg/day (22). The response to corticosteroids is often slow, and several weeks or more of therapy may be required before muscle strength begins to improve. Although corticosteroids remain the mainstay of treatment for the inflammatory myopathies, their use is complicated by many adverse effects. Other immunosuppressive agents, alone or in combination, are being increasingly used for patients with severe disease or treatment-related complications. In patients with very severe, acute disease, particularly those in whom constitutional signs are prominent, intravenous bolus methylprednisolone in doses of 1 gram or 15 mg/kg often provides more immediate benefit. Methotrexate, either oral or intramuscular, given weekly and/or azathioprine are recommended in patients who fail to completely respond to corticosteroids.

Pulmonary disease remains a serious source of morbidity and mortality in myositis patients. Cyclophosphamide, cyclosporine, and tacrolimus are efficacious in patients with interstitial lung disease.

Intravenous immunoglobulin is not only effective for the cutaneous complications of dermatomyositis but has been helpful in other extramuscular manifestations. In addition, for refractory cases, evaluation for and treatment of an underlying malignancy may lead to improvement in dermatomyositis. Patients with inclusion body myositis tend to respond poorly to drug therapy (23).

In most patients, specific therapies directed at the skin disease are not required, and rashes improve as the muscle inflammation comes under control. Hydroxychloroquine could be considered in patients with severe or progressive skin disease, particularly of the erythematous, photosensitive variety. If dysphagia is present, aspiration precautions are essential. Treatment approaches for osteoporosis prevention and photoprotection are similar to those described for SLE. Therapeutic strategies for calcinosis are identical to that described for similar clinical manifestations in scleroderma.

SJÖGREN'S SYNDROME

Sjögren's syndrome is a chronic disease with insidious onset characterized by an immune-mediated inflammatory process of the salivary, lacrimal, and other exocrine glands, as well as nonglandular organs (24,25). It is generally divided into primary and secondary forms based on whether or not another rheumatic disorder is present, such as rheumatoid arthritis or any of the other connective tissue diseases. Symptoms include dryness of the eyes, mouth, skin, vagina, and other tissues. The management of Sjögren's syndrome requires education, monitoring, and symptomatic therapy; no agent has been shown to slow disease progression.

Diagnosis

The diagnosis of Sjögren's syndrome is based on clinical symptoms of *xerostomia* (dryness of the mouth) and *xerophthalmia* (dryness of the eyes), and the presence of autoantibodies (26). Sjögren's syndrome must be differentiated from other disorders that affect the salivary glands (Table 5). Evaluation

Table 5. Diseases associated with parotid enlargement.

Viral infections (mumps, HIV, Epstein-Barr, others)
Sarcoidosis
Amyloidosis
Hyperlipoproteinemia
Endocrine disorders (acromegaly, diabetes mellitus, hypogonadism)
Chronic pancreatitis
Alcoholism/hepatic cirrhosis
Uremia
Tumors (especially lymphoma)

of patients with suspected Sjögren's syndrome may include biopsy of the minor salivary glands of the lip, functional tests of ocular or oral glands, and testing for autoantibodies. Minor salivary gland biopsy is the only reliable method to diagnose the disease with certainty. Typical pathology consists of focal aggregates of lymphocytes, plasma cells, and macrophages adjacent to and replacing the normal acini.

Schirmer's tear test is used to assess tear secretion by the lacrimal glands. *Keratoconjunctivitis sicca,* the sequelae of decreased tear secretion, is diagnosed using an aniline dye (Rose Bengal) that stains the damaged epithelium of both the cornea and conjunctiva. Slit lamp examination after Rose Bengal staining shows a punctate or filamentary keratitis.

Autoantibodies are commonly detected in patients with Sjögren's syndrome, in particular rheumatoid factors, antinuclear antibodies, and antibodies to extractable nuclear antigens, termed Ro (SS-A) and La (SS-B). These autoantibodies are not specific for Sjögren's syndrome and may be found in other autoimmune diseases, especially SLE.

Clinical Features

Most patients describe ocular and oral dryness; tenderness or swelling of the parotid glands may also be seen. Extraglandular features may have more acute symptoms, such as rash, dysphagia, Raynaud's phenomenon, arthralgias/arthritis, and myalgias. Systemic and major organ manifestations of Sjögren's syndrome are infrequent, but can include interstitial pneumonitis, glomerulonephritis, vasculitis, thyroid disease, and central or peripheral neuropathy. Lymphoproliferative disorders are suspected in patients with Sjögren's syndrome in the setting of persistent lymphadenopathy, asymmetric salivary gland enlargement, organomegaly, or new chest radiographic findings. However, the histologic distinction between pseudolymphoma and lymphoma may be difficult. When present, non-Hodgkin's lymphomas are primarily of B-cell origin.

Management

The treatment of Sjögren's syndrome is largely symptomatic with the goal of keeping the conjunctivae and mucosal surfaces moist. Artificial tears should be used regularly. Available preparations differ primarily in viscosity and preservative. The thicker, more viscous drops require less frequent application, although they can cause blurring and leave residue on the lashes. Less viscous drops require more frequent applications. Soft contact lenses may help protect the cornea, especially in the presence of filamentary keratitis; however, patients must be followed very carefully because of the increased risk of infection. Avoiding windy or low humidity environments is helpful. Cigarette smoking and drugs with anticholinergic side effects such as phenothiazines, tricyclic antidepressants, antispasmodics, and anti-Parkinsonian agents should be avoided whenever possible. In severe cases, punctal occlusion (sealing of lacrimal puncta) is an effective method for maximizing tear preservation.

Treatment of xerostomia is difficult. Most patients become aware of the importance of taking small sips of water frequently, and carry bottles of water with them at all times. Stimulation of salivary flow by chewing sugar-free gum or using lozenges is often helpful. Patients should be instructed to avoid dry food, smoking, or the use of drugs with anti-cholinergic side effects that decrease the salivary flow. Recently available muscarinic agonists may stimulate salivary flow in patients with residual gland function (27). Unfortunately, side effects (sweating, abdominal pain, flushing, increased urination) may limit their use. Periodontal disease and tooth decay are serious problems in patients with xerostomia; thus, patients should be reminded of the importance of brushing their teeth after meals. Topical treatment of the teeth with stannous fluoride enhances dental mineralization and retards damage. In cases of rapidly progressive dental disease, fluoride can be directly applied to the teeth from plastic trays that are used at night. Oral use of nystatin vaginal tablets may help oral pain and inflammation from oral candidiasis. Vaginal dryness is treated with lubricant gels, and dry skin with moisturizing lotions.

Constitutional symptoms, arthralgias/arthritis, and sicca symptoms have been treated with hydroxychloroquine and NSAIDs, but these have not been formally evaluated in clinical trials in Sjögren's patients. Corticosteroids and immunosuppressive drugs, such as oral or intravenous cyclophosphamide, are used for patients with severe, progressive extraglandular disease. Sjögren's patients are at increased risk for the development of lymphoma. Decisions regarding chemotherapy and/or radiation depend on the histologic type, location, and extension of the tumor, and should be guided by experienced oncologists.

The author of this chapter would like to acknowledge the contributions of John H. Klippel, MD, who wrote this chapter in the first edition and whose perspective continues to be reflected here.

REFERENCES

1. Mills J. Systemic lupus erythematosus. N Engl J Med 1994;330:1871–9.
2. Hochberg M. Updating the American College of Rheumatology revised criteria for the classification of systemic lupus erythematosus. Arthritis Rheum 1997;40:1725.
3. Ramsey-Goldman R, Manzi S. Systemic lupus erythematosus. In: Goldman M, Hatch M, editors. Women and health. San Diego: Academic Press; 2000. p. 704–23.
4. DiCesare PE, Zuckerman JD. Articular manifestations of systemic lupus erythematosus. In: Lahita RG, editor. Systemic lupus erythematosus. 3rd ed. San Diego: Academic Press; 1999. p. 793–812.
5. Ramsey-Goldman R, Dunn JE, Huang CF, Dunlop D, Rairie JE, Fitzgerald S, Manzi S. Frequency of fractures in women with systemic lupus erythematosus: comparison with United States population data. Arthritis Rheum 1999;42:882–90.
6. Manzi S. Systemic lupus erythematosus: a model for atherogenesis? Rheumatology 2000;39:353–9.
7. Huong DL, Papo T, Beaufils H, Wechsler B, Bletry O, Baumelou A, et al. Renal involvement in systemic lupus erythematosus. A study of 180 patients from a single center. Medicine (Baltimore) 1999;78:148–66.
8. Esdaile JM, Abrahamowicz M, MacKenzie T, Hayslett JP, Kashgarian M. The time-dependence of long-term prediction in lupus nephritis. Arthritis Rheum 1994;37:359–68.
9. The American College of Rheumatology nomenclature and case definitions for neuropsychiatric lupus syndromes. Arthritis Rheum 1999;42:599–608.
10. Guidelines for referral and management of systemic lupus erythematosus in adults. American College of Rheumatology Ad Hoc Committee on Systemic Lupus Erythematosus Guidelines. Arthritis Rheum 1999;42:1785–96.
11. Maisiak R, Austin JS, West SG, Heck L. The effect of person-centered counseling on the psychological status of persons with systemic lupus erythematosus or rheumatoid arthritis: a randomized, controlled trial. Arthritis Care Res 1996;9:60–6.
12. van Vollenhoven RF, Park JL, Genovese MC, West JP, McGuire JL. A double blind, placebo-controlled, clinical trial of dehydroepidandrosterone in severe systemic lupus erythematosus. Lupus 1999;8:181–7.
13. Silman AJ. Scleroderma. Baillieres Clin Rheumatol 1995;9:471–82.
14. Klippel JH. Raynaud's phenomenon: the French tricolor. Arch Intern Med 1991;51:2389–93.
15. Steen VD. Scleroderma renal crisis. In: Steen VD, editor. Rheumatic disease clinics of North America. Philadelphia: WB Saunders; 1996. p. 861–78.
16. Pope JE. Treatment of scleroderma. In: Steen VD, editor. Rheumatic disease clinics of North America. Philadelphia: WB Saunders; 1996. p. 893–907.
17. Yocum DE, Hodes R, Sundstrom WR, Cleeland CS. Use of biofeedback training in treatment of Raynaud's disease and phenomenon. J Rheumatol 1985;12:90–3.
18. Steen VD, Lanz JK Jr, Conte C, Owens GR, Medsger TA Jr. Therapy for severe interstitial lung disease in systemic sclerosis. A retrospective study. Arthritis Rheum 1994;37:1290–6.
19. Plotz PH, Rider LG, Targoff IN, O'Hanlon TP. NIH conference: myositis: immunologic contributions to understanding cause, pathogenesis, and therapy. Ann Intern Med 1995;122:715–24.
20. Reimers CD, Finkenstaedt M. Muscle imaging in inflammatory myopathies. Curr Opin Rheumatol 1997;4:475.
21. Hicks JE. Rehabilitation of patients with myositis. In: Klippel JH, Dieppe PA, editors. Rheumatology. London: Mosby-Year Book; 1994. p. 6.15.4–6.
22. Oddis CV. Current approach to the treatment of polymyositis and dermatomyositis. Curr Opin Rheumatol 2000;12:492–7.
23. Leff RL, Miller FW, Hicks J, Fraser DD, Plotz PH. The treatment of inclusion body myositis: a retrospective review and a randomized, prospective trial of immunosuppressive therapy. Medicine (Baltimore) 1993;72:225–35.
24. Manthorpe R, Asmussen K, Oxhom P. Primary Sjögren's syndrome; diagnostic criteria, clinical features, and disease activity. J Rheumatol 1997;24(Suppl 50):8–11.
25. Parke AL. Sjögren's Syndrome. In: Goldman MB, Hatch MC, editors. Women and health. San Diego: Academic Press; 2000. p. 740–52.
26. Vitali C, Moutsopoulos HM, Bombardieri C. The European Community Study Group on diagnostic criteria for Sjögren's syndrome: sensitivity and specificity of tests for ocular and oral involvement in Sjögren's syndrome. Ann Rheum Dis 1994;53:637–47.
27. Vivino RB, Al-Hashimi I, Kahn Z, LeVeque FG, Salisbury PL 3rd, Tran-Johnson TK, et al. Pilocarpine tablets for the treatment of dry mouth and dry eye symptoms in patients with Sjögren's syndrome: a randomized, placebo-controlled, fixed-dose, multicenter trial. P92-01 Study Group. Arch Intern Med 1999;159:174–81.

Spondylarthropathies

ANTOINE HELEWA, PT, MSc (epid); and BARBARA STOKES, PT

The spondylarthropathies are a group of inflammatory joint diseases that have their main effects on the axial skeleton. The primary disorder of this group is ankylosing spondylitis, and other conditions in the group include reactive arthritis (the most common example being Reiter's syndrome), psoriatic arthritis, and juvenile ankylosing spondylitis. All the diseases in this group show a tendency to occur in families. The serologic test for rheumatoid factor is characteristically negative, however the histocompatability antigen HLA-B27 is positive in the majority of cases (1).

The prevalence rate of ankylosing spondylitis can vary from 0.2% in white Americans to 1.4% in Norwegians (2). The most frequently reported prevalence is 1 per 1,000 population, and men are disproportionately affected, with a 3:1 male:female ratio (3). Age of onset typically ranges from adolescence to 35 years, peaking around 28 years (2). Estimates of prevalence in Reiter's syndrome are difficult due to the nomadic nature of the young target population and underreporting of venereal diseases. In one study of a military population, Reiter's prevalence was estimated at 4 per 1,000 men per year (4).

ETIOLOGY AND PATHOGENESIS

The cause of the ascending inflammation in ankylosing spondylitis is unknown. Due to genetic and clinical similarities to Reiter's syndrome, etiologic models requiring both bacteria and HLA-B27 support the existence of an enteric pathogen (5). Ankylosing spondylitis begins as inflammation in the sacroiliac joints in nearly all patients, and spreads slowly up the spine. The inflammation affects all joint ligaments of the spine at insertion points into bone (*enthesitis*), as well as the synovium of the spinal arthrodial joints. Inflammation is associated with erosions at the enthesis, followed by a healing phase, transforming fibrous ligaments into bone. The process ends in bony fusion or ankylosis. Inflammation of peripheral entheses is commonly seen at the insertion of the Achilles tendon and plantar fascia on the os calcis, leading to the formation of a painful bony spur. Enthesitis at the patellar tendon insertion is common in young male patients. Peripheral spinal joints are sometimes involved, exhibiting rheumatoid-like synovitis, and are more likely to develop into bony ankylosis than in rheumatoid arthritis (RA).

Reiter's syndrome can be induced by such microbial pathogens as *Shigella, Salmonella,* and *Chlamydia.* The arthropathy of Reiter's is typically acute and asymmetric, involving the toes, ankles, and knees, then ascending to the upper extremities and the axial skeleton (6). Enthesitis, another distinctive feature, commonly affects the sites of insertion of the Achilles tendon and plantar fascia (as in ankylosing spondylitis), as well as the symphysis pubis, iliac crest, greater trochanter, and the anterolateral ribs.

CLINICAL FEATURES AND DIAGNOSIS

The onset of ankylosing spondylitis is insidious; patients in the early stages may not be able to recall exactly when symptoms began or the location of the pain. Reports of alternating pain in one buttock then the other, radiating down the thigh, is indicative of sacroiliitis but is often misdiagnosed as hip disease or sciatica. In contrast to mechanical low back pain, low back pain and stiffness in ankylosing spondylitis patients are worse after a period of rest or on waking up in the morning (the gel phenomenon) and improve after exercise, a hot bath, or a shower.

Initially, stiffness may be due to muscle spasm associated with underlying joint inflammation. In the later stages, however, the apophyseal joints may develop fibrous or bony ankylosis, and fusion between vertebrae may limit all movements of the spine to a few degrees of flexion or extension in the upper cervical region (1). An early abnormality revealed on physical examination is tenderness on palpation of the sacroiliac joints, or pain in the same area following hip hyperextension. The straight leg-raising test is negative, and deep tendon reflexes are normal (7,8).

More objective findings occur with longer disease duration, showing loss of lumbar lordosis and restrictions of movements in all planes of the lumbar spine. Schöber's test of lumbar flexion is significantly reduced and the patient is unable to touch fingers to floor by a considerable distance. With ascending spinal inflammation, chest expansion is reduced due to costovertebral joint fusion, and the normal kyphosis of the thoracic spine is accentuated, resulting in a stooped-shoulder appearance. Eventually the inflammation spreads to the cervical spine and is followed by a decreased ability to extend and rotate the neck (Table 1).

Early radiologic changes in the sacroiliac joints may consist of blurring of the joint margins, with erosive changes and sclerosis of the underlying bone. Later, the sclerosis becomes more marked, and there is narrowing of the joint space as cartilage is lost. In the later stages, the sacrum and ilium are joined by bony fusion. There is squaring of the vertebral bodies of the lumbar spine and the development of erosions at the anterior margins. The periphery of the annulus fibrosis becomes calcified and then ossified, and the vertebral bodies become linked with syndesmophytes. The ossification will extend to the posterior longitudinal ligament and the interspinous ligaments. In the final stages, these changes produce the radiologic appearance known as *bamboo spine* (Figure 1).

Nonarticular manifestations of ankylosing spondylitis in the early stages include features of systemic illness, such as fever, weight loss, fatigue, and sometimes a raised erythrocyte sedimentation rate (ESR). In other cases, iritis leading to scarring of the uveal tract with secondary glaucoma may be seen. Aortic insufficiency may develop in 10% of patients and pulmonary fibrosis in 5%.

Table 1. Comparison of rheumatoid arthritis and spondylarthropathies.*

Clinical characteristics	RA	AS	IBD	Psoriatic	Reiter's
M:F	1:3	3:1	1:1	1:1	10-20:1
Genetic	HLA-Dw4	HLA-B27	HLA-B27 with spondylitis only		HLA-B27
Distribution (joints)	Symmetric Peripheral	Axial and hips Peripheral	AS-like	AS-like and/or RA-like, or DIPs only	AS-like and/or RA-like
Sacroiliac involvement	None	Symmetric	Symmetric	Usually asymmetric	
Eye	Episcleritis Scleritis	Uveitis	Uveitis Episcleritis Conjunctivitis	Conjunctivitis Episcleritis Iritis	Conjunctivitis Uveitis Keratitis
Rash	Vasculitis (rare)	None	Erythema nodosum	Psoriasis	Keratoderma
Rheumatoid factor	>80%	<15%	<5%	<5%	<5%

* Reprinted from Association of Rheumatology Health Professionals Teaching Slide Collection, copyright 1997. RA = rheumatoid arthritis; AS = ankylosing spondylitis; IBD = inflammatory bowel disease.

In chronic Reiter's syndrome, sacroiliitis of the lower half of one or both sacroiliac joints is seen in 40–60% of cases (6). This progresses to "pseudo widening" with eventual bony proliferation, sclerosis, and ankylosis. Isolated involvement of the lumbar or thoracic spine may be the initial radiographic finding. Involvement of the cervical spine is uncommon.

Currently accepted criteria for diagnosis of ankylosing spondylitis are based on the New York criteria, modified in 1986, which require the presence of radiographic sacroiliitis and one or more of the clinical symptoms and signs (9).

American College of Rheumatology (ACR) criteria for the diagnosis of Reiter's syndrome are less stringent, reflecting the fact that as many as two-thirds of patients who appear to have the disease do not manifest the classic triad of arthritis, urethritis, and conjunctivitis (10). ACR criteria require the presence of peripheral arthritis of more than one month's duration, occurring in association with urethritis and/or cervicitis (11).

ASSESSMENT

History of Current Illness

Because radiographs are often inconclusive in the early stages of disease, tissue typing is not done routinely, and laboratory tests do not confirm the diagnosis, the history of the illness provides significant clues for diagnosis of spondylarthropathy.

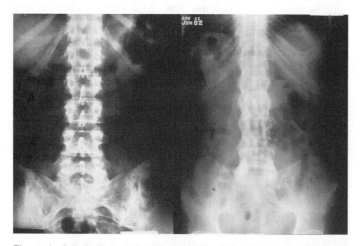

Figure 1. Ankylosing spondylitis: bamboo spine. Reprinted from Association of Rheumatology Health Professionals Teaching Slide Collection, copyright 1997.

Patients with ankylosing spondylitis characteristically report low back pain and stiffness, which can be differentiated from other noninflammatory low back pain by its onset before age 40; insidious, persistent nature; association with morning stiffness; and improvement with exercise (12). Patients may also report chest pain in the costovertebral region of midthoracic areas.

In Reiter's syndrome, the onset is more often acute and is usually associated with asymmetric peripheral joint involvement. Psoriatic arthropathy is variable in its onset; the presence of sacroiliitis is less common and skin or nail involvement is nearly always present.

Painful redness of the eye can occur as acute anterior uveitis in ankylosing spondylitis and conjunctivitis in Reiter's syndrome. Eye involvement is less common in psoriatic arthritis.

In this group of diseases, family history is frequently positive for inflammatory low back pain and other related syndromes, such as inflammatory bowel disease or psoriasis.

Physical and Functional Assessment

Prior to initiation of a treatment program, a full physical and functional assessment is essential to determine the extent of spinal and peripheral joint involvement and to establish a baseline for monitoring the progress of the disease and the response to treatment.

Several indices have been developed to measure physical function in the spondylarthropathies. These can be used in individual patients or as outcome measures of physical function in clinical trials (13–15). Of these, the Bath Ankylosing Spondilitis Functional Index (BASFI) has been shown to be more responsive than the Dougados Functional Index (DFI) and the AS-Specific Health Assessment Questionnaire (15,16). A recent review of 27 clinical trials using the BASFI and the DFI has shown that both are valid and reliable measures of functional capacity in ankylosing spondylitis; however, in physical therapy trials, the BASFI had better responsiveness than the DFI (17) (Table 2).

Two other indices were developed by the Bath group to measure impairment in ankylosing spondylitis: the Bath Ankylosing Spondylitis Disease Activity Index (BASDAI) and the Bath Ankylosing Spondylitis Metrology Index (BASMI). The BASDAI measures symptoms of fatigue, spinal pain, joint pain and swelling, tenderness, and morning stiffness using a visual analog scale. It is self-administered, quick and simple to use, reproducible, and responsive (18). The BASMI is a spinal

Table 2. Bath Ankylosing Spondylitis Functional Index.*

Please place a mark on each line below to indicate your level of ability with each of the following activities during the past week. (An aid is a piece of equipment that helps you perform an action or movement.)

1. Putting on your socks or stockings without help or aids (e.g., sock aid).

   easy —————————————————————————— impossible

2. Bending forward from the waist to pick up a pen from the floor without an aid.

   easy —————————————————————————— impossible

3. Reaching up to a high shelf without help or aids.

   easy —————————————————————————— impossible

4. Getting up out of an armless dining room chair without using your hands or any other help.

   easy —————————————————————————— impossible

5. Getting up off the floor from your back without help.

   easy —————————————————————————— impossible

6. Standing unsupported for 10 minutes without discomfort.

   easy —————————————————————————— impossible

7. Climbing 12–15 steps without using a hand rail or walking aid—**one foot on each step.**

   easy —————————————————————————— impossible

8. Looking over your shoulders without turning your body.

   easy —————————————————————————— impossible

9. Doing physically demanding activities (e.g., physical therapy exercises, gardening, or sports).

   easy —————————————————————————— impossible

10. Doing a full day's activities whether it be at home or at work.

   easy —————————————————————————— impossible

* Reprinted from reference 12, with permission of the Journal of Rheumatology.

mobility index that measures cervical extension using tragus-to-wall distance, lumbar flexion using the modified Schöber's test, cervical rotation using a gravity action goniometer, lumbar side flexion using fingertip-to-floor distance in sitting, and intermalleolar distance to measure bilateral hip abduction. This index was also shown to be reproducible and responsive to treatment effects (18).

In the clinical setting, several assessment measures can be used to assess spinal mobility including the Schöber test, Smythe test, fingertip-to-floor distance, tragus-to-wall distance, lateral flexion and trunk rotation, and intermalleolar distance. Whatever techniques are selected, it is important to standardize the measurement technique and to apply the method consistently, preferably at the same time of day and prior to any exercise the patient might do. Postural alignment, height, and chest expansion should be noted. Hip and shoulder range of motion should also be included, and inflammation or damage of any involved peripheral joints should be assessed (Figure 2).

MANAGEMENT

Pharmacologic Management

Nonsteroidal antiinflammatory drugs (NSAIDs) are usually prescribed in the early stages of ankylosing spondylitis for relief of pain and stiffness, to allow patients to carry out physical activities, or in preparation for exercise. Of the many available NSAIDs, indomethacin as a sustained relief preparation of 75 mg helps reduce night pain and morning stiffness. Naproxen, tolmetin, piroxicam, and diclofenac are also widely used (2). The cyclooxygenase-2 (COX-2) inhibitors celecoxib and rofecoxib are better tolerated than other NSAIDs, due to their lower gastrointestinal side effects.

Sulfasalazine, which reduces the levels of acute-phase reactants, may act as a "disease-modifying" agent. A recent study demonstrated that sulfasalazine achieved a significant improvement in joint pain, tenderness, and swelling in spondylarthropathy patients with peripheral arthritis, but not in patients with spinal manifestations (19).

Immunosuppressive drugs may be used in some severe cases, but their effectiveness has not been established in controlled trials. Infliximab, a biologic agent that blocks tumor necrosis factor (found in sacroiliac joint biopsies of spondylarthropathy patients), was shown to be effective in an open study of 11 patients with ankylosing spondylitis (20). Controlled clinical trials are underway to determine its long-range effects in preventing ankylosis.

Thermal and Other Modalities

Analgesic physical therapy modalities offer short-term relief of pain and muscle spasm lasting from one to several hours. They are often used as a warm-up to relieve muscle tightness in preparation for exercise or physical activities. These include superficial heat or cold in the form of moist hot or cold packs,

Patient's name_____ Date_____

POSTURE (observed in standing)	Yes	No
Hyperextension of cervical spine	___	___
Thoacic Kyphosis	___	___
Diminshed lumbar curve	___	___

RANGE OF MOTION (in cm)

CERVICAL SPINE	R	L
Flex. (chin -sternal notch)	___	___
Ext. (chin -sternal notch)	___	___
Rot. (chin-acromion process)	___	___
Lat. Flex. (tragus -acromion process)	___	___

THORACOLUMBAR SPINE

Flex. (fingertip-floor)	___

Smythe Test
- upper ___
- mid ___
- lower ___

Side flex. (stride sitting	R	L
Fingertip-floor)	___	___

MUSCLE STRENGTH

Muscle group	R		L
_____	_____		_____
_____	_____		_____
_____	_____		_____

** using modified sphygmomanometer

COMMENTS_____

A.M. stiffness _____ hr _____min

Chest expansion _____cm

Intermalleolar distance _____cm

ACTIVE JOINTS

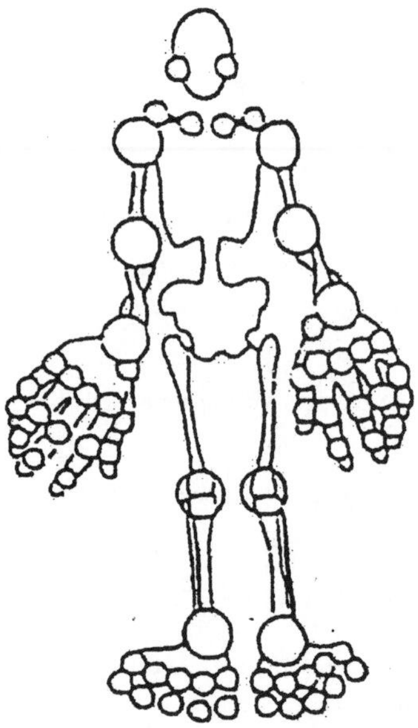

● = active joints
if range is limited, indicate degrees
adjacent to affected joint

Figure 2. Spondylarthropathy assessment form. Reprinted from Stokes B. Ankylosing spondylitis. In: Walker JM, Helewa A, editors. Physical therapy in arthritis. Philadelphia: WB Saunders; 1996, with permission of WB Saunders.

a hot shower or bath in the morning, and transcutaneous eletrical nerve stimulation (TENS). Controlled studies of these modalities on ankylosing spondylitis patients have not been reported. Although patients prefer hot packs, cold packs tend to be more effective when applied to actively inflamed joints.

TENS applied regionally for 30–45 minutes can help relieve pain, but it continues to be a controversial modality in patients with inflammatory arthritis, due to lack of evidence of effectiveness (21). Enthesitis of the Achilles tendon or plantar fascia may respond to local applications of ultrasound, but these effects have not been reported in clinical trials (see also Chapter 27, Physical Modalities).

Rehabilitation

The natural history of the spondylarthropathies is poorly defined and the course of the disease is unpredictable. There is no cure, and there is uncertainty as to whether the course of the disease can be altered. However, studies have shown that early

Table 3. Indications for proprioceptive neuromuscular facilitation techniques.

Indication	Technique
Acute pain/spasm affecting mobility	Hold-relax or rhythmic stabilizations
Chronic or no pain but limited mobility	Contract-relax or slow reversals followed by free active exercise
Decreased rib cage expansion	Slow reversals, resisting rib cage expansion with or without the stretch reflex
Poor postural habits	Rhythmic stabilizations
Limitations of strength	Resisted maximal slow reversals; repeated contractions using stretch, traction, and approximation
Decreased endurance	Low resistance slow reversals

rehabilitation can significantly reduce the impact of disability (22). Disease education, appropriate medical management, regular exercise, and activity modifications are the foundations of a self-management program. The program must be specific to the patient's needs and based on realistic and achievable goals that are mutually agreed upon.

Education about the disease, its manifestations, and appropriate management strategies are key to the development of a rehabilitation program. Due to the familial nature of these conditions, family members may benefit from involvement in the education program, and their participation may also enhance adherence (see also Chapter 23, Patient Education). The importance of self-monitoring, regular exercise, and the role of drug therapy must be emphasized, because the effects of the disease on posture, spinal mobility, and function tend to be insidious and slowly progressive. The patient must assume responsibility for monitoring clinical changes and participating in regular exercise.

Functional limitations are associated with duration of disease, so vocational counseling and job training for patients may reduce the likelihood of long-term disability (22). Workplace assessment and appropriate modifications—along with frequent position changes or stretch breaks—may enhance tolerance of work activities. In a retrospective chart review of 46 patients participating in a trial of the effects of physical therapy on ankylosing spondylitis, the most frequently reported functional difficulties were dressing, body transfers, lifting and carrying, and endurance (23).

A functional assessment can identify problems in activities of daily living (ADL) and lead to a problem-solving process to accommodate loss of motion and facilitate such activities as self care, work, mobility, and endurance. The use of assistive devices is indicated only if restriction of motion is present or safety is at issue. Long-handled devices for dressing and reaching, adjustable swivel chairs with lumbar support, and inclined writing surfaces can be helpful.

The value of teaching patients the principles of proper posture in standing, sitting, and lying cannot be underestimated. Poor posture contributes to fatigue, as even a slight forward inclination of the spine may inhibit the use of the extensor muscles. Exercise alone is not sufficient, and the patient should learn to employ good body mechanics in all daily activities.

Safety is a concern for individuals whose postural changes have affected their balance because of a displacement of the center of mass of the trunk (24). Preventing falls is important. The use of railings, grab bars, and safety mats should be considered for the bathroom. A walking device may assist where balance is impaired or where hip pain and limitation interferes with walking. Patients may have difficulty looking right and left when crossing roads and should use caution. Driving is a challenge to those with restricted neck motion. The seat and headrest should support the neck and back, and wide-angled mirrors can be installed for better peripheral vision (25).

Therapeutic Exercise

Therapeutic exercise, in combination with antiinflammatory therapy, is the cornerstone in the management of the spondylarthropathies. Studies have shown that exercise—whether done individually, in a group, in an inpatient setting, or in the home—improves mobility, posture, and function (23,26–29). There are no definitive answers as to which intervention results in better long-term outcomes or better cost-effectiveness, although one study suggests that there are advantages to group physical therapy through mutual encouragement, reciprocal motivation, exchange of experience, and socialization (30).

The current health care environment in North America does not provide for intensive inpatient therapy, nor does it support outpatient physical therapy over many months. Thus, it is imperative that instruction in self-monitoring and in appropriate self-administered exercise be provided by a skilled health professional. The exercises must respect the learning style and individual exercise preference of the patient. Clear written instructions with illustrations can be of great assistance to patients in remembering specific exercises and positioning.

Relief of pain and stiffness can be achieved by improving the mobility of the spine and involved peripheral joints, and should be undertaken prior to the introduction of a muscle-strengthening component. Spinal mobility may be reduced due to acute pain, muscle spasm, soft tissue contracture, or ankylosis. The large peripheral joints may be restricted due to enthesopathy, soft tissue contracture, or ankylosis, and can be a cause of significant functional limitation.

Before exercising, a warm shower or application of moist heat to the affected areas followed by light arm movement or walking is advised. Patients should plan to exercise at a time of day when they are least tired and have less pain.

Stretching exercises can lengthen the anterior short muscles of the neck, the muscles of the pectoral girdle, the spinal rotators, the hamstrings, and the hip adductors and flexors. Proprioceptive neuromuscular facilitation techniques and patterns were used effectively in one study (23). They can be applied to achieve relief of acute muscle spasm, limited mobility, decreased rib cage expansion, and decreased endurance, as well as to facilitate improved posture (31). The techniques may need to be modified to accommodate established deformity or painful peripheral joints. The techniques outlined in Table 3 will assist in selecting manually applied exercises, which can also be taught to a partner or adapted for the patient to self-administer.

At the beginning of treatment, modified proprioceptive neuromuscular facilitation techniques are emphasized, and a self-administered program of free, active exercise designed to increase mobility, strength, and endurance is introduced. The hands-on component can be decreased and the self-administered program increased over several weeks.

Postural change and inflammation of the costochondral joints may inhibit deep breathing. The use of heat and pain medication may be helpful in preparation for deep breathing exercises. Full rib cage expansion should be encouraged. Using a towel or the patient's own hands, resistance to expansion can be applied and the lower ribs pulled down towards midline on expiration.

Strengthening of the hip and back extensors can be addressed through therapist-applied exercise techniques, alteration of the exercise position, and increasing repetitions, speed, or the intensity of the exercise through the use of weights or elastic resistance materials.

The major muscle groups that require strengthening include the postural muscles, back and neck extensors, shoulder retractors, and hip extensors and abductors. If no peripheral joint inflammation is present, muscles can be strengthened through the use of exercise equipment in fitness facilities. Weight training equipment can be used for specific muscle groups, but the patient should be supervised, and the importance of maintaining an erect posture must be emphasized.

Exercise in water is an enjoyable activity to most patients and offers a number of advantages. Warm water (81–86° F or 27–30° C) can promote relaxation and reduce the discomfort of stretching through the assistance of buoyancy and the support offered to joints. It can strengthen muscles by providing resistance against buoyancy or turbulence or by the use of flotation devices. It also offers a cardiovascular conditioning benefit and can improve endurance. Patients with ankylosing spondylitis who have cardiac involvement are advised to have an exercise tolerance test and medical approval prior to undertaking a pool program. Avoidance of chlorinated pools may be necessary for individuals with psoriasis.

Posture

Maintaining or improving postural alignment is one of the primary treatment goals. Patients should understand the functions of the spine and the benefits of maintaining correct posture. It is important that they learn to monitor changes resulting from the disease process or the treatment program.

Fundamental assessment techniques, such as standing against a wall with heels, buttocks, and shoulders touching the wall, or maintaining the chin parallel to the floor while attempting to touch the occipital protuberance to the wall, provide a basis for monitoring changes. Checking body posture using mirror feedback or measuring body height on a regular basis are simple and fast methods to monitor body posture.

Patients should be educated about performing regular posture checks throughout the day, so they can learn to avoid positions that encourage a stooped posture, such as slouching in chairs or leaning over a work surface for prolonged periods. While working at a desk, posture checks and simple stretches should be carried out frequently. Working on a drafting table with a slight tilt from the horizontal may facilitate an upright posture.

Attention should be given to the sleeping position and the use of pillows. The patient should achieve as much extension of the cervical spine as possible and be provided with adequate support to painful or restricted areas without overuse of pillows. A commercially available contoured pillow that maintains cervical extension while supporting the head may be helpful. Advice from a health professional should be obtained with respect to neck support. Frequent position changes are recommended. Poor posture or sleep hygiene can lead to sleep disturbances (see also Chapter 38, Sleep Disturbance).

To assist with maintenance of hip extension, a 15-minute period of prone lying is recommended daily. If the patient is unable to lie flat in the prone position, a pillow or folded towel under the abdomen may help. Inability to turn the head to the side can be accommodated by placing a rolled towel under the forehead. Lying supine with the buttocks at the edge of the bed and hips extended is an alternative.

The reciprocal patterns of normal gait may be lost in ankylosing spondylitis due to stiffness and loss of spinal rotation or hip motion. Patients should be encouraged to maintain normal, reciprocal arm swing and rotational movements of the lower spine and pelvis.

LEISURE AND RECREATIONAL ACTIVITIES

Recreational activities and sports are often very important to patients with spondylarthropathies. While they are a useful adjunct to the management program, they do not replace therapeutic exercise.

Activities that enhance cardiovascular fitness are beneficial and should be explored with a knowledgeable health professional. Exercise considerations and precautions should be identified; some activities should generally be avoided, such as high-impact sports or those that encourage flexion. Because the spine is less able to absorb shock, there is greater risk of injury and fracture from a fall. Generally, sports activities that encourage spinal extension and rotation are advised. Swimming is an excellent choice because of the therapeutic properties of water; however, snorkels and masks may have to be used for breathing if neck movements are restricted. Badminton, walking, and cross-country skiing can be good choices. Some activities that result in a forward posture can be adapted; examples are shortening the golf swing or raising the handlebars on a bicycle.

Guidance should be provided in the selection of footwear to reduce the impact of some activities on the spine or to accommodate heel spurs. A warm-up period and a cool-down must be carried out to decrease the likelihood of injury and to help relieve stiffness. As mentioned above, a patient with cardiac involvement should be assessed by a physician prior to beginning an exercise/fitness program or sport. Straight Talk on Ankylosing Spondylitis, published by the Spondylitis Association of America, contains excellent guidance in selecting suitable recreational activities (32).

ADHERENCE

Accepting responsibility for managing one's own condition and adhering to the many recommendations regarding medication use, environmental and lifestyle modifications, and exercise can be challenging. This is compounded by the nature of the disease and its fluctuating, often unpredictable course. It is unrealistic to expect patients to adhere to a rigid, time-consuming, and often boring exercise program. An understanding of how to respond to changes in disease symptoms or postural changes by adjusting the exercise program is essential. The health professional, by educating patients and engaging them in the process, can provide them with the knowledge and skills to self-monitor and self-manage their condition.

A recent study (33) on exercise in ankylosing spondylitis showed that the individuals most likely to follow the treatment regime are those who believe exercise to be of benefit, are followed by a rheumatologist, and have a higher education level. Problem solving, negotiating, and respecting a patient's values and beliefs can be instrumental in enhancing adherence to treatment strategies and subsequently improving quality of life (34). Strategies for adherence to treatment regimes are addressed in greater detail in Chapter 41.

SURGICAL INTERVENTION

The most common surgical procedure required by patients with ankylosing spondylitis is total hip arthroplasty. A prospective review of 130 hip replacements showed a high success rate after a mean followup of 7.5 years (35). Occasionally, heterotopic bone formation around the prosthesis may require a course of postoperative radiation. Patients with severe postural deformities may require osteotomy of the lumbar spine, but this procedure is fraught with hazard. Spinal fusion may be necessary in cases of a painful pseudoarthrosis, or to stabilize an atlantoaxial subluxation.

RESOURCES

Patients adjusting to the demands of a chronic disease and the associated lifestyle modifications frequently need assistance in accessing appropriate information or programs to assist them in adhering to the treatment recommendations. There are disease-specific associations in the United States and Canada that provide excellent information in the form of books, pamphlets, videos, and audiotapes. A nominal fee is charged for membership and benefits include regular newsletters, bulletins, information about conferences, and new educational materials. The Ankylosing Spondylitis Association website, www.spondylitis.org, and The Arthritis Society (Canada) website, www.arthritis.ca, have information about resources and programs, and provide links to other arthritis-related organizations.

At the local level, patients need information about where to purchase equipment and supportive footwear and the locations of recreational facilities and warm pools. They may also need information on how to access financial assistance or disability benefits.

REFERENCES

1. Verrier-Jones J. Diagnosis and management of arthritic conditions. In: Walker JM, Helewa A, editors. Physical therapy in arthritis. Philadelphia: WB Saunders; 1996. p. 60–4.
2. Arnett FC. Ankylosing spondylitis. In: Koopman WJ, editor. Arthritis and allied conditions. Baltimore: Williams & Wilkins; 1996. p. 1198–9.
3. Will R, Edmunds L, Elswood J, Calin A. Is there sexual inequality in ankylosing spondylitis? A study of 498 women and 1202 men. J Rheumatol 1990;17:1649–52.
4. Noer HR. An experimental epidemic of Reiter's syndrome. JAMA 1966;198:693–8.
5. Mielants H, Veys EM, Groemaere S, Gothals K, Cuvelier C, Devos M. Gut inflammation in the spondyloarthropathies: clinical, radiologic, biologic and genetic features in relation to the type of histology: a prospective study. J Rheumatol 1991;18:1542–51.
6. Cush JJ, Lipskey PE. Reiter's syndrome and reactive arthritis. In: Koopman WJ, editor. Arthritis and allied conditions. Baltimore: Williams & Wilkins; 1996. p. 1211–2.
7. Blackburn WD Jr, Alarcon JS, Ball JV. Evaluation of patients with back pain of suspected inflammatory nature. Am J Med 1998;85:766–70.
8. Gran JT. An epidemiological survey of the signs and symptoms of ankylosing spondylitis. Clin Rheumatol 1985;4:161–9.
9. Bennett PH, Wood PH. Proceedings of the third international symposium on population studies of the rheumatic diseases. Amsterdam: Excerpta Medica; 1968.
10. Arnett FC. Seronegative spondyloarthropathies. Bull Rheum Dis 1987;37:1–12.
11. Wilkins RF, Arnett FC, Bitter T, Calin A, Fisher L, Ford DK, et al. Reiter's syndrome. Evaluation of preliminary criteria for definite disease. Arthritis Rheum 1981;24:844–9.
12. Van der Linden S, van der Heijde D. Ankylosing spondylitis. Rheum Dis Clin North Am 1998;24:663–76.
13. Calin A, Garrett S, Whitelock H, Kennedy LG, O'hea J, Mallorie P, Jenkinson T. A new approach to defining functional ability in ankylosing spondylitis: the development of the Bath Ankylosing Spondylitis Functional Index. J Rheumatol 1994;21:2281–5.
14. Dougados M, Gueguen A, Nakache JP, Mery C, Amor B. Evaluation of a functional index and an articular index in ankylosing spondylitis. J Rheumatol 1988;15:302–7.
15. Daltroy LH, Larson MG, Roberts WN, Liang MH. A modification of the Health Assessment Questionaire for the spondyloarthropathies. J Rheumatol 1990;17:946–50.
16. Ruof G, Sangla O, Stucki G. Comparative responsiveness of 3 functional indices in ankylosing spondylitis. J Rheumatol 1999;26:1959–63.
17. Ruof G, Stucki G. Comparison of the Dougados Functional Index and the Bath Ankylosing Spondylitis Functional Index. A literature review. J Rheumatol 1999;26:955–60.
18. Calin A. The individual with ankylosing spondylitis: defining disease status and the impact of illness. Br J Rheumatol 1995;34:663–72.
19. Clegg DO, Reda DJ, Abdellatif M. Comparison of sulfasalazine and placebo for the treatment of axial and peripheral articular manifestations of the seronegative spondylarthropathies: a Department of Veterans Affairs cooperative study. Arthritis Rheum 1999;42:2325–9.
20. Brandt J, Haibel H, Cornely D, Golder W, Gonzalez J, Redding J, et al. Successful treatment of ankylosing spondylitis with the anti-tumor necrosis factor alpha monoclonal antibody infliximab. Arthritis Rheum 2000;43:1346–52.
21. Helewa A. Physical therapy management of patients with rheumatoid arthritis. In: Walker JM, Helewa A, editors. Physical therapy in arthritis. Philadelphia: WB Saunders; 1996. p. 247–50.
22. Khan MA. Ankylosing spondylitis. In: Calin A, editor. Spondyloarthropathies. Orlando: Grune and Stratton; 1984, p. 69–117.
23. Kraag G, Stokes B, Groh J, Helewa A, Goldsmith C. The effects of comprehensive home physiotherapy and supervision on patients with ankylosing spondylitis. J Rheumatol 1990;17:228–33.
24. Bot SDM, Caspers, M, Van Royen BJ, Toussaint HM, Kingma I. Biomechanical analysis of posture in patients with spinal kyphosis due to ankylosing spondylitis: a pilot study. Rheumatology 1999;38:441–3.
25. Eriendsson J. Car driving with ankylosing spondylitis. East Sussex, UK: The Ankylosing Spondylitis International Federation and The National Ankylosing Spondylitis Society of Great Britain.
26. Hidding A, van der Linden, de Witte L. Therapeutic effect of individual physical therapy in ankylosing spondylitis related to disease duration. Clin Rheumatol 1993:334–340.
27. Viitanen JV, Suni J, Kautiainen H, Liimatainen M, Takala H. Effect of physiotherapy on spinal mobility in ankylosing spondylitis. Scand J Rheumatol 1992;21:38–41.
28. Helliwell PS, Abbott CA, Chamberlain MA. A randomized trial of three different physiotherapy regimes in ankylosing spondylitis. Physiotherapy 1996;82:85–90.
29. Band D, Jones SD, Kennedy LG, Garrett SL, Porter J, Gay L, et al. Which patients with ankylosing spondylitis derive most benefit from an inpatient management program? J Rheumatol 1997;24:2381–4.

30. Hidding A, van der Linden S, Boers M, Gielen X, de Witte L, Kester A, et al. Is group physical therapy superior to individualized therapy in ankylosing spondylitis? A randomized controlled trial. Arthritis Care Res 1993;6:117–25.

31. Voss DE, Ionta MK, Myers BJ. Proprioceptive neuromuscular facilitation, 3rd ed. Philadelphia: JB Lippincott; 1985.

32. Spondylitis Association of America. Straight talk on ankylosing spondylitis, 2nd ed. Sherman Oaks, CA: Spondylitis Association of America; 1993.

33. Santos H, Brophy S, Calin A. Exercise in ankylosing spondylitis: how much is optimum? J Rheumatol 1998;25:2156–60.

34. Jensen GM, Lorish CD. Promoting patient cooperation with exercise programs: linking research, theory and practice. Arthritis Care Res 1994;7:181–9.

35. Calin A, Elswood J. The outcome of 130 total hip replacements and 2 revisions in ankylosing spondylitis: high success rate after a mean followup of 7.5 years. J Rheumatol 1989;16:955–8.

Additional Recommended Reading

Gall V. Spondylarthropathies. In: Wegener ST, Belza, B, Gall EP, editors. Clinical care in the rheumatic diseases. Atlanta: American College of Rheumatology; 1996, p. 171–5.A

Spondylitis Association of America (quarterly newsletter). P.O. Box 5872 Sherman Oaks, CA 91413.

Gall V. Exercise in the spondyloarthropathies. Arthritis Care Res 1994;7:215–20.

Stokes B. Ankylosing spondylitis. In: Walker JM, Helewa A, editors. Physical therapy in arthritis. Philadelphia: WB Saunders; 1996. p. 287–99.

Osteoarthritis

CARLOS J. LOZADA, MD; and ROY D. ALTMAN, MD

Osteoarthritis (OA) is the most common and probably the oldest documented articular disease. OA affects more than 20 million individuals in the United States alone. This high prevalence entails significant costs to society. If both direct costs (such as physician visits, medications, surgery) and indirect costs (time lost from work, inability to perform self care) are taken into consideration, the economic impact of OA has been estimated at 30 times that of rheumatoid arthritis (RA) (1). As the U.S. population ages over the next few decades, the need for better understanding and better therapeutic alternatives for OA will continue to grow.

OA is no longer considered a "degenerative" or "wear and tear" arthritis, but rather one that involves dynamic biomechanical, biochemical, and cellular processes. There are several factors, such as trauma, infection, and obesity, that may predispose to the development of OA and can potentially be altered. Specific preventive measures are directed at altering these risk factors. Guidelines for the management of OA have been developed and reported (2,3). The therapeutic program, however, needs to be tailored to individual patients and their circumstances, taking into account potential adverse events related to the therapeutic choices.

There is no cure for OA. Therapy is directed at relieving pain, the most common symptom causing patients to seek assistance. Symptom-modifying agents may be prescribed for short-term benefit (e.g., nonsteroidal antiinflammatory drugs [NSAIDs]) or longer-term benefit (e.g., intraarticular hyaluronate).

The ideal therapy for OA would slow or halt the progression of the disease. No proven structure- or disease-modifying agents currently exist, although compounds are being investigated that could potentially prevent, arrest, or reverse OA. Some alternative therapies are also being tested in clinical trials to determine their symptom or structure/disease modifying potential.

PATHOLOGY AND PATHOGENESIS

There is no single identifiable cause for OA. In all likelihood, OA is a heterogeneous group of disorders in which biomechanical, biochemical, and genetic factors lead to phenotypic expression of a common end result.

OA involves the entire joint, including subchondral bone. There is increasing appreciation of the role of inflammation in OA, with expression of cytokines and metalloproteinases in synovium and cartilage. Therefore, the term *degenerative joint disease* is no longer considered appropriate when referring to OA.

Cartilage is initially affected with fibrillation and ulcerations. In many patients, there is accompanying focal synovial membrane inflammation and release of such cytokines as tumor necrosis factor α and interleukin 1β. This stimulates the production of matrix metalloproteinases that proceed to degrade cartilage collagen and proteoglycans.

This damage eventually leads to cartilage loss and bony eburnation. There is subchondral bone formation and eventual appearance of bony spurs (osteophytes). Disease progression is characteristically slow, over several years or decades.

CLINICAL SYMPTOMS

Pain is the most common symptom that leads a patient with OA to be evaluated by a physician. Nevertheless, for unclear reasons, only 40% of patients with severe radiographic OA (Kellgren and Lawrence grade III and IV) have pain (4,5). Even when present, the source of the pain is often not known. Pain in OA has many potential causes, which the history and physical examination should attempt to identify. When the cause is identified, therapy can be more logically directed.

Damage to articular cartilage is the key feature of OA, but articular cartilage does not generate a pain response, because it lacks nerve endings. Menisci similarly do not contain nerves, except away from compressive forces on their outer third, and do not directly account for pain. Nevertheless, articular cartilage, menisci, and even synovial fluid can indirectly cause pain in OA. These are among the many possible etiologies of pain in OA, which include stretching of the joint capsule, increased vascular pressure in subchondral bone, surrounding muscle spasm, release of inflammatory cells in the synovium, and others. The presence of crystals, such as calcium pyrophosphate dihydrate (CPPD), can aggravate inflammation and pain.

Joint pain is also related to the perception of the individual's environment and unique ethnic, cultural, and personal circumstances. Pain is also complicated by the presence of dysthymia, other forms of depression, bipolar disorder, and secondary gains such as a patient seeking Worker's Compensation or disability benefits.

Pain usually occurs during activity and is relieved by rest. Eventually, patients can develop pain at rest and at night. There can be morning stiffness in the joint(s), commonly lasting less than 30 minutes. *Gelling* (stiffness after periods of inactivity) may develop. As the disease progresses, with narrowing of joint space and bony hypertrophy, patients may complain of the "bony" appearance of their joints. They may also report that their knees "lock" or "give way." Muscles may atrophy because of lessened use secondary to pain and the patient may experience weakness or instability.

PHYSICAL EXAMINATION

The joints most commonly involved in OA are weight-bearing joints such as the knee or hip, and central joints in the cervical and lumbosacral spine (Table 1). In patients with hip or knee

Table 1. Common sites of involvement in osteoarthritis.

Cervical spine
First carpometacarpal joint
Distal interphalangeal joints
Proximal interphalangeal joints
Lumbar spine
Hips
Knees
First metatarsophalangeal joint

Table 2. Radiographic features of osteoarthritis.

Joint space narrowing
Osteophyte formation
Subchondral sclerosis
Subchondral cysts

pain, the presence of trochanteric or anserine bursitis should be ruled out.

Affected joints in the hand commonly include the first carpometacarpal joints, distal interphalangeal joints (DIP), and proximal interphalangeal (PIP) joints. Findings on physical examination include bony enlargement and malalignment, depending on disease severity. Heberden's and/or Bouchard's nodes—bony overgrowths at the medial and dorsolateral aspects of the DIP or PIP joints, respectively—may be present. These nodes usually develop slowly over time. Occasionally, there is rapid growth with gelatinous cysts preceding the nodes.

An effusion may be present, but erythema and warmth are usually absent or minimal. Pain can be elicited on both active and passive range of motion of the affected joints. *Crepitus* (a grating sensation upon joint motion) is characteristic on range of motion testing of larger joints, such as the knees. There can be periarticular muscle atrophy, perhaps secondary to disuse. Limitation of joint motion may be present in more advanced cases.

Specific Joint Involvement

Hip. Symptoms are usually insidious in onset. A characteristic limp away from the OA hip (antalgic gait) is characteristic. There is groin pain and reduced motion, particularly in internal rotation. Reports of pain in the trochanteric region, buttocks, sciatic region, or even knee are not uncommon. Pain with tenderness on the lateral aspect of the upper thigh may represent trochanteric bursitis.

Spine. Severe OA of the facet joints of the lumbar spine can result in spinal stenosis. Symptoms of pseudo intermittent claudication can occur with intermittent or constant pain in the legs, worsened by exercise and relieved by sitting down.

Diffuse idiopathic skeletal hyperostosis (DISH) is characterized by flowing ossification along the anterolateral aspect of the vertebral bodies, particularly the anterior longitudinal ligament. There is no associated disc space narrowing or anterior vertebral body squaring.

Hand. Erosive OA of the hand is a variant in which there is prominent DIP and/or PIP involvement. Inflammatory flares result in joint erosion, deformity, and subsequent ankylosis.

Knee. Teenagers and young adults (particularly women) may present with anterior compartment or patellar pain due to *chondromalacia patellae*. This mostly self-limited condition, also referred to as patellofemoral syndrome, is most symptomatic when sitting in a movie theater, walking uphill, or walking up stairs. Although it is often grouped with OA, it can result from a variety of problems, including abnormal quadriceps angle and trauma. Isometric exercises for the quadriceps muscles and avoidance of overuse are of benefit.

LABORATORY AND RADIOGRAPHIC FINDINGS

There are no laboratory abnormalities specific for OA. Acute phase reactants such as erythrocyte sedimentation rate (ESR) are not elevated, and synovial fluid analysis usually indicates a white cell count of less than 2,000/mm^3.

The classic radiographic findings of OA are bony spurs at the joint margins, called *osteophytes*. Other findings include asymmetric joint space narrowing, subchondral sclerosis, and subchondral cyst formation. Radiographic severity of OA correlates with the clinical severity of disease in less than half of patients (Table 2).

DIFFERENTIAL DIAGNOSIS

The diagnosis of OA is clinical and can usually be made based on history and physical examination. Radiographic findings help confirm the clinical impression. The initial goal is to differentiate OA from another arthritis, such as RA.

RA, unlike OA, affects wrists and metacarpophalangeal (MCP) joints but uncommonly affects the DIP joints and lumbosacral spine. RA is typically associated with prominent morning stiffness (lasting more than 1 hour). Radiographic findings in RA are those of bone erosion (periarticular osteopenia, marginal erosions of bone) rather than bone formation. Laboratory findings in RA include elevated acute phase reactants (ESR, C-reactive protein) and a positive serum rheumatoid factor in many. Joint fluid has a substantially elevated white blood cell count with polymorphonuclear cell predominance.

Secondary forms of OA must be considered in individuals with chondrocalcinosis, joint trauma, metabolic bone disorders, hypermobility syndromes, and neuropathic diseases. Spondylarthropathies (such as Reiter's syndrome, ankylosing spondylitis, or psoriatic arthritis) with sacroiliac and lumbosacral spine involvement can be differentiated by clinical history and characteristic radiographic findings.

PREVENTION

The single most important modifiable risk factor for OA is obesity. Obesity in women has been linked to OA of the knees (6). Furthermore, it has been associated with the later development of hip OA (7). Modest weight loss in OA has been accompanied by a decrease in symptoms (8), with a suggestion of reduced radiographic progression. Other studies have shown that a reduction in percent body fat, rather than weight, may be significant in reducing pain from OA of the knee (9).

The role of repetitive, relatively minor, trauma in development of OA is not clear. However, occupations involving considerable bending and lifting seem to be related to OA of the knees. Preventive measures may be indicated, including changes in certain repetitive motions, reduced significant trauma, and reduced bending. Weakness of the quadriceps muscles relative to body weight has been listed as a possible risk factor for OA of the knees (10). Several studies have shown OA of the hip and knee to be associated with muscle weakness, implying a benefit to preventive therapeutic intervention.

TREATMENT

The goals in the treatment of OA are to relieve pain, improve function, and prevent disability. An individualized therapeutic program should be designed after assessing the patient for the causes of pain. The most effective symptomatic therapy combines several approaches and may be more effective if a multidisciplinary team (e.g., rheumatologist, physiatrist, orthopedist, physical therapist, occupational therapist, psychologist, psychiatrist, nurse/nurse coordinator, dietitian, and social worker) is involved in care.

The therapeutic program should include a combination of patient education, physical measures, psychosocial interventions, drugs, and surgical interventions.

Patient Education

Patients should be educated about OA. Misconceptions often exist about this disease, and patients may be concerned about possible rapid progression to disability. This is particularly so in retirees who are no longer living near the rest of their families.

There should be an emphasis on the common nature of OA and its typical slow progression. Discuss therapeutic options that emphasize lifestyle changes, such as exercise and weight control, that might be helpful in altering the natural history of the disease. Alternative or unproven therapies should be objectively discussed as well. A significant number of patients will already have taken one or more prior to seeking the help of modern medicine, but they often do not mention these therapies unless directly asked. Educational pamphlets, such as those available through the Arthritis Foundation, may help.

Continuing emotional support is important as well. It need not be achieved through frequent doctor visits. Data suggest that telephone contact with the patient between visits, even by nonprofessionals, can improve outcomes (11).

Physical Measures

Many physical modalities are available for relieving pain, reducing stiffness, and limiting muscle spasm. Physical measures make up an integral part of any successful therapeutic program for OA. They can be subdivided into exercise, supportive devices, alterations in activities of daily living (ADLs), and thermal modalities.

Exercise. Exercise is the most commonly employed physical measure. Patients with OA should be encouraged to exercise – the myth that any exercise worsens arthritis should be dispelled. Indeed, muscle weakness may precede the development of symptomatic OA. In patients with OA, exercise programs have been linked to pain reduction and function improvement (12). Strengthening of the quadriceps muscles in a patient with knee OA often improves function and decreases pain. In theory, improved muscle support of the joint may retard the progression of OA. (See also Chapter 26, Rest and Exercise.)

Care should be taken to choose exercises that maximize muscle strengthening and minimize stress on the affected joints. Involvement in some particular sport or activity may need to be curtailed or replaced. Swimming is particularly effective in that it exercises multiple muscle groups without placing undue stress on joints. There are exceptions where specific exercises may actually worsen symptoms: chondromalacia patella may be worsened by bicycle riding; lumbar facet OA may be worsened by hyperextension of the spine, such as in swimming.

A supervised program of fitness walking and education improves functional status without worsening OA of the knee. The intensity of the exercise program should be graded. If the regimen is advanced too quickly, symptoms may worsen. The patient should be advised that worsening pain during exercise is a warning sign that exercise tolerance has been reached and rest is needed.

Supportive Devices. Supportive devices can unload joints, improve balance, and decrease pain. They include canes, crutches, walkers, corsets, collars, and shoe orthotics. Canes, when properly used, can increase the base of support, decrease loading, and reduce demands on the lower limb and its joints (13). The cane can unload an affected hip by as much as 60%. The total length of a properly measured cane should be equal to the distance between the upper border of the greater trochanter of the femur and the bottom of the heel of the shoe, resulting in elbow flexion of about 20°. The cane should be held in the hand contralateral to, and moved together with, the affected limb. The healthier limb should precede the affected limb when climbing up stairs. However, when climbing down stairs, the cane and the affected limb should be advanced first.

Proper footwear, including orthotic shoes, is often of great value. A heel and/or sole lift can reduce symptoms of a short leg, which may accentuate lumbar pain and scoliosis. An orthotic device, or orthotic shoe insert, may help the patient with subluxed metatarsophalangeal joints (14). Walking ability and pain from medial compartment OA of the knee can be lessened by the use of a lateral heel-wedged insole. Athletic shoes with good mediolateral support, good medial arch, and calcaneal cushion can reduce pain and provide support.

A knee brace or cage may be of use in patients with tibiofemoral disease, especially those with lateral instability and those with a tendency for the knee to "give out." These are not of value when significant valgus or varus deformities are present.

Supports and orthotics are intended to improve patient activity, improve adherence, and allow the patient to retain functional independence. Use of the devices should be monitored. For example, initial use of a cervical collar should be intermittent, and it should be checked for proper sizing and proper orientation. Cane/crutch tips should be changed when worn, in order to avoid slipping on smooth or wet surfaces.

Alteration in ADLs. Altering activities of daily living may decrease symptoms. For example, raising the level of a chair or toilet seat can be helpful because the hip and knee are subjected to the highest pressures during the initial phase of rising from the seated position.

Thermal Modalities. Thermal modalities can be particularly effective. The use of heat, cold, or alternating heat and cold are based on patient preference and not on any scientific superiority. Traditionally, the more acute the process, the more likely cold applications will be of benefit (reduction in blood flow and pain). Cold is mostly used in the form of cold packs or vapocoolant sprays to relieve muscle spasm, decrease swelling in acute trauma, and relieve pain from inflammation.

The use of heat can be subdivided into superficial and deep, with no proven advantage of one over the other. Hot packs, paraffin baths, hydrotherapy, and radiant heat are vehicles for providing superficial heat. Ultrasound can provide deep heat, usually for larger joints such as hips. The therapeutic value of applying heat includes decreasing joint stiffness, alleviating pain, relieving muscle spasm, and preventing contractures. The use of heat is contraindicated over tissues with inadequate vascular supply, bleeding, or cancer. Heat should also be avoided in areas close to the testicles or near developing fetuses. The range of temperatures used is 40–45°C (104–113°F) for 3–30 minutes (15).

Several miscellaneous physical modalities, with as yet unproven or limited value, include massage, yoga therapy, acupressure, acupuncture, magnets, pulsed electromagnetic fields, transcutaneous neural stimulation (TENS), and spa therapy. (See also Chapter 27, Physical Modalities.)

Psychosocial Measures

Psychosocial factors are integrated with the perception of pain and associated disability. Depression needs to be identified and treated. Other factors that can complicate the clinical picture include older age, lower educational level, lower income, and unmarried status, which have been linked to the tendency to become disabled in patients with musculoskeletal complaints (16).

Reassurance, counseling, and education may minimize the interference of psychosocial factors. Patients who participate in their care and understand their disease are more likely to accept and adapt to the challenges of living with OA. As mentioned above, periodic telephone support has been found to reduce symptoms in patients with OA.

Another potential use for psychosocial intervention is with obese patients, for whom weight loss groups and a stable social support system may be helpful.

Pharmacologic Therapy

Medications used to treat symptoms in OA include topical agents, systemic oral agents, adjuvant therapies (such as antispasmodics and psychoactive drugs) and intraarticular agents. These are often used in combination.

There is a growing need for superior therapies. It is now understood that inflammation has an important role in OA and that it is a disease of the entire joint, not just of cartilage. This shift in paradigm has led to new ideas on how to achieve structure/disease modification in OA, and could lead to clinical use of the first of these drugs within the next decade.

Topical Agents. Topical agents have a role in the treatment of OA. Capsaicin, derived from capsicum, the common pepper plant, has been of value in controlled trials (17). It is available as a nonprescription agent in 2 strengths. It is applied 2–4 times daily and is often accompanied by a sensation of heat or burning for several days, until the nerve endings are depleted

of substance P (a neurotransmitter). Care should be taken to avoid the inadvertent application of capsaicin in the eyes.

Other topical analgesic agents include menthol and salicylate-based over-the-counter topical preparations; however, there are no published trials showing benefit in OA. Topical nonsteroidal antiinflammatory drugs (NSAIDs) are in common use in many parts of the world, but no consistent data support their use.

Systemic Oral Agents. Acetaminophen has been as effective as ibuprofen for the treatment of pain in OA of the knee in some trials (18). In contrast, NSAIDs (including cyclooxygenase-2 [COX-2] inhibitors) have been found to be superior in other trials, particularly in patients with more severe pain (19,20). Acetaminophen appears free of gastrointestinal adverse effects, but hepatotoxicity can occur when ingested at high doses, especially with alcohol. There is epidemiologic evidence for possible renal toxicity even when ingested at the recommended dose (21).

Tramadol has mild suppressive effects on the μ opioid receptor and also inhibits the uptake of norepinephrine and serotonin (22). It appears to have a place in the therapy of OA, and in one study had NSAID-sparing properties. Tramadol is not a controlled substance, but there have been isolated reports of abuse by opioid-dependent patients. Seizures and allergic reactions have also been reported, usually at high doses. Tramadol can produce nausea and central nervous system side effects that can be reduced by starting with 25 mg once daily for 3 days and slowly escalating the dose to the maximum, or until the desired pain relief is achieved.

The pain of OA is generally responsive to narcotic analgesics. Mildly potent and minimally addictive narcotic analgesics, such as codeine and propoxyphene, have been used effectively in patients with OA, especially in combination with non-narcotic analgesics such as acetaminophen. However, propoxyphene should be avoided in the elderly. The chronic nature of the pain in OA and the addictive potential of the stronger opiates and opioids test the skill of the physician in the use of these agents. However, there is a role for narcotics in such chronic noncancer pain as that experienced by people with OA.

Antiinflammatory Drugs. NSAIDs are the most commonly prescribed agents for treatment of both pain and inflammation in OA. In-depth discussions of the pharmacology and potential differences between these agents have been published elsewhere (23).

Traditional NSAIDs are nonselective COX inhibitors, although specific and selective COX-2 inhibitors are now in common use. With most traditional NSAIDs, analgesia can be achieved at smaller doses than are needed for antiinflammatory effects. Since inflammation is usually not severe in OA, lower doses of NSAIDs can be tried initially. The NSAID should then be titrated to the lowest effective dose. Also, since the pain of OA is often intermittent, the use of NSAIDs in OA can similarly be intermittent.

The major adverse effects associated with nonselective NSAIDs are gastrointestinal (peptic ulcer disease, gastritis) and renal (interstitial nephritis, prostaglandin inhibition-related renal insufficiency). These adverse effects are more prevalent in the elderly—the population with the highest prevalence of OA. Effective strategies to reduce the gastrointestinal toxicity of NSAIDs include the use of nonprostaglandin-inhibiting substituted salicylates, co-administration of misoprostol (24) or a proton pump inhibitor (25) with an NSAID, or use of specific

COX-2 inhibitors. Although effective for symptoms, other agents such as H2 blockers have not been effective at gastroprotection (26). There has been no proven value to antacids or sucralfate in this setting.

Patients vary in their benefit and adverse reactions to various NSAIDs. Difference in half-lives of the NSAIDs may influence patient adherence and dosing.

The discovery of 2 isoforms of COX has quickly led to the development of novel therapeutic modalities. Outcome studies have demonstrated a significant reduction in gastrointestinal symptoms and serious gastrointestinal adverse events, such as symptomatic ulcers, bleeds, perforations, and obstructions with specific COX-2 inhibitors when compared to nonselective NSAIDs (27). In addition, platelet aggregation and bleeding time are not affected by specific COX-2 inhibition. These drugs, however, can have similar renal adverse event profiles to nonselective NSAIDs.

The initially available specific COX-2 inhibitors are celecoxib and rofecoxib. Celecoxib has shown superiority to placebo and equivalent clinical efficacy to NSAIDs in relieving the pain of OA and RA (28,29). Rofecoxib has been approved for acute pain and for the pain of OA (30).

Nutraceuticals. *Nutraceuticals* are nutritional supplements with potential pharmacologic value. Patients with OA have used numerous nutraceuticals in the absence scientific support. More attention has recently been paid to some of these compounds in an attempt to bridge the existing information gap relative to conventional therapies (see also Chapter 33, Complementary and Alternative Treatments).

Glucosamine sulfate has been tested orally and intramuscularly, mostly in Europe. Its mechanism of action is unknown, and reports of clinical effect have been received with skepticism. In OA of the knee, oral glucosamine sulfate (1500 mg/day) has shown symptomatic benefit equivalent to analgesic doses of ibuprofen (1200 mg/day) but with slower onset of action (31). Glucosamine sulfate was generally well tolerated. In one European multicenter study, statistically significant structure modification, as measured by x-rays of the knee, was demonstrated at 3-year followup (32). If the findings are confirmed, glucosamine could be the first structure/disease-modifying drug for OA.

Oral chondroitin sulfate has shown ability to relieve pain in small European trials. There is characteristically a slow onset of effect; patients taking NSAIDs had more rapid pain relief. No data exist on chondroitin sulfate and disease/structure modification.

A meta-analysis and quality assessment of the studies of glucosamine and chondroitin in OA of the hip or knee concluded that insufficient information about study design and conduct was provided to allow for a definitive evaluation of either agent (33). Larger studies with longer followup periods are needed. There is also a need for studies on the combination of glucosamine and chondroitin. An NIH-sponsored study is currently in progress.

S-adenosylmethionine (SAM-e), a methyl group donor and oxygen radical scavenger, has been used by intravenous loading and oral maintenance. In one study, 2 centers reported differing results. One center reported reductions in overall pain and resting pain compared with placebo; the other showed no significant difference between the test group and placebo, but included patients with more severe OA.

MSM (methylsulfonylmethane) has been touted as a "sulfate donor" (especially through the Internet). This "natural" product is actually chemically manufactured. It is related to DMSO, a solvent that has also been proposed as a remedy for several different conditions. There is minimal, if any, information on MSM's efficacy and/or toxicity in the peer-reviewed scientific literature.

Still other nutraceuticals are entrenched in popular culture—such as "cat's claw" and shark cartilage—and are being used with increasing frequency. They are sold over-the-counter in pharmacies and health food stores, as well as over the Internet. There are no carefully performed trials to support their use.

Adjuvant Agents. Tricyclic antidepressants can potentiate the effects of the other analgesics. In addition, they may benefit patients having sleep disturbances due to nocturnal myoclonus and fibromyalgia-like complaints.

Antispasmodics are useful in reducing muscle pain and spasm in OA. Although the main treatment for muscle spasm involves the physical modalities noted above, pain associated with muscle spasm may be reduced with an injection of lidocaine with or without a depot corticosteroid. The value of oral medications in relieving the pain of muscle spasm is controversial. Clinical trials have not convincingly demonstrated any medication to be superior to placebo. However, centrally acting agents may be helpful for their sedating qualities and potential for disrupting neurologic transmission of the pain sensation.

Intraarticular Therapy. Oral corticosteroids are not indicated for the treatment of OA. In contrast, intraarticular depot corticosteroids may be of value when synovial inflammation is present. Synovial effusions should be removed prior to injection. Depot corticosteroids may also be helpful in periarticular soft tissue complications, such as anserine bursitis. They have not been consistently helpful in facet joints for treatment of chronic low back pain, but have been useful in many patients as epidural injections for symptomatic spinal stenosis. In spite of the impression of many clinicians that intraarticular corticosteroids are of benefit in OA, few published trials support their benefit over aspiration alone. Some trials have shown short-term benefit (34). In general, depot corticosteoroid use should be limited to 4 injections to any single joint per year. Complications such as septic arthritis are rare if proper aseptic technique is employed.

Synthetic and naturally occurring hyaluronan derivatives are administered intraarticularly. They are only approved for use at the knee, although trials are ongoing for hips and shoulders. At this point there is conflicting evidence on efficacy. Current studies may provide additional insights. In general, hyaluronan derivatives are reported to reduce pain for more prolonged periods of time than other intraarticular therapies and potentially to improve mobility (35). They are administered through a series of 3–5 injections into the knee joint, one week apart.

Structure/Disease-Modifying Agents. The term "structure/disease-modifying agents" for OA refers to medications that are intended to retard the progression of OA and/or enhance a normal reparative process. It is difficult to establish the value of a structure/disease-modifying drug in a disease that progresses at variable rates and has no definable clinical or laboratory marker of activity or progression. Measures used to identify structure/disease modification include radiographic assessment of joint space or magnetic resonance imaging (36). Although several agents are being evaluated for these properties, none have been established as effective. Agents with structure/disease-modifying potential can be categorized as follows: 1) growth factors and cytokines; 2) sulfated and non-sulfated sugars; 3) hormones and other steroids; and 4) enzyme inhibitors. Particularly intriguing areas of investigation include glucosamine sulfate (see above); metalloproteinase inhibitors, such as the tetracyclines; growth factors and cytokines; and chondrocyte/stem cell transplantation.

Tetracyclines, apart from any antimicrobial effect, are inhibitors of tissue metalloproteinases. Doxycycline has reduced the severity of OA in canine models. A multicenter controlled trial using doxycycline for structure modification in obese women with OA of the knee is ongoing. Other compounds with collagenase-inhibiting properties are being developed and investigated as structure/disease-modifying agents not only for OA, but for rheumatoid arthritis as well.

Structure/disease modification has yet to be achieved in OA and any claims are premature until well-designed, double-blind, placebo-controlled trials are undertaken. Trials currently underway could provide an answer as to whether this is a realistic goal.

Surgical Intervention

The primary reason for elective orthopedic surgery is intractable pain. A secondary reason is restoration of compromised function. Interventions include removal of loose bodies, stabilization of joints, redistribution of joint forces (e.g., osteotomy), relief of neural impingement (spinal stenosis, herniated disc), and joint replacement.

Total hip and knee arthroplasties have improved the morbidity and probably the indirect mortality of OA. Most series report good to excellent long-term results in more than 90% of patients undergoing either hip or knee replacement, with 85% success rates at 20 years followup of the Charnley total hip prosthesis. These procedures appear cost effective when the improved quality of life and the alternatives are considered.

Osteotomies may serve as alternatives to arthroplasty in younger, overweight patients and in unicompartmental disease of the knee. This may delay progression of disease. However, only 50% of patients with knee osteotomies have satisfactory results at 10 years (37). Hip osteotomies have less certain long-term results.

Arthroscopic intervention should be limited to patients in whom an additional diagnosis is suspected. Surgical arthroscopy is useful for repair and for partial removal of damaged menisci. The value of synovectomy and debridement has not been established in OA.

Arthroscopic lavage has also been tried, with some success. Large-bore needle lavage with saline may be effective in the relief of knee pain in OA for up to 6 months in selected patients (34).

REFERENCES

1. Kramer JS, Yelin EH, Epstein WV. Social and economic impacts of four musculoskeletal conditions: a study using national community-based data. J Rheumatol 1983;26:901–7.
2. Recommendations for the medical management of osteoarthritis of the hip and knee: 2000 update. American College of Rheumatology Subcommittee on Osteoarthritis Guidelines. Arthritis Rheum 2000;43:1905–15.
3. Pendleton A, Arden N, Dougados M, Doherty M, Bannwarth B, Bijlsma JWJ, et al. EULAR recommendations for the management of knee osteoarthritis: report of a task force of the Standing Committee for International Clinical Studies Including Therapeutic Trials (ESCISIT). Ann Rheum Dis 2000;59:936–44.
4. Kellgren JH, Lawrence RC. Radiological assessment of osteoarthrosis. Ann Rheum Dis 1957;16:494–501.
5. Hochberg MC, Lawrence RC, Everett DF, Cornoni-Huntley J. Epidemiologic associations of pain in osteoarthritis of the knee: data from the National Health and Nutrition Examination Survey and the National Health and Nutrition Examination-I Epidemiologic Follow-up Survey. Semin Arthritis Rheum 1989;18(Suppl 2):4–9.
6. Hochberg MC, Lethbridge-Cejku M, Scott WW Jr, Reichle R, Plato CC, Tobin JD. The association of body weight, body fatness and body fat distribution with osteoarthritis of the knee: data from the Baltimore Longitudinal Study of Aging. J Rheumatol 1995;22:488–93.
7. Karlson EW, Mandl LA, Grodstein F, Sangha O, Liang MH, Speizer FE. Risk factors for severe hip osteoarthritis in a large female cohort study. Arthritis Rheum 2000;43(9 suppl):S224.
8. Felson DT, Zhang Y, Anthony JM, Naimark A, Anderson JJ. Weight loss reduces the risk for symptomatic knee osteoarthritis in women. The Framingham Study. Ann Intern Med 1992;116:535–9.
9. Toda Y, Toda T, Takemura S, Wada T, Morimoto T, Ogawa R. Change in body fat, but not body weight or metabolic correlates of obesity, is related to symptomatic relief of obese patients with knee osteoarthritis after a weight control program. J Rheumatol 1998;25:2181–6.
10. Slemenda C, Heilman DK, Brandt KD, Katz BP, Mazzuca SA, Braunstein EM, et al. Reduced quadriceps strength relative to body weight: a risk factor for knee osteoarthritis in women? Arthritis Rheum 1998;41:1951–9.
11. Weinberger M, Tierney WM, Cowper PA, Katz BP, Booher PA. Cost-effectiveness of increased telephone contact for patients with osteoarthritis. A randomized, controlled trial. Arthritis Rheum 1993;36:243–6.
12. van Baar ME, Dekker J, Oostendorp RA, Bijl D. The effectiveness of exercise therapy in patients with osteoarthritis of the hip or knee: a randomized clinical trial. J Rheumatol 1998;25:2432–9.
13. Blount WP. Don't throw away the cane. J Bone Joint Surg 1956;38A:695–708.
14. Thompson JA, Jennings MB, Hodge W. Orthotic therapy in the management of osteoarthritis. J Am Podiatr Med Assoc 1992;82:136–9.
15. Basford JR. Physical agents and biofeedback. In: DeLisa JA, et al., editors. Rehabilitation medicine - principles and practice. Philadelphia: JB Lippincott; 1988, p. 257–75.
16. Cunningham LS, Kelsy JL. Epidemiology of musculoskeletal impairments and associated disability. AJPH 1984;74:574–9.
17. McCarthy GM, McCarthy DJ. Effect of topical capsaicin in the therapy of painful osteoarthritis of the hands. J Rheumatol 1992;19:604–7.
18. Bradley JD, Brandt KD, Katz BP, Kalasinski LA, Ryan SI. Comparison of an antiinflammatory dose of ibuprofen, an analgestic dose of ibuprofen, and acetaminophen in the treatment of patients with osteoarthritis of the knee. N Engl J Med 1991;325:87–91.
19. Geba GP, Weaver AL, Schnitzer TJ, Fleischmann RM, Polis AB, Matzura-Wolfe DM, et al. A comparison of rofecoxib to celecoxib and acetaminophen in the treatment of osteoarthritis. Arthritis Rheum 2000; 43(9 suppl):S384.
20. Altman RD, IAP Study Group. Ibuprofen, acetaminophen and placebo in osteoarthritis of the knee: a six-day double-blind study. Arthritis Rheum 1999;41(9 suppl):S403.
21. Perneger TV, Whelton PK, Klag MJ. Risk of kidney failure associated with the use of acetaminophen, aspirin, and nonsteroidal antiinflammatory drugs. N Engl J Med 1994;331:1675–9.
22. Raffa RB, Friederichs E, Reimann W, Shank RP, Codd EE, Vaught JL. Opioid and nonopioid components independently contribute to the mechanism of action of tramadol, an "atypical" opioid analgesic. J Pharmacol Exp Ther 1992;260:275–85.
23. Brooks PM, Day PO. Nonsteroidal antiinflammatory drugs—differences and similarities. N Engl J Med 1991;324:1716–25.
24. Graham DY, Agrawal NM, Roth SH. Prevention of NSAID-induced gastric ulcer with misoprostol: multicenter, double-blind, placebo-controlled trial. Lancet 1988;2:1277–1280.
25. Hawkey CJ, Karrasch JA, Szczepanski L, Walker DG, Barkun A, Swannell AJ, et al. Omeprazole compared with misoprostol for ulcers associated with nonsteroidal antiinflammatory drugs. Omeprazole versus Misoprostol for NSAID-induced Ulcer Management (OMINUM) Study Group. N Engl J Med 1998;338:727–34.
26. Yeomans ND, Tulassay Z, Juhasz L, Racz I, Howard JM, van Rensburg CJ, et al. A comparison of omeprazole with ranitidine for ulcers associated with nonsteroidal antiinflammatory drugs. Acid Suppression Trial: Ranitidine versus Omeprazole for NSAID-associated Ulcer Treatment (ASTRONAUT) Study Group. N Engl J Med 1998;338:719–26.
27. Silverstein FE, Faich G, Goldstein JL, Simon LS, Pincus T, Whelton A, et al. Gastrointestinal toxicity with celecoxib vs nonsteroidal anti-inflammatory drugs for osteoarthritis and rheumatoid arthritis: the CLASS study: a

randomized controlled trial. Celecoxib Long-term Arthritis Safety Study. JAMA 2000;284:1247–55.

28. Hubbard R, Geis GS, Woods E, Yu S, Zhao W. Efficacy, tolerability and safety of celecoxib, a specific COX-2 inhibitor, in osteoarthritis. Arthritis Rheum 1998;41(9 suppl):S196.

29. Geis GS, Stead H, Morant S, Naudin R, Hubbard R. Efficacy and safety of celecoxib, a specific COX-2 inhibitor, in patients with rheumatoid arthritis. Arthritis Rheum 1998;41(9 suppl):S316.

30. Ehrich E, Schnitzer T, Kivitz A, Weaver A, Wolfe F, Morrison B, et al. MK-966, a highly selective COX-2 inhibitor, was effective in the treatment of osteoarthritis (OA) of the knee and hip in a 6-week placebo controlled study. Arthritis Rheum 1997;40(9 suppl):S85.

31. Muller-Fabender H, Bach GL, Haase W, et al. Glucosamine sulfate compared to ibuprofen in osteoarthritis of the knee. Osteoarthritis and Cartilage 1994;2:61–9.

32. Reginster J-Y, Deroisy R, Paul I, Lee RL, Henrotin Y, Giacovelli G, et al. Glucosamine sulfate significantly reduces progression of knee osteoarthritis over 3 years: a large, randomised, placebo-controlled, double-blind, prospective trial. Arthritis Rheum 1999;42(9 suppl):S400.

33. McAlindon TE, Gulin J, Felson DT. Glucosamine (GL) and chondroitin (CH) treatment for osteoarthritis (OA) of the knee or hip: meta-analysis and quality assessment of clinical trials. Arthritis Rheum 1998;41(9 suppl):S198.

34. Ravaud P, Moulinier L, Giraudeau B, Ayral X, Guerin C, Noel E, et al. Effects of joint lavage and steroid injection in patients with osteoarthritis of the knee: results of a multicenter, randomized, controlled trial. Arthritis Rheum 1999;42:475–82.

35. Peyron JG. Intraarticular hyaluronan injections in the treatment of osteoarthritis: state-of-the art review. J Rheumatol 1993;20(Suppl 39):10–15.

36. Lozada CJ, Altman RD. Chondroprotection in osteoarthritis. Bull Rheum Dis 1997;46(7):5–7.

37. Oldenbring S, Egund N, Knutson K, Lindstrand A, Larsen ST. Revision after osteotomy for gonarthrosis: a 10–19 year follow-up of 314 cases. Acta Orthop Scand 1990;61:128–30.

Osteoporosis

MICHAEL J. MARICIC, MD

Osteoporosis is "a disease characterized by low bone mass and microarchitectural deterioration of bone tissue, leading to enhanced bone fragility and a consequent increase in fracture risk" (1) (Figure 1). Osteoporosis is a major medical, economic, and social health problem in the United States that results in significant pain, functional disability, and increased mortality. Approximately 1.2 million fractures attributable to osteoporosis occur each year in persons aged 45 years and older (2), including 600,000 vertebral crush fractures and 250,000 fractures of the hip. Forty to fifty percent of white women over age 50 will suffer an osteoporotic fracture, and one-sixth will sustain a fracture of the hip. The risk of hip fracture begins to rise after age 45, and then rises exponentially, doubling for every 5 years of age.

Hip fracture in the elderly is associated with a 12–20% excess mortality rate in the next year due to complications of immobilization (pneumonia, pulmonary embolus). Approximately half of elderly patients with hip fractures never regain the same level of functional independence, and 25% require long-term institutional care. The total direct and indirect annual costs for osteoporosis approach $10 billion per year.

The etiology of osteoporosis is multifactorial. Genetics accounts for 60–80% of the variance in bone mass. Peak bone mass is usually attained by age 20–25, and then remains relatively stable until menopause. A 2–3% decline in bone mass (mainly trabecular) may then occur for a period of approximately 5 years (Figure 2). Gonadal deficiency, lifelong calcium deficiency, chronic alcohol and nicotine use, immobilization, and medications such as corticosteroids, anticonvulsants, and excessive thyroid supplementation all may contribute to accelerated bone loss. Chronic corticosteroid use accelerates bone loss through a variety of mechanisms (Table 1), and is associated with high fracture rates, particularly in patients with rheumatic disease.

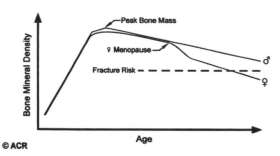

Changes in Bone Density with Age

Figure 2. Peak bone mass is usually higher in males than in females, and is reached by the middle of the third decade of life. There is a slow decline in bone mass in both sexes, with rapid acceleration during the first years following menopause in women.

CLINICAL ASPECTS AND DIAGNOSIS

Although assessing a patient's clinical risk factors for osteoporosis should be a routine component of the history, these risk factors are unreliable for predicting an individual patient's bone density—the most important predictor of future fracture risk. Therefore, an essential component of diagnosis, prediction of fracture risk, and measurement of the response to treatment involves bone density measurement. DEXA (dual energy x-ray absorptiometry) is currently the gold standard because of its accuracy and precision. Bone density measurement is essential for the diagnosis of low bone mass (3) and is an excellent method for assessing future fracture risk (Figure 3) and for determining efficacy of therapy (4).

PREVENTION AND TREATMENT

The ultimate goal of prevention and/or treatment is to minimize the incidence of osteoporotic fractures. A number of important pharmacologic advances have improved our ability to prevent and manage osteoporosis. The current challenges are to identify which patients are candidates for treatment, to choose the most appropriate therapy based on the complete patient profile, and to ensure long-term adherence to therapy.

Therapies approved for the prevention or treatment of osteoporosis are listed in Table 2. If a postmenopausal woman

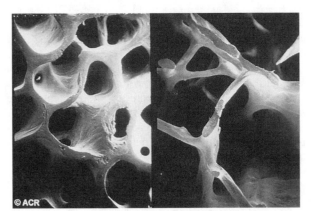

Figure 1. The image on the left shows normal trabecular bone. The image on the right displays a decreased amount of bone and loss of trabecular connectivity, 2 cardinal features of osteoporosis.

Table 1. Effects of corticosteroids on bone metabolism.

Direct inhibitory effect on osteoblasts
Decreased calcium absorption
Increased calcium excretion
Secondary increase in parathyroid hormone level
Decreased estrogen and testosterone production

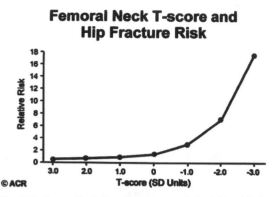

Figure 3. This figure illustrates the exponential relationship between declining T-score and relative risk of hip fracture. For each decrease of 1.0 SD, there is a 2.5- to 2.7-fold increased risk of fracture.

Table 3. National Osteoporosis Foundation risk factors for osteoporotic fractures.

Nonmodifiable
  Personal history of fracture as an adult
  History of fracture in first-degree relative
  Caucasian race
  Advanced age
  Female sex
  Dementia
  Poor health/fragility

Potentially modifiable
  Current cigarette smoking
  Low body weight (<127 lbs)
  Estrogen deficiency
  Early menopause (<age 45) or bilateral ovariectomy
  Prolonged premenopausal amenorrhea (>1 year)
  Low lifelong calcium intake
  Impaired eyesight despite adequate correction
  Recurrent falls
  Inadequate physical activity
  Poor health/frailty

has already suffered an osteoporotic fracture, one would usually prescribe a drug that has documented efficacy for reducing fracture risk. Preventive intervention is a more complex decision that involves consideration not only of the patient's T-score (–2.0 in the absence of additional risk factors and –1.5 if risk factors are present, according to National Osteoporosis Foundation [NOF] guidelines [2]), but also the cost and adverse effects of the medication and likelihood of long-term use by the patient.

Successful management of osteoporosis is based on a combination of nonpharmacologic and pharmacologic approaches. Reducing modifiable risk factors, along with ensuring adequate calcium and vitamin D intake, should be considered essential prior to pharmacologic intervention.

NONPHARMACOLOGIC MANAGEMENT

Although few prospective, well-controlled studies document a beneficial effect of physical activity on bone mass, weight-bearing exercise nonetheless plays a role in the prevention and treatment of osteoporosis by maintaining muscle mass and promoting strength, coordination, and balance (5). To maximize long-term adherence, the exercise should be individualized to the patient's overall physical ability, health status, and preferences. Lifestyle modifications that help counteract osteoporosis are summarized in Table 3.

Reducing Risk of Falls

There are several ways to reduce the likelihood of falls, which are an important risk factor for fracture in the elderly patient with osteoporosis. Treating such comorbidities as dementia, gait disorders, decreased vision, and decreased

Table 2. FDA-approved agents for prevention and treatment of postmenopausal osteoporosis.

Prevention		Treatment	
Agent	Dose	Agent	Dose
Estrogens	Varied	Calcitonin-salmon nasal spray	200 IU/day
Raloxifene	60 mg/day	Raloxifene	60 mg/day
Alendronate	5 mg/day	Alendronate	10 mg/day
Risedronate	5 mg/day	Risedronate	5 mg/day

strength may prevent falls. The use of such drugs as sedatives, tranquilizers, and other medications that affect central nervous system function should be reduced. Phyisical hazards in the home environment, such as throw rugs, should be removed, and sturdy railings and adequate lighting should be installed where needed. Finally, patients should be educated about their risk of falling and strategies to improve home safety.

Calcium and Vitamin D

The role of dietary calcium in the prevention and treatment of osteoporosis has been investigated (6–8). The National Institutes of Health has formulated recommendations for the optimal daily intake of bioavailable calcium, which vary with age and gender. The elderly need more calcium as a result of altered calcium homeostasis—including an age-related decline in intestinal calcium absorption (6).

Because the recommended dose of calcium is usually not obtained through diet alone, calcium supplementation is often required. Calcium supplements are available in several different salt forms, dosage forms, and strengths. Calcium carbonate and calcium citrate contain a calcium composition of 40% and 22%, respectively. Calcium carbonate is well absorbed when taken after an acid-generating meal, and is usually the preparation of choice due to its low cost. In patients who are achlorhydric, calcium citrate is preferred because calcium carbonate would not be absorbed.

The physiologic effects of vitamin D include an increase in calcium and phosphorus absorption from the small intestine, a reduction in urinary calcium excretion, and maintenance of muscle strength, which may play a very important role in protection against falls. Elderly patients are often deficient in 1,25-dihydroxyvitamin D, the metabolically active form of vitamin D, because of low intake, inadequate sunlight exposure, and impaired renal synthesis of calcitriol.

Consuming 400–800 IU/day of vitamin D improves calcium balance and reduces the risk of fractures in the elderly (7,8). In a study that evaluated the effect of calcium and vitamin D_3 in 445 community-dwelling men and women 65 years of age and older, 500 mg of calcium and 700 IU of vitamin D_3 moderately reduced bone loss measured in the femoral neck, spine, and total body, and reduced the incidence of nonvertebral fractures (7). In another study, the effects of 1500 mg calcium and 800 IU vitamin D per day were compared with placebo in a large population of assisted care residents in France. After 18 months, hip fractures were reduced by 43% (8). As a substantial proportion of this population was vitamin D deficient, the results may not be applicable to the U.S. population. Nevertheless, the results of these trials support the proposal that calcium and vitamin D should be an integral component of any osteoporosis management program.

PHARMACOLOGIC MANAGEMENT

Estrogen Replacement Therapy

Until a few years ago estrogen replacement therapy (ERT) was the agent of choice to prevent and treat osteoporosis, based on a wealth of retrospective data suggesting that women who took estrogen experienced fewer fractures and derived such extraskeletal benefits as a reduction in cardiovascular events and mortality. Recently, both assumptions have been challenged, and in 2000, the FDA withdrew its approval of estrogen replacement for the treatment of osteoporosis. Estrogen continues to be approved for the prevention of bone loss in postmenopausal women.

Most of the data regarding the effect of estrogen on fractures comes from case-control and cohort epidemiologic studies. In these studies, ERT increased bone mineral density (BMD) and reduced the risk of vertebral and nonvertebral fractures (9,10). The beneficial effect of ERT appears to be greatest among current or recent users; once estrogen is discontinued, benefits diminish.

Observational studies also had suggested a protective effect of estrogen against various cardiovascular diseases. However, results from the Heart and Estrogen/Progestin Replacement Study demonstrated that the overall rate of coronary heart disease (CHD)-related events in postmenopausal women with established coronary disease was not reduced (11). Therefore, the role of estrogen in the secondary prevention of CHD events remains controversial. ERT is associated with other benefits, such as the alleviation of menopausal and urogenital symptoms (hot flashes, vaginal dryness), and potential cognitive benefits.

Despite the benefits of ERT, long-term adherence is poor because of concerns over short-term adverse events, such as breakthrough bleeding, and potential long-term risks, such as breast cancer. The incidence of breast cancer may be increased in patients taking ERT (12), although clinical trial results do not consistently support this. Currently, ERT is not recommended for patients with a known or suspected carcinoma of the breast, unless the benefits outweigh the risks.

Without the addition of a progestin at least 12 days per month, estrogen increases the risk of endrometrial hyperplasia and adenocarcinoma (13). Women with an intact uterus must take cyclic or continuous progestin with estrogen. Another disadvantage of ERT is an increased risk of venous thromboembolism, particularly in the first year of use.

ERT is easily administered and available in several dosages. The various schedules (cyclic, daily combined) and routes of administration (oral, transdermal) all have similar effects on the skeleton. The dosage of estrogen delivered, rather than the route of administration, is the important determinant of skeletal effects.

As with other medications, the benefits and risks of ERT must be individually considered before starting treatment. Sociodemographic factors, (geographic region and education level), may be more influential than clinical factors, (risk for cardiovascular disease) when deciding whether to choose ERT (14). An understanding of these sociodemographic variations is essential in helping to choose the best candidates for ERT.

Raloxifene

Raloxifene belongs to a class of drugs known as selective estrogen receptor modulators (SERMs) and appears to have tissue-specific estrogen agonist and antagonist actions. Raloxifene was the first SERM approved for the prevention and treatment of osteoporosis. Its approval as a preventive agent is based on studies in perimenopausal women demonstrating prevention of bone loss (15).

The efficacy of raloxifene in the treatment of osteoporosis was demonstrated in the Multiple Outcomes of Raloxifene Evaluation (MORE) study, a double-blind, placebo-controlled, trial of over 7700 people with osteoporosis (16). Approximately one-third of patients entered the study with prevalent vertebral fractures; the others had low bone mass without fractures. The 3-year final analysis of the MORE study results showed that 60 mg/day of raloxifene reduced the relative risk for new vertebral fractures by 30% in postmenopausal women who had at least one baseline vertebral fracture, and by 50% in those who had no prevalent vertebral fracture. There was no significant reduction of hip fractures; however, the study was not powered to demonstrate such an effect.

Raloxifene does not cause endometrial proliferation, and it beneficially affects the lipid profile by decreasing total and LDL cholesterol (17). Raloxifene's effects on cardiovascular events and mortality is the focus of a current prospective study. Although the MORE study demonstrated a significant decrease in the risk of new breast cancers in patients taking raloxifene compared to placebo (18), risk reduction for breast cancer was not a primary endpoint. Therefore, a prospective double-blind study comparing raloxifene to tamoxifene for breast cancer prevention is currently underway.

The most common adverse events associated with raloxifene include hot flashes (which are more common in perimenopausal rather than late postmenopausal women) and leg cramps. Raloxifene also increases the risk of venous thromboembolic events, and therefore should not be used in patients with an active or past history of such episodes.

Raloxifene is administered as a single daily dose of 60 mg/day with adequate calcium and vitamin D supplementation.

Calcitonin

Calcitonin is a 32-amino acid polypeptide hormone that directly suppresses osteoclast activity. In the U.S., calcitonin-salmon nasal spray is indicated for osteoporosis treatment, but not prevention, in women who are at least 5 years postmenopausal.

Calcitonin-salmon nasal spray reduces postmenopausal bone loss and decreases the risk of new vertebral fractures. A large placebo-controlled study to evaluate the efficacy and safety of calcitonin-salmon nasal spray in reducing the rate of new vertebral fractures in postmenopausal osteoporotic women showed a 33% reduction ($P = 0.03$) in risk of new vertebral fractures in patients receiving 200 IU calcitonin-salmon nasal spray over a 5-year period (19). However, the study was not designed to assess the effect of calcitonin-salmon nasal spray on hip or other nonvertebral fractures.

Calcitonin is generally well tolerated. With the exception of allergy to calcitonin-salmon nasal spray or any of its components, there are no contraindications to this therapy. Adverse events associated with calcitonin-salmon nasal spray involve local irritation of the nasal mucosa, such as rhinitis, and other nasal symptoms.

The recommended dosage in postmenopausal osteoporotic women is 200 IU/day (1 spray) administered intranasally in alternative nostrils.

Bisphosphonates

Bisphosphonates bind to the surface of bone undergoing active reabsorption and inhibit the maturation and function of osteoclasts. Bisphosphonates are classified in at least 2 groups, each of which has a different mode of action. Non-nitrogen containing bisphosphonates such as etidronate enhance osteoclastic cell death (apoptosis) by being incorporated into cytotoxic adenosine triphosphate (ATP) analogs. Nitrogen-containing bisphosphonates such as alendronate and risedronate inhibit the conversion of geranyl-pyrophosphate and farnesyl-pyrophosphate synthetase in the cholesterol pathway. These enzymatic steps are involved in protein prenylation, a process necessary for cytoskeleton organization, vesicle transport, membrane ruffling, and apoptosis of osteoclasts.

Bisphosphonates are poorly absorbed when taken orally. The oral bioavailability with an overnight fast and dosing 2 hours before breakfast with water is approximately 1%. Strict adherence to the dosing regimen is necessary to maximize absorption. Alendronate or risedronate, for example, must be taken on an empty stomach following an overnight fast with 6-8 ounces of plain water only. The patient must not consume anything for 30 minutes following dosing, and must remain upright for at least 30 minutes to reduce the risk of esophageal irritation.

Bisphosphonates are effective for preventing and treating both corticosteroid-related and postmenopausal osteoporosis. Alendronate has also been demonstrated to be effective in preventing bone loss in men with osteoporosis.

Etidronate. Etidronate was the first bisphosphonate to become clinically available for the treatment of metabolic bone disease. In a randomized clinical trial, etidronate (400 mg/day for 14 days) followed by calcium carbonate (500 mg/day for 74 days) significantly reduced the relative risk of spine fractures at 2 years. When these patients were followed for a third year, there was no significant reduction in vertebral fractures, except in patients who had the lowest baseline BMD at study entry (20).

Etidronate is not approved in the U.S. for treatment of women with postmenopausal osteoporosis, although it is approved in many countries throughout the world. When prescribing etidronate for osteoporosis, it is imperative that a rigorous cycling of treatment (as described above) be followed. Continuous, long-term treatment with etidronate (greater than 6 months) introduces the risk of demineralization and the development of osteomalacia.

Alendronate. Indicated for the treatment of corticosteroid-induced osteoporosis and for the prevention and treatment of postmenopausal osteoporosis, alendronate increases BMD and reduces the risk of new fractures. The recommended dosages are 5 mg/day for prevention and 10 mg/day for the treatment of postmenopausal osteoporosis.

In an initial study, alendronate reduced the relative risk of spine fracture by 48% compared with placebo over 3 years (21). A subsequent study assessed the effect of alendronate in 2027 women with low BMD and at least one preexisting vertebral fracture (22). Alendronate reduced the risk of new vertebral fractures by 47% and the risk of hip and wrist fractures by 51% and 48%, respectively.

Recent data support the therapeutic equivalency of alendronate, 70 mg once weekly, 35 mg twice weekly, and 10 mg/day (23). In this study, increases in lumbosacral, hip, and total body BMD were identical among the 3 patient groups receiving these dosages. The rate of bone turnover suppression was also identical. The once weekly dose was well tolerated with an incidence of gastrointestinal (GI) side effects similar to that of daily administration.

Alendronate has also been approved for the treatment of men with osteoporosis and for the treatment of corticosteroid-induced osteoporosis, based on studies demonstrating its efficacy in preserving bone density at the hip and spine (24,25).

Although virtually all clinical trials with alendronate have indicated an overall incidence of GI effects similar to placebo, rare cases of esophagitis and ulcers have occurred in post-marketing surveillance. Therefore, alendronate should not be given to patients with active, symptomatic upper GI disease or esophageal abnormalities that delay esophageal emptying, such as stricture of achalasia.

Risedronate. Risedronate, a nitrogen-containing bisphosphonate, has recently been approved for prevention and treatment of both corticosteroid-induced (26) and postmenopausal osteoporosis. A randomized, double-blind, placebo-controlled trial was undertaken to examine how much risedronate reduced the risk of new vertebral fractures in 2458 postmenopausal women (younger than 85) who had at least 1 vertebral fracture at baseline (27). Over 3 years, treatment with risedronate at 5 mg/day decreased the cumulative incidence of new vertebral fractures by 41%. A fracture reduction of 65% was observed after the first year. The cumulative incidence of nonvertebral fractures was reduced by 39% over 3 years. Risedronate also significantly increased BMD in the lumbosacral spine, femoral neck, and midshaft of the radius.

In a large study of almost 10,000 postmenopausal women, risedronate showed a 39% reduction of hip fractures compared with placebo in a subgroup of patients less than 80 years old who had low femoral neck bone mineral density (T < −3.0) and at least one additional risk factor for hip fracture (28). In patients who had both low femoral neck bone density and at least one prevalent vertebral fracture, risedronate reduced the risk of hip fracture by 58%. However, in a subgroup of women at least 80 years old who were entered into the study on the basis of risk factors for hip fracture rather than low bone density, no significant reduction in hip fractures was observed.

In all trials, the adverse event profile of risedronate, including GI events, was similar to that of placebo. However, the same prescribing precautions apply as for alendronate. The patient must take risedronate with 8 ounces of water on an empty stomach 30 minutes before the first meal. Caution should be utilized in patients with active reflux disease or esophageal dysmotility. Risedronate is given at a dosage of 5 mg/day. It is not yet known whether risedronate can be administered at less frequent intervals (e.g., once-weekly).

FUTURE TREATMENTS

Currently, all available treatments for osteoporosis work by inhibiting bone resorption. It is likely that in the future, medications that directly stimulate bone formation, combination therapies, and specific biologic mediators of bone turnover will enter the therapeutic arena. Several combinations of the available therapies have been tried. Combinations of estrogen with etidronate or alendronate, and alendronate with raloxifene have all been demonstrated to increase bone density in an additive or synergistic fashion compared to either single agent alone (29). No study has yet demonstrated additive fracture protection. Currently, combination therapy is usually reserved for patients who experience fracture despite being treated with a single agent.

Preliminary results of vertebral fracture reduction with injectable parathyroid hormone (PTH) suggest the potential for substantial increases in bone density and corresponding reduction in vertebral fractures. In a recent trial of 1637 women with postmenopausal osteoporosis, recombinant PTH significantly reduced new vertebral fractures and nonvertebral fractures for both the 20 μg/d and 40 μg/d groups, respectively, for a mean of 21 months (30). Barriers to widespread use of injectable PTH may include cost and the injectable nature of the medication.

Similar to the basic science breakthroughs in rheumatoid arthritis that have led to the tumor necrosis factor inhibitors, exciting discoveries regarding cytokine control and cross talk between osteoblasts and osteoclasts have led to the development of specific biologic inhibitors of bone turnover. Osteoprotegerin, a natural inhibitor of osteoclast activation, is being produced by recombinant technology and undergoing human trials in osteoporosis (31). In the future, osteoporosis treatments may be based on this type of specific biologic mediator rather than the nonspecific type currently used.

REFERENCES

1. Kanis JA, Melton LJ, Christiansen C, Johnston CC, Khaltaev N. Perspective: the diagnosis of osteoporosis. J Bone Min Res 1994;8:1137–1141.
2. National Osteoporosis Foundation. Physician's Guide to Prevention and Treatment of Osteoporosis. Washington, DC: National Osteoporosis Foundation; 1998.
3. Genant HK, Engelke K, Fuerst T, Gluer CC, Grampp S, Harris ST, et al. Noninvasive assessment of bone mineral and structure: state of the art. J Bone Miner Res 1996;11:707–30.
4. Miller PD, Bonnick SL, Rosen CJ. Consensus of an international panel on the clinical utility of bone mass measurements in the detection of low bone mass in the adult population. Calcif Tissue Int 1996;58:207–14.
5. Krall EA, Dawson-Hughes B. Walking is related to bone density and rates of bone loss. Am J Med 1994;96:20–6.
6. NIH Consensus Conference. Optimal calcium intake. NIH Consensus Development Panel on Optimal Calcium Intake. JAMA 1994;272:1942–8.
7. Dawson-Hughes B, Harris SS, Krall EA, Dallal GE. Effect of calcium and vitamin D supplementation on bone density in men and women 65 years of age or older. N Engl J Med 1997;337:670–6.
8. Chapuy MC, Arlot ME, Duboeuf F, Brun J, Crouzet B, Arnaud S, et al. Vitamin D$_3$ and calcium to prevent hip fractures in elderly women. N Engl J Med 1992;327:1637–42.
9. Cauley JA, Seeley DG, Ensrud K, Ettinger B, Black D, Cummings SR. Estrogen replacement therapy and fractures in older women. Study of Osteoporotic Fractures Research Group. Ann Intern Med 1995;122:9–16.
10. Kiel DP, Felson DT, Anderson JJ, Wilson PW, Moskowitz MA. Hip fracture and the use of estrogens in postmenopausal women. The Framingham Study. N Eng J Med 1987;317:1169–1174.
11. Hulley S, Grady D, Bush T, Furberg C, Herrington D, Riggs B, et al. Randomized trial of estrogen plus progestin for secondary prevention of coronary heart disease in postmenopausal women. Heart and Estrogen/Progestin Replacement Study (HERS) Research Group. JAMA. 1998;280:605–13.
12. Colditz GA, Hankinson SE, Hunter DJ, Willett WC, Manson SE, Stampfer MJ, et al. The use of estrogens and progestins and the risk of breast cancer in postmenopausal women. N Engl J Med 1995;332:1589–93.
13. The Postmenopausal Estrogen/Progestins Interventions (PEPI) Trial. Effects of estrogen or estrogen/progestin regimens on heart disease risk factors in postmenopausal women. JAMA 1995;273:199–208.
14. Keating NL, Cleary PD, Rossi AS, Zaslavsky AM, Ayanian JZ. Use of hormone replacement therapy by postmenopausal women in the United States. Ann Intern Med 1999;130:545–53.
15. Delmas PD, Bjarnason NH, Mitlak B, Ravoux A, Shah AS, Huster WJ, et al. Effects of raloxifene on bone mineral density, serum cholesterol concentrations, and uterine endometrium in postmenopausal women. N Engl J Med 1997;337:1641–7.
16. Ettinger B, Black D, Mitlak BH, Knickerbocker RK, Nickelsen T, Genant HK, et al. Reduction of vertebral fracture risk in postmenopausal women with osteoporosis treated with raloxifene: results from a 3-year randomized clinical trial. JAMA 1999;282:637–45.
17. Walsh BW, Kuller LH, Wild RA, Paul S, Farmer M, Lawrence JB, et al. Effects of raloxifene on serum lipids and coagulation factors in healthy postmenopausal women JAMA 1998;279:1445–51.
18. Cummings SR, Eckert S, Krueger KA, Grady D, Powles TJ, Cauley JA, et al. The effect of raloxifene on risk of breast cancer in postmenopausal women: results from the MORE randomized trial. Multiple Outcomes of Raloxifene Evaluation JAMA 1999;281:2189–97.
19. Chesnut CH 3rd, Silverman S, Andriano K, Genant H, Gimona A, et al. A randomized trial of nasal spray salmon calcitonin in postmenopausal women with established osteoporosis: the prevent recurrence of osteoporotic fractures study. PROOF Study Group. Am J Med 2000;109:267–76.
20. Harris ST, Watts NB, Jackson RD, Genant HK, Wasnich RD, Ross P, et al. Four year study of intermittent cyclic etidronate treatment of postmenopausal osteoporosis: three years of blinded therapy followed by one year of open therapy. Am J Med 1993;95:557–67.
21. Liberman UA, Weiss SR, Broll J, Minne HW, Quan H, Bell NH, et al. Effect of oral alendronate on bone mineral density and the incidence of fractures in postmenopsusal osteoporosis. The Alendronate Phase III Osteoporosis Treatment Study Group. N Engl J Med. 1995;333:1437–1443.
22. Black DM, Cummings SR, Karpf DB, Cauley JA, Thompson DE, Nevitt MC, et al. Randomised trial of effect of alendronate on risk of fracture in women with existing vertebral fractures. Fracture Intervention Trail Research Group. Lancet 1996;348:1535–41.
23. Schnitzer T, Bone HG, Crepaldi G, Adami S, McClung M, Kiel D, et al. Therapeutic equivalence of alendronate 70 mg once-weekly and alendronate 10 mg daily in the treatment of osteoporosis. Alendronate Once-Weekly Study Group. Aging (Milano). 2000;12:1–12.
24. Orwoll E, Ettinger M, Weiss S, Miller P, Kendler D, Graham J, et al. Alendronate for the treatment of osteoporosis in men. N Engl J Med 2000;343:604–10.
25. Saag KG, Emkey R, Schnitzer TJ, Brown JP, Hawkins F, Geomaere S, et al. Alendronate for the prevention and treatment of glucocorticoid-induced osteoporosis. Glucocurticoid-Induced Osteoporosis Intervention Study Group. N Engl J Med 1998;339:292–9.
26. Cohen S, Levy RM, Keller M, Boling E, Emkey RD, Greenwald M, et al. Risedronate therapy prevents corticosteroid-induced bone loss: a twelve-month multicenter, randomized, double-blind, placebo-controlled, parallel group study. Arthritis Rheum 1999;42:2309–18.
27. Harris ST, Watts NB, Genant HK, McKeever CD, Hangartner T, Keller M, et al. Effects of risedronate treatment on vertebral and nonvertebral fractures in women with postmenopausal osteoporosis: a randomized controlled trial. JAMA 1999;282:1344–52.

28. McClung MR, Geusens P, Miller PD, Zippel H, Bensen WG, Roux C, et al. Effect of risedronate on the risk of hip fracture in elderly women. Hip Intervention Program Study Group. N Engl J Med 2001;344:333–40.

29. Wimalawansa SJ: Prevention and treatment of osteoporosis: efficacy of combination of hormone replacement therapy with other antiresorptive agents. J Clin Densitom 2000;3:187–201.

30. Neer RM, Arnaud C, Zanchetta JR, Prince R, et al. Recombinant human PTH [rhPTH(1-34)] reduces the risk of spine and non-spine fractures in postmenopausal osteoporosis. The Endocrine Society. June 2000. Abstract 193.

31. Hofbauer LC, Khosla S, Dunstan CR, Lacey D, Boyle WJ, Riggs BL. The roles of osteoprotegerin and osteoprotegerin ligand in the paracrine regulation of bone resorption. J Bone Miner Res 2000;15:2–12.

Acute Inflammatory Arthritis

H. RALPH SCHUMACHER, Jr., MD

Patients often think of arthritis as a chronic, slowly progressive disorder. However, it can also first present as a new, acute symptom (1–3). This should raise consideration of infection, crystal disease, and trauma, although it can also be the first sign of many other joint and systemic diseases. The possibilities can be narrowed with a careful history and physical examination. Characteristics may not match a textbook-defined type of arthritis, so making a definitive diagnosis can be difficult in the early days or weeks after onset. However, early attempts at classification of the arthritis are essential.

CLINICAL FINDINGS

History

Taking the patient's family history can help, because gout, rheumatoid arthritis (RA), systemic lupus erythematosus (SLE), and the spondylarthropathies often run in families.

Symptoms that precede acute arthritis may provide important clues. Back pain that is worse in the morning may suggest spondylarthropathy. Pharyngitis suggests rheumatic fever, neisserial or viral infection, or Still's disease. Urethritis or pelvic inflammatory disease may indicate gonococcal arthritis or *Chlamydia*- or *Ureaplasma*-related reactive arthritis. Diarrhea may suggest reactive arthritis or the arthritis of inflammatory bowel disease. Any preceding infection can be the origin of an organism causing infectious arthritis. A previous joint procedure also suggests possible infection. Residence in endemic areas raises concern about Lyme disease, which can be further suggested by a history of recent tick exposure, rash, palpitations, or Bell's palsy.

A history of trauma can suggest the occurrence of a fracture or an internal derangement of ligament or cartilage, but minor trauma can also precipitate acute gout or introduce infection. Medications used may also provide clues, as they can affect the results of tests and influence the choice or outcome of therapy.

Physical Examination

The physical examination must distinguish arthritis (an inflammation in the articular space) from processes that affect the periarticular area, such as a bursitis, tendinitis, or cellulitis. Deep, axial joints such as the hips and sacroiliac joints are particularly difficult to evaluate.

An effort should be made to look for signs at extraarticular sites suggesting specific causes, such as pustules in gonococcemia, and mouth ulcers in Behçet's syndrome, reactive arthritis, and SLE. Small patches of psoriasis may be found between the buttocks or behind the ears. The keratoderma blennorrhagicum of reactive arthritis can be subtle and often affects only the feet. Erythema nodosum may suggest the presence of SLE, sarcoidosis, or inflammatory bowel disease. Skin ulcerations can be a source of infection. Splinter hemorrhages suggest bacterial endocarditis. Tophi of gout usually do not antedate arthritis, but they can be seen over joints, at Achilles tendons, and in olecranon bursae or over the extensor surface of the forearms. Fever occurs with several types of arthritis, including gout and pseudogout, but raises concern about infection.

Tenderness, some limitation of function, and soft-tissue swelling can virtually always be detected in true arthritis upon careful examination of the joint. An important early step is differentiating the joint inflammation of arthritis from symptoms caused by periarticular disease or degenerative or mechanical problems. Only true joint disease should produce the overt swelling and tenderness around the circumference of the joint. Tenderness that is localized at one side of the joint raises concerns of tendinitis, bursitis, bone disease, or cellulitis. Pain on a single motion, such as abduction at the shoulder, suggests bursitis.

Sometimes, inflammatory arthritis is only a minor feature of a potentially serious systemic disease; even mild arthritis should prompt a full and careful general evaluation. Among systemic diseases that may have mild inflammatory arthritis as the first clue are SLE, Wegener's granulomatosis and other types of vasculitis, polymyositis, scleroderma, subacute bacterial endocarditis, sarcoidosis, hemochromatosis, hyperparathyroidism, leukemia, lymphoma, and other malignant tumors. Classifying the pattern of joint swelling, as described below, may narrow the diagnostic possibilities.

Monarthritis. Swelling and pain in a single joint is the most common presentation of infectious arthritis and requires evaluation without delay. Monarthritis is also a common presentation of crystal-induced arthritis, hemarthrosis from trauma or other causes, exacerbations of osteoarthritis, and occasionally of foreign bodies, tumors, avascular necrosis, Lyme disease, or other systemic diseases.

Oligoarthritis. Involvement of several joints can occasionally occur with any infection, but this is more likely in immunosuppressed hosts, persons with antecedent joint disease, and abusers of intravenous drugs. Oligoarthritis is a characteristic presentation of Lyme disease, reactive arthritis, and other seronegative spondylarthropathies. It is not uncommon in crystal diseases, especially after the early bouts. Lower extremity, asymmetric, and large joint involvement are often most prominent in the spondylarthropathies, but they are also seen in some patients who are difficult to classify and tend to have a better prognosis. Tuberculosis involves 2 or 3 joints in 10–15% of cases.

Gonococcal arthritis is especially likely to produce migratory arthritis and tendinitis before lodging in one joint. Rheumatic fever and Lyme disease also can cause migratory arthritis. Palindromic rheumatism involves a series of joints in sequence, with symptom-free intervals between attacks.

Polyarthritis. Rheumatoid arthritis is the most common

cause of persistent polyarthritis, but viral arthritis and other systemic diseases must be considered early. Distinguishing early RA from viral arthritis, SLE, and other systemic rheumatic diseases may be impossible unless other clues are detected on history and physical examination. Inflammation of many joints, symmetric joint involvement, involvement of metacarpophalangeal joints, and long duration of morning stiffness tend to predict RA. Subcutaneous nodules provide strong evidence of RA, but they usually do not occur early, and occasionally require aspiration or biopsy for definitive diagnosis.

Up to 25% of patients with recent-onset polyarthritis have a transient disease that resolves without diagnosis. The more acute the onset and the fewer prognostic factors for RA present, the more likely that the polyarthritis is not RA, and that resolution will occur.

RADIOGRAPHIC FINDINGS

Radiographs of the involved joint are often not helpful in establishing the cause of acute arthritis. However fractures, tumors, or signs of antecedent chronic disease such as osteoarthritis can be seen on plain radiographs. Chondrocalcinosis in the involved joint suggests, but does not prove, that the acute arthritis is pseudogout. Periarticular calcifications suggest apatite crystal disease. In suspected acute septic arthritis, there are usually no radiologic findings other than soft-tissue swelling, but a film can help exclude other causes and provide a baseline for future comparisons. Magnetic resonance imaging is probably overused but may help identify early sacroiliac involvement. Magnetic resonance imaging can help localize an infectious or inflammatory process to the joint, its surrounding tissue, or bone; it may also be useful in characterizing joint problems during pregnancy.

LABORATORY TESTING

The use of cultures and Gram stains of blood, skin lesions or ulcers, cervical or urethral swabs, urine, or any other possible source of microorganisms is important in suspected infectious arthritis. This is especially true for gonococcal arthritis, because synovial fluid cultures are positive in only approximately 25% of patients. Tests for HIV and Lyme antibodies may be appropriate, but no single serologic test can establish the cause of any acute arthritis. The test for rheumatoid factor can be positive not only in RA but in many diseases associated with arthritis, including sarcoidosis, hepatitis C infection, and subacute bacterial endocarditis. Measurements of serum uric acid during the acute phase of arthritis are notoriously misleading, and the results must be interpreted with caution. Other tests should be done as indicated by each specific disease under consideration. Analysis of synovial fluid is often considered the single most useful test (4,5).

Arthrocentesis and Synovial Fluid Analysis

Arthrocentesis provides crucial information and can be performed at the bedside or in the office with almost no complications, as long as sterile techniques are used. Arthrocentesis should be performed in virtually every patient with acute arthritis and certainly in those with monarthritis (6), especially if infection is suspected. It may be difficult to aspirate fluid from some joints, such as the hips or the sacroiliac joints, and the procedure may need to be done under the guidance of ultrasonography, computed tomography, or fluoroscopy. Most of the important information from synovial fluid analysis is obtained through the total leukocyte count and differential count, cultures, Gram stain, and examination of a wet preparation for crystals and other microscopic abnormalities. All these studies can be performed with only 1–2 ml of fluid; often only a few drops are needed. Failure to use synovial fluid analysis was one of the major factors that led to misdiagnoses and prolonged hospital stays in one study (2).

Gross Examination. Important clues can be obtained from gross examination of the joint fluid. Bloody fluid suggests fracture, tumor, coagulation abnormalities, destructive arthritis of any kind, or rare problems such as scurvy. Cloudy yellow fluid suggests one of the inflammatory arthritides and must be investigated further. Absolutely clear transparent fluid with no color or pale yellow is most often due to noninflammatory causes of effusion. Opaque material may be pus, but it may occasionally be due to urate or apatite crystals.

Leukocyte Counts and Differentials. Normal synovial fluid contains fewer than 180 cells/mm^3, most of which should be mononuclear. Fluid is considered to be "noninflammatory" if it contains fewer than 2,000 cells/mm^3, although most samples of synovial fluid from patients with osteoarthritis contain fewer than 500 cells/mm^3. In general, as the leukocyte count increases, so does the suspicion of infection. Effusions containing more than 100,000 leukocytes/mm^3 are considered septic until proved otherwise. The wide spectrum of leukocyte counts in both sterile and septic inflammatory arthritis makes strict classification imprudent. Differential leukocyte counts can help; a finding of more than 90% polymorphonuclear cells should prompt concern about infection or crystal-induced disease.

Wet Drop Preparation and Crystal Identification. Careful examination of a single drop of synovial fluid under a cover slip to identify crystals can establish a diagnosis early and avoid unnecessary hospital admissions for the treatment of suspected infectious arthritis (5,7). Although most easily seen as brightly negatively birefringent needles on compensated polarized light microscopy, monosodium urate crystals can also be seen and tentatively identified by normal light microscopy. Calcium pyrophosphate dihydrate (CPPD) crystals are less intensely birefringent than monosodium urate crystals and are more rod-shaped or rhomboid with positive birefringence on compensated polarized light microscopy. These crystals may be small and difficult to see on normal light microscopy. Other less common crystals should be considered if findings are atypical (5). Among those that can cause acute arthritis are the pyramidal oxalates or the maltese crosses of lipid liquid crystals. Wet preparations of all synovial fluids should be examined not only for crystals but also for other particles such as fat droplets and blood. Large fat droplets in synovial fluid suggest a fracture involving the marrow space. Small lipid droplets, which can occur in pancreatic fat necrosis or fractures, can be misread by Coulter counters as leukocytes.

Cultures. The presence of crystals does not exclude infection, as antecedent abnormalities such as gout may increase the likelihood of septic arthritis. Cultures should be performed on samples of synovial fluid if there is any concern about infection, even if crystals are present. Cultures and Gram stain are obligatory when infection is suspected. Gram-positive bacteria can be seen on a well prepared slide of culture-positive fluids approximately 80% of the time. Gram-negative bacteria are seen less frequently, and *Neisseria gonorrhoeae* and *N. meningitidis* are rarely seen. Special stains and cultures for mycobacteria and fungi are sometimes appropriate. Most microbiology laboratories prefer to receive fluid promptly in a capped syringe and with instructions as to which organisms are suspected.

Synovial Biopsy, Arthroscopy, and Special Techniques. Needle biopsy of the synovial membrane or a biopsy obtained during arthroscopy is seldom practical as an initial step. However, culture of synovial tissue may have a greater yield than a synovial fluid culture in certain settings, such as when gonococcal or mycobacterial disease is suspected or when no fluid is available for culture. Biopsies can identify infiltrative diseases such as amyloidosis, sarcoidosis, pigmented villonodular synovitis, or tumor. Recent use of polymerase chain reaction and immuno-electron microscopy may allow diagnosis of some difficult to identify infections (8,9).

SEPTIC ARTHRITIS

Etiology and Pathogenesis

Acute infections in joints can be caused by virtually any microbial agent (10). Entry into the joint can be via the circulation from a site of infection elsewhere or by direct penetration after a wound, surgery, or local infection. Gonococcal arthritis is probably the most common septic arthritis, although the frequency varies among populations. Women are affected 2 to 3 times as often as men. A migratory tendinitis or arthritis often precedes gonococcal monarthritis. The response to therapy is usually rapid and complete; thus, this form of infectious arthritis is much less destructive than staphylococcal arthritis.

Nongonococcal bacterial infections are the most serious (11). Large joints such as the knee or hip are the most frequently affected, but any joint can be involved. Sternoclavicular joint infection is more common among intravenous drug users.

Approximately 80–90% of nongonococcal bacterial infections are monarticular. Polyarticular involvement occurs more often in the presence of a predisposing condition such as RA. The discovery of a primary site of infection can be an important clue to the infectious agent involved. By far the most common agents are Gram-positive aerobes (approximately 80%). *Staphylococcus aureus* accounts for 60%; non-group A, β-hemolytic streptococci for 15%; and *Streptococcus pneumoniae* for 3%. Gram-negative bacteria and anaerobes are increasingly frequent causes due to drug use and the rising number of immunocompromised hosts. Anaerobic infections are also more common in patients who have wounds of an extremity or gastrointestinal cancers.

Although tuberculosis and fungal arthritis are more likely to be chronic, acute mycobacterial arthritis has been reported. Atypical mycobacteria can involve multiple joints and may even mimic recent onset RA (12). Acute monarthritis associated with herpes simplex virus and other viruses has also been described.

The characteristic acute oligoarthritis of Lyme disease occurs months after the initial infection, and may occur in as many as 60% of untreated patients. Large joints such as the knee are usually involved and tend to be more swollen than painful. Acute monarthritis can also be caused by other spirochetes, such as *Treponema pallidum*, and some subacute infectious synovitis can be due to *Chlamydia* and *Ureaplasma* organisms that are especially difficult to culture.

Incidence and Risk

Although septic arthritis is less common than other types of acute inflammatory arthritis, its potential impact is greater. Early diagnosis and treatment are essential. Risk factors that should increase concern about septic arthritis include infection elsewhere in the body, very old or young age, presence of other systemic diseases, recent arthrocentesis or surgery, prosthetic joints, immunosuppression, and intravenous drug abuse.

Clinical Aspects

Infected joints are painful, tender, and limited in motion; the classic hot, red, dramatic swelling is often but not invariably present, and some signs may be masked by partial treatment or use of immunosuppressive drugs. Single joint involvement is most common, but multiple joints can be involved. Alternatively, a single joint can be infected in a patient with RA or other types of arthritis in other joints. Fever is usually present but may be low grade in up to 50% of cases or even absent in patients taking aspirin or acetaminophen. Shaking chills are especially suggestive of infection.

The most useful diagnostic test is arthrocentesis for cultures, Gram and/or acid fast staining, and full synovial fluid analysis as described above. Cultures of blood and other possible sites of infection plus complete blood counts looking for leukocytes with a left shift are required. Radiographs provide a baseline to compare for later evidence of erosions or osteomyelitis, or to look for evidence of gas-forming organisms. In joints that cannot be aspirated easily, gallium or indium scans can help identify infection.

Course and Prognosis

The prognosis is excellent if diagnosis is established during the first several days and appropriate treatment is started. Acute gonococcal or streptococcal septic arthritis often resolve completely within 2 weeks. Resolution may be much slower with staphylococcal and Gram-negative infections. Some improvement should be noted within 1 week with appropriate therapy. Prognosis is worse in previously diseased joints, with late treatment, and when immunosuppression, polyarticular disease, and other high risk factors are present.

Treatment

Initial treatment includes prompt aspiration of the joint and repeated aspiration daily or more often to keep the joint free of the destructive exudate. Guided by clinical and joint fluid clues, broad spectrum parenteral antibiotic coverage for Gram-positive and (if any clues) for Gram-negative organisms is usually needed until culture and sensitivity reports are obtained. Initial coverage should include a drug for methicillin-resistant staphylococci, if this is suggested by such factors as acquisition of infection in the hospital. If diagnosis or treatment are delayed, if the joint is less accessible to needle drainage, or if the patient is not responding, arthroscopic or surgical drainage may be needed. Splinting can reduce pain, but passive then active range of motion should be started as soon as tolerated to prevent contractures and loss of strength.

Duration of antibiotic therapy is determined by response and associated factors. Parenteral antibiotics are usually continued until the joint is virtually normal. Oral antibiotics are then used for an additional period. Staphylococcal infection in an RA joint may require at least 6 weeks of antibiotic treatment.

GOUT

Etiology and Pathogenesis

Gout is the deposition of monosodium urate crystals in joints and other connective tissues. This deposition is the result of hyperuricemia, with elevated serum uric acid levels causing supersaturation of extracellular fluids. As defined, gout can be asymptomatic when crystals are precipitated and detected only coincidentally. Most often gout is identified when urate crystal deposition causes acute or chronic arthritis, *tophi* (deposits visible over joints or in connective tissue or seen in radiographs), gouty nephropathy, or renal stones.

Increased uric acid in the serum and in total body stores can result from overproduction or underexcretion of uric acid. Many genetic and environmental factors influence an individual's uric acid level. Some of the potentially treatable causes of hyperuricemia include underexcretion of uric acid due to diuretics, low-dose aspirin, cyclosporine, acidosis, or renal insufficiency. Overproduction of uric acid can be due to enzyme abnormalities, but also occasionally to hematologic malignancies and other causes of rapid turnover of cells. Alcoholism contributes to gout both by increased production and decreased excretion of urate.

Whatever the cause, when sufficient levels are present deposition of monosodium urate (MSU) crystals can occur in joints and other connective tissues, including those of the kidney. If there is overexcretion, uric acid can precipitate in the renal collecting system and can cause stones.

Monosodium urate crystals in the joint can cause acute or chronic inflammation by stimulating the release of chemotactic factors and a variety of other mediators of inflammation. Crystals can also exist in the joint without causing inflammation; several groups are investigating how various proteins bound to the crystals and cytokines generated by the crystals affect the presence and pattern of inflammation.

Incidence and Risk

The prevalence of gout has increased over the last few decades in the U.S. and in a number of other countries with a high standard of living. Gout is predominantly a disease of adult men, with a peak incidence in the fifth decade. Although less common in women, gout should be considered after menopause and with the use of diuretics. Premenopausal women with renal failure or using cyclosporine may also develop gout (13). In 1986, the prevalence of self-reported gout in the U.S.

was estimated at 13.6/1,000 men, and 6.4/1,000 women. Thus, gout is the most common cause of inflammatory arthritis in men over age 30 and probably the second most common form of inflammatory arthritis in the U.S. (14). In addition, gout frequently results in significant short-term disability, occupational limitations, and utilization of medical services, making the disease a significant public health problem.

Clinical Aspects

As with the other crystal diseases, gout can take several forms. Asymptomatic hyperuricemia is not strictly considered gout, as by no means all patients with hyperuricemia will develop clinical signs of gout.

The acute arthritis of gout is the most common early clinical manifestation. The metatarsophalangeal joint of the first toe is involved most often, and is affected at some time in 75% of patients. The ankle, tarsal area, and the knee are also commonly involved. A wrist or finger joint is less often involved during early attacks. The first episode of acute gouty arthritis may begin abruptly in a single joint, often during the night, so that the patient awakes with dramatic unexplained joint pain and swelling. Affected joints are usually warm, red, and tender. The diffuse periarticular erythema that often accompanies these attacks can be confused with cellulitis.

Early attacks tend to subside spontaneously over 3–10 days, even without treatment. Desquamation of the skin overlaying the affected joint may occur when the inflammation subsides. Patients are often completely free of symptoms after an acute attack. Subsequent episodes may occur more frequently, involve more joints, and persist longer. Polyarticular gout occasionally occurs in patients having their first attack. Usually, patients with more than one inflamed joint are those with more prolonged disease and suboptimal management. Acute attacks may be triggered by a specific event such as trauma, alcohol, drugs, swings in uric acid levels, surgical stress, or acute medical illness.

The intervals between attacks constitute the intercritical stage of gout. Even during an asymptomatic period, MSU crystals can often be aspirated from previously involved joints or from joints that have never been overtly affected. Because crystal deposition persists between attacks, a definitive diagnosis can still be made even during this asymptomatic period (15).

Clinically evident subcutaneous MSU crystal-containing tophi occur only in fairly advanced gout, although microtophi appear to be present in the synovial membrane even at an early stage. On average, tophi are first noted 10 years after the first episode of arthritis. Deforming arthritis can develop as a result of the erosion of cartilage and subchondral bone caused by crystal deposition and the chronic inflammatory reaction. Chronic gouty arthritis can mimic RA, although it tends to be less symmetric than typical rheumatoid disease and it can involve any joint.

Radiographs are usually normal except for soft tissue swelling with early acute gout. The bony cysts or erosions that can occur in chronic gout are round or oval and are surrounded with a sclerotic margin.

The demonstration of MSU crystals is now generally considered to be mandatory for establishing the diagnosis of gout as an explanation for acute arthritis, because serum urate levels can be misleading. Only a single drop of fluid is necessary for the detection of crystals. The crystals, which are either intra-or extracellular and are typically rod- or needle-shaped (3–20 μ), are usually visible with a light microscope. A polarizing microscope shows the characteristic bright negative birefringence.

The value of serum uric acid levels in the diagnosis of the acute attack is limited. Serum uric acid levels can be normal at the time of acute gouty arthritis. Some normal levels are explained by high doses of aspirin or recent institution of a uricosuric agent. Whatever the reasons, a normal serum uric acid level does not exclude the diagnosis of acute gout. In almost all patients, serum uric acid levels will be elevated at some time. Serum urate measurements are important in following treatment. Some people without gout may have elevated serum uric acid due to drugs or other causes.

Course and Prognosis

Initial acute attacks subside spontaneously over days to a week. If gout is inadequately treated, episodes become more frequent and chronic tophaceous gout can develop. Over 20 years, more than 50% of untreated patients would develop overt chronic disease.

Treatment

Acute gout can be managed with one of several drugs, but resting the acutely inflamed joint will make any regimen more effective. Use of a nonsteroidal antiinflammatory drug (NSAID) in doses at or near the maximum recommended is probably the most common regimen in patients with no contraindications to these agents. Colchicine is used less often, but 2–3 tablets (0.5 mg each) can be dramatically effective if given at the first sign of an attack. When given in the often recommended regimen of 0.5 mg every hour until 8 pills or intolerance, side effects such as nausea, vomiting, or diarrhea are common. Because many patients with gout have contraindications to NSAIDs or colchicine, or have severe attacks that are less responsive, adrenocorticosteroids or adrenocorticotrophic hormone (ACTH) have been used increasingly. Prednisone can be given at 20–40 mg/day and then gradually tapered as the attack subsides. ACTH can be given as 40–80 IU subcutaneously. If only 1–2 joints are involved, depot corticosteroids can be injected intraarticularly once infection has been excluded. Intravenous colchicine is also a useful alternative in patients who are not taking medication orally.

If patients have recurrent attacks or tophi, plans must be made for long-term treatment with urate lowering agents, such as the uricosuric probenecid, or allopurinol.

CALCIUM PYROPHOSPHATE DIHYDRATE CRYSTAL DEPOSITION DISEASE

Etiology and Pathogenesis

Calcium pyrophosphate dihydrate crystal deposition disease can be defined as illness related to the presence of these crystals in joints, bursae, or other periarticular tissues (16). Deposition primarily occurs in cartilage and menisci, and is initially asymptomatic. Crystal deposition can also occur as a late result of osteoarthritis. In this situation the role of the CPPD is not clear.

Acute inflammation is thought to result from a dose-related response to release of CPPD crystals from deposits in cartilage or other tissues into the joint space. Phagocytosis of crystals (as occurs with urates in gout) releases inflammatory mediators causing the acute symptoms.

Radiographs showing calcific densities in articular hyaline or fibrocartilaginous tissues are diagnostically helpful. The most characteristic sites for this chondrocalcinosis are in the knees and wrists, so these may be radiographed for screening. Joints with extensive joint space narrowing may not show chondrocalcinosis but may still contain CPPD.

Incidence and Risk

Although common, clinically symptomatic CPPD-associated disease is about half as frequent as gout. Incidence is nearly equal in men and women, but CPPD deposition dramatically increases with age. Nearly 50% of people have radiographic evidence of chondrocalcinosis (almost always due to CPPD) in their 80s, and risk of CPPD-associated disease clearly increases with age. Some associated diseases that should be considered in younger patients are hyperparathyroidism, hemochromatosis, ochronosis, myxedematous hypothyroidism, hypophosphatasia, hypomagnesemia, and familial hypocalciuric hypercalcemia.

Clinical Aspects

A variety of clinical presentations are seen with CPPD, including acute arthritis often called "pseudogout," chronic RA-like inflammatory arthritis, osteoarthritis, and a very destructive arthritis (16). Acute arthritis is the pattern in about 25% of cases.

Acute attacks occur in one or more joints and can last for several days or weeks. Attacks are self-limited but can be as abrupt in onset and as severe as true acute gout; however, the average attack is less painful than in gout. The knee is the site of almost half of all attacks, although any other joint, including the first metatarsophalangeal joint, can be involved. Provocation of acute attacks by surgery or other acute illness is common. Patients are usually asymptomatic between acute attacks.

Definitive diagnosis is only by identification of the classic rod- or rhomboid-shaped crystals described above. Infection can coexist with CPPD disease, so should be excluded. Some patients with CPPD disease develop fevers that cause confusion. Younger patients with CPPD should receive a thorough examination as well as serum tests for iron, transferrin, thyroid stimulating hormone, calcium, phosphorus, and magnesium levels. Some CPPD deposits result from previous traumatic arthritis or meniscectomy and are localized to a single joint.

Course and Prognosis

There is no known treatment to eliminate CPPD crystal deposits. In most cases, deposition gradually increases unless an underlying metabolic cause is corrected. Recurrent attacks or chronic arthritis often develop, although disabling disease is uncommon. Associated diseases can be life-threatening if not detected and treated.

Treatment

Acute attacks in large joints can be treated by thorough aspiration alone or combined with injection of a depot corticosteroid. NSAIDs or cyclooxygenase-2 (COX-2) inhibitors are often effective. Colchicine given intravenously may be used in patients who cannot take NSAIDs. In addition, 0.5 mg of colchicine given 1–2 times per day is often successfully used to prevent attacks.

APATITE CRYSTAL DISEASE

Etiology and Pathogenesis

Apatite crystals and other associated calcium phosphates commonly deposit in tendons, other soft tissues around joints, and synovia. Most cases are idiopathic, although local trauma or some systemic diseases may be factors. As with urates and CPPD, these deposits can be asymptomatic until aggregates of crystals are released into joint or bursal spaces to be phagocytized and cause acute inflammation (17,18).

Incidence and Risk

There are no accurate studies of incidence of either periarticular calcifications or acute attacks. This cause of acute arthritis or bursitis may be even more common than gout but may be missed because of the difficulty of diagnosis. One survey showed that 5% of all adult shoulders had periarticular calcifications. Calcifications can be transient and disappear after attacks. Adults of all ages can be affected, and incidence increases with age. Risk factors for apatite deposition are renal failure treated with chronic dialysis and associated with hyperphosphatemia, the renal phosphate retaining syndrome of tumoral calcinosis, local deposition from corticosteroid injections, central nervous system insults, collagen disease, and milk alkali syndrome. As with CPPD disease, there are familial cases, increased occurrence with OA, and a destructive arthritis at large joints.

Clinical Aspects

Acute inflammation due to apatite crystals is often localized to a bursa or tendon sheath, suggesting this diagnosis. However, the entire joint may also be involved. There may be erythema, swelling, and tenderness; fever can occur. Pain on motion stressing the involved structure may also be severe with less objective evidence of inflammation. Common sites include the shoulders, fingers, wrists, hips, and even the first metatarsophalangeal joints.

Diagnosis depends on classic findings: radiographic evidence of calcification in soft tissue at the site of pain and, ideally, crystal identification by aspiration of synovial or bursal fluid.

Course and Prognosis

Unless an underlying cause of correctable hyperphosphatemia or hypercalcemia can be detected, most patients will remain at risk of further attacks. Disabling chronic disease is generally rare in idiopathic cases.

Treatment

Acute attacks can be treated with NSAIDs or with oral or intravenous colchicine, as used for gout. Aspiration of the calcific deposit and injection of a depot corticosteroid can also be very effective. Rest during the most acute pain should be followed as symptoms improve by range of motion exercise to prevent residual stiffness.

MANAGEMENT OF UNDIAGNOSED ACUTE ARTHRITIS

Management decisions often must be made before all the results of tests are available. For instance, a patient with synovial fluid indicating a highly inflammatory process, a negative Gram stain, and no obvious source of infection requires antibiotic coverage, although it is wise to obtain several cultures first. Needle aspiration at least once daily is mandatory in suspected cases of septic arthritis, as long as fluid is present. If cultures are negative and the arthritis persists, antibiotics are often discontinued and more extensive tests are performed. Although NSAIDs are often useful for symptomatic treatment, it may be best to withhold them at least for a few days to avoid obscuring the natural disease course and any fever. In culture-negative patients, all fluid removed should be examined for crystals, even if no crystals were seen in the first specimen aspirated. A response to colchicine, although initially considered a diagnostic test for gout, does not prove this diagnosis.

Local heat or cold applications are usually not needed. However, cold packs may occasionally be helpful when carefully used over acute gouty joints. Local protection with a splint or wrap may alleviate symptoms during evaluation. A cast should not be put on an acutely inflamed joint.

EDUCATION

Brochures, such as those available from the Arthritis Foundation, about specific suspected diseases can be used to initiate patient education. Adherence to treatment regimens may be especially critical in suspected septic arthritis and gout. Using a team approach to patient education did make an important difference in adherence and outcome in one study involving patients with gout (19). Reassurance is often in order as soon as it becomes apparent that one is dealing with a self-limited and less dangerous form of acute arthritis. Patients are often already aware of the worst possibilities and may be concerned about something so rare as malignancy as a cause.

REFERENCES

1. Baker DG, Schumacher HR. Acute monoarthritis. N Engl J Med 1993; 329:1013–20.

2. Panush RS, Carias K, Kramer N, Rosenstein ED. Acute arthritis in the hospital. J Clin Rheum 1995;1:74–80.

3. Schumacher HR. Arthritis of recent onset. A guide to evaluation and initial therapy for primary care physicians. Postgrad Med 1995;97:52–63.

4. Eisenberg JM, Schumacher HR, Davidson PK, Kaufmann L. Usefulness of synovial fluid analysis in the evaluation of joint effusions. Use of threshold analysis and likelihood ratios to assess a diagnostic test. Arch Intern Med 1984;144:715–9.

5. Schumacher HR, Reginato AJ. Atlas of synovial fluid analysis and crystal identification. Philadelphia: Lea & Febiger, 1991.

6. American College of Rheumatology Ad Hoc Committee on Clinical Guidelines. Guidelines for the initial evaluation of the adult patient with acute musculoskeletal symptoms. Arthritis Rheum 1996;39:1–8.

7. Paul H, Reginato AJ, Schumacher HR. Alizarin red S staining as a screening test to detect calcium compounds in synovial fluid. Arthritis Rheum 1983;26:191–200.

8. Inman RD, Whittum-Hudson JA, Schumacher HR, Hudson AP. Chlamydia and associated arthritis. Current Opin Rheum 2000;12:254–62.

9. Stahl HD, Seidl B, Hubner B, Altrichter S, Pfeiffer R, Pustowoit B, et al. High incidence of parvovirus B19 DNA in synovial tissue of patients with undifferentiated mono- and oligoarthritis. Clin Rheumatol 2000;19:281–6.

10. Goldenberg DL, Reed JI. Bacterial arthritis. N Engl J Med 1985;312:764–71.

11. Mahowald M: Infectious disorders. A. Septic arthritis. In: Klippel JH, Weyand CM, Wortmann RL, editors. Primer on the rheumatic diseases. 11th ed. Atlanta: Arthritis Foundation; 1997, pp 196–200.

12. Kanik KS, Greenwald DP. Mycobacterium avium/mycobacterium intracellulare complex associated arthritis masquerading as seronegative rheumatoid arthritis. J Clin Rheum 2000;6:154–7.

13. Park YB, Park YS, Song J, Lee WK, Suh CH, Lee SK. Clinical manifestations of Korean female gouty patients. Clin Rheumatol 2000;19:142–6.

14. Lawrence RC, Hochberg MC, Kelsey JL, McDuffie FC, Medsger TA Jr, Felts WR, et al. Estimates of the prevalence of selected arthritic and musculoskeletal diseases in the United States. J Rheumatol 1989;16:427–41.

15. Pascual E. Persistence of monosodium urate crystals and low-grade inflammation in the synovial fluid of patients with untreated gout. Arthritis Rheum 1991;34:141–5.

16. Ryan LM. Calcium pyrophosphate dihydrate crystal deposition. In: Klippel JH, Weyand CM, Wortmann RL, editors. Primer on the rheumatic diseases. 11th ed. Atlanta: Arthritis Foundation; 1997, pp 226–9.

17. McCarty DJ, Gatter RA. Recurrent acute inflammation associated with local apatite deposition. Arthritis Rheum 1966;9:804–19.

18. Fam AG, Rubenstein J. Hydroxyapatite pseudopodagra. A syndrome of young women. Arthritis Rheum 1989;32:741–7.

19. Murphy-Bielicki B, Schumacher HR. How does patient education affect gout? Clin Rheum in Prac 1984;2:77–80.

CHAPTER 20

Fibromyalgia

CAROL S. BURCKHARDT, RN, PhD

Fibromyalgia is a common syndrome of chronic, widespread pain. Diagnosis is based on the American College of Rheumatology (ACR) 1990 criteria for classification of fibromyalgia, which require a history of widespread pain lasting for at least 3 months and a physical finding of pain in 11 of 18 specified tender points. Pain is considered widespread if it is present in the axial skeleton on the left and right sides of the body and above and below the waist (1). Although these criteria were originally developed for research purposes, they have since come into clinical use.

The typical fibromyalgia patient is a woman between 30 and 50 years of age. Prevalence studies in the United States indicate that fibromyalgia affects about 3–5% of adult women and about 0.5% of adult men (2). Prevalence increases with age but the syndrome is also seen in children. Most patients attribute the onset of fibromyalgia to a stressor, such as an acute injury, febrile illness, surgery, or long-term psychosocial stresses. Onset is usually gradual over a period of months or years during which localized or regional pain becomes widespread, although some patients begin with widespread pain after a febrile illness. Why some persons are vulnerable to the progression of localized pain to generalized pain is not well understood, although a genetic predisposition, early childhood trauma, and prolonged stress have been implicated (3,4).

The impact of fibromyalgia can be severe. Patients report lower quality of life than patients with rheumatoid arthritis, systemic lupus erythematosus, type 1 diabetes, or chronic obstructive pulmonary disease (5). Routine tasks take longer to accomplish, and adaptations that patients must make to minimize pain and fatigue can have a negative impact on employment and on leisure activities (6).

ETIOLOGY AND PATHOGENESIS

A single etiologic mechanism is unlikely to produce the complexity of fibromyalgia symptoms. It is likely that fibromyalgia represents a complex hyperalgesic pain syndrome, in which abnormalities of central sensory processing interact with peripheral pain generators and psychoneuroendocrine dysfunction to produce a wide spectrum of symptoms (7). Central sensitization includes a reduction in pain threshold (allodynia), an increased response to painful stimuli (hyperalgesia), and an increase in the duration of pain after the stimulation. Patients experience muscle tension or contraction as pain in such a way that low or moderate muscle exertion leads to postexertional pain. Pain that inhibits maximal muscle contraction results in decreased muscle strength and endurance and deconditioning (8).

Some evidence suggests that the pain of fibromyalgia is related to disordered central processing of pain stimuli. Pressure pain thresholds as well as the point at which patients experience pain with heat and cold application are decreased (9). Changes in the neurotransmitter systems of substance P and serotonin are both implicated in the pain amplification. Substance P is believed to facilitate pain signals, while serotonin may modulate the signals (10). Low growth hormone levels are believed to contribute to postexertional muscle pain (11). Imaging techniques have detected decreased regional blood flow in the thalamus and caudate nuclei (structures involved in the processing of pain stimuli) (12). Numerous abnormalities in the hypothalamus–pituitary–adrenal axis have been identified (13).

CLINICAL FEATURES

Pain

The core symptom of fibromyalgia is chronic, widespread pain. The pain is usually perceived as arising from muscle but many patients also report joint pain, probably because of the morning stiffness they experience. Patients commonly describe their pain as tender, aching, stiff, throbbing, and sore. Their use of affective words is usually confined to tiring, troublesome, and annoying. Although constant, pain may wax and wane over days or weeks, with flares occurring in response to cold weather, psychosocial stressors, poor sleep, systemic infections, or increased exertion. Patients sometimes report feeling less pain during a part of the day, usually about 3 hours after arising and lasting 3 to 4 hours. The pain is worst in one or two locations, often in the neck, shoulders, and back, but it appears to migrate around the body in a seemingly unpredictable fashion (7).

Disordered Sleep

Persons with fibromyalgia report disturbed sleep and most feel exhausted even after a night of sleep. Typically, they perceive their sleep as light and unrefreshing and are easily aroused by auditory stimuli. Many patients have a disordered sleep physiology characterized by alpha intrusion on non-REM sleep which disrupts sleep stages 3 and 4, causing periodic limb movements and dysregulated biological circadian rhythm (14). Unlike most adults in whom the deepest sleep comes at the beginning of the sleep cycle, the best sleep for fibromyalgia patients usually occurs in the hour or two immediately before morning awakening. Although almost all patients have sleep disturbances, most do not report insomnia. Restless leg syndrome, which by definition occurs during the daytime, is nearly always associated with periodic limb movement during sleep and is characterized by feelings of numbness, tingling, and crawling sensations that necessitate constantly moving the legs.

Fatigue

Chronic fatigue and easy fatigability are characteristic of fibromyalgia and may be more debilitating than pain. The etiology is complex, with nonrestorative sleep, deconditioning, endocrine dysfunction, and depression all contributing to an experience that is both physical and emotional (1,15). Many patients appear to meet criteria for chronic fatigue syndrome (CFS) although they tend not to have low-grade fevers or adenopathy.

Associated Disorders

Fibromyalgia patients often have problems other than pain and fatigue. Irritable bowel syndrome, irritable bladder syndrome, paresthesia, dizziness, tension and migraine headaches, temporomandibular joint dysfunction, and neurally mediated hypotension are all found in higher percentages in fibromyalgia patients than in the general population (16). Most of these symptoms are believed to occur as a result of the abnormal sensory processing described above.

Individuals with fibromyalgia often report stiffness upon arising in the morning. Although the stiffness tends to dissipate, they may retain a sensation of joint swelling. There is no clinical evidence of joint deformity, fluid accumulation, increased warmth, or erythema in the joints of patients with fibromyalgia. However, in some cases there may be fluid retention in soft tissue leading to a general sense of bloating (17).

Cognitive dysfunction is among the most distressing symptoms. Patients often worry that forgetfulness and inability to think clearly or work effectively are signs of early neurodegenerative disease. However, the cause of these problems is more likely fatigue, unrefreshing sleep, chronic pain, and psychological distress. The problem nearly always gets better when patients' sleep quality improves. Factors that may exacerbate symptoms of fibromyalgia include noise, noxious smells, cold intolerance, weather changes, stress, and too much or too little exercise.

Psychological Distress

The multiplicity of patient symptoms, together with normal laboratory test results, has led practitioners unfamiliar with fibromyalgia to label patients as psychologically disturbed. Early reports found increased rates of hypochondriasis, hysteria, and depression on standardized measures such as the Minnesota Multiphasic Personality Inventory (MMPI). However, the validity of the MMPI for patients with chronic pain from any source has been questioned. Depressive and anxious symptoms can be normal reactions to persistent chronic pain and fatigue. Unfortunately, these symptoms have often been confused with psychiatric diagnoses, leading some researchers and clinicians to believe that most or all fibromyalgia patients have a mental disorder. Psychiatric disorders are more common in persons with fibromyalgia who become patients (18); however these patients are not necessarily characteristic of the general population. Psychological distress—in particular, anxiety and worry about the illness—is more often a consequence of pain, uncertainty about diagnosis, and ineffective treatment than a specific trait of the individual.

Table 1. Major treatment strategies and instruments for measuring outcomes.

Treatment strategies	Outcome measures
Patient education	Individually designed knowledge Tests based on content
Medications	Fibromyalgia Impact Questionnaire (FIQ) (28)
	Visual analog scales (0–10) for pain, sleep, and fatigue (contained within the FIQ)
	Beck Depression Inventory (29)
	Center for Epidemiological Studies-Depression (CES-D Scale) (30)
Exercise	Flexibility tests (31)
	6-minute walk time (32)
	Health Assessment Questionnaire (HAQ) (33)
Coping skills training	FIQ (28)
	Coping Strategies Questionnaire (34)

Fibromyalgia is not common in patients with major depressive disorder and even those patients with depression who complain of pain are not likely to have multiple tender points (19). Nevertheless, because psychological distress and psychiatric disorders can be disabling, they need to be taken seriously and treated in an effective, compassionate manner when present.

COURSE AND PROGNOSIS

Long-term followup studies of fibromyalgia patients have yielded conflicting results. Early studies of patients in tertiary care indicated that symptoms persisted over many years and did not respond well to treatment (20). However, more recent studies of children, adult patients in primary care, and patients who have been treated with multidisciplinary approaches indicate that many of these individuals do get better (21–23).

Fibromyalgia does not appear to progress or become more severe over time, nor is it a prodrome of other rheumatic or nonrheumatic diseases. In fact, the opposite may be true. A recent study found that older women with fibromyalgia had fewer and less severe symptoms than did younger women with fibromyalgia (24). Also, patients with inflammatory diseases, such as systemic lupus erythematosus, develop fibromyalgia secondary to their primary disease (25).

TREATMENT

Successful treatment of fibromyalgia involves an individualized, comprehensive, and goal-oriented approach (26). The patient must believe that providers recognize the syndrome as a documented, legitimate disorder, that the symptoms are real, and that effective treatment is available. Persons with fibromyalgia face permanent changes in lifestyle, threats to dignity and self-esteem, disruption of normal life roles, and decreasing resources of which providers should be aware. Although close interaction with a primary provider is important, patients can benefit greatly from treatment by a multidisciplinary team (23,27). Table 1 summarizes major categories of treatment and supplies a list of instruments for measuring outcomes (28–34).

Pharmacologic Treatment

Drug therapy in fibromyalgia focuses on the management of pain and sleep disturbances. Tricyclic antidepressants in small doses were among the first drugs studied for their effects on sleep. Overall, the tricyclics in doses of about one-fifth that of an anti-depressant dose are useful for improving sleep quality. This effect is thought to be due to the drugs' effects on inhibiting serotonin reuptake and for their antihistamine effect. Amitriptyline in doses of 10–50 mg at bedtime is commonly prescribed (35). Unfortunately, many tricyclics have undesirable side effects, such as dry mouth, constipation, and weight gain, even in small doses. It is worth giving a patient a 6-night trial of several different medications with somewhat different side effect profiles; for instance, one might first try amitriptyline 10 mg, then nortriptyline 10 mg, and, finally, trazadone 25 mg (a non-tricyclic), with a 1-night washout between them. These medications may stop working after a few weeks or months but patients can be advised to take a "drug holiday" of a week or so, after which they may again be effective. Short-acting hypnotic agents, such as zolpidem (Ambien) or zaliplon (Sonata), have been found to be helpful for some patients, particularly those who are intolerant of the "hangover" effects of the tricyclics. However, these medications should be used sparingly, not more than 2–3 times in a week, because they can be habit-forming.

Specific causes of sleep problems, such as sleep apnea, bruxism, reflux, and periodic limb movement, should be identified so that appropriate treatment can be initiated. Either carbidopa/levodopa (Sinemet) 10/100 or clonazepan (Klonopin) 0.5 to 1.0 substantially helps restless legs and periodic limb movements when taken in the evening. Overweight patients and particularly male patients with fibromyalgia may have a potentially serious mechanical sleep apnea. This problem should be assessed and treated with continuous positive airway pressure (C-PAP) or by surgical procedures (7).

Effective medication management for chronic pain is an inexact science. Usual pain medications, such as nonsteroidal antiinflammatory drugs and acetaminophen, rarely provide effective control when taken alone. Prednisone has been shown to be ineffective. Tramadol (Ultram), a non-narcotic analgesic, has been found to be moderately effective (36), due to its dual action: it inhibits reuptake of norepinephrine and has a weak affinity for μ-opioid receptors. The usual dosage is 50–100 mg every 4–6 hours and should be taken routinely rather than when pain is escalating. The dose should be titrated gradually to avoid adverse effects such as dizziness, nausea, headache, and constipation. The risk of seizures, while rare, may be increased in patients taking tricyclic antidepressants, selective serotonin reuptake inhibitors (SSRIs), or opioids.

The use of opioids is gaining credibility for treating chronic nonmalignant pain. While not the first choice, opioids should be considered after less powerful analgesics have failed. However, initial research has found that only a subgroup of fibromyalgia patients responds to opioids (37). Patients must be educated on the use of opioids, especially on the differences between physical dependence and addiction.

Recently, more emphasis has been placed on treating pain with SSRIs and other newer anti-depressants, such as fluoxetine (Prozac), nafazodone (Serzone), or venlafaxine (Effexor). These drugs are sometimes called "adjuvant analgesics" because they act indirectly to relieve pain. Current evidence is insufficient for making specific recommendations for the use of these antidepressants for pain relief because the extant trials are inadequate in sample size, therapeutic dose, and duration to test efficacy. However, fibromyalgia patients who report depression should be treated with a therapeutic dose and adequate duration of an antidepressant. Those with histories of mood and anxiety disorders may be more responsive to antidepressant treatment of fibromyalgia symptoms; thus, an adequate trial at therapeutic dosage and sufficient duration should be offered to them also (35). If patients experience insomnia associated with these drugs, they should be taken in the morning and a sedating antidepressant, such as trazodone, given at night.

Nonpharmacologic Treatment

Nonpharmacologic treatments that target pain, stress, and physical and psychological dysfunction using a variety of physical, cognitive, behavioral, and educational strategies are essential components of multidisciplinary treatment programs. The majority of nonpharmacologic strategies are based on self-management where patients are the decision-makers about when to initiate a strategy, how long to adhere to it, and how to determine efficacy. For patients to successfully carry out the work of self-management, they need state-of-the-art knowledge regarding the strategy description, procedures, and expected efficacy. Physical therapists, occupational therapists, nurses, health educators, psychologists, and others play important roles in educating and instructing patients. Other nonpharmacologic interventions include acupuncture, chiropractic, physical therapy modalities, massage, and other forms of body work.

Exercise

Exercise as a treatment for fibromyalgia was among the first nonpharmacologic strategies advocated. Individuals with fibromyalgia were noted to be physically unfit (38); thus, physical therapists and other clinicians promoted aerobic exercise. Studies have shown significant changes in aerobic capacity, pain, and physical function associated with aerobic exercise programs. One controlled trial focused on muscle strength training as the primary treatment; it showed that the 2 groups receiving this training and flexibility training (the attention control) improved significantly on muscle strength and physical function variables.

An appropriate exercise prescription for patients with fibromyalgia must take into account their deconditioned state. Training at too high a level of aerobic intensity or strength training with weights that are too heavy can cause muscle microtrauma, which in turn will result in increased muscle pain, further sleep disruption, and deconditioning. Exercise programs should follow guidelines that take into account these risks as well as the well-known benefits of exercise. Exercise prescription should fit the person's current level of fitness. As a general rule, patients should be encouraged to start at a level below what they think can be accomplished. Not only is success a powerful motivator, but the risk of injury is lessened and the likelihood of continuation is increased (39).

The goal of stretching is to release tightened muscle bands and provide pain relief. Stretching should be done at least once a day or in short bouts several times a day. Developing routine stretch breaks during the day can be very helpful in decreasing pain. Warming the muscle by active gentle movement or by warm water prior to the initial stretching bout will enable stretching without muscle damage. The patient should be encouraged to stretch to the point of feeling slight resistance (like a tight rubber band) and then hold for 10–15 seconds initially. A stretch should never be held to the point of pain, as that will cause a contraction of muscle fibers—the opposite of the desired effect. Identifying the stopping point may be easier with the eyes closed. As the patient progresses in a stretching program, the stretch can be held longer (up to 1 minute).

Strength training is the second part of a comprehensive exercise program. Most people with fibromyalgia have lost strength, which makes their muscle more vulnerable to exertional muscle damage. Strength training should be undertaken in a way that reduces eccentric muscle work (where the muscle is lengthened while contracting) and increases the time between contractions so that the muscle can fully relax. Patients should pause for a count of 4 between repetitions of any strengthening exercise. An effective strength training component alternates days so that upper body work is done one day, followed by a day of no strength training, then a day of lower body strengthening followed by a day of no strength training (40). Strength training should minimize any work done above the head and shoulders, as the shoulder girdle is extremely sensitive to muscle damage, especially in women.

Aerobic endurance training can be accomplished in several ways. Patients should be encouraged to incorporate activities they enjoy into an endurance program. Walking requires no special skills or place. It can be done in short bouts of 3–10 minutes at a time over the course of a day. Patients need to understand that they can derive benefit from short bouts of exercise that fit into their daily schedule. Alternatively, they can do a longer bout of 20–30 minutes once a day. In either case, walking should be done at a moderate pace so that after exercise patients feel that they could have done more. Duration and intensity should increase only gradually. For example, increasing time by 1 or 2 minutes per week may be a pace that is sustainable and prevents injury.

Water aerobics performed in a warm pool provide a good alternative to walking. Local chapters of the Arthritis Foundation are good resources for identifying such programs. In these programs also, patients should perform the exercises while keeping their arms below their shoulders. Exercise equipment, such as treadmills, rowing machines, and stationary bicycles are also potential methods of aerobic exercise. Patients should use the same general principles discussed above when developing an aerobic program. An exercise history or diary can help identify other forms of exercise in which they engage on a regular basis, such as gardening, stair climbing, or dancing. These can also be considered part of an exercise program if performed regularly. Whatever program is chosen, it should be low-impact and enjoyable.

Coping Skills Training

Individuals with fibromyalgia must learn a variety of skills to help them cope with and manage persistent, unpleasant, and painful symptoms. Self-management is based on the assumption that individuals are capable of controlling and changing their thoughts, feelings, behaviors, and physiological responses. Strategies include the following: 1) education that increases their knowledge of the scientific understanding of the fibromyalgia disease process, what treatments are available and how they work, and where to obtain resources; 2) pacing

to maximize energy for valued activities and to allow effective time management; 3) monitoring current coping and self-management efforts so that they can see how use of different strategies affects their disease; 4) specific techniques, such as relaxation, visualization, and cognitive restructuring, can help the individual cope with pain, fatigue, anxiety, and depression (see also Chapter 24, Cognitive Behavioral Interventions).

One powerful strategy is to help the patient learn to think non-negatively. Negative self-talk implies helplessness, hopelessness, and victimization. Simple procedures, such as having patients ask themselves if a particular thought is useful, or visualizing a stop sign when they start to catastrophize, can begin the restructuring process. Learning to stop, become aware of their bodies, and take deep breaths when anxious or tense can decrease symptoms. If patients respond to these simple techniques, they should be given resources for cognitive behavioral therapy where they can learn more. Meditation, prayer, or other spiritual practices can support patients' efforts to regain a sense of peacefulness and purpose in their lives.

Measuring Outcomes of Treatment

Learning to recognize change is an important skill. Simple scales on which patients measure changes in pain, fatigue, sleep, anxiety, or mood from day to day can help them take a more "scientific" approach to symptoms and notice when self-management techniques are working. These scales can also be useful for providing information and feedback to health professionals. The Fibromyalgia Impact Questionnaire (FIQ) is currently the most widely used clinical and research instrument for measuring symptom impact and change as a result of treatment (28). The FIQ and numerous other validated instruments for measuring health status and quality of life are available online through such sites as www.qlmed.org.

REFERENCES

1. Wolfe F, Smythe HA, Yunus MB, Bennett RM, Bombardier C, Goldenberg DL, et al. The American College of Rheumatology 1990 criteria for the classification of fibromyalgia: report of the Multicenter Criteria Committee. Arthritis Rheum 1990;33:160–72.
2. Wolfe F, Ross K, Anderson J, Russell IJ, Hebert L. The prevalence and characteristics of fibromyalgia in the general population. Arthritis Rheum 1995;38:19–28.
3. Buskila D, Neumann L. Fibromyalgia syndrome (FM) and nonarticular tenderness in relatives of patients with FM. J Rheumatol 1997;24:941–4.
4. Boisset-Pioro MH, Esdaile JM, Fitzcharles M-A. Sexual and physical abuse in women with fibromyalgia syndrome. Arthritis Rheum 1995;38:235–41.
5. Burckhardt CS, Clark SR, Bennett RM. Fibromyalgia and quality of life: a comparative analysis. J Rheumatol 1993;20:475–9.
6. Henriksson C, Liedberg G. Factor of importance for work disability in women with fibromyalgia. J Rheumatol 2000;27:1271–6.
7. Bennett RM. Fibromyalgia. In: Wall PD, Melzack R, editors. Textbook of pain. Edinburgh: Churchill Livingstone; 2000. p. 570–600.
8. Sorensen J, Graven-Nielsen T, Henriksson KG, Bengtsson M, Arendt-Nielsen L. Hyperexcitability in fibromyalgia. J Rheumatol 1998;25:152–5.
9. Kosek E, Ekholm J, Hensson P. Sensory dysfunction in fibromyalgia patients with implications for pathogenic mechanisms. Pain 1996;68:375–83.
10. Russell IJ. Neurochemical pathogenesis of fibromyalgia syndrome. J Musculoskeletal Pain 1999;7:183–91.
11. Bennett RM, Clark SR, Campbell SM, Burckhardt CS. Low levels of somatomedin C in patients with the fibromyalgia syndrome: a possible link between sleep and muscle pain. Arthritis Rheum 1992;35:1113–6.

12. Mountz JM, Bradley LA, Modell JG, Alexander RW, Triana-Alexander M, Aaron LA, et al. Fibromyalgia in women: abnormalities of regional cerebral blood flow in the thalamus and the caudate nucleus are associated with low pain threshold levels. Arthritis Rheum 1995;38:926–38.

13. Crofford LJ, Pillemer SR, Kalogeras KT, Cash JM, Michelson D, Kling MA, et al. Hypothalamic–pituitary–adrenal axis perturbations in patients with fibromyalgia. Arthritis Rheum 1994;37:1583–92.

14. Moldofsky H. Chronobiological influences on fibromyalgia syndrome: theoretical and therapeutic implications. Baillieres Clin Rheumatol 1994; 8:801–10.

15. Bennett RM, Cook DM, Clark SR, Burckhardt CS, Campbell SM. Hypothalamic-pituitary-insulin-like growth factor-1 axis dysfunction in patients with fibromyalgia. J Rheumatol 1997;24:1384–9.

16. Clauw DJ. Fibromyalgia: more than just a musculoskeletal disease. Am Fam Physician 1995;52:843–51,853–4.

17. Deodhar AA, Fisher RA, Blacker CV, Woolf AD. Fluid retention syndrome and fibromyalgia. Br J Rheumatol 1994;33:576–82.

18. Aaron LA, Bradley LA, Alarcón GS, Alexander RW, Triana-Alexander M, Martin MY, et al. Psychiatric diagnoses in patients with fibromyalgia are related to health care–seeking behavior rather than to illness. Arthritis Rheum 1996;39:436–45.

19. Fassbender K, Samborsky W, Kellner M, Muller W, Lautenbacher S. Tender points, depression and functional symptoms: comparison between fibromyalgia and major depression. Clin Rheumatol 1997;16:76–9.

20. Wolfe F, Anderson J, Harkness D, Bennett RM, Caro XJ, Goldenberg DL, et al. Health status and disease severity in fibromyalgia: results of a six-center longitudinal study. Arthritis Rheum 1997;40:1571–9.

21. Siegel DM, Janeway D, Baum J. Fibromyalgia syndrome in children and adolescents: clinical features at presentation and status at follow-up. Pediatrics 1998;101:377–82.

22. Granges G, Zilko P, Litteljohn GO. Fibromyalgia syndrome: assessment of the severity of the condition 2 years after diagnosis. J Rheumatol 1994;21:523–9.

23. Bennett RM, Burckhardt CS, Clark SR, O'Reilly CA, Wiens AN, Campbell SM. Group treatment of fibromyalgia: a 6 month outpatient program. J Rheumatol 1996;23:521–8.

24. Burckhardt CS, Clark SR, Bennett RM. Pain coping strategies and quality of life of women with Fibromyalgia: does age make a difference? J Musculoskeletal Pain. 2001;9(2):5–18.

25. Middleton GD, McFarlin JE, Lipsky PE. The prevalence and clinical impact of fibromyalgia in systemic lupus erythematosus. Arthritis Rheum 1994;37:1181–8.

26. Masi AT. Management of fibromyalgia syndrome: a person-centered approach. J Musculoskeletal Med 1994;11:27–37.

27. Mease PJ, Driscoll P, Uslan D, Blair J, London C, Belza B, et al. Multidisciplinary self-management and treatment program for patients with fibromyalgia/chronic fatigue syndrome [abstract]. Arthritis Rheum 1995;38 Suppl 9:S271.

28. Burckhardt CS, Clark SR, Bennett RM. The Fibromyalgia Impact Questionnaire: development and validation. J Rheumatol 1991;18:728–35.

29. Beck AT, Rush AJ, Shaw BF, Emery G. Cognitive therapy of depression. New York: Guilford Press; 1979.

30. Radloff LS. The CES-D scale: a self-report depression scale for research in the general population. J Appl Psychological Measure 1977; 1:385–401.

31. Mannerkorpi K, Burckhardt CS, Bjelle A. Physical performance characteristics of women with fibromyalgia. Arthritis Care Res 1994;7:123–9.

32. King S, Wessel J, Bhambhani Yl, Maikala R, Sholter D, Maksymowych, W. Validity and reliability of the 6 minute walk in persons with fibromyalgia. J Rheumatol 1999;26:2233–7.

33. Fries JF, Spitz P, Kraines RG, Holman HR. Measurement of patient outcome in arthritis. Arthritis Rheum 1980;26:137–45.

34. Rosenthiel AK, Keefe FJ. The use of coping strategies in chronic low back pain patients: relationship to patient characteristics and current adjustment. Pain 1983;17:33–44.

35. Arnold LM, Keck PE, Welge JA. Antidepressant treatment of fibromyalgia: a meta-analysis and review. Psychosomatics 2000;41:104–13.

36. Biasi G, Manca S, Manganelli S, Marcolongo R. Tramadol in the fibromyalgia syndrome: a controlled clinical trial versus placebo. Int J Clin Pharmacol Res 1998;18:13–9.

37. Sorensen J, Bengtsson A, Ahlner J, Henriksson KG, Ekselius L, Bengtsson M. Fibromyalgia–are there different mechanisms in the processing of pain? A double blind crossover comparison of analgesic drugs. J Rheumatol 1997;24:1615–21.

38. Bennett RM, Clark SR, Goldberg L, Nelson D, Bonafede RP, Porter J, et al. Aerobic fitness in patients with fibrositis: a controlled study of respiratory gas exchange and [133]xenon clearance from exercising muscle. Arthritis Rheum 1989;32:454–60.

39. Clark SR. Prescribing exercise for fibromyalgia patients. Arthritis Care Res 1994;7:221–5.

40. Clark SR, Jones KD, Burckhardt CS, Bennett R. Exercise for patients with fibromyalgia: risks versus benefits. Curr Rheumatol Rep 2001;3:135–40.

Periarticular Rheumatic Diseases

ANTHONY M. REGINATO, MD, PhD; and ANTONIO J. REGINATO, MD

The majority of patients who present to their primary health care provider with musculoskeletal pain have a soft-tissue disorder rather than less common crippling forms of articular rheumatism. Soft-tissue rheumatism is one of the most common and misunderstood categories of disorders, but it usually has a benign course and an excellent response to therapy (1). These conditions may involve anatomic regions such as the hand, wrist, elbow, shoulder, spine, hip, knee, ankle, heel, midfoot, and forefoot. Overuse, repetitive strain or trauma, acute and chronic infections, foreign bodies, entrapment neuropathies, aging, and crystal deposition play an important pathological role in their development.

The keys to diagnosis of soft-tissue rheumatism are the history and, more importantly, the precise physical examination of the anatomic structures involved and identification of precipitating and aggravating factors. Diagnostic musculoskeletal ultrasonography, underutilized in the United States, is a cost-effective way to determine periarticular soft-tissue integrity and improve the accuracy of needle placement for diagnostic and therapeutic purposes (2).

The practitioner should not overlook clues to systemic disorders, because conditions as varied as infection (gonococcemia, secondary syphilis, mycobacterial and fungal infections), rheumatoid arthritis (RA), ankylosing spondylitis, reactive arthritis, psoriatic arthritis, crystal-induced arthritis, sarcoidosis, and amyloidosis can lead to quite similar soft-tissue rheumatism syndromes, as shown in Table 1.

BURSITIS

Bursae are closed sacs, often with lining that resembles the synovial membrane lining of the diarthrodial joints, which secrete and absorb bursal fluid. The bursae provide the gliding mechanism between 2 musculoskeletal structures, such as skin over bone, muscle over muscle, and tendon over bone (3). There are approximately 150 such structures in the body, and new ones, called *adventitious bursae*, may develop at pressure points such as bunions or the site of amputation.

Inflammation of a bursa may be superficial (such as those present in the shoulder, trochanter, elbow, and knee, Figure 1) or deep (such as ischial tuberosity, iliopsoas, popliteal and anserine bursae). Bursitis is rarely seen in patients younger than 20 years and becomes common in middle-aged and older individuals. The superficial structures are vulnerable because they are interposed between the skin and the underlying bony structures. The various etiologic types of subcutaneous bursitis are summarized in Table 1.

The development of bursitis is a function of repetitive physical stresses and the condition of the bursae and surrounding tissues. Idiopathic or traumatic bursitis is characterized by noninflammatory effusion from repetitive local trauma. In septic bursitis, reduced skin gliding over bony prominences results

Table 1. Etiology of acute and chronic bursitis and tendinitis.

Common
  Bacterial
    Staphylococcus aureus
    S. pyogens
    Gonococcemia
  Crystal-induced
    Monosodium urate
    Calcium pyrophosphate
    Apatite
  Traumatic
  Rheumatoid arthritis
Uncommon
  Septic
  Fungal
    Sporothrix scheckii
  Mycobacterias
    Mycobacterium tuberculosis
    M. marinum
    M. gordonae
    M. leprae
  Spirochetes
    Syphilis
  Dialysis elbow
  Foreign bodies
  Reiter's syndrome
  Seronegative spondylarthropathy
  Scleroderma
  Systemic lupus erythematosus
  Amyloidosis
  Sarcoidosis
  Hemochromatosis
  Hypertrophic osteoarthropathy
  Giant cell tumor
  Pigmented villonodular synovitis
  Synovial sarcoma

in the abrasion, fissuring, and translocation into the bursal sac of bacteria normally present in the skin. The same mechanical factors favor formation of tophaceous deposits in crystal-induced arthritis and rheumatoid nodules. In fact, superficial bursae and independent adjacent diarthrodial joint synovitis may coexist in such conditions as RA and crystal-induced arthritis.

Certain bursae are common sites of inflammation. In the upper extremity, the most frequently affected are the subacromial and the olecranon bursae (Figure 1A). In the lower extremity, trochanteric, prepatellar (Figure 1B and 1C), anserine, gastrocnemius-semimembranosus (Figure 2A), and retrocalcaneal bursae are most frequently involved. Inflammation of the deeper bursae may impinge on vascular or neural structures and result in limb edema, ischemia, and compression neuropathies. Alternatively, inflammation may cause rupture of the bursa to the soft tissues, inducing a pseudo-thrombophlebitis syndrome. These are well-known complications of the iliopsoas and popliteal bursitis, or Baker's cyst (Figure 2B). Isolated bursal effusions are usually limited to children. Several deep bursae connect to the adjacent joints, and the bursitis

A

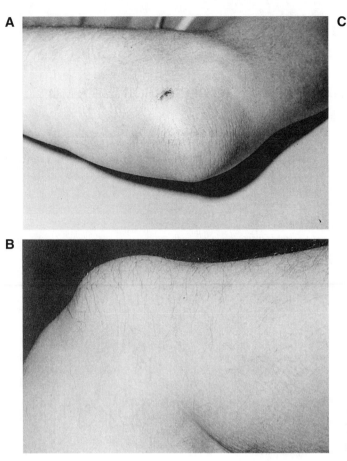

B

C

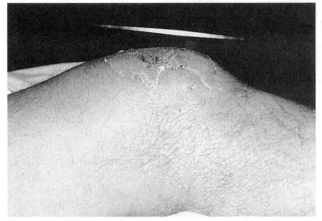

Figure 1. **A,** Staphylococcal olecranon septic bursitis showing skin abrasion, redness, and edema. **B,** Traumatic prepatellar bursitis showing noninflammatory changes. **C,** Prepatellar septic bursitis showing skin abrasion, erythema, and skin desquamation.

might represent a pathological process secondary to the neighboring joint. This is true for the subacromial, iliopsoas, and Baker's cyst.

Patients with acute bursitis present with abrupt onset of localized pain aggravated by any movement of the structures adjacent to the bursae. The pain is usually described as deep, aching discomfort. Features that suggest bursitis include sudden onset of swelling, redness, or tenderness after repetitive activity that is localized to the bursa and not the joint. Infection is suggested by the presence of fever, chills, and fluctuant swelling of the bursae, in association with redness, local heat, exquisite point tenderness, and sometimes significant edema over the underlying skin (Figure 1A). Fever should suggest infection, but it can also be present with crystal-induced bursitis. The absence of fever does not exclude infection, as only one-third of patients with olecranon septic bursitis present with fever (4).

Aspiration, which is easily accomplished when the bursa is superficial, can rule out infection and allow crystal identification. Bursal or joint fluid with white blood cell counts greater than 1,000/mm^3 indicates inflammation; fewer than 1,000 white blood cells is characteristic of traumatic noninflammatory fluids. Olecranon bursal infections tend to give higher white cell counts (though not as high as those seen with septic arthritis) with a mean of 13,500 white cells/mm^3 (5). In about 40% of these patients, the count is below 10,000 white cells (6). Bursitis due to RA and gout can produce similarly elevated white blood cell counts.

Gram and acid fast stains, pertinent cultures, and examination of fresh preparation of bursal fluid under polarized light are essential to identify infectious agents and different crystals (7). Patients presenting with fever and chills should also have blood cultures. Most cases of septic bursitis are caused by *Staphylococcus aureus*, but the Gram stain is positive in only 65% (4). If the stain shows no bacteria, or if Gram-positive cocci are found, then a penicillinase-resistant anti-staphylococcal drug should be used. If Gram-negative organisms are found, an extrabursal site of infection should be sought.

The choice of an antibiotic should be based on the most likely organism causing the extrabursal infection. Penicillin-resistant *Staphylococcus aureus* should always be considered in the diabetic, intravenous drug abuser, or immunocompromised patient. Septic bursitis always requires therapy with parenteral antibiotics. Patients with more serious underlying conditions may require intravenous antibiotics and hospitalization and, rarely, surgical drainage and bursectomy. At initiation of therapy, the bursal contents should be drained through a 16- or 18-gauge needle—a process that may need to be repeated 2–3 times over the course of the first week of treatment. The duration of antibiotic therapy averages 3–4 weeks. Antibiotics should be continued for an additional 5 days after the bursal fluid has cleared or become sterile. Nonseptic bursitis can be managed with rest, cold compresses, nonsteroidal antiinflammatory drugs (NSAIDs), and corticosteroid injections. As septic bursitis may occur with a noncharacteristic clinical presentation and clear noninflammatory bursal fluid, the cor-

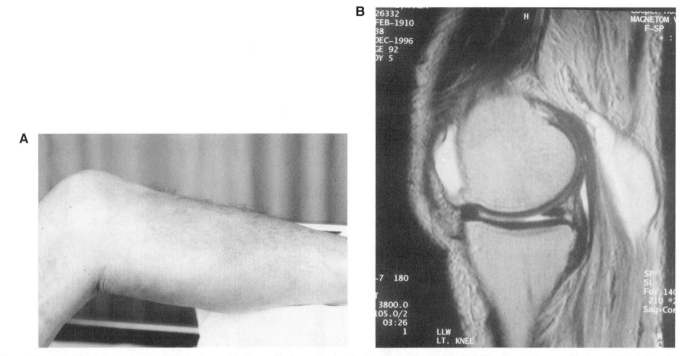

Figure 2. A, Inflamed and ruptured Baker's cyst in the calf of a patient with rheumatoid arthritis. B, MRI showing knee effusion and leaking of cyst into the calf.

ticosteroid injection should be delayed until the results of the bursal fluid cultures show no growth for at least 48 hours.

TENDINITIS

The term *tendinitis* refers to inflammation of the peritendinous tissues or synovial sheaths (tenosynovitis). Tenosynovitis most often occurs from exercise, overuse, unaccustomed activity, puncture wound, or foreign body penetration. When tenosynovitis is identified in the absence of trauma, a systemic disease should always be suspected as part of a systemic inflammatory process, as seen in bursitis (Table 1) (Figure 3). If these diseases are present, the recommended therapy for them should be followed. Disseminated gonococcemia or secondary syphilis should be suspected in sexually active individuals with inflammation involving the tendons of the ankle or wrist in the setting of monarthritis or polyarthritis, fever, and skin rash (Figure 3B). Needle aspiration of the tendon sheath might yield a few drops of fluid for culture and crystal analysis. The correct point of aspiration can be easily detected using ultrasonography (8).

REGIONAL FORMS

Several forms of bursitis and tendinitis are particularly common; their unique aspects will be described using a regional approach.

Hand and Wrist

Dupuytren's Contracture. Dupuytren's contracture, a fibrous thickening of the palmar fascia, affects predominantly middle-aged males and older individuals of Northern European decent. It is inherited as an autosomal dominant trait with variable penetrance and is associated with tobacco smoking, diabetes mellitus, local trauma, heavy manual work, alcohol abuse, and the long-term use of anti-epileptic medications with or without associated reflex sympathetic dystrophy. It usually is bilateral and involves proliferation of the hand palmar fascia with thickening and formation of tender fibrotic nodes and cords. As the disease progresses, flexion contracture of the metacarpophalangeal (MCP), proximal interphalangeal (PIP), and rarely, distal interphalangeal joints can occur. The ring and little fingers are most commonly involved.

In some patients, the disease progresses with rapid palmar fibrosis and fibrotic lesions elsewhere. These patients tend to exhibit disease earlier in life (in their 20s or 30s), have a positive family history, and show bilateral involvement. In patients with diabetes mellitus, Dupuytren's contracture has been described in association with trigger fingers, carpal tunnel syndrome, lateral epicondylitis, and frozen shoulder. It can also develop in the aftermath of sympathetic dystrophy.

Progression of Dupuytren's contracture is unpredictable, and multiple medical treatments have been tried without much success (9). Selective fasciectomy is the surgical procedure most commonly used; results depend on the stage and severity of the disease (10). Although surgical excision does not cure the disease, it may delay progression. Recurrences are more frequent in patients with nodular stage disease. Indications for surgery can be guided by a positive *table top test*, i.e., when the patient can no longer place the hand completely flat on a hard surface, correlated with greater than 30° flexor contractures at the PIP joints. As the disease becomes more aggressive, complete surgical correction becomes less likely.

Trigger Finger or Finger-Stenosing Tenosynovitis. *Trigger finger* is the locking of one or several fingers in flexion, resulting in painful clicking and popping during extension of

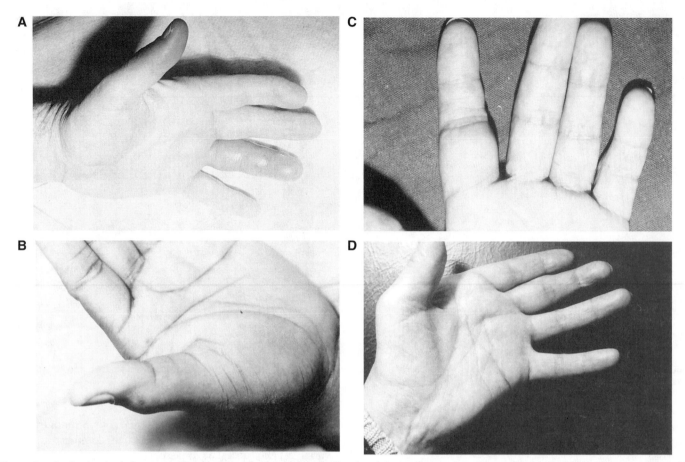

Figure 3. **A,** Acute staphylococcal annular finger flexion tenosynovitis showing swelling and erythema. **B,** Acute thumb flexor tenosynovitis observed in a patient with disseminated gonococcemia. **C,** Granulomatous index finger tenosynovitis in a patient with lupus pernio due to sarcoidosis. **D,** Giant cell tumor or pigmented villonodular synovitis of the middle finger flexor tendon sheath in a patient with rheumatoid arthritis.

the digit. On physical examination, the patient usually localizes the pain to the volar aspect of the MCP joint. The trigger may be subtle (a simple give in the tendon) or dramatic (permanent locking of the finger in flexion). Trigger finger is common in young children, middle-aged women, and older individuals. When more than 3 digits are affected, the condition may be idiopathic or may indicate other systemic conditions. Trigger finger should be distinguished from tendon involvement seen in systemic inflammatory conditions such as RA and psoriatic arthritis, in which the sheath is diffusely thickened and the trigger phenomenon is unusual.

Spontaneous improvement occurs in only 15−20% of cases. If untreated, permanent contracture can develop. Nonsurgical treatment includes splinting, NSAID administration, and corticosteroid injections. These injections into the tendon sheath provide pain relief in more than 95% of cases (11); however, they have a lower rate of success in diabetic patients (12). Complications such as infection and tendon rupture are rare, and subcutaneous fat atrophy and depigmentation may occur at the site of injection. After 2 injections without relief of symptoms, surgical release of the pulley system is highly successful, with minimal morbidity and low recurrence rate (13,14).

DeQuervain's Tenosynovitis. DeQuervain's tenosynovitis, or stenosing tenosynovitis of the first dorsal compartment of the hand, is a common cause of wrist and thumb pain in women 30−50 years of age (15). Patients report disabling pain in the radial aspect of the wrist or forearm over several weeks to months, often associated with recent pregnancies and/or repetitive use of the thumb or wrist. The patients drop objects from their hands, and activities such as lifting a baby or changing diapers cause excruciating pain.

Diffuse or localized swelling over the first extensor compartment along the radial styloid is seen on physical exam. The patients may notice crepitation during adduction/abduction motions of the thumb. A positive Finkelstein's test usually reproduces the pain when the examiner performs ulnar flexion of the wrist while the remaining four fingers encircle and grasp the thumb. This condition can be confused with osteoarthritis or chondrocalcinosis of the first carpometacarpal joint, which can coexist with DeQuervain's tenosynovitis. Swelling and tenderness are noted along the sheath of the abductor pollicis longus, which spreads distally over the base of the first metacarpal, and the extensor pollicis brevis, which inserts at the base of the distal phalanx of the thumb.

Nonsurgical treatment includes NSAIDs, a splint that partially or totally immobilizes the thumb during certain activities that exacerbate pain, and corticosteroid injections. The injection may be repeated twice, if necessary. Lack of response may be due to anatomic variation of the sheath (16). If symptoms persist, surgical release of the first compartment is indicated.

Acute, Subacute and Chronic Digital Flexor Tenosynovitis. Digital flexor tenosynovitis results from inflammation of the synovial sheath of the flexor digital tendon (Figure 3). Acute septic tenosynovitis is usually caused by *Staphylococcus* *aureus* or *Streptococcus pyogenes* from direct inoculation. Abrasions, fissures, puncture injuries, and foreign body penetration are likely to cause suppurative tenosynovitis (17). Gonococcemia, meningococcemia, and secondary syphilis (18) may give rise to acute or subacute synovial and tenosynovial infection of the fingers and wrist. Mycobacteria or fungi (especially sporotrichosis) may cause subacute or chronic tenosynovitis. Calcific tenosynovitis due to apatite crystal deposition often occurs idiopathically or in patients with scleroderma, mixed connective tissue disease, or systemic lupus erythematosus (SLE). Patients with digital ulcers have an increased risk of developing a suppurative tenosynovitis.

The patient usually presents with exquisite tenderness over the entire flexor sheath, while the digit is maintained in an antalgic, semiflexed position, with pain on extension of the finger, and swelling of the digit (Figures 3A and 3B). If untreated, suppurative tenosynovitis may spread to the palmar spaces and wrist when the first and fifth digits are involved. Hand surgery consultation should immediately be obtained for surgical drainage, debridement, and biopsy. Wide-spectrum parenteral antibiotics must be administered pending Gram stain and cultures. Subacute tenosynovitis with intact skin and calcific tendinitis may be treated conservatively with NSAIDs and splints. Failure to improve should trigger surgical drainage and biopsy, with further workup and treatment as suppurative or proliferative tenosynovitis. Calcific tendinitis improves slowly, and the hand should be protected for 1−2 weeks.

Proliferative Tenosynovitis. Chronic multiple tenosynovitis usually results from systemic disease such as RA, rheumatoid nodulosis, scleroderma, mixed connective-tissue disease, SLE, and psoriatic arthritis. Single sheath tenosynovitis usually represents foreign body tenosynovitis (most commonly seen in children, farmers, gardeners, fishermen, and divers), sarcoidosis (Figure 3C), pigmented villonodular synovitis (PVNS) or giant cell tumors (19) (Figure 3D), tuberculosis, synovial chondromatosis, and even the deadly synovial sarcomas. Proliferative synovitis may also be caused by mycobacterias, fungi, algae, and tophaceous crystalline deposits, mainly monosodium urate crystals (20). Patients witness the slow growth of a small eccentric, elongated painless lump. Some of these conditions may cause erosive damage of adjacent bones and joints.

Local corticosteroid injections are useful in treating tenosynovitis caused by systemic diseases. In single sheath tenosynovitis, surgical exploration is mandatory for both tissue diagnosis and treatment. The tissue requires proper bacteriologic studies for indolent microorganisms such as acid-fast organism and fungi, as well as absolute alcohol fixation and compensated light microscopy to look at crystal and foreign bodies. Tenosynovectomy is curative for PVNS or giant cell tumor, fibroma of the tendon sheath, and synovial chondromatosis; it is diagnostic for synovial sarcoma.

Carpal Tunnel Syndrome (CTS). CTS, one the most common compression neuropathies, is caused by impingement of the median nerve at the carpal tunnel (21). It occurs more frequently in women, often accompanying pregnancy, menopause, Colles' fracture, RA, diabetes mellitus, and trauma (22). CTS results from an increase or change in pressure within the carpal tunnel, which encloses the median nerve. Increased pressure with flexion or extension of the joint (Phalen's sign) explains nocturnal and early morning worsening of symptoms. Acute CTS occurs in a rapidly expanding lesion within the carpal tunnels and is seen in fractures, hematomas (anticoagulation and hemophiliac), necrotizing fasciitis, tumoral calci-

nosis, crystal-induced inflammation, and other systemic inflammatory conditions.

Most patients present with paresthesias and/or pain in one or both hands. The thumb, index, and middle finger are most commonly involved, but the whole hand may be numb. Activities that flex the wrists, such as driving or holding the telephone, may increase numbness. Clumsiness and pain radiating up the arm to the shoulder are commonly reported. Differential diagnosis includes cervical radiculopathy, diabetic neuropathy, and compression of the median nerve at proximal locations. The anterior interosseous nerve syndrome is characterized by weakness of the thumb, index, and middle fingers. In the pronator syndrome, the pain is localized on the proximal forearm, with paresthesias in the three and one-half digits supplied by the medial nerve. Percussion at the pronator muscle may reproduce the paresthesias while the Phalen's test is negative.

Provocative tests include *Tinel's sign* (light percussion at the wrist) and *Phalen's sign* (flexing of the wrist passively) resulting in increased paresthesia within 60 seconds and an electrical sensation radiating to the thumb, index finger, or middle finger respectively. Tinel's sign is less sensitive and more specific than Phalen's sign, with a 6% false-positive rate (23). *McMurthry's sign*, manual pressure on the nerve at the carpal tunnel, reproduces the painful symptoms and/or paresthesias. Decreased sensitivity and thenar atrophy occur in patients with longstanding median nerve compression. Electrodiagnostic testing is helpful in evaluating additional compressive sites and confirms the diagnosis before surgery. Sensory abnormalities are seen earlier than motor abnormalities because the median nerve is composed mostly of sensory fibers at the level of the wrist. A positive electrodiagnostic test is often required for surgical approval in workers' compensation claims.

Conservative measures, including NSAIDs, resting volar splints that hold the wrist in a neutral position, and corticosteroid injections, are the mainstay of nonsurgical therapy. The splints should be worn at night and during activities that exacerbate the symptoms. Surgery should be considered when permanent symptoms are present and in acute CTS, with the exception of crystal-induced synovitis, which responds to conservative treatment. Both open and endoscopic carpal tunnel release are highly effective to relieve symptoms (24). Pathologic studies of wrist flexor tendon sheaths are useful to detect granulomatous synovitis, PVNS, synovial sarcomas, and amyloidosis.

Elbow

Olecranon Bursitis. Olecranon bursitis is the inflammation of the bursa that overlies the olecranon process of the ulna. It is commonly related to infection, repetitive trauma, or underlying rheumatic process such as gout or RA. It is directly or indirectly related to repetitive direct pressure or repetitive activities on the bursa. The patient presents with pain at the posterior aspect of the elbow that is aggravated by flexion of the elbow past 90°, local swelling or bogginess, erythema, and tender olecranon bursa with normal range extension of the elbow joint (Figure 1A). This finding may help differentiate olecranon bursitis from an effusion within the joint itself. Aspiration of the bursa is necessary to exclude infection. The most common cause of infection is *S. aureus*, requiring antibiotic treatment.

A compression bandage is recommended to prevent recurrence in nonseptic bursitis. In traumatic and crystal-induced bursitis, an injection of corticosteroid should also be considered if the Gram stain and 48-hour culture results are negative. This usually induces dramatic improvement of symptoms. Periodic applications of ice and the use of an elbow pad can prevent recurrence and offer protection against infection. Rarely, if infection persists or bursitis becomes recurrent, surgical excision may be required.

Lateral Epicondylitis (Tennis Elbow). Tennis elbow or lateral epicondylitis is common in middle-aged people. It is more often related to work (electricians, machine operators, switchboard operators, and bricklayers) than to tennis. Tennis elbow results from overuse of the extensor carpi radialis brevis, the wrist dorsiflexors that span the lateral epicondyle and the base of the third metacarpal. Patients present with lateralized pain over the soft tissue just distal to the epicondyle. The pain is reproduced by resisted dorsiflexion of the wrist, and passive elbow range of motion is normal. Any degree of restriction in motion should raise the possibility of an intraarticular process such as inflammatory synovitis, osteoarthritis, chondrocalcinosis, osteochondromas, aseptic bone necrosis, and osteochondritis dissecans. Radiographs are useful to detect these conditions as well as calcific tendinitis and exostosis.

Tennis elbow may resolve spontaneously with time and rest of the affected arm. Total immobilization is discouraged so as to reduce muscle atrophy and loss of strength. A counterforce forearm brace is widely used for pain relief and should be worn during activities. Ice packs, capsaicin cream, and NSAIDs can be used to control pain and inflammation. Isometric and range of motion exercises for the upper extremity should be implemented. Local corticosteroid injections can be added if treatment progresses slowly or if the patient is unable to participate in physical therapy due to residual inflammation and pain. Such injections are relatively safe, and more than 80% of patients experience short-term relief (25). About 10% of patients develop chronic symptoms despite medical treatment and may require surgery if other causes of elbow pain are excluded.

Golfer's Elbow. Similar to tennis elbow but much less common, golfer's elbow affects the medial epicondyle. Medial epicondylitis occurs in golf players as well in manual workers such as bricklayers. The condition is caused from repetitive traction stress at the medial epicondyle attachment of the pronator teres or flexor carpi radialis muscles. Patients present with pain at the medial aspect of the elbow that increases with resistance to wrist flexion and forearm pronation. Local tenderness at the medial epicondyle or slightly distal to it confirms the diagnosis. Ulnar paresthesias from associated compressive neuropathy may be present in up to 30% of the cases.

The treatment for golfer's elbow is similar to that for tennis elbow. Because the ulnar nerve runs behind the medial epicondyle, corticosteroid injections should be administered with care to avoid nerve injury and transient hand weakness due to the anesthesia.

Shoulder

The shoulder consists of many joints including the acromioclavicular, sternoclavicular, glenohumeral, and scapulothoracic muscular joints (26). To accurately diagnose and treat disorders of the shoulder, it is necessary to understand the anatomy and function of the shoulder structures. The rotator cuff, a soft-tissue structure composed of various tendons from four muscle groups (supraspinatus, subscapularis, teres minor, and infraspinatus) provides stability during shoulder motion. Different sites for corticosteroid injections and their anatomic structures are shown in Figure 4. Inflammation or tears of the rotator cuff tendons may occur after repetitive use or overuse, secondary to trauma including impingement and aging with calcification due to apatite crystal deposition. These deposits are the most common cause of shoulder discomfort leading to secondary inflammation of the subacromial bursae and the bicipital tendon.

Clinical diagnosis of the shoulder problem can be made from the patient's history and physical examination, including ultrasonography. A careful examination of the shoulder joint should help differentiate between arthritis, tendinitis, bursitis, and a frozen shoulder. In elderly patients, it is mandatory to obtain a shoulder radiograph in internal and external rotation to exclude underlying bone disease and look for calcific tendinitis.

Rotator Cuff Tendinitis. Rotator cuff tendinitis is the most common cause of localized shoulder pain in athletes. It usually arises from small tears and inflammation of the rotator cuff tendon—in particular the supraspinatus, near the insertion into the greater tuberosity of the humerus. Tendinitis, with resultant inflammation and swelling of the rotator cuff tendon, causes impingement of the cuff beneath the coracoacromial arch. This further aggravates the tendinitis, which may become chronic. Rotator cuff tendinitis can be associated with subacromial bursitis, further decreasing the subacromial space. Active shoulder movement is restricted by pain. The inflammation of the tendon (or overlying bursa) causes the typical impingement sign or "painful arc" on raising the shoulder, as the inflamed and edematous tendon impinges on the undersurface of the acromion and coracoacromial ligament at approximately 90°. The pain, which is severe and incapacitating, is made worse by use of the arm when the patient is supine, resulting in loss of sleep and inability to work. It may refer into the upper arm, causing the patient to insist that the problem is in the arm, not the shoulder. Radiographs usually appear normal and are not necessary in typical cases, but they are important in the elderly to exclude multiple myeloma or metastatic carcinoma.

Treatment should consist of 2 parts. First, treatment of the tendinitis includes avoidance of aggravating activity, local application of ice, NSAIDs, and electrotherapeutic modalities to reduce pain and inflammation. If these regimens have limited results, corticosteroid injections into the subacromial space may reduce the patient's symptoms sufficiently to allow rehabilitation. The second part involves physical therapy to correct anatomic abnormalities that may cause an impingement syndrome, glenohumeral instability, muscle weakness or incoordination, or soft-tissue tightness.

Calcific Tendinitis. This condition, which occurs in 8% of the population, is characterized by the deposition of apatite crystals in the tendon and also may be associated with calcium deposits elsewhere (27). Calcifications may exist in the absence of symptoms. In other cases, deposits may provoke an acute inflammatory reaction accompanied by swelling, pain, tenderness, and fever, resembling a gouty attack or septic arthritis. In such cases, radiographs and ultrasonography may help in the diagnosis. Administration of NSAIDs and corticosteroid injections are effective in most patients.

Bicipital Tendinitis. Tendinitis of the long head of the biceps commonly occurs in conjunction with primary impingement or inflammation of the rotator cuff. Patients have a history of repetitive overhead arm use and anterior shoulder

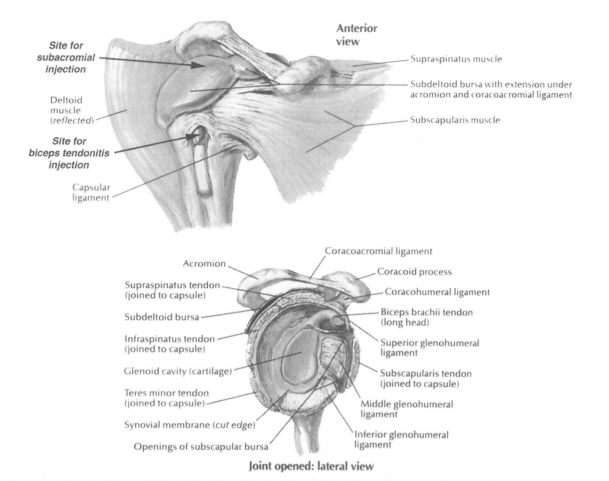

Site for subacromial injection

Deltoid muscle *(reflected)*

Site for biceps tendonitis injection

Capsular ligament

Anterior view

Supraspinatus muscle

Subdeltoid bursa with extension under acromion and coracoacromial ligament

Subscapularis muscle

Coracoacromial ligament

Acromion

Coracoid process

Supraspinatus tendon (joined to capsule)

Coracohumeral ligament

Subdeltoid bursa

Biceps brachii tendon (long head)

Infraspinatus tendon (joined to capsule)

Superior glenohumeral ligament

Glenoid cavity (cartilage)

Subscapularis tendon (joined to capsule)

Teres minor tendon (joined to capsule)

Middle glenohumeral ligament

Synovial membrane *(cut edge)*

Inferior glenohumeral ligament

Openings of subscapular bursa

Joint opened: lateral view

Figure 4. Structures of the shoulder and their relationships. Note that the subdeltoid bursa lies next to the supraspinatus tendon, but separate from the shoulder joint. Note the acromion and the coracoacromial ligaments, which may impinge on the supraspinatus tendon upon abduction of the arm. (Anterior and lateral views modified from Rheumatology Illustrations by Frank H. Netter, MD, Novartis Pharmaceuticals Corporation).

pain. Tenderness is found in the bicipital groove on the anterior humerus and moves as the arm is abducted and externally rotated. Pain is provoked by shoulder rotation and elevation and may be reproduced by supination of the forearm against resistance (*Yergason's maneuver*). Alternatively, pain may be reproduced at the bicipital groove when the patient places his hands on the head and abducts the arms (*Ludington's sign*) or when he flexes the shoulder against resistance with the elbow extended (*Speed's test*). Tendons of the long head of the biceps may rupture, resulting in the "Popeye sign" caused by rolling up of the contracted biceps belly.

Patients respond to rest, moist heat, therapeutic ultrasound, and NSAIDs. Gentle physical therapy should be initiated slowly. Corticosteroid injection into the bicipital tendon sheath may be considered; however, the potential risk of tendon rupture makes this somewhat risky. Alternatively, corticosteroid injections into the subacromial bursa may reduce the risk and provide some benefit. Bicipital tendinitis can occur in conjunction with rotator cuff tendinitis, and therapy should be designed to treat both.

Subacromial-Subdeltoid Bursitis. Subacromial-subdeltoid bursitis is difficult to differentiate from the inflamed underlying rotator cuff tendons, and isolated bursitis is rare. Acute pain and associated tenderness occur in the lateral aspect of the shoulder and inferior tip of the acromion, sometimes with radiation distally and proximally. The impingement sign is present along with limited range of motion secondary to pain. Subdeltoid septic bursitis and septic rotator cuff tendinitis are uncommon but have been described in intravenous drug users. Treatment of nonseptic subacromial bursitis is similar to treatment for other types of tendinitis of the shoulder.

Senile Tendinosis and Milwaukee Shoulder. Shoulder pain in the elderly is often multifactorial and may include age-related rotator cuff tendinosis, rotator tears, impingement from acromioclavicular joint osteoarthritis, spurs, and cervical spondylosis (27). Rotator cuff tendon degeneration increases with age and is common in the aging population. Recurrent rotator cuff tendinosis is followed by progressive shoulder limitation, superior subluxation, intraarticular calcification, and large bloody effusions. Disability in activities of daily living and sleep disturbance are frequent in rotator cuff disease in the elderly. *Milwaukee shoulder* represents the most serious complication of rotator cuff disease. In cases with full-thickness tears, arthroscopic anterior acromionectomy and debridement are effective in reducing pain and improving function (28). Hemiarthroplasty has been shown to be effective for pain relief.

Frozen Shoulder (Adhesive Capsulitis). Frozen shoulder is a condition of the glenohumeral joint characterized by severe pain and reduced active and passive range of motion (29). The condition may appear spontaneously or following minor shoulder trauma, cervical radiculopathy, hemiparesis, lung cancer, cardiac catherization, or myocardial infarction. Patients develop gradual or abrupt severe, deep, aching pain that is experienced anteriorly along the biceps muscle; such pain can be severe at night.

The mainstay of treatment is active mobilization physiotherapy. All patients should be instructed on range of motion exercises. Subacromial or intraarticular corticosteroid injection may be helpful, but the response is not as dramatic as in the acute phase (30). Most cases resolve with physical therapy over 12−24 months. Refractory cases of frozen shoulder improve remarkably with manipulation under anesthesia or arthroscopic release of the anterior and inferior capsular structures, alone or in combination.

Hip and Buttock

Trochanteric Bursitis. Trochanteric bursitis results from abnormal gait caused by leg-length discrepancy; nerve paralysis; apatite deposits; painful conditions of the foot, knee, and hip; spinal disorders; lumbar spondylosis; and dorsal scoliosis. Iliotibial band shortening may be a contributing factor. Patients present with pain over the greater trochanter while walking and lying in bed on the affected side. Pain is aggravated by internal rotation of the hip. Trochanteric bursitis may be secondary, or associated with hip disease. Resisted abduction reproduces the pain in a minority of cases. The classic finding is point tenderness at the posterior aspect of the greater trochanter.

Treatment includes local measures for symptom relief, rest, heat or cold applications, NSAIDs, and corticosteroid injections. Failure to respond to conservative treatment should be evaluated by the orthopedist for simple longitudinal release of the iliotibial band or arthroscopic bursectomy.

Ischial Bursitis. Patients with ischial bursitis report buttock pain that persists throughout the day and find it difficult to sit on one side of the buttock. On physical examination, point tenderness is demonstrated at the ischial tuberosity. Treatment consists of NSAIDs, hamstring stretching exercises, aspiration of the bursa, and corticosteroid injections.

Iliopsoas Bursitis. Iliopsoas bursitis involves a variety of pain syndromes and compressive syndromes caused by distention of the iliopsoas bursa. The iliopsoas bursa is the largest bursa in humans and separates the anterior aspect of the coxofemoral joint from the iliopsoas muscle. The bursa may become distended in hip conditions such as RA, osteoarthritis, synovial chondromatosis, and septic arthritis.

Small bursal distention may be asymptomatic; however, larger distention can compress adjacent structures such as the femoral vein, artery, or nerves. The resulting symptoms of leg edema, limb ischemia, quadriceps weakness, and sensory deficits can be appreciated in the anterior thigh. Radiographs aid in recognition of chronic hip joint abnormalities. Ultrasonography and magnetic resonance imaging may be helpful in patients with compressive syndromes. Patients with septic arthritis of the hip may also develop an iliopsoas bursal abscess.

Irritative iliopsoas bursitis features groin pain that radiates to the buttock or anterior thigh, mimicking coxofemoral arthritis. Passive hip flexion triggers the pain. Unlike in hip arthritis, passive hip rotation is painless. Obturator nerve entrapment syndrome is an important cause of hip pain in athletes and should be considered in the differential diagnosis. The pain occurs on the adductor origin of the pubic bone and is aggravated by exercise. As the patient exercises, the pain radiates

down the medial aspect of the thigh towards the knee. The patient has adductor muscle weakness, spasm, and paresthesias along the medial distal thigh. Irritative iliopsoas bursitis resolves with rest and NSAIDs. In recalcitrant cases, a corticosteroid injection may be considered under fluoroscopy. Large distended iliopsoas bursae may be treated indirectly by treating the hip condition responsible for the effusion.

Knee

Prepatellar Bursitis. Prepatellar bursitis, known as housemaid's knee, frequently occurs after trauma or after persistent kneeling or praying (Figure 1B). Patients present with swelling and mild pain at the lower aspect of the patella that extends proximal to the tibial tuberosity. It may be misdiagnosed as a knee effusion. In contrast to acute arthritis, however, patients with acute prepatellar bursitis keep the knee in full extension or tolerate gentle passive knee extension without pain. Large, relatively painless, cold effusion is characteristic of traumatic bursitis. Aspiration should be performed to rule out infection. Bursal gout may be the first manifestation of the disease; acute arthritis may coexist. Similarly, septic prepatellar bursitis may coexist with gout. In RA, prepatellar bursitis is more rare than olecranon bursitis, but may occur in patients with prepatellar rheumatoid nodules.

Treatment of traumatic bursitis consists of preventing recurrent trauma with protective kneepads. Spontaneous regression can be expected to occur in weeks to months. Conservative measures are recommended, but if they fail and infection has been excluded, corticosteroid injections are effective.

Patellar Tendinitis. Patellar tendinitis, also known as jumper's knee, results from repetitive overloading of the patellar tendon. Patients present with pain at the inferior aspect of the knee that is aggravated by stair climbing and running. Physical examination reveals tenderness of the patellar tendon at the inferior pole of the patella. Treatment consists of rest, NSAIDs, quadriceps stretching exercises, and lower extremity strengthening.

Anserine Bursitis. Anserine bursitis is the most common cause of medial knee pain. Patients tend to be middle-aged or older women with mild patellofemoral osteoarthritis, obesity, and valgus angulations of the knee. Two closely related bursae can be found near the insertion of the tendons of the gracilis, sartorius, and semimembranous muscles on the anterior-medial area of the knee. Patients report pain over the affected area. On examination, an area of exquisite point tenderness is found 2 inches below the knee joint space, medial to the tibial tuberosity.

Management includes rest, ice, NSAIDs, strengthening exercises of the hamstrings, and weight reduction. Local injection of corticosteroid can be effective in relieving pain. If conservative treatment fails, the bursal sac may be resected.

Two additional bursae in the medial knee may cause occasional symptoms. One is the collateral ligament bursa (known as the "no name, no fame bursa") located between the anterior portion of the medial collateral ligament and the joint capsule. The other is the more posteriorly located semimembranous bursa, saddled around the semimembranous tendon. Patients with no name, no fame bursitis have medial knee pain and tenderness following trauma or overexercise. Tenderness increases with flexion. Involvement of the semimembranous bursa results in swelling at the posterior edge of the medial femoral condyle.

Popliteal or Baker's Cyst. Popliteal cysts represent distended gastrocnemius and semimembranous bursae usually associated with a knee effusion and commonly secondary to chronic RA, osteoarthritis, or internal derangement of the knee (Figure 2A and 2B). It is less commonly seen in septic arthritis, hemarthrosis during anticoagulant therapy, crystal-induced arthritis, ankylosing spondylitis, and Reiter's syndrome. Although most cysts are asymptomatic, a variety of complications have been reported, including persistent leg edema, rupture of or dissection into the calf with a pseudothrombophlebitic syndrome, popliteal vein thrombosis, and popliteal arterial occlusion. Ultrasonography allows detection of the knee effusion and dissecting or ruptured cyst, and excludes the presence of associated thrombophlebitis and deep vein thrombosis.

Bed rest and measures to decrease the knee effusion with intra-articular corticosteroid injection in nonseptic synovitis are effective. Septic arthritis requires parenteral antibiotics and joint drainage.

Iliotibial Band Syndrome. Iliotibial band syndrome is a common cause of lateral knee pain in runners, cyclists, football players, and military recruits. The iliotibial band is a thick condensation of the tensor fascia lata, gluteus maximus, and gluteus medius. The band acts to maintain the knee in the extended position and stabilizes the knee during weight bearing.

Patients present with lateral knee pain upon walking and running, which is aggravated by climbing stairs or walking uphill and relieved by walking with the knee fully extended. Pain is localized over the lateral femoral condyle on flexion and extension movements, while pressure applied over the lateral epicondyle reproducibly causes pain. Treatment consists of temporarily halting or decreasing activity, local heat, and NSAIDs for 2 weeks.

Ankle and Foot

Achilles Tendinitis. Pain associated with tenderness and swelling of the Achilles tendon or near its attachment is often seen in chronic strain resulting from recreational athletics. It may be associated with spondylarthropathy, such as ankylosing spondylitis, psoriatic arthritis, or reactive arthritis, but is rarely seen with gout. All patients should be examined to rule out associated systemic conditions. Examination reveals localized swelling or thickening of the Achilles tendon and tenderness on palpation. Loss of dorsal flexion strength or discomfort with resisted motion can occur. Peritendinitis can be distinguished from Achilles tendinitis by the painful arc sign. Peritendinitis involves the tendon sheath, and as the foot is moved through dorsiflexion to plantar flexion, the area of tenderness is unchanged; whereas with tendinitis, the area of tenderness moves with the foot.

Treatment includes the use of a heel lift in the shoe and avoidance of irritating activity. Occasionally, a short course of cast immobilization provides relief of symptoms. A removable walking cast can be employed. Once symptoms resolve, the patient should follow a gentle program of gastrocnemius-soleus stretching and strengthening. Injections are generally not recommended due to the possibility of tendon rupture. Surgical intervention is rare, with the exception of tendon rupture.

Surgical debridement of the degenerated thickened tendon may be an indication in patients who fail to respond to 6 months of conservative treatment.

Plantar Fasciitis and Heel Pain. Heel pain is a frequent complaint in medical practice and can be frustrating to treat. Plantar fasciitis is associated with disabling plantar heel pain, which is worse with weight bearing and usually severe during the first steps in the morning or after prolonged sitting. The pain may be sharp, dull, or burning in nature. Tenderness is typically located over the plantar aspect of the medial calcaneal tuberosity, and sometimes, the anterior plantar fascia may be tender. Calcaneal spurs may or may not be present. Plantar fasciitis may be a clinical clue to underlying spondylarthropathy.

Time often relieves this condition, and use of soft silicone heel pads with a gel insert may be all that is needed. Initial treatment includes stretching, a heel cup, and NSAIDs. Patients should be taught to stretch the heel cord by leaning against a wall, feet flat and turned slightly inward, for 30 seconds with multiple repetitions. Orthotic devices may help correct anatomic or biomechanical abnormalities. However, when disability is pronounced, injection of the tender spot with a mixture of corticosteroid and lidocaine, using a medial or lateral approach to avoid heel fat-pad atrophy, can result in rapid cure. Multiple injections increase the chance of rupture of the plantar fascia. Cast immobilization may be used to break the chronic pain cycle. The American Orthopaedic Foot and Ankle Society recommends 6–12 months of conservative treatment before considering surgery. More than 90% of patients respond to medical treatment within this time frame (31). Surgical procedure consists of partial plantar fascia release with or without decompression of the nerve of the abductor digiti minimi.

Myofascial Pain Syndromes. Myofascial pain syndrome is marked by myofascial trigger points, which are defined as a small area within a tight band of skeletal muscle fiber that gives rise to characteristic referred pain. Spraying with ethylchloride, followed by active or passive stretching exercises for the involved muscles, may be beneficial. Trigger point injections of a local anesthetic, such as lidocaine, should be considered in highly irritable trigger points.

REFERENCES

1. Canoso JJ. Musculoskeletal conditions. In: Rheumatology in primary care. Philadelphia: WB Saunders; 1997. p. 20–96.
2. Canoso JJ. Ultrasound imaging: a rheumatologist's dream. J Rheumatol 2000;27:2063–2064.
3. Canoso JJ. Bursae, tendons and ligaments. Rheum Dis Clin North Am 1981;7:189–221.
4. Ho G Jr, Tice AD, Kaplan SR. Septic bursitis in the prepatellar and olecranon bursae: an analysis of 25 cases. Ann Intern Med 1978;89:21–7.
5. Canoso JJ. Bursal membrane and fluid. In: Cohen AS, editor. Laboratory diagnostic procedures in rheumatic diseases. New York: Grune and Stratton; 1985. p. 55–76.
6. Ho G Jr, Mikolich DJ. Bacterial Infection of the superficial subcutaneous bursae. Clin Rheum Dis 1986;12:437–57.
7. Schumacher HR, Reginato AJ. Atlas of synovial fluid analysis and crystal identification. Philadelphia: Lea & Febiger; 1991.
8. Koski JM. Ultrasound guided injections in rheumatology. J Rheumatol 2000;27:2131–8.
9. Hurst LC, Badalamente MA. Nonoperative treatment of Dupuytren's disease. Hand Clin 1999;15:97–107.
10. Benson LS, Williams CS, Kahle M. Dupuytren's contracture. J Am Acad Orthop Surg 1998;6:24–35.
11. Anderson B, Kaye S. Treatment of flexor tenosynovitis of the hand ('trigger finger') with corticosteroids. A prospective study of the response to local injection. Arch Intern Med 1991;151:153–6.

12. Chammas M, Bousquet P, Renard E, Poirier JL, Jaffiol C, Allieu Y. Dupuytren's disease, carpal tunnel syndrome, trigger finger, and diabetes mellitus. J Hand Surg 1995;20:109–14.
13. Benson LS, Ptaszek AJ. Injection versus surgery in the treatment of trigger finger. J Hand Surg 1997;22:138–44.
14. Turowski GA, Zdankiewicz PD, Thomson JG. The results of surgical treatment of trigger finger. J Hand Surg 1997;22:145–9.
15. Bahm J, Szabo Z, Foucher G. The anatomy of de Quervain's disease. A study of operative findings. Int Orthop 1995;19:209–11.
16. Nagaoka M, Matsuzaki H, Suzuki T. Ultrasonographic examination of de Quervain's disease. J Orthop Sci 2000;5:96–9.
17. Reginato AJ, Ferreiro JL, O'Connor CR, Barbasan C, Arasa J, Bednar J, et al. Clinical and pathologic studies of twenty-six patients with penetrating foreign body injury to the joints, bursae, and tendon sheaths. Arthritis Rheum 1990;33:1753–62.
18. Reginato AJ, Schumacher HR, Jimenez S, Maurer K. Synovitis in secondary syphilis. Clinical, light, and electron microscopic studies. Arthritis Rheum 1979;22:170–6.
19. Reginato A, Martinez V, Schumacher HR, Torres J. Giant cell tumour associated with rheumatoid arthritis. Ann Rheum Dis 1974;33:333–41.
20. Kostman JR, Rush P, Reginato AJ. Granulomatous tophaceous gout mimicking tuberculous tenosynovitis: report of two cases. Clin Infect Dis 1995;21:217–9.
21. Allieu Y, Chammas M. Carpal tunnel syndrome. Etiology, diagnosis. Rev Prat 2000 15;50:661–6.
22. Stevens JC, Beard CM, O'Fallon WM, Kurland LT. Conditions associated with carpal tunnel syndrome. Mayo Clin Proc 1992;67:541–8
23. Gellman H, Gelberman RN, Tan Am, Botte MJ. Carpal tunnel syndrome: an evaluation of the provocative diagnostic tests. J Bone Joint Surg Am 1986;68:735–7.
24. Brown RA, Gelberman RH, Seiler JG 3rd, Abrahamsson SO, Weiland AJ, Urbaniak JR, et al. Carpal tunnel release. A prospective, randomized assessment of open and endoscopic methods. J Bone Joint Surg Am 1993;75:1265–75.
25. Hay EM, Paterson SM, Lewis M, Hosie G, Croft P. Pragmatic randomised controlled trial of local corticosteroid injection and naproxen for treatment of lateral epicondylitis of elbow in primary care. BMJ 1999;319:964–8.
26. Huang HH, Qureshi AA, Biundo JJ Jr. Sports and other soft tissue injuries, tendinitis, bursitis, and occupation-related syndromes. Curr Opin Rheumatol 2000;12:150–4.
27. Daigneault J, Cooney LM Jr. Shoulder pain in older people. J Am Geriatr Soc 1998;46:1144–51.
28. Rochwerger A, Franceschi JP, Viton JM, Roux H, Mattei JP. Surgical management of calcific tendinitis of the shoulder: an analysis of 26 cases. Clin Rheumatol 1999;18:313–16.
29. Noel E, Thomas T, Schaeverbeke T, Thomas P, Bonjean M, Revel M. Frozen shoulder. Joint Bone Spine 2000;67:393–400.
30. de Jong BA, Dahmen R, Hogeweg JA, Marti RK. Intra-articular triamcinolone acetonide injection in patients with capsulitis of the shoulder: a comparative study of two dose regimens. Clin Rehabil 1998;12:211–5.
31. Chou LB, Oloff LM, Bocko AP. The painful foot and ankle; viewpoints from orthopaedics and podiatry. In: Harris ED Jr, Genovese MC, editors. Primary care rheumatology. Philadelphia: WB Saunders; 2000. p. 213–7.

Polymyalgia Rheumatica

STEPHEN A. PAGET, MD, FACP, FACR

Polymyalgia rheumatica (PMR) is a systemic inflammatory disorder that occurs in individuals over 50 years of age, commonly associated with an elevated erythrocyte sedimentation rate and anemia. Patients often report constitutional symptoms; proximal aches and pains; and stiffness and soreness in the neck, shoulders, and pelvic girdle. The syndrome is defined by its clinical presentation and by the exclusion of other disorders that can mimic it, including hypothyroidism, malignancy, connective tissue disorders such as systemic lupus erythematosus and rheumatoid arthritis (RA) in the elderly, and infectious disorders. Once established, diagnosis is confirmed by the rapid and nearly miraculous response to low-dose corticosteroids (1–4).

PMR is one part of a spectrum of inflammatory disorders, with the other component being a systemic vasculitis known as giant cell arteritis (GCA) or temporal arteritis. GCA is a granulomatous vasculitis of the large- and medium-sized vessels and can, in its most virulent form, lead to occlusive vascular disease and its attendant ischemic aftermaths such as blindness and stroke. Approximately 50% of patients with GCA have aches and pain characteristic of PMR; conversely, 10% of PMR patients either have or develop concomitant GCA. This scope of possible disease presentations has important diagnostic, therapeutic, and pathogenetic implications (5,6).

INCIDENCE

PMR is a descriptive term that was first suggested by Barber in 1957 to describe a syndrome of aching in elderly patients that could not be attributed to defined rheumatic, infectious, or neoplastic disorders. It is estimated to affect approximately 1 in 1,000 persons in the United States population over 50 years of age, with peak incidence between the ages of 60 and 80. However, there are well-documented reports of PMR (usually in association with GCA) in patients in their forties. Sixty percent of patients are female. While the sedimentation rate is usually elevated, this is not invariable and the diagnoses of PMR and GCA are *clinical* ones, supported by, but not totally defined by, laboratory tests (1–4).

PATHOPHYSIOLOGY

PMR is probably a multifactorial disease, with both environmental and genetic factors contributing to susceptibility and severity. To date, the only genetic associations found relate to genes in the HLA complex (HLA–DR4). Environmental factors such as infectious agents have been linked to the development of PMR and GCA. The senescence of the immune system may also play a role in a disorder that presents primarily in the elderly. Musculoskeletal symptoms appear to be linked to a nonerosive articular and extraarticular synovitis. The specific cytokine production by the involved tissues may influence clinical disease. Cytokine profiles for PMR and GCA have been shown to be different. Because the inflammatory response is regulated by a delicate balance between pro- and antiinflammatory cytokines, immunologic findings in these syndromes will help to establish the actual defects causing PMR and GCA and will eventually lead to better understanding of the disease pathogenesis and more focused therapeutic options (7,8).

CLINICAL ASPECTS

Patients with PMR frequently report malaise and fatigue, as if they had a severe viral illness. Both PMR and GCA can present with fevers of unknown origin. Fever is usually low, but temperatures may reach 102° F. Anorexia and weight loss may be prominent features and suggest malignancy. While no direct association between PMR and neoplasm has been proven, malignancy can mimic PMR and thus an age-appropriate and symptom- and sign-focused malignancy assessment is mandatory (3).

Other symptoms of PMR include chronic, symmetric aching and stiffness of the proximal muscles, soft tissues, and joints. These symptoms are most prominent in the shoulder and pelvic girdles and neck. Aching and stiffness are worse in the morning and on exertion and can be incapacitating. Muscles may be tender; disuse may lead to atrophy, and contractures can occur. Muscle strength is often difficult to evaluate because pain is present; however, it should be normal when pain is taken out of the picture (9,10).

The majority of patients have poorly localized tenderness over their joints, especially prominent over the shoulders and hips, low back, and buttocks. The original description of PMR excluded synovitis as a feature; however, while proximal symptoms and signs dominate the clinical picture, synovitis of the hands, wrists, and knees can be present and patients can have carpal tunnel syndrome due to flexor tenosynovitis. Inflammatory joint disorders in the elderly have many overlapping features. One-third of individuals diagnosed with RA are over 60 years of age. In that age group, the joint presentation can be either the characteristic symmetric polyarthritis of the small joints of the hands and feet or proximal findings more characteristic of PMR. In fact, some rheumatologists have speculated that PMR and RA in the elderly are the same disorder (11,12).

LABORATORY STUDIES

An elevated Westergren erythrocyte sedimentation rate (ESR) is a laboratory hallmark of PMR; it is usually in excess of 50

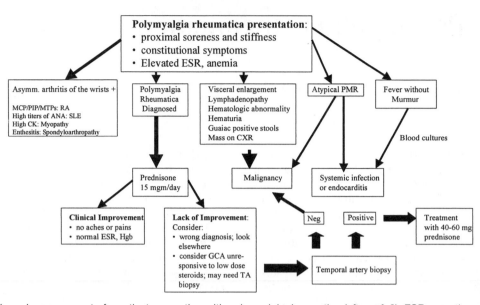

Figure 1. The diagnosis and management of a patient presenting with polymyalgia rheumatica (after ref. 3). ESR = erythrocyte sedimentation rate; asymm. = asymmetric; MCP = metacarpophalangeal; PIP = proximal interphalangeal; MTP = metatarsophalangeal; RA = rheumatoid arthritis; ANA = antinuclear antibodies; SLE = systemic lupus erythematosus; CK = creatine kinase; CXR = chest x-ray; PMR = polymyalgia rheumatica; Hgb = hemoglobin; GCA = giant cell arteritis; TA = temporal artery; neg = negative.

mm/hour and may exceed 100 mm/hour. Some physicians employ the C-reactive protein (CRP) as their guide to the state of the inflammatory process. It must be noted, however, that the diagnosis of PMR is a clinical one and is only supported, not defined, by an elevated ESR or CRP. A low or normal ESR may be seen in patients who are treated with corticosteroids for another disorder. The ESR should normalize within 7–10 days after initiating therapy with low-dose steroids. As steroids are tapered, the ESR may gradually rise again. However, treatment changes should be based on the return of clinical signs and symptoms of disease activity and not solely on increased ESR (13).

Normocytic normochromic anemia is seen in approximately 50% of patients and may serve as an indicator of clinical response to corticosteroids or of disease exacerbation when steroids are tapered. Thrombocytosis is commonly seen when disease is active, normalizes when steroids have suppressed the clinical manifestations, and can be similarly employed as a sign of active or inactive disease. Leukocytosis is common with white blood cell counts in the 12,000–16,000 range. Counts over 25,000–30,000 should alert the clinician to the possibility of an infection or malignancy.

The frequency of rheumatoid factors, antinuclear antibodies, and other autoreactive antibodies is not higher than that of age-matched controls. In those cases where the clinical picture lies in the center between PMR and RA, a positive rheumatoid factor may support the latter.

Muscle enzyme levels (creatine kinase) are normal as are electromyograms. Muscle biopsies may show type II fiber atrophy but do not demonstrate an inflammatory cell infiltrate. The latter two tests are not commonly performed in the setting of a diagnosis of PMR.

Bone scintigraphy has demonstrated high uptake in the region of the shoulders consistent with joint or periarticular inflammation. Plain x-rays are normal. Synovial fluid analysis may show a mildly elevated white blood cell count between 1,000 and 8,000 with a predominance of lymphocytes. Mild synovial proliferation with a slight lymphocytic infiltration has been found on biopsy of synovial tissue. Other studies include TSH to rule out hypothyroidism and immunoelectrophoresis to exclude multiple myeloma. An age-appropriate malignancy evaluation is mandatory in this age group, due to the rare malignancy as the cause of the syndrome.

Differential Diagnosis

When symptoms suggestive of PMR are present, clinical entities such as neoplasias, infections, muscle diseases, and other rheumatic disorders must be considered and ruled out with the appropriate clinical and laboratory testing (see Figure 1) (3,13). The clinician should be guided by a complete individual and family history and physical exam. Not every patient needs an extensive work-up for each differential diagnosis.

TREATMENT

The initial treatment for PMR is 15 mg of prednisone in a dosing schedule of 5 mg three times a day with meals. A prompt and dramatic clinical response is considered by some to be an absolute criterion for the diagnosis. Most symptoms resolve in 48–72 hours and the ESR, anemia, and thrombocytosis should normalize after 7–10 days. If the anticipated dramatic improvement does not occur within a week's time, alternative diagnoses should be considered, such as RA, an underlying giant cell arteritis that is not responsive to a low dose of prednisone, malignancy, or infection. Symptoms and signs that may indicate GCA include headache, visual symptoms (however mild and transient), and scalp tenderness or abnormal temporal arteries on examination. Malignancy may be associated with a prominent weight loss, physical findings such as a breast mass or visceral symptoms, or laboratory findings such as guaiac-positive stools or hematuria. Infections may present with a prominent fever with chills and leukocytosis, as well as local symptoms such as cough or dysuria. Significant clinical overlap occurs between these disorders, and PMR and GCA patients can present as diagnostic enigmas (4,5,13).

Once disease manifestations are controlled, the dose of corticosteroid should be slowly tapered to the lowest level that controls the symptoms. A typical tapering schedule would be to decrease prednisone by 1–2.5 mg every 7–10 days with close observation for symptom return. While serial ESR measures and complete blood counts are part of the monitoring, therapeutic decisions are based on signs and symptoms, not solely on an elevation of the ESR or CRP. Thus, the dose of prednisone should be increased only for recurrence of symptoms.

PMR, in most patients, lasts for 1–2 years and during that time the dose of corticosteroids needed to control symptoms may fluctuate. Up to 40% of PMR patients may have their disease for as long as 7 years. While the dose of steroid will inexorably decrease during the course of the illness, minor elevations of prednisone of 1–2.5 mg may be necessary to re-set the inflammatory thermostat and control a recurrence of aches and pains and/or fatigue.

Guidelines for the treatment of PMR include the following:

1. The lowest dose of corticosteroid that controls the disorder is the optimal one. The cumulative negative effect of steroid therapy should always be considered, especially in an elderly population of women who are likely to have postmenopausal osteoporosis.
2. PMR patients should be made aware that they could develop giant cell arteritis during the year after their PMR diagnosis was made. Thus, they should report to the physician immediately any visual symptoms, severe and persistent headache, scalp tenderness, jaw pain with eating, or limb claudication. Such symptoms may reflect impending vascular occlusion due to inflammation and may demand an immediate increase in corticosteroid dosage to 60 mg/day or more.
3. When chronic steroids are prescribed, prophylaxis against the likely long-term side effects of these drugs in an elderly patient population with many comorbidities must be considered, including:
   a. Immunizations against influenza and pneumococcus.
   b. Close monitoring for infections, diabetes, hypertension, depression, myopathy, and gastrointestinal problems such as ulcers and diverticulitis. Remember that an elevated ESR could be due to causes other than PMR and thus an increase in steroid dose based on an elevated ESR may further suppress a cholecystitis, diverticulitis, or urinary tract infection.
   c. Osteoporosis monitoring and treatment. This includes yearly bone density measurements, the daily institution of 1,500 mg of calcium and 800 units of vitamin D3, and

consideration for the prophylactic or therapeutic use of bisphosphonates such as alendronate and risedronate. The use of estrogen replacement in women and assessment for testosterone replacement in men with osteopenia is appropriate.
   d. Often, as steroids are tapered, patients re-develop significant aches and pains and fatigue that limit function. Increasing the dose of corticosteroid by a few milligrams usually controls the inflammation. If patients continue to need prednisone doses over 10 mg/day or develop increasing side effects from the cumulative doses, steroid-sparing drugs are considered. These include nonsteroidal antiinflammatory drugs (be aware of an increased rate of side effects in this elderly population) or weekly methotrexate. Although there is little in the literature to support the use of methotrexate in PMR, rheumatologists sometimes use it in the setting where one cannot easily differentiate between PMR and elderly-onset RA.
   e. Close partnership with a rheumatologist is helpful when treating patients with more refractory disease, those who have GCA, and patients with many side effects from chronic steroid use.

REFERENCES

1. Spiera H, Davison S. Long-term follow-up of polymyalgia rheumatica. Mt Sinai J Med 1978;45:225–9.
2. Bahlas S, Ramos-Remus C, David P. Clinical outcome of 149 patients with polymyalgia rheumatica and giant cell arteritis. J Rheumatol 1998; 25:99–104.
3. Gonzalez-Gay MA, Garcia-Porrua C, Salvarani C, Olivieri I, Hunder GG. Polymyalgia rheumatica manifestations in different conditions mimicking polymyalgia rheumatica. Clin Exp Rheumatol 2000;18:755–9.
4. Chuang T-Y, Hunder GG, Ilstrup DM, Kurkland LT. Polymyalgia rheumatica: a 10-year epidemiologic and clinical study. Ann Intern Med 1982;97:672–80.
5. Leibowitz E, Paget S. Giant cell arteritis. 2001; emedicine.com
6. Hamilton CR Jr, Shelley WM, Tumulty PA. Giant cell arteritis: including temporal arteritis and polymyalgia rheumatica. Medicine (Baltimore) 1971;50:1–27.
7. Weyand CM, Hicok KC, Hunder GG. Tissue cytokine patterns in patients with polymyalgia rheumatica and giant cell arteritis. Ann Intern Med 1994;212:484–91.
8. Wagner AD, Goronzy JJ, Weyand CM. Functional profile of tissue-infiltrating and circulating CD 68+ cells in giant cell arteritis: evidence for two components. J Clin Invest 1994;94:1134–40.
9. Salvarani C, Cantini F, Macchioni P, Olivieri I, Niccoli L, Padula A, et al. Distal musculoskeletal manifestations in polymyalgia rheumatica: a prospective followup study. Arthritis Rheum 1998;41:1221–6.
10. Salvarani C, Cantini F, Olivieri I, Hunder GG. Polymyalgia rheumatica: a disorder of extra-articular synovial structures. J Rheumatol 1999;26:517–21.
11. Healey LA, Sheets PK. The relation of polymyalgia rheumatica to rheumatoid arthritis. J Rheumatol 1988;15:750–2.
12. Healey LA. Polymyalgia rheumatica and seronegative rheumatoid arthritis may be the same entity. J Rheumatol 1992;19:270–2.
13. Stern R. Polymyalgia rheumatica and temporal arteritis. In: Paget SA, Gibofsky A, Beary JF III. Manual of rheumatology and outpatient orthopedic disorders: diagnosis and therapy. 4th ed. Philadelphia: Lippincott Williams & Wilkins; 2000. p. 181–6.

SECTION D: CLINICAL INTERVENTIONS

CHAPTER

23

Patient Education for Arthritis Self-Management

MICHELE L. BOUTAUGH, BSN, MPH; and TERESA J. BRADY, PhD, LP, OTR

The American College of Rheumatology guidelines for the treatment of rheumatoid arthritis (RA) and osteoarthritis (OA) include patient education to enhance self-management as a first line of treatment (1,2). Educating patients for self-management involves not only transmitting information but also using multiple strategies to foster healthy beliefs, behaviors, and skills. This chapter provides an overview of characteristics of quality patient education, a review of studies on the effectiveness of various forms of arthritis education, and advice for incorporating theory-based principles of education into clinical practice.

WHAT IS QUALITY PATIENT EDUCATION?

Patient education is defined in the Arthritis and Musculoskeletal Patient Education Standards as "planned, organized learning experiences designed to facilitate voluntary adoption of behaviors or beliefs conducive to health" (3). Quality education for patients with chronic conditions like arthritis is designed to foster *self-management*, or the beliefs and behaviors that persons with arthritis use to manage their condition and to achieve or maintain optimal health status or quality of life (4).

Traditional patient education is based on the premise that increased knowledge leads to behavior change, which in turn leads to improved health outcomes. However, there is growing recognition that although increased knowledge is necessary, it usually is not sufficient to bring about desired changes in health behaviors and health outcomes. Patient education that focuses primarily on transmitting information has less impact than forms of education that focus on helping patients incorporate behavior change into their lifestyles. A meta-analysis of patient education clinical trials demonstrated that interventions including behavioral techniques demonstrated greater changes in pain, functional disability, and tender joints than interventions that relied solely on information dissemination (5).

Self-management enhancing education programs differ dramatically from traditional patient education programs, which primarily use didactic methods to inform patients about arthritis and its treatment. Self-management education uses interactive methods to increase patients' confidence and skills in day-to-day management of their arthritis. With less emphasis on arthritis content, self-management education builds generalizable skills such as decision-making, problem-solving, self-monitoring, and communicating with health care providers.

Self-management education generally uses participatory methods such as discussion, brainstorming, and developing self-contracts for trials of small behavior changes.

Education to foster self-management can be provided through group classes or individualized instruction that incorporates behavioral techniques. Other interventions that may contain self-management-enhancing education include group exercise and education classes, telephone support programs, mediated instruction, and cognitive behavioral therapy. (Chapter 24 describes cognitive behavioral interventions, which will not be reviewed in this chapter.) Table 1 describes the other common types of educational interventions used in arthritis and lists their capabilities and limitations.

IMPACT OF ARTHRITIS EDUCATION

Effectiveness of the Arthritis Self-Management Program

Healthy People 2010 (www.health.gov/healthypeople), the nation's goals and objectives for health improvement for the years 2000–2010, includes an objective related to arthritis education: "Increase the proportion of persons with arthritis who have had effective, evidence-based arthritis education as an integral part of the management of their condition" (6). The arthritis education program with the most extensive and robust data supporting its effectiveness is the Arthritis Self-Management Program (ASMP) developed by Lorig and colleagues at Stanford University. In the United States, the ASMP was adopted by the Arthritis Foundation and has been disseminated nationwide as the Arthritis Self-Help Course. Four-month followup of the original ASMP participants demonstrated decreased pain and increased arthritis knowledge, frequency of exercise, and relaxation, compared with a control group. A cost-benefit study found a persistent 20% decrease in pain, along with a 43% reduction in physician visits, resulting in an estimated savings of $189 for an OA patient and $648 for an RA patient over the 4 years of the study (7). A subsequent cost-effectiveness analysis (8) determined that the program saved costs at the same time that it reduced pain.

The ASMP has been disseminated internationally; studies in the United Kingdom (9), Canada (10), the Netherlands (11), and Australia (12) have generally replicated the positive short-

Table 1. Types of educational interventions/programs.

Type/references	Characteristics	Capabilities/advantages	Limitations
Self-management/ self-help group programs (7,9,10–14)	Group class series with sessions usually lasting about 2–2.5 hours for 5–7 weeks. Emphasis on interactive methods/experiential learning and strategies to improve self-efficacy (via goal-setting, contracting, feedback, use of positive role models, reinterpretation of symptoms, persuasion). Content focuses on how to adopt new behaviors and problem-solving skills.	Promotes peer support and problem-solving skills. Ideally taught by trained lay leaders who provide modeling and can be low cost. Efficient; able to educate up to 15 patients at a time. Solid evidence on effectiveness.	Time- and labor-intensive for course leaders and participants. Classes not always available in desired locations and times. Training required for course leaders. Some patients dislike groups. Not tailored to individual needs.
Individual/one-to-one instruction (16–18,20)	Verbal instruction by individual practitioner or team of health professionals. Typical content is disease and treatment information. Effectiveness can be enhanced if combined with other educational/behavioral strategies (e.g., use of print materials and other media/technology, demonstration and practice of recommended skills, telephone support, etc.).	Can be personalized to meet needs of patients. Can be individualized to patient's readiness to change. Can be incorporated into clinical practice.	Verbal instruction alone and leaflet alone have minimal impact beyond increased knowledge. Difficult to coordinate comprehensive education if multiple providers are involved.
Exercise/education classes (skill practice) (34)	Group class series that includes exercise demonstration, practice, and educational discussion. May include self-efficacy enhancing strategies, problem-solving discussions and other activities to promote long-term maintenance of exercise.	Can be taught in community by fitness professionals. Ongoing class series can help support long-term behavior change. Promotes peer support.	Lack of availability. Requires commitment of course leaders and participants to time-intensive activity.
Telephone support (19,27,28)	Proactive, structured telephone contacts by trained laypersons or professional counselors. Content may include monitoring of symptoms, medication adherence and side effects, barriers to medical care/appointment-keeping, and self-care activities.	Can be used to reinforce professional instruction and reduce face-to-face clinical encounters. Can be low-cost when delivered by lay persons. Evidence of effectiveness.	One-to-one contact can be labor-intensive. Lack of nonverbal cues reduces ability to gauge reactions of the patients and effectiveness of communication.
Mediated instruction/technology based (21–23)	Format may include personalized, self-paced instruction using self-instructional workbooks and audiovisual aids, computer-assisted instruction and/or computer tailored print materials or Internet programs. Content may be focused on one issue such as stress management or total joint replacement, or may include a variety of self-management and/or cognitive behavioral topics and strategies.	Can reduce need for professional time; can reinforce professional instruction. Can be delivered at home or via the Internet; allows for broad dissemination. Tailored content is more persuasive and effective.	Cost varies depending upon the type of media used. Media can be costly and difficult to keep up-to-date. Excludes peer support. Minimal human interaction.

term changes in self-efficacy, diet, exercise, and cognitive symptom management, although the long-term results were less significant in some studies. In addition to modifications of the ASMP for different countries, adaptations have been tested for other languages and for shortened versions of the course. Two groups have found positive changes in pain, disability, and self-efficacy from a Spanish-language version of the ASMP (13,14).

To address administrator concerns about course length, Lorig and colleagues (15) tested shortened versions of the ASMP. Results suggested a dose-response pattern. In all variables, the 6-week course was more effective than the 3-week course, and the 3-week course did not change health care utilization. A 1.5-hour version produced some changes in knowledge, pain, self-efficacy, and possibly, increased contact with the Arthritis Foundation.

Effectiveness of Individual Education Strategies

The effectiveness of educational leaflets or booklets appears to be limited to knowledge changes, whereas individualized in-

struction has produced broader but inconsistent results. In one study, patients receiving an educational booklet showed an increase in knowledge at 6 weeks but no change in clinical or functional status (16). In a similar study evaluating the effects of an educational leaflet at 3-week and 6-month followup, the experimental group demonstrated an increase in knowledge at 3 weeks that was maintained at 6 months (17).

Evaluation of individual one-to-one instruction programs has produced mixed results. Some studies of individual instruction from a health professional showed no effect, whereas others showed positive effects, particularly if the instruction was accompanied by educational materials and behavioral strategies. A study in which the experimental group received 30–60 minutes of individual instruction along with an educational leaflet showed no difference in outcomes, compared to a group that only received the leaflet (16). When 2 educational interventions (one group received educational materials, the second received the same materials plus health professional instruction) were compared with a control group, neither experimental group demonstrated significant changes in self-efficacy, health behaviors, or health status (18). The study authors note, however, that despite receiving training, materials, and a protocol to follow, professionals had difficulty providing educational discussions as part of their routine practice.

In contrast, there is growing evidence that individual instruction can be effective when combined with behavioral strategies and other reinforcement activities. In inner city patients with knee OA, a brief (30–60 minute) individualized learning session provided by an arthritis nurse specialist and supplemented by 2 follow-up telephone calls reduced resting knee pain and significantly improved functional status (19). These benefits persisted at 12 months along with a significant reduction in primary care visits.

In an observational study of exercise by elderly women with hip or knee OA, only 42% of the women recalled receiving medical advice to exercise (20). While 63% of those who recalled receiving the recommendation did exercise, most exercised at subtherapeutic levels. When the exercise recommendation was accompanied by instructional materials, demonstration of the exercises, and monitoring of adherence, both the percentage of women exercising and the frequency of exercising at a therapeutic level increased.

Alternative Delivery Methods and Use of Technology

Although group-based self-management programs have been shown to be efficacious, and individual instruction enhanced with behavioral techniques shows some benefits, the need to reach broader audiences and maximize program cost-effectiveness has led to the development and testing of many alternative methods of program delivery. A home study program that incorporated audiocassettes, illustrated print materials and telephone contacts by trained community coordinators achieved positive changes in self-care behaviors, and decreased helplessness, pain, depression, and disability (21). However, when the trained community coordinators and supportive phone calls were removed from the program to reduce costs, behavioral changes were achieved but changes in health outcomes were not.

Advances in computer technology present new and convenient means for patient education. A computer-assisted instruction program was found to be effective in increasing appropriate use of medication and self-efficacy in patients with hip and knee OA (22). Computers are now being used to tailor the education provided to patients. A computer-tailored, mail-delivered, self-management program that allows for education to be individualized to each consumer's needs resulted in positive changes in function, pain, vitality, frequency of exercise, and self-efficacy, as well as a significant decrease in doctor visits (23). The Arthritis Foundation is currently offering a similar Internet-based tailored program, *Connect and Control: Your Online Arthritis Action Guide*. Participants access this program on the web (www.arthritis.org). After completing an online questionnaire, participants receive tailored self-management education based on a variety of different variables, including demographic characteristics, health beliefs (e.g., perceived benefits and barriers), self-efficacy, stage of change, valued life activities, priority problems, and functional status.

Impact of Quality Arthritis Patient Education

Several reviews have yielded important observations about the impact of quality arthritis patient education. First, arthritis education can be effective in producing positive changes in knowledge about arthritis, behavior, psychosocial status, and other health outcomes (24). A meta-analysis of psycho-educational interventions in arthritis found that experimental groups had significantly greater improvements in pain (16%), depression (22%), and disability (8%), compared with control groups (25). A more recent meta-analysis of 34 studies demonstrated positive effect sizes (a standardized measure of change) for knowledge, behavior, psychological status, pain, or functional status (26).

Second, because most of these studies involved subjects who were already receiving medical care, these results suggest that formal education programs can achieve clinically significant health outcomes beyond the improvement provided by medical care. A comparison of patient education studies in OA and RA patients taking nonsteroidal antiinflammatory drug (NSAID) therapy showed that patient education interventions are 20–30% as efficacious as NSAID treatment for pain relief in OA and RA, 40% as efficacious for improvement in functional ability in RA, and 60–80% as efficacious in reducing painful joint counts in RA (5). These positive effects from education are in addition to the benefits participants received from their medications.

Third, there is growing evidence that arthritis patient education can affect health care utilization and costs. Two studies of the Arthritis Self-Management Program have demonstrated reduction of physician visits and costs (7,9). In a telephone support intervention, the annual costs of a 1-unit improvement in pain were found to be $31, and in function, $71 (27). Reduced physician visits were also demonstrated in a telephone treatment/counseling program for OA patients (28) and a brief self-care education session supplemented by 2 followup telephone calls (19). In another cost-benefit study evaluating 3 experimental interventions for OA patients in a health maintenance organization, all 3 groups (education, social support, and combined education/support) achieved an average savings of $1,279 per participant per year in year 3 (29). In summary, there is robust evidence supporting the effectiveness of group education models, evidence that individual instruction supplemented by behavioral methods or telephone followup can influence health behaviors, and evidence that leaflets or booklets can increase knowledge but are not likely to influence behavior or health status. Technology-enhanced education shows promise in arthritis. Evidence also supports the cost-effectiveness of both group education models and enhanced individual education.

ENHANCING SELF-MANAGEMENT IN CLINICAL PRACTICE

Four Critical Activities

Some have questioned whether it is feasible for busy clinicians to provide self-management enhancing patient education in the midst of their routine clinical practice. However, practitioners play a crucial role in preparing the patient for and supporting self-management. Even in the minimal time available in the

Table 2. Basic self-management enhancing activities for clinical practice.

1. **Reinforce** the value of self-management activities.
   Before patients are likely to respond to recommendations and referrals to self-management education programs, they must recognize the importance of self-management and their role in managing their condition. It is crucial for professionals to repeatedly stress the improvements in symptoms and health status resulting from self-management activities until the patient also recognizes their value.
2. **Recommend** strongly that patients participate in self-management activities.
   The American College of Rheumatology guidelines for the management of osteoarthritis and rheumatoid arthritis list the Arthritis Self-Management Program and physical activity among the initial steps in a management plan. Patients need to receive clear recommendations to participate in these activities.
3. **Refer** patients to self-management resources.
   Recommendation alone is not likely to be enough. Patients will need specific information about what to do and where to go. People with arthritis have different needs for self-management support. Some may gain the confidence and skills they need from reading appropriate books and pamphlets; others will require community programs like the Arthritis Self-Management Program. At a minimum, professionals should give the patient specific contact information for the programs they recommend. The Arthritis Foundation is a key resource for patient information and services. Local chapters of the Arthritis Foundation have information brochures available, including a listing of services offered.
4. **Reconsider** your approach to engaging your patients in self-management activities.
   Patients may not readily engage in recommended self-management activities, especially those that require sustained effort. Professionals will need to assess whether their patients with arthritis are engaged in self-management activities that will improve their symptoms and function. If not, professionals may need to reconsider their approach and match their recommendations with a patient's readiness to act on them.

most time-pressured clinical practice, practitioners can influence their patients' beliefs about self-management and refer patients to other resources that build confidence and skills in self-management.

Brady et al outline 4 critical activities designed to enhance patient self-management that most practitioners can incorporate into clinical practice (4). Practitioners need to 1) *recognize and reinforce* the importance of self-management and the patient's role in arthritis management; 2) *recommend* strongly (and repeatedly, if necessary) that patients participate in specific self-management activities such as the Arthritis Self-Management Program and physical activity or exercise programs; 3) *refer* patients to appropriate self-management resources; and if necessary, 4) *reconsider* their approach to engaging patients in self-management activities if patients appear to have difficulty adopting self-management behaviors. Further detail is provided in Table 2.

Strategies to Enhance Self-Management in Clinical Practice

The literature is not yet clear about what types or combinations of educational interventions are most effective and what mechanisms contribute to their efficacy. Nevertheless, the Arthritis and Musculoskeletal Patient Education Standards (3) and several literature reviews (5,11,21,26) confirm common features of high-quality patient education, and there is a need to apply what *is* known to current practice. Successful education is a continuous, active process; it is not something done *to* the patient, but rather must be done *with* the patient as an active participant. Current effective approaches to self-management education are based on theories that have been described elsewhere (30,31). The following are several theory-based strategies that may be useful for practitioners who have the time and resources to move beyond the 4 critical activities described in the previous section. While not all practitioners will have the time and resources to provide extensive education, all should have the capacity to support self-management and refer to other resources as necessary.

Identify the Patients' Perspective. One of the first steps of effective education is to identify the patients' perspective: their needs and problems, goals and expectations, and relevant health beliefs and practices (32). Patients can feel over-

whelmed at the time of diagnosis or whenever their symptoms worsen. Education at this time should be aimed at mitigating fears and suggesting support resources. Because readiness to learn is usually oriented to current problems, eliciting patients' key concerns or problems allows you to capitalize on teachable moments and to individualize the educational messages and recommendations. A patient whose main perceived problem is pain or the inability to perform a valued activity may be more likely to adopt an exercise program if it is framed as a way to help manage pain or as a way of achieving the desired activity. A quick way of determining patients' concerns is to ask, "What are the most important problems or concerns you are having now as a result of your arthritis?" Encourage patients to bring a list of their concerns or problems with them to visits.

It is also important to identify and accommodate patients' beliefs about the cause of their condition and symptoms and their expectations about treatment (e.g., "What do you expect will happen—good or bad—if you do this recommended treatment/behavior? What have you already done to help improve your condition/symptoms?") In this electronic age, patients are likely to already have some information about treatment options, particularly alternative and complementary remedies, that may be inaccurate or unbalanced. Although it is important to clarify unrealistic expectations, misconceptions, and harmful practices, it is also imperative to recognize that trying to change deeply rooted cultural or religious beliefs or practices will likely meet with resistance. It may be more useful to expand their possible explanations for a problem (see section on building self-efficacy) or suggest adding a new behavior rather than initially trying to eliminate old ones. For example, if weight is a problem, suggest adding some exercise instead of recommending major dietary changes initially. When patients make an informed decision not to do a recommended behavior, show respect and keep the door open by offering to help in the future.

Identify Readiness to Change. Recognize that patients vary in their readiness to change behaviors. In a study of the readiness of RA or OA patients to adopt self-management strategies, 44% were categorized as "precontemplative" (not intending to take action in the foreseeable future), 11% "contemplative" (thinking about a change but undecided about when), and 22% in "preparation" (getting ready to take action). Another 6% were classified as being in "unprepared action" (those who were making overt changes in behavior but who had not really thought about or prepared for action), and 17% were in "maintenance" (33).

A simple way to gauge patients' readiness to change is to ask whether they have ever considered doing the behavior, are thinking about changing, or are ready for action. Having this information allows the provider to tailor the intervention, such as prescribing exercise. Patients who are in the precontemplative stage will probably not respond well to traditional interventions such as providing detailed instruction about how to make exercising a regular habit. Instead, it may be better to spend time raising the patient's awareness about how exercising is relevant to personal goals. Patients in the contemplative stage can be assisted to start exercising through such techniques as using a decision-making worksheet to weigh the pros and cons of exercising. Patients in the preparation phase can be helped by suggesting that they set a specific date to begin exercising, share their commitment with family or friends, and take small steps such as signing up for an exercise class or joining a health club. Once a person has moved into the action phase, behavioral control strategies become appropriate (see section on using behavioral techniques).

Use a Multifaceted Approach. As noted earlier, self-management often requires that the patient learn a variety of information, attitudes, and skills. It also necessitates that the practitioner use multiple strategies to engage the patient. The effectiveness of verbal instructions can be enhanced by being specific and by using lay language to inform patients about their diagnosis and about *why, what, how,* and *when* to do a recommended behavior (32). Posters, anatomical models, supplementary videotapes, and other audiovisuals can be used to reinforce key messages. To help retention, summarize conclusions and instructions at the end of the visit. Write down the diagnosis and provide supplementary print materials, such as those available from the Arthritis Foundation or Lupus Foundation of America.

Another approach is to use a CD-ROM-based system to print patient-specific brochures on demand. Useful CD-ROMs are available from the American Academy of Family Physicians, as well as other sources. Patients can also be referred to various Web sites for up-to-date patient information; for example, the Arthritis Foundation's site, www.arthritis.org, and the Missouri Arthritis Rehabilitation Research and Training Center site, www.muhealth.org/~arthritis.

When teaching skills, allow time to demonstrate the skill and provide opportunities for repetitive practice and feedback. Check understanding by having patients recall what, when, and how often they plan to do the agreed-upon regimen. Ask them to demonstrate any needed skills.

Use Behavioral Techniques. A variety of behavioral techniques can help patients adopt a recommended treatment or achieve and maintain their desired behavior changes (32,34). Help patients build new habits by mentioning ways that they could use environmental cues to prompt and motivate behaviors. For example, suggest the linking of new behaviors to old behaviors (e.g., riding their stationary bicycle while watching their favorite soap opera).

Self-monitoring tools, such as an exercise, medication, or food diary, can remind about and reinforce behaviors. Suggest that patients put their tools in places relevant to the behavior (e.g., place a food diary on the refrigerator). Reinforce progress by reviewing such tools during clinical visits.

Use nonthreatening questions to identify potential barriers to behavioral changes and to assess progress. ("Many of my patients find it difficult to follow all of their exercise program. What problems do you expect might keep you from doing your exercises as scheduled?" "Many people miss taking their medication at times. Was there any dose that you were likely to miss? What made it difficult to take medications at that time?")

To help patients maintain behaviors over time, teach contracting (see section on building self-efficacy). Reassure patients that missing an exercise session or other lapses in behavior are inevitable but should be treated as temporary setbacks and not as reasons for stopping the behavior altogether. (See Chapter 41, Adherence, for additional ideas.)

Model Problem-Solving Skills. Practitioners can help patients become more active partners in their care by teaching them how to solve problems rather than by providing solutions (30). When patients present a problem—for example, a situation in which they have not followed through on a mutually agreed-upon behavior—ask them to generate a list of potential solutions, including any they have used in the past to deal with similar problems. Then have them examine the pros and cons of each option before selecting one to try.

Build Self-Efficacy. Self-efficacy is the degree of confidence in one's ability to execute a behavior regularly. The addition of self-efficacy enhancing strategies to the ASMP increased the course's effectiveness (30). Many of these self-efficacy enhancing strategies can easily be incorporated into clinical practice. To promote self-efficacy, remember to break down skills and behaviors into easily mastered components. Self-efficacy can also be enhanced through short-term goal-setting/contracting and feedback; reinterpretation of symptoms; and modeling and persuasion.

Have patients set realistic, short-term goals to accomplish something they want to achieve. To determine what is practical, identify what patients are doing now and then suggest that they set a goal to do just a little more. Once patients have experienced success, other components can gradually be added. Strengthen commitment by having patients write down their goals in a contract that includes a clear description of the activity, how long it will be done, how many times, and how often. Then ask how confident they are that they can carry out their contract on a scale of 0 (not at all sure) to 10 (totally sure). If they don't feel confident (a rating of less than 7), help them modify the goal so that it is achievable or problem-solve to address any perceived barriers. During followup contacts, monitor progress on goals and provide praise and positive feedback for progress.

Help patients reinterpret the causes of their symptoms by explaining possible reasons for symptoms like pain and fatigue. When patients understand that their symptoms can be due to multiple causes beyond the disease process (e.g., deconditioning, stress, or depression), their motivation to consider other nonpharmacologic strategies may increase.

A powerful way to influence patient levels of self-efficacy and to motivate behavior change is to provide positive role models. People with arthritis who are successfully managing their condition can be used as lay instructors or mentors. Modeling also can be provided through the media. To increase the effectiveness of print and audiovisual materials, use visuals and real-life vignettes of people that represent the patient's age and ethnic diversity. Practitioners also need to be aware that they will be observed and that they need to practice what they preach about exercise, weight control, smoking, and other recommended behaviors. Use credible people to persuade pa-

Table 3. Arthritis self-management education topics.

Specific arthritis information
    Nature and course of disease—what to expect
    Medical treatment/medications; how to take medications appropriately
    Importance of self-management
    Nonpharmacologic management strategies
        Balancing activity and rest
        Exercise: range of motion, conditioning, and strengthening
        Activity and environmental modification, assistive devices, bracing and
          footwear
        Relaxation and other stress management techniques
        Use of heat/cold and other pain reduction techniques
    Role of surgery in arthritis management
    Assessment of complementary and alternative therapies and unproven
      remedies
Generic self-management skills
    Goal-setting and contracting
    Problem-solving
    Decision-making
    Communicating with health care professionals
    Cognitive symptom modification
    Appropriate use of health professionals and the health care system

tients to change specific behaviors. For many people, physicians have the most credibility; for others, peer educators may be more influential.

Mobilize Support Systems. Nurture natural support networks by asking patients which family members or significant others are most likely to help them with their self-management and then clarify what kind of help is desired (30). This may include doing the recommended behavior with the patient (e.g., exercise), providing praise or other positive consequences, giving reminders, or engaging in other supportive activities (34). Encourage significant others to participate in clinical visits and patient education activities if the patient wishes them to be involved. Refer patients to self-management classes and support groups that are structured to encourage participants to help each other. Encourage patients who are successfully managing their disease to mentor new patients. For example, link people who have had successful joint replacement surgery with those considering such surgery. Face-to-face contact is not always necessary. The telephone is often overlooked as an easy way to reinforce information and provide practical support (19,27,28).

Content to Enhance Self-Management

In addition to understanding facts about arthritis and its management, people with arthritis must develop specific self-management skills, the judgment to modify their self-management activities in response to changing disease status or circumstance, and the confidence to be an effective self-manager. Table 3 outlines arthritis-specific content to be covered in effective arthritis education, as well as generic self-management skills. Health professionals may find it useful to create arthritis education records or checklists to document which topics have been discussed and to create an orderly flow of information from visit to visit. However, the education provided must be driven by patient need, not professional protocol; individual instruction must incorporate the essentials of good educational practice. Much of the literature reviewed highlights the fact that the educational processes used to provide the information are at least as important as the specific information provided.

SUMMARY

Arthritis patient education programs have been effective in producing significant changes in knowledge, behaviors, and psychological and health outcomes. The improvement in health status is above and beyond the improvement provided by traditional medical care. Trends in arthritis patient education include more of an emphasis on theory-based programs, training in generic skill development, targeting to a broader range of people with rheumatic diseases, and more innovative, cost-effective methods of program delivery. Effective, empirically proven, and theory-based patient education techniques can be integrated into routine clinical practice and should be considered an essential part of the management of rheumatic diseases.

REFERENCES

1. Recommendations for the medical management of osteoarthritis of the hip and knee: 2000 update. American College of Rheumatology Subcommittee on Osteoarthritis Guidelines. Arthritis Rheum 2000;43:1905–15.
2. Guidelines for the management of rheumatoid arthritis. American College of Rheumatology Ad Hoc Committee on Clinical Guidelines. Arthritis Rheum 1996;39:713–22.
3. Burckhart CS, Lorig K, Moncur C, Melvin J, Beardmore T, Boyd M, et al. Arthritis and musculoskeletal patient education standards. Arthritis Foundation. Arthritis Care Res 1994;7:1–4.
4. Brady TJ, Sniezek JE, Conn DL. Enhancing patient self-management in clinical practice. Bull Rheum Dis 2001;49:1–4.
5. Superio-Cabuslay E, Ward MM, Lorig KR. Patient education interventions in osteoarthritis and rheumatoid arthritis: a meta-analytic comparison with non-steroidal antiinflammatory drug treatment. Arthritis Care Res 1996;9:292–301.
6. U.S. Department of Health and Human Services (HHS). Healthy People 2010 summary of objectives. Available at: http://www.health.gov/healthy-people//Document/HTML/Volume1/02Arthritis.htm. Accessed July 17, 2001.
7. Lorig KR, Mazonson PD, Holman HR. Evidence suggesting that health education for self-management in patients with chronic arthritis has sustained health benefits while reducing health care costs. Arthritis Rheum 1993;36:439–46.
8. Krueger JM, Helmick CG, Callahan LF, Haddix AC. Cost-effectiveness of the arthritis self-help course. Arch Intern Med 1998;158:1245–9.
9. Barlow JH, Turner AP, Wright CC. A randomized controlled study of the Arthritis Self-Management Programme in the UK. Health Educ Res 2000; 15:665–80.
10. McGowan P, Green L. Arthritis self-management in native populations of British Columbia: An application of health promotion and participatory research principles in chronic disease control. Can J Aging 1995; 14(Suppl):201–12.
11. Taal E, Riemsma RP, Brus HL, Seydel ER, Rasker JJ, Wiegman O. Group education for patients with rheumatoid arthritis. Patient Educ Couns 1993;20:177–87.
12. Lindroth Y, Bauman A, Brooks PM, Priestley D. A 5-year follow-up of a controlled trial of an arthritis education programme. Br J Rheumatol 1995;34:647–52.
13. Lorig K, Gonzalez VM, Ritter P. Community-based Spanish language arthritis education program: a randomized trial. Med Care 1999;37:957–63.
14. Wong AL, Lau VP, Harked Sylmar JO. Preliminary evaluation of the Arthritis Foundation Orange County Spanish self-empowerment program. Arthritis Rheum 2000;43(Suppl):S331.
15. Lorig K, Gonzalez VM, Laurent DD, Morgan L, Laris BA. Arthritis self-management program variations: three studies. Arthritis Care Res 1998;11:448–54.
16. Maggs FM, Jubb RW, Kemm JR. Single-blind randomized controlled trial of an educational booklet for patients with chronic arthritis. Br J Rheumatol 1996;35:775–7.
17. Barlow JH, Wright CC. Knowledge in patients with rheumatoid arthritis: A longer-term follow-up of a randomized controlled study of patient education leaflets. Br J Rheumatol 1998;37:373–6.
18. Riemsma RP, Taal E, Brus HL, Rassker JJ, Wiegman O. Coordinated

individual education with an arthritis passport for patients with rheumatoid arthritis. Arthritis Care Res 1997;10:238–49.

19. Mazzuca SA, Brandt KD, Katz BP, Hanna MP, Melfi CA. Reduced utilization and cost of primary care clinic visits resulting from self-care education for patients with osteoarthritis of the knee. Arthritis Rheum 1999;42:1267–73.

20. Dexter PA. Joint exercises in elderly persons with symptomatic osteoarthritis of the hip or knee. Performance patterns, medical support patterns, and the relationship between exercising and medical care. Arthritis Care Res 1992;5:36–41.

21. Goeppinger J, Lorig K. Interventions to reduce the impact of chronic diseases. Annu Rev Nurs Res 1997;15:101–22.

22. Edworthy SM, Devins GM. Improving medication adherence through patient education distinguishing between appropriate and inappropriate utilization. Patient Education Study Group. J Rheumatol 1999;26:1793–801.

23. Fries JF, Carey C, McShane DJ. Patient education in arthritis: randomized controlled trial of a mail-delivered program. J Rheumatol 1997;24:1378–83.

24. Hirano PC, Laurent DD, Lorig K. Arthritis patient education studies, 1987-1991: a review of the literature. Patient Educ Couns 1994;24:9–54.

25. Mullen PD, Laville E, Biddle A, Lorig K. Efficacy of psychoeducational interventions on pain, depression and disability in people with arthritis: A meta-analysis. J Rheumatol 1987;15:33–9.

26. Hawley DJ. Psycho-educational interventions for the treatment of arthritis. Baillieres Clin Rheumatol 1995;9:803–23.

27. Weinberger M, Tierney WM, Cowper PA, Katz BP, Booher PA. Cost-effectiveness of increased telephone contact for patients with osteoarthritis. Arthritis Rheum 1993;36:243–6.

28. Maisiak R, Austin J, Heck L. Health outcomes of two telephone interventions for patients with rheumatoid arthritis or osteoarthritis. Arthritis Rheum 1996;39:1391–9.

29. Cronan TA, Hay M, Groessl E, Bigatti S, Gallagher R, Tomita M. The effects of social support and education on health care costs after three years. Arthritis Care Res 1998;11:326–34.

30. Gonzalez VM, Goeppinger J, Lorig K. Four psychosocial theories and their application to patient education and clinical practice. Arthritis Care Res 1990;3:132–43.

31. Boutaugh ML, Brady TJ. Patient education for self-management. In: Melvin JL, Jenson GM, editors. Rheumatologic rehabilitation series: assessment and management. Bethesda: American Occupational Therapy Association; 1998. p. 219–58.

32. Daltroy LH. Doctor-patient communication in rheumatological disorders. Baillieres Clin Rheumatol 1993;7:221–39.

33. Keefe FJ, Lefebvre JC, Kerns RD, Rosenberg R, Beaupre P, Prochaska J, et al. Understanding the adoption of arthritis self-management: stages of change profiles among arthritis patients. Pain 2000;87:303–13.

34. Allegrante JP, Kovar PA, MacKensie CR, Peterson MG, Gutin B. A walking education program for patients with osteoarthritis of the knee: theory and intervention strategies. Health Educ Q 1993;20:63–81.

Additional Recommended Reading

Green LW, Kreuter MW. Health promotion planning: an educational and ecological approach. 3rd ed. London: Mayfield Publishing; 1999.

Lorig K, Holman H. Arthritis self-management studies: a twelve-year review. Health Educ Q 1993;20:17–28.

Lorish CD, Boutaugh ML. Patient education in rheumatology. Curr Opin Rheumatol 1997;9:106–11.

Cognitive Behavioral Interventions

FRANCIS J. KEEFE, PhD; DAVID S. CALDWELL, MD; and ANN ASPNES, BA

Rheumatic disease patients may be similar in disease severity yet vary substantially in their pain, physical disability, and psychological disability. Patients with rheumatoid arthritis (RA), for example, who feel helpless about being able to cope with their disease and who have little social support from friends or family may report severe pain and become quite disabled in the face of mild to moderate disease. Other patients with the same degree of disease severity may report little pain and lead active and productive lives. Such variations in response to rheumatic disease cannot be explained by biomedical models that view arthritis pain and disability as primarily due to disease activity. Newly developed cognitive behavioral models maintain that cognitive factors (that is, beliefs, coping strategies, or appraisals) and behavioral factors (home or work environment) may be just as important as biomedical factors in understanding how individuals adjust to chronic diseases. These models have led to innovative treatments that have been shown to be effective in managing pain and disability in rheumatic disease patients (1–4).

ELEMENTS OF COGNITIVE BEHAVIORAL THERAPY

Cognitive behavioral therapy for rheumatic disease patients has 3 basic elements: a rationale for treatment, coping skills training, and training in methods for maintenance of coping skills to prevent setbacks in coping efforts.

Rationale for Treatment

The rationale for cognitive behavioral therapy should be introduced at the start of treatment, prior to any training in pain coping skills. The goals of therapy are: 1) to educate patients about the influence of cognitive and behavioral factors on pain and other arthritis symptoms, 2) to emphasize the role that coping skills can play in managing symptoms and reducing physical and psychological disability, and 3) to enhance a sense of control over their disease.

Most programs use an adaptation model to help patients understand the interrelationships between arthritis symptoms and patterns of adjustment. To introduce this model, patients are typically asked to describe how the symptoms of their rheumatic disease, such as pain, stiffness, or fatigue, have affected the behavioral, cognitive, and affective areas of functioning. Patients often can identify a variety of problematic behaviors (e.g., reduced tolerance for activities, decreased involvement in pleasurable activities, and increased dependence on others), cognitions (negative thoughts about self, others, and the future), and affective responses (depression, guilt, or anxiety). In discussion with patients, the emphasis is on increasing awareness of how problematic patterns develop and are learned over time, as well as on helping patients recognize the connections between their thoughts, feelings, and behaviors.

An important tenet of the cognitive behavioral model is that learned patterns of adjustment to rheumatic disease can be changed by learning new cognitive and behavioral coping skills. Patients are systematically trained to use a variety of cognitive coping skills, such as imagery and cognitive restructuring, and behavioral coping skills, such as activity pacing and goal setting. Cognitive behavioral therapy thus encourages patients to take an active role in managing and controlling their symptoms and disease. While this is effective in reducing pain and related symptoms, it will not allow patients to achieve total control over a rheumatic disease such as RA. In providing a treatment rationale, the therapist helps patients understand that they can significantly increase their ability to control symptoms while acknowledging that, at times, there may be disease flares and symptoms that are beyond their control.

Coping Skills Training

In cognitive behavioral therapy, each treatment session is structured to maximize the learning of cognitive and behavioral coping skills. The individual is first instructed in a coping skill and is guided by the therapist through a brief practice session. The therapist then provides corrective feedback and suggestions for applying the skill in controlling arthritis symptoms. Coping skills are practiced in order of difficulty, starting with the least difficult (e.g. relaxation training) and proceeding to the more difficult and complex (cognitive restructuring).

A hallmark of cognitive behavioral therapy is that it provides training in a wide variety of coping skills. The skills are grouped together on a list or "menu" to highlight the fact that patients have multiple coping options and can mix and match skills to deal with different problems.

Relaxation Training. Relaxation training is one of the most important and basic coping skills for rheumatic disease patients. It is typically introduced early because it is easy to learn and is very effective in controlling patients' symptoms. Training in relaxation methods provides several benefits. First, it can reduce muscle tension that may contribute to pain or tension. Second, it makes patients more aware of increases in their level of tension so that they can intervene early before tension causes increased pain or fatigue. Third, when patients relax they are able to shift their attention away from arthritis symptoms, which often reduces pain. Finally, learning to relax can improve patients' abilities to rest and sleep.

Although there are a variety of methods for teaching relaxation, including meditation, autogenic training, and biofeed-

Table 1. Recording form: 5-column method.

Situation	Automatic thoughts	Feelings	Restructured thoughts	Modified feelings and responses
Flare in my arthritis	It is hopeless, I am never going to get better.	Depressed and discouraged	My last flare only lasted a few days. I made it through that one.	More optimistic. Takes it easy for a few days.
Criticism from a co-worker	No one understands what it is like to have arthritis.	Anger	Maybe this had nothing to do with my arthritis. Maybe she is just having a bad day.	Empathy. Finds out how the coworker is feeling.
Inability to do all the housework. Husband had to help out.	I should be able to pull my own weight.	Guilt	I don't have to do everything myself. It's OK for us to work together.	Relieved. Plans to do more housework together.

back, most cognitive behavioral training programs use a progressive relaxation method similar to that of Bernstein and Borkovec (5). Progressive relaxation involves a series of exercises in which patients are asked to alternately tense and relax major muscle groups throughout the body. The exercises focus on muscles in the legs, arms, trunk, shoulders, neck, and face. The individual repeats each exercise slowly while attending to the sensations that accompany tension and relaxation. Instructions are often recorded, and patients are encouraged to listen to the 15–20-minute audiotape twice a day. After 2–3 weeks of daily practice, most patients show an excellent ability to relax when in a quiet and comfortable environment. Training then shifts to the application of learned relaxation skills to more physically demanding activities such as walking or climbing stairs. Patients can be taught abbreviated relaxation methods in which they briefly (for 30 seconds) scan major muscle groups, identifying and then relaxing any areas of excessive tension. These abbreviated relaxation methods can be done while the patient is engaged in other activities such as eating, talking on the phone, or driving. They provide an excellent means of generalizing the benefits of relaxation to a variety of home and work activities.

Imagery Training. Imagery is a useful method of diverting attention away from pain and other rheumatic disease symptoms. Imagery is often introduced as an adjunct to relaxation training. Many types of imagery are used in cognitive behavioral therapy, but probably the most common is pleasant imagery, for example, imagining oneself reclining on a sunny beach. The instructions emphasize the need to focus on the imagined scene for a specific period of time (usually a few minutes) and encourage the individual to involve as many sensory modalities as possible. The patient might, for example, try to imagine feeling the warmth of the sand on the beach, seeing the blue sky, hearing the sounds of the waves breaking and seagulls flying overhead, and even tasting the slight salty taste that might be on one's lips after a brief swim. It is important to emphasize that the patient is in control of the image. Patients can select an appropriate scene and can switch to a new scene or stop focusing on the image whenever they want. This reduces patients' concerns that the therapist is controlling their thoughts or hypnotizing them. Asking patients to close their eyes and relax deeply usually helps them concentrate more fully on the imagery.

Activity–Rest Pacing. Persons with rheumatic diseases often have difficulty pacing their activities. Many patients report a cycle in which they overdo daily activities, experience increased pain and fatigue, and then require a prolonged period of rest to recover. When this cycle is repeated over the course of months and years, it has many negative consequences including a decreased tolerance for activity, a belief that one is incapable of being active, and a restricted lifestyle that provides few diversions from pain or other symptoms. Arthritis patients who cope with pain by decreasing activity have substantially higher psychological distress and pain and report that arthritis interferes more with their involvement in activities of daily living (6). Activity–rest pacing is designed to break this maladaptive pattern by teaching patients to plan their daily schedule so that moderate periods of activity are followed by limited periods of rest (see also Chapter 26, Rest and Exercise). For example, a patient with RA who experiences severe joint pain after 2 hours of working at a computer terminal can alter her work schedule so that she works no longer than 30 minutes before taking a 5-minute break. Over a period of weeks the duration of the activity phase of the cycle is gradually increased from 30 to 40 and then 50 minutes of typing, and the rest phase of the cycle is decreased. This enables patients to gradually increase their activity without increasing their symptoms. Benefits of using the activity–rest cycle include a reduction in pain and fatigue, increased tolerance for activities of daily living, and an enhanced sense of control over rheumatic disease symptoms.

Cognitive Restructuring. In cognitive restructuring patients are taught to identify, challenge, and modify negative automatic thoughts that may contribute to pain or emotional distress. Individuals with rheumatic disease who are depressed or anxious or who have severe pain typically have negative thoughts about themselves, others, and the future. These negative thoughts represent how they view their situation and do not reflect the actual situation. When erroneous and distorted, these thoughts can trigger emotional responses such as depression or anxiety. Some arthritis patients cope with pain by engaging in catastrophizing, a behavior associated with much higher levels of pain, pain behavior, and psychological and physical disability (7,8). The goal of cognitive restructuring is to help the patient become aware of negative thoughts and to restructure underlying attitudes and beliefs. Because the negative thoughts occur spontaneously for brief periods of time, patients need to systematically monitor them. A common form of monitoring is the 5-column method that asks patients to record the situation, their thoughts, and feelings (Table 1). Patients are encouraged to recognize the connection between the situations, their automatic thoughts, and their feelings. The therapist works with the patient to examine the evidence for negative thoughts and to develop alternative ways of appraising the situation, such as "I've been through flares in the past. They are difficult, but I know my symptoms will improve with time." When patients change their negative automatic thoughts, they report substantial improvements in mood. They are also better able to adhere to and maintain the use of other cognitive and behavioral coping skills.

Training in Maintenance Enhancement Methods

The daily use of coping strategies appears to be an important mediator of the long-term outcome of cognitive behavioral therapy. Patients with RA who use coping skills frequently have much better outcomes 12 months after completing cognitive behavioral training than those who do not (9). However, individuals who are faced with flares in disease activity or other stressful life events may question the effectiveness of their coping abilities and may reduce or curtail their coping efforts. To prevent such setbacks, most programs include training in maintenance enhancement methods. Comprehensive training in maintenance enhancement has been used to prevent relapse from disorders such as smoking, obesity, and alcoholism and has recently been extended to rheumatic disease patients (10).

These programs have several important features. First, they use cognitive therapy methods to increase patient awareness of potential relapse situations. These methods include developing a list of high-risk situations likely to lead to setbacks, identifying early warning signs of relapse, and cognitively rehearsing how one might cope with different relapse situations. Second, maintenance enhancement programs use behavioral rehearsal to develop a sense of self-efficacy in managing arthritis symptoms. In behavioral rehearsal, the patient identifies a high-risk situation such as an emotionally demanding life event that might lead to a setback or relapse. The therapist then models coping strategies that could be used, has the patient rehearse these strategies, and provides feedback. Finally, maintenance enhancement emphasizes training in self-control skills in order to maintain frequent practice of coping skills. Patients may be taught to use diaries and calendars to monitor important target behaviors such as the frequency of relaxation practice or early warning signs of a setback. They are also trained to use self-reinforcement to reward the appropriate use and practice of coping skills.

showed lower levels of disease progression, medication intake, depression, anxiety, and helplessness compared with controls (13). Many RA patients are able to maintain their gains over 12 months (9,14). Long-term improvements in pain and functional status are most clearly apparent in patients who continued to frequently practice coping skills (9).

Research has also demonstrated that cognitive behavioral training is more effective than an arthritis education condition or standard care in reducing pain and psychological disability in patients with osteoarthritis (OA) of the knees (15). The efficacy of an intervention that combined cognitive behavioral therapy with educational information about arthritis has been tested in a large sample of patients, 85% of whom had OA (16). Results indicated significant reductions in pain and psychological disability. A followup study of these patients found that they were able to maintain improvements in pain and depression up to 4 years after completing treatment (17).

The effects of cognitive behavioral therapy on fibromyalgia have been evaluated in controlled studies; several have shown that training can produce improvements in pain and functional disability (3). However, only 3 controlled studies have compared cognitive behavioral interventions to a condition that controls for therapist attention and other nonspecific factors. Only one of these studies found that training was more effective than an attention control condition (18). A recent meta-analysis of 49 treatment outcome studies compared the effects of nonpharmocologic treatments for fibromyalgia to those of pharmacologic treatments such as antidepressants, muscle relaxants, and nonsteroidal antiinflammatory drugs (19). The results showed that nonpharmacologic treatments (including such psychological interventions as biofeedback, relaxation, and cognitive behavioral therapy, as well as physically-based treatments and combined psychological and physical treatments) were superior to pharmacologic treatments alone in reducing self-report symptoms of fibromyalgia and improving daily function.

OUTCOMES OF COGNITIVE BEHAVIORAL THERAPY

Controlled studies have evaluated the efficacy of cognitive behavioral therapy in rheumatic disease patients. The design of most of these studies is similar. Patients are randomly assigned to receive cognitive behavioral training or one or more control conditions. The cognitive behavioral interventions are typically carried out in group sessions that last from 1.5 to 2 hours for 6–10 weeks. Outcome is evaluated using a comprehensive set of pain, physical disability, and psychological disability measures administered before and after treatment. Many studies have included a long-term followup assessment in order to evaluate the maintenance of therapeutic improvements.

Patients with RA who received cognitive behavioral training have shown significant reductions in pain, pain behavior, anxiety, and depression when compared to patients in a social support control condition (11). In other studies, training was found to improve outcome significantly in terms of pain relief, coping, and function in persons with RA (3,4,9,12). Interestingly, a recent study tested the effectiveness of cognitive behavioral therapy in 55 unselected patients with RA who were consecutive referrals to a rheumatology clinic. Results indicated that patients receiving cognitive behavioral therapy

PATIENT REFERRAL

Cognitive behavioral therapists are often clinical psychologists (or members of other health care disciplines) who have training in cognitive and behavioral psychology and are experienced in working with medical patients. Cognitive behavioral therapy is one of the most popular therapeutic techniques; thus, many teaching hospitals have trained therapists on their faculty or staff.

Many patients with rheumatic disease are reluctant to accept a referral to a psychologist or mental health professional because they view this as a sign that their symptoms are not being taken seriously. It is therefore important to prepare the patient before making the referral. Individuals should be reassured about the reality of their diagnosis and symptoms and told that cognitive behavioral training is designed to help them cope with their disease. It may be helpful to emphasize that this therapy focuses on coping in the "here and now" and does not dwell on early childhood conflicts or underlying unconscious conflicts. Patients who are overly skeptical or otherwise concerned about cognitive behavioral therapy can be encouraged to pursue treatment on a trial basis. At the end of a 3-session trial, most patients have become quite involved in treatment and choose to continue.

Several skills used in cognitive behavioral training are also taught at an introductory level in the Arthritis Self-Management Program developed by the Arthritis Foundation, which may provide another option for referral. After completing the program, patients who require additional intervention can be referred to a therapist who has more extensive formal training in cognitive behavioral therapy.

COGNITIVE BEHAVIORAL THERAPY AND ONGOING MEDICAL MANAGEMENT

Cognitive behavioral therapy is designed to complement the medical treatment of rheumatic diseases, not replace it. Although some patients may reduce their use of pain medications during treatment, most patients continue with important components of their treatment regimen such as the use of medications or physical therapy.

Cognitive behavioral training methods may actually be useful in enhancing rheumatic disease patients' adherence to medical regimens. Consider, for example, the RA patient who becomes depressed during a major disease flare and decides to stop taking methotrexate. By applying coping methods such as cognitive restructuring and relaxation, the patient may be able to calm himself, reduce emotional distress, and make a more rational choice about the need for arthritis medication.

Some rheumatic disease patients tend to consider their symptoms from either a purely medical or a purely psychological viewpoint. Patients who see their disease as simply a medical problem are willing to pursue medical treatment options but view psychological treatments as irrelevant. Conversely, patients who respond quite well to psychologically based treatments may downplay the significance of medical treatments. To circumvent this problem it is important to help patients adopt a biobehavioral model of their disease that acknowledges the relevance of both biologic and behavioral factors in the understanding and treatment of disease.

Gate Control Theory

A simplified version of the gate control theory (20) can help patients adopt a more biobehavioral perspective on their pain. This theory can be presented by drawing a schematic diagram that illustrates basic elements of the traditional pain pathway, such as pain receptors in a joint, a neural pathway through the spinal cord, and sensory centers in the brain. Discussion should focus on how this traditional model of pain sensation fails to account for many clinical pain phenomena such as the persistence of pain after amputation, the absence of pain during sports or wartime injuries, or the fact that surgical interruption of the pathway often fails to abolish persistent pain.

The gate control theory is then introduced as an alternative explanation. This theory maintains that there is a gating mechanism in the spinal cord, which regulates the flow of neural impulses from the site of disease or injury to the brain. When the gate is closed, pain signals are blocked at the level of the spinal cord and thus do not reach the brain. When the gate is open, however, the signals are free to pass through to centers of the brain responsible for pain sensation. Research findings indicate that centers of the brain responsible for cognition (e.g., thoughts, memories, and expectations) and emotions (depres-

sion, anxiety) can influence whether the gate is open or closed (21,22). The role of the patient's own coping efforts in controlling problematic cognitive and emotional responses is then discussed. Arthritis patients respond positively to the gate control theory and report that it helps them better understand the connections between cognitive behavioral interventions and their own disease symptoms.

INVOLVEMENT OF FAMILY

It is important to remember that patients have symptoms that occur in a social context. The way that a spouse or family member responds to the individual can have an important impact on treatment outcome. There has been growing interest in involving spouses or significant others in cognitive behavioral treatment programs. Involving these individuals may help the patient acquire coping skills, increase the frequency of coping skills practice, and enhance treatment outcome.

When the patient's spouse or family is included in treatment, they should actively participate rather than passively observe the treatment process. A spouse, for example, can be taught relaxation techniques along with the patient, and the couple can then be encouraged to practice together at least once a week. Family members can also be encouraged to prompt and reinforce the use of coping skills. A family member could accompany the patient to an exercise session and encourage the patient to pace the exercise or to use imagery techniques to reduce pain or stiffness following vigorous exercise. Training in communication skills can be provided to help patients and family members communicate more effectively about newly learned coping techniques.

Although there are few controlled studies on the effects of family involvement in cognitive behavioral programs for arthritis, available evidence suggests that this approach may be quite effective. For example, some of the largest effects of cognitive behavioral training on pain and pain behavior were obtained in a study that incorporated spouses or family members in the treatment program (14). Only one published study (23) has directly compared a spouse/family assisted cognitive behavioral intervention with an arthritis information control condition that involved a spouse or family member. Results indicated that cognitive behavioral intervention was significantly more effective in reducing the severity of pain and number of swollen joints. A year later, patients receiving spouse-assisted cognitive behavioral training had significantly higher levels of self-efficacy and tended to show improvements in physical disability when compared to controls (24). Patients who showed the largest increases in self-efficacy during the intervention were much more likely to show long-term improvements in physical disability. Patients who showed the largest increases in marital adjustment were more likely to show long-term improvements in psychological disability, physical disability, and pain behavior.

VARIABLES AFFECTING TREATMENT OUTCOME

Patients vary in their response to cognitive behavioral therapy. Some show substantial improvements in pain and functional status, while others show more modest gains. Recent studies suggest that several variables might explain these variations in treatment outcome. Self-efficacy appears to be one of the most important variables associated with positive outcomes in cognitive behavioral training. Self-efficacy can be defined as the belief that one has the ability to engage in a course of action sufficient to attain a desired outcome (25). Patients who show substantial increases in self-efficacy over the course of training are much more likely to show improvements in pain, psychological distress, and physical disability (26). Daily coping is another variable that may relate to the outcome of cognitive behavioral interventions. Patients who continue to practice the coping skills learned in cognitive behavioral training have shown much better long-term outcomes. Daily diaries provide an excellent means of analyzing changes in coping that occur as a result of treatment. Daily recordings of coping and coping efficacy have several advantages, including the ability to track rapidly changing processes closer to their real time, reduction of biases due to recall or memory, and the ability to apply powerful within-person analyses that provide a test of causal relations between coping and arthritis outcomes (27). One study found that increases in the daily use of pain reduction efforts and relaxation strategies by RA patients led to an improvement in next-day pain and positive mood (28).

Arthritis patients also may vary in their readiness to engage in self-management efforts. We have identified 5 distinct clusters among arthritis patients based on their responses to a readiness to change questionnaire: 1) precontemplation—patients appeared to lack motivation to action and scored low on a measure of active coping; 2) contemplation—patients intended to take action in the future but scored quite low on a measure of active coping; 3) preparation—patients appeared to be at a transition in which they were both thinking about change and making some overt behavior changes; 4) unprepared action—patients reported taking action but did not appear to have thought about or prepared for action; and 5) prepared maintenance—patients appeared to be working the hardest to cope and were coping with more severe pain and physical and psychological disability (29). These same 5 clusters were identified in both RA and OA patients (30) and may have important implications for arthritis patients' willingness to participate in cognitive behavioral therapy or other self-help interventions. It is possible that the efficacy of training could be improved by tailoring the intervention to the patients' particular stage of readiness for change.

USE AS AN EARLY INTERVENTION

Patients are usually referred for cognitive behavioral therapy late in the course of their disease. Most published studies have been conducted with patients with disease duration of 6–12 years. However, this therapy need not, and probably should not, be reserved as a treatment of last resort. Early intervention could have many benefits in the management of rheumatic disease patients such as reducing pain and emotional distress, enhancing the effects of ongoing treatment, improving treatment adherence, and possibly slowing the progression of disease. Only one recent study has systematically evaluated the efficacy of cognitive behavioral training in patients with recent-onset RA (<2 years of disease history) (31). Patients receiving cognitive behavioral therapy had a significant decrease in depressive symptoms and a reduction in C-reactive

protein levels. At 6 months followup, these patients had fewer actively inflamed joints. Taken together, these findings suggest that cognitive behavioral therapy may have a role to play in the early treatment of RA.

REFERENCES

1. Keefe FJ, Dunsmore J, Burnett R. Behavioral and cognitive-behavioral approaches to chronic pain: recent advances and future directions. J Consult Clin Psychol 1992;60:528–36.
2. Young LD. Psychological factors in rheumatoid arthritis. J Consult Clin Psychol 1992;60:619–27.
3. Bradley LA, Alberts KR. Psychological and behavioral approaches to pain management for patients with rheumatic disease. Rheum Dis Clin North Am 1999;25:215–32.
4. Keefe FJ, Smith SJ, Buffington ALH, Gibson J, Studts J, Caldwell DS. Recent advances and future directions in the biopsychosocial assessment and treatment of arthritis. J Consult Clin Psychol. In press.
5. Bernstein DA, Borkovec TD. Progressive relaxation training: a manual for the helping professions. Champaign (IL): Research Press; 1973.
6. Van Lankveld W, Naring G, van't Pad Bosch P, van de Putte L. The negative effect of decreasing the level of activity in coping with pain in rheumatoid arthritis: an increase in psychological distress and disease impact. J Behav Med 2000;23:377–91.
7. Sullivan MJ, Thorn B, Haythornthwaite JA, Keefe F, Martin M, Bradley LA, et al. Theoretical perspectives on the relation between catastrophizing and pain. Clin J Pain 2001;17:52–64.
8. Keefe FJ, Lefebvre JC, Egert JR. The relationship of gender to pain, pain behavior, and disability in osteoarthritis patients: the role of catastrophizing. Pain 2000;87:325–34.
9. Parker JC, Frank RG, Beck NC, Smarr KL, Buescher KL, Phillips LR, et al. Pain management in rheumatoid arthritis patients: a cognitive-behavioral approach. Arthritis Rheum 1988;31:593–601.
10. Keefe FJ, van Horn Y. Cognitive—behavioral treatment of rheumatoid arthritis pain: maintaining treatment gains. Arthritis Care Res 1993;6:213–22.
11. Bradley LA, Young LD, Anderson KO, Turner RA, Agudelo CA, McDaniel LK, et al. Effects of psychological therapy on pain behavior of rheumatoid arthritis patients: treatment outcome and six-month followup. Arthritis Rheum 1987;30:1105–14.
12. Applebaum KA, Blanchard EB, Hickling EJ, Alfonso M. Cognitive behavioral treatment of a veteran population with moderate to severe rheumatoid arthritis. Behav Ther 1988;19:489–502.
13. Leibing E, Pfingsten M, Bartmann U, Rueger U, Schuessler G. Cognitive-behavioral treatment in unselected rheumatoid arthritis outpatients. Clin J Pain 1999;15:58–66.
14. Bradley LA, Young LD, Anderson KO, Turner RA, Agudelo CA, McDaniel LK, et al. Effects of cognitive-behavior therapy on rheumatoid arthritis pain behavior: one year follow-up. In: Dubner R, Gebhart G, Bond M, editors. Proceedings of the Vth World Congress on Pain. Amsterdam: Elsevier; 1988. p. 310–4.
15. Keefe FJ, Caldwell DS, Williams DA, Gil KM, Mitchell D, Robertson D, et al. Pain coping skills training in the management of osteoarthritic knee pain: a comparative study. Behav Ther 1990;21:49–62.
16. Lorig K, Lubeck D, Kraines RG, Seleznick M, Holman HR. Outcomes of self-help education for patients with arthritis. Arthritis Rheum 1985;28:680–5.
17. Holman H, Mazonson P, Lorig K. Health education for self-management has significant early and sustained benefits in chronic arthritis. Trans Assoc Am Physicians 1989;102:204–8.
18. Buckelew SP, Conway R, Parker J, Deuser WE, Read J, Witty TE, et al. Biofeedback/relaxation training and exercise interventions for fibromyalgia: a prospective trial. Arthritis Care Res 1998;11:196–209.
19. Rossy LA, Buckelew SP, Dorr N. A meta-analysis of fibromyalgia treatment interventions. Ann Behav Med 1999;21:180–91.
20. Melzack R, Wall P. Pain mechanisms: a new theory. Science 1965;50:971–9.
21. Melzack R. The challenge of pain. London: Penguin Press; 1999.
22. Keefe FJ, France CR. Pain: biopsychosocial mechanisms and management. Curr Dir Psychol Sci 1999;8:137–41.
23. Radjovec V, Nicassio PM, Weisman MH. Behavioral intervention with and without family support for rheumatoid arthritis. Behav Ther 1992;23:13–30.
24. Keefe FJ, Caldwell DS, Baucom D, Salley A, Robinson E, Timmons K, et

al. Spouse-assisted coping skills training in the management of knee pain in osteoarthritis: long-term followup results. Arthritis Care Res 1999;12: 101–11.

25. Bandura A. Self-efficacy: toward a unifying theory of behavioral change. Psychol Rev 1977;84:191–215.
26. Keefe FJ, Bonk V. Psychosocial assessment of pain in patients having rheumatic diseases. Rheum Dis Clin North Am 1999;25:81–103.
27. Tennen H, Affleck G, Armeli S, Carney MA. A daily process approach to coping: linking theory, research, and practice. Am Psychol 2000;55:626–36.
28. Keefe FJ, Affleck G, Lefebvre JC, Starr K, Caldwell DS, Tennen H. Pain coping strategies and coping efficacy in rheumatoid arthritis: a daily process analysis. Pain 1997;69:35–42.
29. Keefe FJ, Lefebvre JC, Kerns RD, Rosenberg R, Beaupre P, Prochaska J, et al. Understanding the adoption of arthritis self-management: stages of change profiles among arthritis patients. Pain 2000;87:303–13.
30. Prochaska JO, Diclemente CC. The transtheoretical approach: towards a systematic eclectic framework. Homewood (IL): Dow Jones, Irwin; 1984.
31. Sharpe L, Sensky T, Timberlake N, Ryan B, Brewin CR, Allard S. A blind, randomized, controlled trial of cognitive-behavioral intervention for patients with recent onset rheumatoid arthritis: preventing psychological and physical morbidity. Pain 2001;89:275–83.

Resources

The Association for the Advancement of Behavior Therapy (305 Seventh Avenue, New York, NY 10001-6008, tel. 212-647-1890) also maintains a referrals service for the general public that can provide the names of CBT therapists in the patient's local area along with a pamphlet offering guidelines on choosing a therapist.

CHAPTER 25

Pharmacologic Interventions in the 21st Century

DONALD R. MILLER, PharmD

In the last few years an explosion of novel drugs for rheumatic diseases has led to new options and strategies for treatment. The 1990s saw the introduction of several innovative therapies, and combinations of drugs in rheumatoid arthritis (RA) became common, even in early disease, with the idea of attempting nearly complete disease suppression before joint damage occurs. Evidence is accumulating that most disease-modifying drugs are safe when used in early RA and, more importantly, that early use can delay joint damage. On the other hand, nonsteroidal antiinflammatory drugs (NSAIDs) are regarded now as relatively dangerous drugs. These developments have led to strategies that rely less on controlling symptoms of RA and more on limiting joint destruction and other long-term complications. American College of Rheumatology (ACR) guidelines stress starting disease-modifying drugs within 3 months for patients with an established diagnosis of RA and ongoing symptoms despite NSAID treatment (1). New guidelines are available for osteoarthritis as well (2). All health care professionals need to recognize the expected therapeutic and adverse effects of antirheumatic drugs so they can participate in patient assessment and monitoring of drug effects.

The decision to use any drug is based on the expected ratio of risk versus benefit in a specific patient. The intensity of treatment should reflect the type and severity of arthritis. It is inappropriate to use corticosteroids in osteoarthritis (OA), for example, but these drugs may be essential in dealing with life-threatening complications of systemic lupus erythematosus (SLE). Drug regimens should be used in adequate doses and for a long enough time to see benefits before changing or adding another. Some drugs require 3–6 months to show full efficacy. Successful therapy often combines drugs having different mechanisms of action and toxicity.

ANALGESICS

Because a cardinal manifestation of all types of arthritis is pain, analgesic drugs play a central role in therapy. Analgesics alone are a therapeutic mainstay in noninflammatory arthritis such as OA, but they are insufficient where inflammation is prominent.

Acetaminophen

One of the safest drugs available, acetaminophen is known by several nonprescription brand names, including Tylenol, Panadol, and Anacin-3. According to American College of Rheumatology guidelines, acetaminophen as needed up to 4 gm/day should be the first-line pharmacologic therapy for OA, based on cost, efficacy, and safety (2). Acetaminophen does not cause gastrointestinal bleeding and has minimal toxicity in recommended doses. Doses higher than 4 gm/day may risk liver toxicity with no increase in benefit. Acetaminophen has been found to be better than placebo and as good as NSAIDs when used in OA patients. It can be used alone to treat osteoarthritis or as an adjunct to NSAIDs. Unfortunately, there is a ceiling to its analgesic effect, and it has no antiinflammatory effect.

Narcotics

Weak narcotic drugs such as propoxyphene (Darvon), codeine, and oxycodone (OxyContin, Percocet) are frequently used for acute musculoskeletal pain or as chronic adjunct therapy with NSAIDs. Tramadol (Ultram) is a drug with some opioid properties that is not scheduled as a controlled substance. The updated ACR guidelines for OA suggest that tramadol, propoxyphene, codeine, or oxycodone can be appropriate for long-term use in patients with moderate to severe pain and poor response or contraindications to other oral therapy (2). Tramadol should be used first due to lower risk of abuse.

Opioids reduce the perception of pain in the central nervous system. They are additive to NSAIDs in analgesia and have no ceiling effect. Thus their mechanism is different from, and complementary to, the peripheral mechanism of other analgesics. Occasional doses may induce sleepiness, dizziness, or constipation but otherwise are safe for short-term use.

Chronic narcotic use is controversial due to the potential for inducing physical and psychological dependence. However, in 1997, the American Academy of Pain Management and the American Pain Society published a joint consensus statement that encourages a more liberal role for opioids in chronic nonmalignant pain. The American Geriatric Society guidelines for chronic nonmalignant pain, published in 1998, also address the underuse of opioids to treat chronic pain. The guidelines emphasize that fear of tolerance or addiction for patients with physiologic pain is grossly exaggerated and leads to undertreatment.

A decision to prescribe and take these drugs regularly should be based on the severity of pain, lack of effect of other drugs, and a clear understanding by the patient of permissible maximum daily doses. Preferably, opioids should be prescribed in controlled release dosage forms that do not contain other analgesics so that dosage titration is simplified. Individual dosage titration and appropriate management of side effects are important components of therapy. With careful supervision, use of these drugs is a reasonable option for certain patients.

Table 1. Nonsteroidal antiinflammatory drugs.*

	Starting dose	Maximum approved dose	Half-life (hours)	Generic/OTC	COX selectivity
Aspirin	650 mg qid	1,300 mg qid	3–20†	yes/yes	COX-1
Celecoxib	200 mg qid	200 mg bid	12	no/no	COX-2
Choline salicylate	870 mg qid	1,740 mg qid	3–20†	no/yes	COX-2
Diclofenac	50 mg bid	75 mg tid	2	yes/no	none
Diflunisal	250 mg bid	500 mg tid	12	no/no	none
Etodolac	300 mg bid	400 mg tid	7	no/no	COX-2 preferential
Fenoprofen	300 mg tid	800 mg qid	3	yes/no	none
Flurbiprofen	50 mg qid	300 mg tid	6	yes/no	none
Ibuprofen	300 mg qid	800 mg qid	2	yes/yes	none
Indomethacin	25 mg bid	50 mg qid	4	yes/no	none
Ketoprofen	50 mg qid	75 mg qid	3	yes/yes	none
Meclofenamate	50 mg tid	100 mg qid	2	yes/no	none
Meloxicam	7.5 mg qd	15 mg qd	20	no/no	COX-2 preferential
Nabumetone	1 gm qd	1 gm bid	24	no/no	COX-2 preferential
Naproxen	250 mg bid	500 mg tid	13	yes/yes	none
Oxaprozin	600 mg qd	1,800 mg qd	42	no/no	none
Piroxicam	10 mg qd	20 mg qd	45	yes/no	none
Rofecoxib	12.5 mg qd	25 mg qd	17	no/no	COX-2
Salsalate	500 mg tid	1,000 mg tid	3–20†	yes/no	COX-2
Sulindac	150 mg bid	200 mg bid	18	yes/no	none
Tolmetin	200 mg tid	400 mg tid	1–5†	yes/no	none

* OTC = over-the-counter; COX = cyclooxygenase; qd = once daily; bid = twice daily; tid = three times daily; qid = four times daily. Reproduced with permission from Miller DR. Osteoarthritis. In: Mueller B, Bertch K, Dunsworth T, et al, eds. Pharmacotherapy self-assessment program. 4th ed. Rheumatology module. Kansas City, MO: American College of Clinical Pharmacy; 2001. p. 231.
† Dose-related half-life.

Capsaicin

Capsaicin, available in a topical cream in 0.025%, 0.075%, and 0.25% concentrations (Zostrix, Dolorac and others), is a derivative of red chili peppers that depletes peripheral sensory nerves of a neurotransmitter called substance P. Initially capsaicin causes stinging or burning sensations as it displaces substance P. After a few days, however, pain perception is reduced. One study in OA demonstrated that capsaicin decreased pain and tenderness by about 40% when applied to specific joints 4 times daily for a month (3). A high strength (0.25%) formulation of capsaicin can be applied twice a day and has been shown to provide faster and stronger pain relief than a 0.025% preparation.

Glucosamine and Chondroitin

Glucosamine and chondroitin have become highly popular "nutritional supplements" for OA. Glucosamine is a hexosamine sugar used as a building block for glycosaminoglycans (GAGs) that make up cartilage. Chondroitin is the most abundant GAG in human articular cartilage and is believed to work by competitively inhibiting the degradative enzymes in articular cartilage.

A meta-analysis of the efficacy of both glucosamine and chondroitin in symptomatic management of knee and/or hip OA found sufficient evidence from clinical trials to support the use of these supplements (4). Also, a recent 3-year study found that glucosamine alone at 1,500 mg/day improved symptoms and reduced the loss of radiologic joint space in knee OA (5). No significant side effects were noted.

Recent data on safety and efficacy support the use of these supplements in OA. The 2000 update to the ACR osteoarthritis guidelines made no recommendation regarding them. However, in a recent press release, the ACR has stated that it is "not

unreasonable" for physicians to concur in the use of the products after discussion with patients. Appropriate doses are 1,500 mg of glucosamine and 1,200 mg of chondroitin per day. Symptomatic benefits should be evident within 2 months. Health professionals should be sure that self-treating patients are using the products for OA and not for another form of arthritis.

NONSTEROIDAL ANTIINFLAMMATORY DRUGS

The NSAIDS are a large group of drugs that have peripheral analgesic and antiinflammatory effects. These drugs are often divided into several classes based on chemical category, but such classification is arbitrary and is not helpful in choosing a specific drug. Selectivity for the cyclooxygenase enzyme is a more useful classification (6). The prototype NSAID is aspirin (acetylsalicylic acid), which is converted to salicylic acid after absorption. Several other nonacetylated salicylate derivatives are available. These differ from aspirin in their inability to inhibit prostaglandin synthesis, as discussed below. A complete list of NSAIDs currently available in the United States is provided in Table 1.

NSAIDs inhibit the enzyme cyclooxygenase (COX), which converts a precursor molecule into various prostaglandins. Prostaglandins are ubiquitous, locally synthesized chemicals that have a role in inflammation as well as numerous other body processes. The nonspecific inhibition of prostaglandin synthesis throughout the body explains the wide range of adverse effects that are caused by NSAIDs. However, the nonacetylated salicylates are very weak inhibitors of prostaglandin synthesis.

In 1990 it was discovered that 2 different forms of COX exist. COX-1 is present at low levels in many organs, including platelets, kidneys, and the gastrointestinal (GI) tract, while under basal conditions COX-2 is present in a much more limited distribution. However, COX-2 is induced up to 20-fold by inflammatory cytokines during tissue injury, and thus generates prostaglandins that cause pain and inflammation. Therefore, it appears that the therapeutic activity of NSAIDs is due to COX-2 inhibition, while certain toxicities (particularly GI and antiplatelet toxicities) are primarily the result of COX-1 inhibition. All of the older NSAIDs have activity against both forms of COX. Some drugs, including nabumetone, etodolac, and meloxicam, appear to be somewhat COX-2 preferential. Only celecoxib and rofecoxib meet the strict criterion for being COX-2 selective—which is the lack of COX-1 inhibition in platelets *in vivo* at therapeutic doses (6).

The analgesic action of NSAIDs occurs at lower doses than antiinflammatory effects. Thus, low doses may be adequate in OA. The analgesia occurs peripherally by inhibition of prostaglandin synthesis. Prostaglandins sensitize afferent sensory nerves to the effect of pain-inducing chemical stimuli. Antiinflammatory effects of NSAIDs occur near the high end of their dosage range. The antiinflammatory mechanism may be due to several effects. In addition to inhibiting prostaglandin synthesis, NSAIDs have multiple independent effects such as altering macrophage and neutrophil function. Although NSAIDs provide symptomatic relief of arthritis, they have no effect on underlying disease processes. This is one reason why many physicians start additional drug therapy at early stages of rheumatic disease.

When NSAIDs are compared in clinical trials, there is little difference between them in effectiveness or tolerance. None, including the COX-2 selective drugs, is superior to aspirin in efficacy. However, patient response is variable and highly individual. A patient may respond to one drug in the class despite no benefit from another. This unpredictability means that drug selection is essentially a trial and error process. To prevent patients from becoming discouraged, they may be told at the onset that several drugs may have to be tried before finding one that is effective. Although pain relief will be obtained quickly with NSAIDs, it may take 2–4 weeks before full antiinflammatory effect is achieved. Thus, patients are usually given a 1-month trial before deciding to alter therapy.

Two areas in which NSAIDs differ are duration of action and frequency of dosing. Longer-acting drugs may be useful for patients who have difficulty remembering to take frequent doses. All NSAIDs are well absorbed; taking with food may delay but does not reduce absorption. Normally, NSAIDs are taken with meals to reduce GI distress. These drugs also differ significantly in cost. Because they are comparably effective, it is reasonable to try a lower-cost NSAID or a generic version in most patients before moving to more expensive drugs.

Gastrointestinal problems are the most common side effect of NSAID use. Nausea and abdominal distress may be reduced by taking medication with food. All NSAIDs may cause GI bleeding and ulcers, but bleeding does not always correlate with subjective patient reports. Gastrointestinal bleeding may be due to 2 separate effects. First, almost all NSAIDs are weak acids capable of disrupting GI mucosa by direct topical actions. This effect may be reduced by putting an enteric (delayed release) coating on the drug tablet or by giving nonacidic NSAIDs. Second, NSAIDs inhibit synthesis of prostaglandins in the GI tract, rendering it less able to protect and repair itself. This is why the COX-2 selective drugs have minimal GI toxicity.

Some older NSAIDs may cause ulcers less commonly than others. In large, population-based studies, nonacetylated salicylates, ibuprofen, and enteric-coated forms of aspirin appear safer. COX-2 preferential drugs such as nabumetone, etodolac, and meloxicam also appear to be somewhat safer. However, the COX-2 selective drugs—celecoxib and rofecoxib—have the greatest gastrointestinal safety and are the NSAIDs of choice for patients at high risk of GI bleeding (7,8).

Patients at high risk of GI ulcers include the elderly, those with a previous history of ulcers, smokers, those taking concurrent corticosteroids or anticoagulants, and those with severe arthritis or other disability (8). Higher NSAID doses also increase risk. Patients with 2 or more risk factors for GI bleeding should receive COX-2 selective drugs or, if COX-2 selective drugs are not effective, take a concurrent therapy to prevent GI bleeding. Misoprostol, an orally active prostaglandin analog, and proton pump inhibitors (such as omeprazole or lansoprazole) have been shown to prevent both gastric and duodenal ulcers. Histamine-2 receptor antagonists like cimetidine and ranitidine prevent development of duodenal ulcers but not gastric. When an ulcer does develop from an NSAID, it will heal with normal ulcer therapies. If the NSAID must be continued, proton pump inhibitors heal most ulcers even during concomitant NSAID therapy (8).

Central nervous system toxicities may also occur with NSAID use. Dizziness, headache, drowsiness, or ringing in the ears will sometimes develop. Indomethacin is particularly likely to cause headaches.

NSAIDs may affect kidney function in patients who already have some intrinsic renal dysfunction or who have reduced renal blood flow (e.g., patients with congestive heart failure and the elderly). The kidneys synthesize prostaglandins to help maintain blood flow in situations where perfusion is reduced. Some patients develop retention of sodium and water resulting in weight gain or mild leg edema; others develop worsening of hypertension. Occasionally, NSAIDs may cause acute renal failure. These drugs can also cause an interstitial nephritis that is unpredictable and allergic in nature. Safer alternatives for patients at risk of renal toxicity include nonacetylated salicylates, which are very weak prostaglandin inhibitors, and sulindac, which is not excreted by the kidney in active form. It was hoped that COX-2 selective drugs would be safer for the kidney, but COX-2 is present in renal tissue and celecoxib and rofecoxib have effects on renal blood flow similar to older NSAIDs (9).

Some patients develop pseudo-allergic reactions to NSAIDs. A syndrome of wheezing, nasal rhinitis, and laryngeal edema has been described. This syndrome is prostaglandin-mediated, so patients who react to one NSAID may react to others. A nonacetylated salicylate may be cautiously tried. A second type of reaction to aspirin involves urticaria and angioedema, and patients are more likely to cross-react to other salicylates as well as NSAIDs.

Nonsteroidal drugs cause minor elevations of liver enzyme levels in up to 15% of patients. Serious liver toxicity is rare, but both hepatocellular and cholestatic reactions, with occasional deaths, have been reported. Cases of agranulocytosis and aplastic anemia have been reported rarely, mostly with phenylbutazone and indomethacin use. Most NSAIDs, except nonacetylated salicylates and COX-2 specific drugs, inhibit platelet aggregation. Aspirin irreversibly acetylates platelets, while other NSAIDs inhibit platelet function only while they are in the bloodstream.

Patients taking NSAIDs should be monitored regularly for efficacy and safety. If little or no benefit is obtained within 1 month, it is reasonable to try an alternative NSAID. Combining 2 or more NSAIDs is not beneficial and increases the risk of toxicity. Monitoring for safety usually includes complete blood counts to watch for anemia as a sign of GI bleeding, serum creatinine and potassium to assess renal impairment, and possibly liver enzyme tests to watch for liver problems.

HYALURONIC ACID DERIVATIVES

Hyaluronan (hyaluonic acid, HA) is a large glycosaminoglycan that in solution forms an extensive network that enables joint fluid to act as a viscous lubricant at rest or on gentle movement of a joint, and as an elastic solid shock absorber at high shear rates. In OA, the concentration and molecular weight of HA are reduced, compromising the viscoelastic properties of joint fluid. Thus, injection of exogenous HA into the joint may restore some of the normal protective properties of endogenous HA (10). Technically, hyaluronan products are classified as medical devices because of their purported mechanism as lubricating agents. Clinicians can choose from 3 products. Hyalgan and Supartz are sodium hyaluronate, and Synvisc is hylan G-F 20, a longer-acting polymer of hyaluronate. Hyalgan or Supartz are administered in a series of 5 joint injections, Synvisc in 3.

Clinical trials have found that HA preparations reduced OA symptoms for an average of 8 months. HA normally flows through the joint with a half-life of only 12 to 24 hours in animals, so the reason for its long-lasting therapeutic effects is unknown. Clinical trials in OA of the knee have demonstrated that the products relieve pain and improve function better than placebo for several months. Good responses typically occur in 75% or more of studied patients and benefits have lasted an average of 8 months. Although differences between HA and placebo have not been large, the benefits are comparable to relief from NSAIDs. The best responses occurred in patients with milder changes on radiographs. Compared with intraarticular steroids, HA injections have less dramatic but longer-lasting effects. Two studies have found intraarticular hyaluronic acid to be superior to methylprednisolone, and one study found hylan G-F 20 to be better than lower molecular weight hyaluronan.

Hyaluronan preparations appear to be safe; local reactions at the injection site (pain, swelling) are generally mild and transient. The candidates include patients with residual knee symptoms despite pharmacologic therapy, those with poor adherence to oral medication, patients at risk of GI complications from NSAIDs, those who need corticosteroid injections, and patients with early, milder OA who fail acetaminophen therapy. Courses of treatment can be repeated approximately every 6 months for several years if effective, although limited data are available on the effectiveness of multiple courses.

CORTICOSTEROIDS

Corticosteroids are analogs of cortisone, a natural antiinflammatory hormone first isolated in the 1940s. They were heavily used as "wonder drugs" during the 1950s until their adverse effects became apparent. Corticosteroids are still recognized as

Table 2. Comparison of oral corticosteroids.

Drug (trade name)	Equivalent dose (mg)	Relative anti-inflammatory potency
Short acting		
Hydrocortisone (Cortef)	20	1
Cortisone (Cortone)	25	0.8
Intermediate acting		
Prednisone (Deltasone)	5	4
Prednisolone (Delta-Cortef)	5	4
Methylprednisolone (Medrol)	4	5
Triamcinolone (Kenacort)	4	5
Long acting		
Betamethasone (Celestone)	0.6	25
Dexamethasone (Decadron)	0.75	30

the most powerful antiinflammatory drugs available. However, they should be used judiciously in the lowest dose for the shortest possible time in order to avoid long-term adverse effects. Corticosteroids are used only in conditions where inflammation is prominent and not responsive to NSAIDs. These drugs do not alter the course of RA (11). In certain cases of organ inflammation complicating SLE or rheumatoid vasculitis, however, large doses may be life saving. A list and comparison of drugs is shown in Table 2.

The mechanism of action of corticosteroids is complex (12). They alter the distribution and function of white blood cells, suppress both humoral and cell-mediated immune function, and inhibit phospholipase, an enzyme in cell membranes that generates a prostaglandin precursor.

A "physiologic" dose of systemic corticosteroid is considered to be the equivalent of the body's normal daily secretion of 20 to 30 mg of hydrocortisone. Thus, a physiologic dose of prednisone is 5 to 7.5 mg/day. Doses lower than this cause only modest suppression of endogenous hydrocortisone secretion and few adverse effects, whereas larger doses are likely to cause significant adverse effects (13). Prednisone is usually the steroid of choice in rheumatic disease because of its intermediate duration of action, which allows once-daily dosing. However, if given in the morning, prednisone's effect will have diminished by the time the body's endogenous hydrocortisone secretion peaks early the next morning. To further minimize adrenal suppression, prednisone is sometimes given only on alternate days. However, alternate day therapy is not maximally effective and is not suitable for initiating therapy or for controlling highly active disease. Steroids with a long duration of action, like dexamethasone, may suppress the adrenal gland even on alternate day therapy.

Corticosteroids may be given orally, intravenously, or intraarticularly. Local injection into a joint, tendon sheath, or bursa may be used when inflammation is localized, whereas systemic administration is used for generalized inflammation. The most feared complication of articular injection is introduction of bacteria causing an infection. Intraarticular injections should not be repeated more than 3–4 times per year because of a risk of osteonecrosis (14).

Indications for systemic steroids are controversial but usually include short-term treatment of RA while waiting for slow-acting drugs to work, severe synovitis that impairs functional ability, and extraarticular inflammation. Low doses of prednisone (7.5 mg/day or less) are sufficient for articular inflammation, modest doses (10–15 mg/day) are used in polymyalgia rheumatica, and high doses (40–60 mg/day) may be used in SLE or vasculitis. Occasionally, large intravenous boluses (up to 1 gm/day methylprednisolone for 3 days) may be used in severe or refractory extraarticular disease.

Clinical benefit occurs rapidly; patients usually notice improvement within 24 hours. Once improvement has stabilized, the dose is tapered to the minimum effective dose. Monitoring of corticosteroid therapy should include blood counts, serum potassium level, and glucose. Due to the risk of osteoporosis with long-term use, supplemental calcium and vitamin D should be considered.

SLOW-ACTING ANTIRHEUMATIC DRUGS

This heterogenous group of drugs has a delayed onset of action, ranging from 3 weeks to 3 months. They are sometimes referred to as second-line drugs because they were traditionally used only after a trial of several NSAIDs. They appear to work at an earlier stage in the inflammatory process than NSAIDs, and some can retard progression of joint erosion; thus the name "disease-modifying drugs" (DMARDs).

Used alone at later stages of RA, beneficial effects of these drugs are often short-lived, with disease activity returning to baseline shortly after drug discontinuation, and they seldom improve disease enough to cause true remission. Even with continued treatment only half of all patients stay on individual drugs longer than 2 years (14). However, the disappointing long-term efficacy of these drugs may be due in part to the fact that they are started too late in the disease course (15). One reason for this delay has been fear of severe organ toxicity, but data suggest that adverse effects of these drugs are no more severe than those of NSAIDs (16). The current approach is to start the drugs earlier, sometimes in combination. The superiority of this approach is now proven (15,17).

Gold Compounds

Gold compounds were the first disease-modifying drugs to be widely used. There are 2 compounds (gold sodium thiomalate and gold thioglucose) administered by intramuscular injection, and 1 (auranofin) given orally. The parenteral and orally administered drugs are not interchangeable, as they have different profiles of safety and efficacy.

Intramuscular compounds were accidentally discovered to have activity in RA during the 1930s. Their dosage protocols developed empirically. The standard regimen is a 50 mg injection once a week. Lower doses are often given at first to test for tolerance, and less frequent doses (50 mg every 2–4 weeks) are used for maintenance. Injectable gold compounds produce clinical improvement in about 70% of patients; however, it may take 3–6 months for this to occur.

A major drawback to the use of these compounds is their adverse effects, which occur in approximately 30% of patients. The most common reactions are mucocutaneous. A dermatitis may occur in the first weeks of therapy, but it resolves on drug discontinuation. Less frequent reactions include stomatitis, generalized pruritus, gray-blue discoloration of mucous membranes, alopecia, and exfoliative dermatitis. Proteinuria, which occurs in 2–10% of patients, may be mild and transient and not require drug discontinuation. Nephrotic syndrome may occur. Therapy is usually stopped if urinary protein is greater than 1 gm per 24 hours. Blood dyscrasias are another serious adverse effect. Leukopenia, thrombocytopenia, and aplastic anemia

have all been reported. Monitoring of injectable gold should include blood counts and urinalysis every 1–2 weeks prior to the next scheduled injection.

Auranofin is the orally active gold compound. It is given twice daily in 3 mg capsules. Its effectiveness is less than that of injectable gold, which offsets its convenience (18). Adverse effects are similar to injectable gold except that diarrhea is very common with auranofin, while the incidence of renal and hematologic effects may be somewhat lower.

Penicillamine

Penicillamine was first used as a heavy metal chelator and was discovered to have antirheumatic activity in the 1960s. Its mechanism of action is unknown. It is taken orally, starting at 250 mg once daily and increasing to 250 mg three times daily if necessary. Because penicillamine is a metal chelator, it must be taken on an empty stomach, and 2 hours apart from iron salts or antacids, to assure adequate absorption. The effectiveness of penicillamine is similar to that of injectable gold, but adverse effects may be more common.

Many side effects of penicillamine are similar to those seen with gold compounds. Blood counts and urinalysis need to be monitored regularly. Additional effects caused by penicillamine include nausea, changes in taste that may resolve with continued therapy, and, rarely, autoimmune syndromes. Most side effects appear to be dose-related so attempts should be made to keep the dose as low as possible.

Antimalarial Drugs

Chloroquine and hydroxychloroquine were used as antimalarial compounds before their antirheumatic activity was discovered. They are believed to work by raising the pH of cytoplasmic compartments in antigen-processing cells like macrophages, thus diminishing immune response. These drugs are slightly less effective in RA than injectable gold or penicillamine (18) but their safety is far greater (16,18). They are also very useful in treating joint and skin symptoms in SLE.

Antimalarial drugs are well tolerated, occasionally causing significant nausea or dizziness. The major concern is ocular toxicity. The drugs have a high affinity for the retina, and if early signs of retinal damage are not detected it can become irreversible and lead to blindness. If regular ophthalmic exams are done every 6 months, damage is easily detected at an early stage. Patients may report poor distance vision, difficulty reading, night blindness, and small areas of vision loss. The drugs may also deposit in the cornea, but this does not cause serious problems.

Ocular toxicity is dose related. Consequently, dosage is limited to less than 4 mg/kg/day (typically 250 mg/day) for chloroquine and 6.5 mg/kg/day (400 mg/day) for hydroxychloroquine. Overall, the safety and minimal monitoring required make antimalarial drugs a good choice in early RA and SLE.

Sulfasalazine

Although sulfasalazine may be better known for treating inflammatory bowel disease, it has proven efficacy in RA, ankylosing spondylitis, and other spondylarthropathies. It is also FDA approved for use in children with RA. Antibacterial, antiinflammatory, and immunomodulatory effects may contribute to its efficacy but no predominant mechanism has been established. Like other slow-acting drugs, improvement is not seen for at least 8–12 weeks. The dose is 2–3 gm/day in divided doses, although the starting dose is usually smaller to avoid side effects.

Common side effects are nausea, vomiting, headache, or fever. Other potential adverse reactions may include rash, hemolysis, blood dyscrasias, and male infertility. Compared to other slow-acting drugs it is equally efficacious but has a high frequency of side effects (18).

Methotrexate

Methotrexate, an analog of folic acid, is currently the standard treatment for severe RA, although its mechanism of action is unclear. It was believed to inhibit dihydrofolate reductase, an enzyme critical to synthesis of DNA in actively dividing cells. However, other mechanisms such as adenosine release are probably important, as small doses of supplemental folic acid do not interfere with methotrexate's efficacy. Methotrexate has both antiinflammatory and immunosuppressive properties, but antiinflammatory activity predominates at the low doses used in RA.

Methotrexate can be given orally or parenterally in a once-weekly dose. The typical starting dose is 7.5 mg weekly with a maximum of about 25 mg/week. The unusual dosage regimen was developed to minimize the drug's liver toxicity. Methotrexate's effectiveness is at least as high as other slow-acting drugs (18), and some studies find that patients are likely to stay on methotrexate longer (14). Another advantage is a relatively fast onset of action (3–6 weeks).

The adverse effects of methotrexate are usually well tolerated, although some may be life-threatening. Common side effects are nausea, vomiting, diarrhea, mouth ulcers, decreased white blood cell counts, and megaloblastic anemia. Hepatotoxicity is the most worrisome long-term effect. An increase in liver enzymes occurs commonly after a methotrexate dose. A small number of patients develop significant liver fibrosis or cirrhosis, and periodic liver biopsies are advocated by some authors. Patients taking methotrexate should be warned to avoid alcoholic beverages, which increase liver toxicity. Other risk factors are obesity, diabetes, and impaired renal function. Another potentially fatal toxicity of methotrexate is the unpredictable development of pulmonary interstitial inflammation. Methotrexate is teratogenic but is not known to cause malignancy.

Although folate antagonism may not account for methotrexate's therapeutic efficacy, it does cause much of the toxicity. Low-dose folic acid supplements (5 to 27.5 mg/week) lessen adverse effects without altering efficacy (19). On the other hand, the antibiotic trimethoprim, found in Proloprim, Septra, and Bactrim, is also a human folate antagonist and should be avoided.

Leflunomide

Leflunomide (Arava) is a new oral slow-acting antirheumatic drug. It is an antimetabolite that has an antiproliferative effect on T lymphocytes. Leflunomide's active metabolite has a half-life of about 2 weeks, so it takes some time for blood levels to build up or to be reduced. Although other drugs have been shown to retard joint destruction in RA, leflunomide was the first drug to get FDA approval for this indication.

Trials in RA patients found leflunomide to be superior to placebo and comparable to methotrexate or sulfasalazine after 1 year (20). Improvement began as early as 1 month after treatment started. In one study the Sharp x-ray score was essentially unchanged in leflunomide patients compared to a worsening of 1.4 points with sulfasalazine and 5.6 with placebo.

Common adverse effects include diarrhea, rash, and reversible alopecia. Liver enzymes increase in about 10% of patients and anaphylaxis has been reported. Leflunomide must be used cautiously with other hepatotoxic drugs such as methotrexate. Leflunomide is also teratogenic and must be avoided in patients who may conceive. Both men and women who wish to have children must discontinue the drug and should take cholestyramine 8 gm three times daily for 11 days to bind and eliminate the drug.

Because of the long half-life of its metabolite, leflunomide dosage begins with a loading dose of 100 mg/day for 3 days, followed by a maintenance dose of 20 mg/day (or 10 mg/day if 20 mg is poorly tolerated).

Azathioprine

Azathioprine (Imuran) is an immunosuppressive or cytotoxic drug believed to interfere with cell division by inhibiting metabolism and synthesis of proteins and DNA. It has been used in doses of 0.75 to 2.5 mg/kg/day for rheumatic diseases. Dosage is started at the low end and gradually increased as needed. Allopurinol interferes with azathioprine metabolism, necessitating a 50% reduction in dose.

Azathioprine is similar in effectiveness to other slow-acting drugs in treatment of RA (18). The usual lag period is required to see an effect. Side effects include GI intolerance, reduced white blood cell counts with risk of infection, pancreatitis, hepatotoxicity, and long-term risk of malignancy.

Cyclophosphamide

Cyclophosphamide (Cytoxan) is an alkylating agent, which nonspecifically kills cells by chemically reacting with DNA and RNA molecules. It suppresses the immune system by killing lymphocytes. Oral dosage begins at 50–75 mg/day and may be cautiously increased after 8 weeks if poor response is seen. Large intravenous doses may be used for lupus nephritis.

This drug is infrequently used in RA due its considerable toxicity. However, it has an important role in treatment of lupus nephritis and various forms of vasculitis. Nausea, mouth sores, alopecia, and low white blood counts are common. Suppression of ovarian and testicular function may occur with chronic therapy. A unique problem with cyclophosphamide is hemorrhagic inflammation of the urinary bladder, due to accumulation of an irritating drug metabolite. Patients may report painful urination and/or blood in the urine. Bladder cancer can be a long-term adverse effect. These problems are reduced by drinking plenty of fluids and frequently emptying the bladder, especially before bedtime.

Table 3. Unusual doses and key toxicities for antirheumatic drugs.

	Usual dose*	Toxicities that require monitoring
Salicylates, NSAIDs	See Table 1	Gastrointestinal ulceration and bleeding; renal impairment
Corticosteroids	See text and Table 2	Hypertension, hyperglycemia, euphoria, depression, osteoporosis, adrenal suppression, impaired wound healing, cataracts, susceptibility to infection
Analgesics		
Acetaminophen	600 mg to 1 gm qid	Risk of hepatotoxicity in overdose or in chronic alcohol abusers
Capsaicin	Topically bid–qid	Local burning sensation initially
Chondroitin	400 mg tid	
Glucosamine	500 mg tid	Worsening of diabetes
Hyaluronates	2 ml by intraarticular injection once weekly for 3–5 weeks	Local reactions, pain
Oxycodone	5 to 10 mg qid as needed or 10 to 20 mg (sustained release) bid	Dizziness, drowsiness, nausea, low risk of physical and psychological dependence
Propoxyphene	65 mg qid as needed	Dizziness, drowsiness, nausea, low risk of physical and psychological dependence
Tramadol	50 to 100 mg qid as needed	Drowsiness, dizziness, nausea, low risk of physical and psychological dependence
Slow-acting drugs		
Auranofin	3 mg bid	Bone marrow suppression, proteinuria
Azathioprine	50–150 mg/day	Bone marrow suppression, liver toxicity, lymphoproliferative disorders
Cyclosporine	3–5 mg/kg/day	Renal impairment, anemia, hypertension
Gold, injectable	50 mg weekly	Bone marrow suppression, proteinuria
Hydroxychloroquine	200–400 mg/day	Retinal damage
Leflunomide	10–20 mg/day	Liver toxicity, rash
Methotrexate	7.5–15 mg weekly	Bone marrow suppression, liver toxicity, pulmonary toxicity
Minocycline	100 mg bid	Dizziness
Mycophenolate	1 gm bid	Bone marrow suppression
Penicillamine	250–750 mg/day	Bone marrow suppression, proteinuria
Sulfasalazine	1 gm bid	Bone marrow suppression, rash
Biologic agents		
Etanercept	25 mg twice weekly	Local skin reactions, susceptibility to infection
Infliximab	10 mg/kg q 4 weeks	Hypersensitivity reactions, susceptibility to infection

* bid = twice daily; tid = three times daily; qid = four times daily; NSAIDs = nonsteroidal antiinflammatory drugs.

Cyclosporine

Cyclosporine is an immunosuppressive drug used to prevent organ rejection. The drug is available in different dosage forms that are not interchangeable, and only the microemulsion form (Neoral) is FDA approved for treatment of severe RA. It inhibits production and utilization of interleukin-2, a growth factor for lymphocytes, and has the typical 6–12-week lag period before producing benefit. Renal damage, hypertension, gum hypertrophy, and increased body hair are the most common adverse effects. Recommended dosing is 2.5–4.0 mg/kg/day divided into 2 equal doses (21). Higher doses increase the risk of nephropathy. Currently, it is reserved for severe, progressive RA unresponsive to other drugs.

Minocycline

Three double-blinded trials have shown minocycline to have a slow-acting effect in RA, although it is not FDA approved for this indication (22). The benefit appears modest, but may be more pronounced in early RA. Minocycline's mechanism of action is unknown but is probably unrelated to its antibiotic activity. Tetracyclines are known to inhibit matrix metalloproteinases, and potentially may retard loss of joint space in OA as well. Because minocycline is well tolerated except for nausea and dizziness, it is an attractive addition to the drug arsenal.

Mycophenolate Mofetil

Mycophenolate mofetil (CellCept) is a purine antimetabolite currently approved for immunosuppression to prevent organ

rejection. It has been studied in about 600 patients with RA with promising results. It has also been studied as an alternative to cyclophosphamide in treating lupus nephritis. The drug has no liver or renal toxicity and could provide a safer alternative to cyclosporine or azathioprine in immunosuppressive regimens. Gastrointestinal upset is the most common adverse effect.

COMBINATION THERAPY

Combining drugs with different mechanisms of action and different toxicities may provide additional benefits over monotherapy. Early reports found that combining drugs in RA often caused more toxicity than benefit. However, continued research found that several drugs combined with methotrexate have at least additive benefits without intolerable side effects. Safer drugs like hydroxychloroquine and minocycline also may be used together with other slow-acting drugs. Combination therapies give clinicians more options for aggressive treatment.

Some rheumatologists now initiate treatment with combinations of slow-acting drugs and/or steroids and gradually withdraw drugs as improvement in disease occurs (23). More commonly, patients with poor response to initial monotherapy will receive combinations of slow-acting or disease-modifying drugs. Many rheumatologists save combination therapy for patients who fail to respond satisfactorily to methotrexate alone. Table 3 lists the usual doses and key toxicities for the most common antirheumatic drugs discussed in this chapter.

BIOLOGIC AGENTS

A new and exciting approach to treatment of RA is to attack specific parts of the immune system, including the chemical messengers that coordinate the autoimmune process. Two of these key chemicals are interleukin-1 (IL-1) and tumor necrosis factor alpha (TNFα).

Etanercept (Enbrel) and infliximab (Remicade) are the first "biological response modifiers" approved for RA. Tumor necrosis factor alpha (TNFα) is recognized to be a key cytokine responsible for inflammation and bone resorption in RA. It stimulates production of additional inflammatory mediators, leading to perpetuation of chronic inflammation and tissue destruction. TNFα normally binds to receptors on the surface of certain cells. Recombinant DNA technology has allowed production of soluble proteins that mimic the TNF receptor and harmlessly bind to TNF so it is removed from circulation. Etanercept is a soluble receptor of TNF. TNF can also be removed from circulation by specific antibodies produced against it. Infliximab is a monoclonal antibody to TNF made by combining a human immunoglobulin with a binding region produced in mice. Neither of these provides permanent relief but must be used in conjunction with an overall strategy for disease control just as other disease-modifying drugs are.

Etanercept has been approved as initial or as later therapy for moderate to severely active RA and for polyarticular juvenile rheumatoid arthritis. It can be given alone or in conjunction with methotrexate or other slow-acting drugs. Recently it has also been shown to be more rapidly effective than methotrexate in early, severe RA. Etanercept is given by subcutaneous injection in a dose of 25 mg twice a week and can be self-injected after training. Its effects begin within a few weeks but also wear off within 1 month of stopping it. Infliximab has also been studied in double-blind clinical trials (24). Repeated doses of infliximab plus methotrexate were more effective than either infliximab or methotrexate alone, and results suggest that infliximab can be used safely with methotrexate for at least 1 year. It appears that both etanercept and infliximab can slow joint erosion. The response to a single infusion of infliximab lasts a median of 10 weeks (range 1 to 19 weeks) but may decrease with repeated infusions. The FDA has approved infliximab for combination use with methotrexate as a first-line therapy to inhibit the progression of structural damage in patients with moderate-to-severe RA.

The TNF inhibitors have few side effects. Injection site reactions are common with etanercept. Otherwise it is well tolerated and no autoimmune disease has occurred, even though antibodies can develop. With wider use, some cases of pancytopenia and demyelinating syndromes have been reported with etanercept. Infliximab may cause hypersensitivity reactions, including fever, chills, dyspnea, urticaria, and hypotension. Both etanercept and infliximab should be avoided or stopped in patients with infections, as their immune suppressing properties have led to overwhelming infections in some patients.

Other biologic response modifiers are under investigation. An interleukin-1 receptor antagonist (IL-1Ra, anakinra) has been studied as monotherapy and in combination with methotrexate for RA. Preliminary studies suggest that IL-1Ra can significantly slow the rate of joint damage.

Although they represent an exciting new approach to RA, the long-term effects of biologic therapies are unknown. Because TNF is also important in suppressing tumors, TNF antagonists could predispose to cancer. It is possible that combining anti-TNF drugs with other biologic therapies may have synergistic effects. TNF is a critical cytokine in many rheumatic diseases, making it likely that the TNF inhibitors will have applications in other diseases as well.

MEDICATIONS FOR GOUT

Medications used in gout can be divided into 2 groups: those used for treating acute gouty arthritis and those used to prevent long-term complications by lowering uric acid blood levels. The first group includes NSAIDs and corticosteroids, which have been discussed already, and colchicine. The second group includes probenecid, sulphinpyrazone, and allopurinol.

Colchicine

Colchicine has been used in plant form for centuries, but it is less often used today because of its toxicities. It inhibits neutrophil function by an effect on microtubules. The traditional regimen for acute gouty arthritis has been a 0.5 or 0.6 mg tablet of colchicine given orally every hour until relief is obtained, intolerable side effects occur, or a maximum dose of 6 mg is reached. Colchicine may also be given on a chronic basis (1 or 2 tablets daily) to prevent gouty arthritis.

Although effective, most patients complain of significant nausea, vomiting, and diarrhea from colchicine. These side effects can be partly overcome by giving the drug intravenously (up to 3 mg), but this route is more likely to produce organ toxicity such as neuropathy, bone marrow depression, renal and liver toxicity, and shock. The maximum dose should be lowered for the elderly and those with renal or hepatic impairment (25).

Probenecid and Sulfinpyrazone

These two drugs are uricosurics, meaning they increase excretion of uric acid in the urine. The dose range is 500–2,000 mg/day for probenecid and 100–800 mg/day for sulfinpyrazone (25). The dose should start at the lower end for both drugs to avoid precipitation of renal stones, and fluid intake should be increased concomitantly. These drugs are ineffective in patients with poor renal function and can be antagonized by even low doses of aspirin. In the early weeks of therapy they may actually increase the risk of gouty arthritis, so a prophylactic antiinflammatory drug should also be prescribed. The drugs are well tolerated, with occasional rashes or GI distress reported.

Allopurinol

Allopurinol lowers formation of uric acid. The usual dose is 300 mg/day; this should be lowered to 100 mg/day in patients with renal impairment. Allopurinol is more versatile than uricosurics because it is effective at all levels of renal function and also in both overproducers and underexcretors of uric acid. However, it inhibits metabolism of many other drugs and can cause rashes, bone marrow depression, and a multi-organ hypersensitivity syndrome involving fever, severe skin reactions, and renal and hepatic failure. Neither allopurinol nor uricosurics should be used in asymptomatic hyperuricemia.

MUSCLE RELAXANTS

Muscle relaxing drugs such as carisoprodol, cyclobenzaprine, methocarbamol, and chlorzoxazone are used to relieve secondary muscle spasm in back pain and other chronic painful conditions. Cyclobenzaprine (Flexeril) is widely used to manage fibromyalgia. Both cyclobenzaprine and a chemically related antidepressant, amitriptyline, have been shown to improve sleep and relieve pain in patients with fibromyalgia (26). Cyclobenzaprine's dose is 10 mg 1–3 times daily, while amitriptyline is used in low doses (10 to 50 mg) at bedtime. Both of these drugs frequently cause drowsiness and anticholinergic side effects such as dry mouth, constipation, confusion, and urine retention.

REFERENCES

1. American College of Rheumatology Ad Hoc Committee on Clinical Guidelines. Guidelines for the management of rheumatoid arthritis. Arthritis Rheum 1996;39:713–22.
2. American College of Rheumatology Subcommittee on Osteoarthritis Guidelines. Recommendations for the medical management of osteoarthritis of the hip and knee: 2000 update. Arthritis Rheum 2000;43:1905–15.
3. McCarthy GM, McCarty DY. Effect of topical capsaicin in the therapy of painful osteoarthritis of the hands. J Rheumatol 1992;19:604–7.
4. McAlindon TE, Lavalley MP, Gulin JP, Felson D. Glucosamine and chondroitin for treatment of osteoarthritis: a systematic quality assessment and analysis. JAMA 2000;283:1469–75.
5. Reginster JY, Deroisy R, Rovati LC, Lee RL, Lejeune E, Bruyere O, et al. Long-term effects of glucosamine sulfate on osteoarthritis progression: a randomized, placebo-controlled trial. Lancet 2001;357:251–6.
6. Lipsky PE, Abramson SB, Crofford L, Dubois RN, Simon LS, van de Putte LB. The classification of cyclooxygenase inhibitors. J Rheumatol 1998;25:2298–303.
7. Silverstein FE, Faich G, Goldstein JL, Simon LS, Pincus T, Whelton A, et al. Gastrointestinal toxicity with celecoxib vs nonsteroidal anti-inflammatory drugs for osteoarthritis and rheumatoid arthritis: the CLASS study. A randomized controlled study. JAMA 2000;284:1247–55.
8. Wolfe MM, Lichtenstein DR, Singh G. Gastrointestinal toxicity of nonsteroidal anti-inflammatory drugs. N Engl J Med 1999;340:1888–99.
9. Brater DC. Effects of nonsteroidal anti-inflammatory drugs on renal function: focus on cyclooxygenase-2-selective inhibition. Am J Med 1999; 107:65s–71s.
10. Brandt KD, Smith GN Jr, Simon LS. Intraarticular injection of hyaluronan as treatment for knee osteoarthritis: what is the evidence? [review]. Arthritis Rheum 2000;43:1192–203.
11. McDougall R, Sibley J, Haga M, Russell A. Outcome in patients with rheumatoid arthritis receiving prednisone compared to matched controls. J Rheumatol 1994;21:1207–13.
12. Weiss MM. Corticosteroids in rheumatoid arthritis. Semin Arthritis Rheum 1989;19:9–21.
13. Saag KG, Koehnke R, Caldwell JR, Brasington R, Burmeister LF, Zimmerman B, et al. Low dose long-term corticosteroid therapy in rheumatoid arthritis: an analysis of serious adverse events. Am J Med 1994;96:115–23.
14. Pincus T, Marcum SB, Callahan LF. Long term drug therapy for rheumatoid arthritis in seven rheumatology private practices. II. Second line drugs and prednisone. J Rheumatol 1992;19:1885–94.
15. Möttönen T, Paimela L, Ahonen J, Helve T, Hannonen P, Leirisalo-Repo M. Outcome in patients with early rheumatoid arthritis treated according to the "sawtooth" strategy. Arthritis Rheum 1996;39:996–1005.
16. Fries JF. ARAMIS and toxicity measurement. J Rheumatol 1995;22: 995–7.
17. Tsakonas E, Fitzgerald AA, Fitzcharles MA, Cividino A, Thorne JC, M'Seffar A, et al. Consequences of delayed therapy with second-line agents in rheumatoid arthritis: a 3 year followup on the hydroxychloroquine in early rheumatoid arthritis study. J Rheumatol 2000;27:623–9.
18. Felson DT, Anderson JJ, Meenan RF. The comparative efficacy and toxicity of second-line drugs in rheumatoid arthritis: results of two meta-analyses. Arthritis Rheum 1990;33:1449–61.
19. Morgan SL, Baggott JE, Vaughn WH, Austin JS, Veitch TA, Lee JY, et al. Supplementation with folic acid during methotrexate therapy for rheumatoid arthritis: a double blind, placebo-controlled trial. Ann Intern Med 1994;121:833–41.
20. Dunn EC, Small RE. Leflunomide: an immunomodulatory agent for the treatment of rheumatoid arthritis. Formulary 1999;34:21–31.
21. Cush JJ, Tugwell P, Weinblatt M, Yocum D. US consensus guidelines for the use of cyclosporin A in rheumatoid arthritis. J Rheumatol 1999;26: 1176–86.
22. O'Dell JR, Haire CE, Palmer W, Drymalski W, Wees S, Blakely K, et al. Treatment of early rheumatoid arthritis with minocycline or placebo: results of a randomized, double-blind, placebo-controlled trial. Arthritis Rheum 1997;40:842–8.
23. Verhoeven AC, Boers M, Tugwell P. Combination therapy in rheumatoid arthritis: updated systematic review. Br J Rheumatol 1998;37:612–9.
24. Fox DA. Cytokine blockade as a new strategy to treat rheumatoid arthritis. Arch Intern Med 2000;160:437–44.
25. Star VL, Hochberg MC. Prevention and management of gout. Drugs 1993;45:212–22.
26. Carette S, Bell MJ, Reynolds WJ, Haraoui B, McCain GA, Bykerk VP, et al. Comparison of amitriptyline, cyclobenzaprine, and placebo in the treatment of fibromyalgia: a randomized, double-blind clinical trial. Arthritis Rheum 1994;37:32–40.

Additional Recommended Reading

American College of Rheumatology Ad Hoc Committee on Clinical Guidelines. Guidelines for monitoring drug therapy in rheumatoid arthritis. Arthritis Rheum 1996;39:723–31.

Drugs for rheumatoid arthritis. Med Lett Drugs Ther 2000;42:57–64.

Kremer JM. Combination therapy with biological agents in rheumatoid arthritis: perils and promise [editorial]. Arthritis Rheum 1998;41:1548–51.

American Geriatrics Society Panel on Chronic Pain in Older Persons. The management of chronic pain in older persons. J Am Geriatr Soc 1998;46: 635–51.

Web Resources

JointAndBone.org. URL: http://www.jointandbone.org [news on rheumatology including drug therapy].

Clinical Pharmacology 2000. URL: http://cp.gsm.com/ [free, updated information on drugs].

Medscape DrugInfo. URL: http://promini.medscape.com/drugdg/search.asp [free, updated information on drugs].

CHAPTER 26

Rest and Exercise

MARIAN A. MINOR, PT, PhD; and MARIE D. WESTBY, BSc, PT

Finding the correct balance of physical activity and rest in the comprehensive management of rheumatic disease is a historic and continuing challenge. The ability of the person with arthritis to effectively combine rest and exercise plays a crucial role in achieving optimal outcomes. Historically, vigorous physical activity—even weight bearing—was proscribed for a person with acute illness, joint pathology, or traumatic injury. Now, however, there is a growing understanding of the deleterious effects of prolonged physical inactivity. Current knowledge of disease etiology, joint physiology, and the effects of various types of exercise provides evidence for more specific recommendations for rest, and more positive recommendations for exercise.

REST

Rest is a key component of rheumatic disease care. It can be divided into 2 types: general (whole body) rest and rest of specific joints. Adequate general rest, including restorative sleep at night, is necessary for health. During periods of active systemic inflammatory disease, additional rest is recommended to offset the fatigue that may be a physiologic consequence of increased inflammatory activity. Rest also protects involved organs and organ systems (cardiovascular, musculoskeletal, pulmonary, and renal) from pathologic stress that may result from strenuous activity. An adequate prescription of general rest should include instructions for time, place, and proper positioning. Rest is not a benign prescription; unnecessary, prolonged inactivity produces illness and leads to disability.

Rest of specific joints often is necessary in both inflammatory conditions and osteoarthritis (OA). The purpose of specific rest is to avoid activity-related injury, provide periods of joint unloading, and encourage maintenance of function and activity in spite of isolated joint swelling or pain. This type of rest includes activity modifications, use of assistive devices and walking aids, and protective or supportive splinting. Limiting particular activities, using alternate movements to avoid repetitive strain, and avoiding certain activities such as stair climbing, lifting, power gripping, or running are examples of activity modifications. Assistive devices such as jar openers and electric can openers can rest particular joints by passing the activity on to another joint. Similarly, walking aids pass some of the weight-bearing load to the arm. Using splints or orthoses may rest joints by providing support during activity, limiting motion, or assuring proper positioning during rest. Complete immobilization is rarely recommended.

During periods of active inflammation, joint structures (including capsules, ligaments, tendons, and cartilage) should be protected. However, rest alone cannot control the ill effects of inflammation. Additional management, including medication, joint aspiration, and injection, is essential to reduce inflammation and swelling quickly. Inflammation of the joint can lead to stretching or rupture of capsule, ligaments, and tendons. Inflamed joints are unstable and vulnerable to activity-related injuries. Neuromuscular response, muscle strength and endurance, and proprioception necessary for joint protection also can be diminished by pain and swelling.

Recommendations for Rest

General Rest. During periods of acute inflammatory disease, at least 8 to 10 hours of sleep at night and 30- to 60-minute morning and afternoon rest periods are recommended. In some systemic diseases such as polymyositis and polymyalgia rheumatica, acute episodes of muscular inflammation and systemic complications may require periods of bed rest. Total body rest should be prescribed for specific durations and at specific times to avoid extreme fatigue or exhaustion.

Night rest should start with relaxing activities (warm bath or shower, gentle range-of-motion or relaxation exercise) early in the evening, to provide adequate time for sleep. A regular sleep and wake schedule should be encouraged. Pain, stiffness, anxiety, and depression that often accompany rheumatic diseases may disrupt sleep patterns and lead to additional problems related to inadequate rest. Therefore, attention to good sleep habits is an important part of comprehensive care and effective self-management (see also Chapter 38, Sleep Disturbance).

Suggestions for posture and positioning during rest include a firm sleeping surface; egg crate, sheepskin or other mattress covers for comfort; a pillow that supports the head and neck without causing neck flexion and forward shoulders; pillows to maintain body alignment if the patient lies on his or her side (supine with hips and knees extended is preferred); and night splints, if needed.

Joint-Specific Rest. Several methods can be used to rest a specific joint or joints during periods of pain or inflammation. Biomechanical stabilization and support is provided by orthoses or splints to decrease motion and/or loading of specific joints. This type of support is usually recommended for specified rest periods or during potentially stressful activities. Examples include functional wrist splints, finger and thumb splints, resting or night splints, rigid foot orthoses to support and stabilize the foot during weight bearing, and shoe modifications or orthoses to eliminate or reduce metatarsal extension.

Joint loading may be controlled by modifying activities with respect to muscular contraction, weight bearing, and impact forces. Suggested modifications may include restricting stair climbing for persons with hip and knee joint involvement; reducing time spent standing; alternating periods of weight bearing with periods of non–weight bearing; or modifying recreational exercise to low-impact or gravity-reduced activities such as swimming, bicycling, or walking.

Repetitive joint motion and loading should be alternated with rest. This can be achieved with a schedule of regular rest

Table 1. Purpose, components, and recommendations for rest.

General rest	Joint-specific rest
Purpose	
Offset disease-related fatigue	Avoid activity-related injury
Protect involved organs from pathologic stress	Unload joint as needed
	Maintain general function/activity levels
Components	
Nighttime sleep	Assistive devices
Daytime rest periods	Orthoses/splinting
Activity modification	
Recommendations	
8–10 hours nighttime sleep	Modify activities to avoid overuse or deforming joint forces
30–60-minute rest periods during day	Provide biomechanical stabilization and support
Use relaxation techniques	
Proper posture, positioning	Control joint loading and weight bearing
Determine specific times and places to rest	
Establish good sleep practices	Alternate rest with dynamic activity

breaks during repetitive activities such as using a keyboard, sewing, playing an instrument, production line work, walking, or sitting. Conversely, regular exercise periods should be scheduled during the day for joints that are being immobilized by a splint or are otherwise inactive.

In addition to following the recommendations for rest, some self-monitoring method should be chosen to assess effectiveness of the rest prescription. Appropriate indicators include reduced joint swelling, less fatigue, less pain, heightened energy level or mood, or less morning stiffness. The rationale, components, and recommendations for rest in rheumatic disease are summarized in Table 1.

EXERCISE

Persons with arthritis demonstrate limited range of motion, decreased muscle strength and endurance, abnormalities in gait and posture, functional limitations, and general deconditioning. Appropriate regular physical activity and exercise can lead to improvement in these areas, as well as reducing pain, fatigue, and depression (1,2).

Physical activity can be defined as any bodily movement produced by skeletal muscle that results in energy expenditure. Regular physical activity is not only necessary for general health; it also reduces the risk for a number of diseases and decreases dysfunction and disability in arthritis. Exercise consists of planned, structured, and repetitive bodily movement done to improve or maintain one or more components of physical fitness. Therapeutic exercise is often prescribed for the person with arthritis to reduce impairment (range of motion/flexibility, muscular function, pain, fatigue) and maintain or improve function (activities of daily living, locomotion, balance). General fitness and cardiovascular health, also dependent on adequate levels of physical activity or exercise, are addressed in Chapter 40, Deconditioning. Recommendations for physical activity to promote general health and for exercise to achieve cardiovascular and muscular fitness (3) appear in Table 2. Although these recommendations were developed for

the general population, many people with arthritis can safely exercise at these levels to improve health and fitness.

The assumption that exercise causes joint damage has been challenged by a number of research reports. It appears that dynamic exercise, both resisted and non-resisted, can improve range of motion, strength, endurance, function, and gait without exacerbation of disease or increased joint symptoms (4–10). Joint immobilization leads to cartilage and periarticular tissue weakening and pathology, whereas regular joint motion and intermittent weight bearing appear to be protective (11). The type of exercise being performed determines the physiologic and metabolic responses. In persons with knee joint effusions, prolonged isometric contraction of the quadriceps and extreme knee flexion can decrease synovial circulation (12), and maximal contraction of gluteal muscles can increase hip joint contact pressure (13). Conversely, dynamic activities such as cycling and walking increase synovial circulation in the knee, even in the presence of effusion (12).

Too often people with arthritis in hip or knee joints are cautioned against all weight-bearing activities such as walking, running, dancing, and stair climbing. Exercise research and evidence of joint loading and intraarticular pressures in normal and diseased joints provide information to guide appropriate exercise and activity recommendations. In addition to aquatic exercise and stationary bicycling, weight-bearing exercises such as walking and low impact aerobic dance can be performed safely by persons with symptomatic joints. Improvements in flexibility, strength, endurance, function, cardiovascular fitness, and general health status have been documented, with no aggravation of symptoms (1,2,4–10). In persons with rheumatoid arthritis (RA), reduction in joint swelling has been reported in aerobic exercise studies (5,8).

Some weight-bearing activities do increase joint loading and probably should be avoided or minimized. Stair descent and ascent, one-legged stance, and carrying loads greater than 10% of body weight may significantly increase loading of the hip

Table 2. Recommendations for health and fitness in the apparently healthy population.*

Physical activity for general health
Mode:	Whole body, repetitive activities
Frequency:	On most days of the week
Intensity:	Moderate; 55–70% age-predicted maximal heart rate; RPE 12–13/2–4
Duration:	30 minutes *accumulation* (three 10-minute bouts)

Exercise training for cardiovascular fitness
Mode:	Rhythmic, aerobic exercise
Frequency:	3–5 days/week
Intensity:	70–85% age-predicted maximal heart rate; RPE 14–16/4–7
Duration:	20–30 minutes continuous

Exercise training for muscular fitness (strength and endurance)
Mode:	Dynamic, resistance exercise for major muscle groups
Frequency:	2–3 days/week on alternate days
Volume:	8–10 exercises; resistance adequate to induce fatigue after 8–12 repetitions; or 10–15 repetitions if over 50–60 years of age or frail

Exercise for musculoskeletal flexibility
Mode:	Gentle stretching; static or PNF technique
Frequency:	2–3 days/week minimum
Intensity:	Stretch to a position of mild tension/discomfort
Duration:	Hold position for 10–30 seconds for static; 6-second contraction followed by 10–30-second assisted stretch for PNF
Repetitions:	3–4 repetitions for each stretch

* RPE = rating of perceived exertion (original scale 6–20, modified scale 0–10); PNF = proprioceptive neuromuscular facilitation (ref. 3).

(13,14), and faster walking speeds and running increase biomechanical stress at the knee (15). Not all people with hip or knee involvement should avoid these activities, but understanding the biomechanical consequences of these actions does provide the basis for rational choices and modifications.

Range of Motion and Flexibility Exercise

Exercise can relieve stiffness, increase or maintain joint motion, and increase length and elasticity in muscle and periarticular tissues. In arthritis, active and active/self-assisted exercise is recommended. During acute joint inflammation, joint motion should be maintained with at least one complete range of motion exercise daily. It is important not to overstretch inflamed tissues, as tensile strength can be reduced by as much as 50%, and tears and overstretching can occur. Application of cold prior to exercise may reduce pain. When joint symptoms are subacute or chronic, goals can include increasing range of motion with gentle, controlled stretching. A warm-up activity such as walking, or the use of moist heat prior to stretching, may be useful.

Active range-of-motion exercise can produce benefits in addition to maintaining flexibility and joint motion. Gentle exercise performed in the evening can significantly reduce morning stiffness for persons with RA (16). An exercise program of active exercise and relaxation (the ROM or Range of Motion Dance program) has shown significant improvements in self-reported function and pain (17). Table 2 contains recommendations for flexibility exercises for the apparently healthy population.

Recommendations for range of motion/flexibility exercise include the following: 1) exercise daily when stiffness and pain are the least; 2) take a warm shower, or apply heat and/or cold prior to or after exercise; 3) perform gentle range-of-motion exercise in the evening to reduce morning stiffness and in the morning to limber up prior to arising; 4) modify exercises (decrease frequency or adapt movement) to avoid increasing joint pain either during or after the exercise; 5) use self-assistive techniques (such as overhead pulleys or wand exercises) to perform gentle stretching; and 6) reduce number of repetitions when joints are actively inflamed.

Muscle Conditioning Exercise

Decreased muscle strength, endurance, and power in persons with arthritis may be due to intraarticular and extraarticular inflammatory disease processes, side effects of medication, disuse, reflex inhibition in response to pain and joint effusion, impaired proprioception leading to decreased protective muscular reflexes, and loss of mechanical integrity around the joint. Muscle conditioning programs can improve strength, endurance, proprioception, and function without exacerbating pain or disease activity (9,10,18,19). Table 3 outlines the purpose and recommendations for isometric and dynamic muscle conditioning exercise for people with arthritis.

Isometric Exercise. Isometric exercise is often suggested prior to or in conjunction with dynamic resistive and aerobic exercise programs. Initially, isometric exercise may be indicated to improve muscle tone, static endurance, and strength, and to prepare joints for more vigorous activity. This type of exercise involves muscle contraction without joint movement.

Table 3. Purpose and recommendations for isometric and dynamic muscle conditioning exercise.*

Isometric	Dynamic
Purpose	
Minimize atrophy	Maintain/increase dynamic strength/endurance
Improve tone	
Maintain/increase static strength/endurance	Increase muscle power
	Improve function
Prepare for dynamic and weight bearing activity	Enhance synovial blood flow
	Promote strength of bone and cartilage
Recommendations	
Perform at functional joint angles	Able to perform 8–10 repetitions against gravity before additional resistance
Breath normally; do not hold breath	
Intensity: ≤ 70% one MVC	
Duration: 6 seconds	Use functional movements
Frequency: 5–10 repetitions daily	Progressive resistance regimen
	Modify ACSM guidelines as needed
Precautions	
Decreased muscle blood flow	May increase biomechanical stress on unstable or malaligned joint
May increase intraarticular pressure	Need for power grip
May increase blood pressure	

* MCV = maximum voluntary contraction; ACSM = American College of Sports Medicine.

Isometric contractions performed at 70% of the maximal voluntary contraction, held for 6 seconds and repeated 5 to 10 times daily, can increase strength significantly. Although isometric exercise avoids the concerns associated with joint motion and mechanical irritation, it can produce other unwanted effects. Isometric exercise at more than 50% maximal voluntary contraction constricts blood flow through the exercising muscle, which can produce unnecessary post-exercise muscle soreness. Also, the increased peripheral vascular resistance produces increased blood pressure. In the knee and hip, high intensity isometric contraction has been shown to increase intraarticular pressure (12,13).

Dynamic Exercise. Dynamic exercise is repetitive muscle contraction and relaxation involving joint motion and changes in muscle length. It includes both shortening (concentric) and lengthening (eccentric) contractions. Dynamic exercise can improve strength and endurance. Resistance (physiologic overload) can be supplied by weight of the body part or external resistance in the form of free weights, elastic bands, or a variety of resistive exercise equipment. An informed and cautious approach to resistance training is recommended to protect unstable or inflamed joints from damage.

Adequate neuromuscular warm up and a cool down with gentle stretching of the exercised muscles enhance safety and comfort. If exercise is painful in the outer range of motion, the exercise should be performed within the pain-free range. Exercise of 8–10 anti-gravity repetitions should be well tolerated before additional resistance is added. Maximum benefit and maintenance are achieved by incorporating functional movements and body positions in the recommended exercise routine. The patient should learn to perform exercises rhythmically with well-controlled movement toward the outer part of the range. Resistance, repetitions, or frequency can be modified as needed.

Gradual progression of resistance and repetitions is recommended. Intensity, frequency, or motion should be reduced if joint swelling or pain occurs. Loads of up to 70% 1 repetition maximum, used in a circuit resistance training program of persons with controlled RA, demonstrated significant improvements in strength and function with no exacerbation in joint symptoms (10). In persons with knee OA, muscular training, including isometric, isotonic, and functional exercises, resulted in improved strength, proprioception, and function, as well as decreased pain (9).

Aerobic Exercise. Regular physical activity improves health for people of all ages and with various chronic conditions. Although arthritis is one of the most common reasons reported for limiting physical activity; a number of well-controlled studies suggest that people with arthritis can safely exercise regularly and vigorously enough to improve cardiovascular fitness and endurance (1,2,4–7,20). The training regimens of these studies generally have incorporated the guidelines for cardiovascular fitness described in Table 2. For individuals who are currently sedentary, the physical activity recommendation for accumulating 30 minutes of moderate activity on most days of the week is an appropriate goal. As activity tolerance and fitness improve, progressing to the more demanding fitness guidelines may become an option.

Aquatic Exercise. Water provides an ideal environment in which to exercise. Pain often decreases while in water due to a number of factors including increased sensory input from the pressure and temperature, muscle relaxation, and decreased joint compression (21). Water can be used to support, assist, or resist movement permitting all types of exercise to be performed. Improvements in joint tenderness, activity level, functional status, grip strength, exercise tolerance, and mood have been shown with aquatic fitness programs (5,8,20). Additional social benefits have been reported with participation in the Arthritis Foundation's Aquatic Program (AFAP). Other forms of exercise in water such as swimming and deep water running may prove beneficial; however, there are no published intervention studies in the arthritis population. A single session of deep water running using a flotation vest resulted in successful achievement of target exercise heart rate with no exacerbation of symptoms in 8 women with RA (22).

Recommendations for aquatic exercise include the following: 1) select a pool with water temperature of 84°F–92°F (29°C–33°C); 2) exercise in sufficiently deep water to minimize joint compression (mid-chest to shoulder level); 3) use nonslip, padded footwear to reduce foot discomfort; 4) choose aquatic exercise programs specifically designed for people with arthritis; and 5) receive instruction in proper technique before starting a swimming or deep water running program.

Implementing an Exercise Program

The most important requirements for the successful design, implementation, and maintenance of an exercise program are to: 1) establish reasonable goals, 2) understand how and when to adapt and modify the exercise program, and 3) monitor for effectiveness.

Establish Reasonable Goals. Reasonable goals emerge when patient and professional collaborate to assess and prioritize needs. For persons with few involved joints, mild disease, and recent onset, this process is fairly straightforward. For the person with multiple joint involvement, fluctuating or severe disease, and functional loss, the decision-making process is more complex. An exercise prescription of reasonable length and complexity, designed to reduce impairments and increase functions important to the patient, will more likely be maintained than a complex, time-consuming program.

Each exercise prescription should include a functional assessment, either by patient self-report or through observed performance, and a determination of joint protection needs. Assessment must extend beyond active disease. For example, joint disease in one knee is often accompanied by decreased range of motion and strength in hip and ankle on the involved side, and in lower extremity joints on the opposite side. Disturbed gait kinetics and kinematics also occur. Hand and wrist pain may easily result in decreased motion and strength in elbows and shoulders and poor head and upper body posture.

Adapt or Modify Program. Self-management skills are essential for exercise maintenance. The person with arthritis must make day-to-day decisions about exercise adaptation and modification. Pain, joint swelling, and fatigue are good markers to use in this decision-making; they are important, well known experiences and they have clinical relevance. Increases in these markers may indicate increased disease activity, overexertion, or aggravation of symptoms from other daily activities. The appropriate response is modification of current exercise until the problem subsides or additional treatment is undertaken. The person with arthritis should be encouraged to readily discuss changes in pain, swelling, or fatigue with a knowledgeable health care provider.

Monitor Effectiveness. Both the health care provider and the person with arthritis need to monitor program success. Effectiveness can be evaluated with measures of disease activity such as joint swelling or stiffness; measures of impairment such as range of motion, strength, endurance, pain, or fatigue; or functional assessments such as gait, activities of daily living, or depression. An exercise program may also affect physical activity levels, occupational performance, or social factors. When the exercise recommendation is based on clear goals that are important to both health professional and patient, and the program is designed to achieve those goals, the choice of evaluation tools is relatively simple. When and how often to evaluate are important considerations that should be based on a determination of when changes can be expected.

Simple self-tests can be used to show improvements in strength, endurance, range of motion, or function. For example, a meaningful self-test in an exercise program to increase shoulder motion could be to periodically mark vertical reach on a wall or attempt to reach an object placed on a higher shelf. If increased ankle motion is an exercise goal, the patient could measure ankle dorsiflexion by the thickness of books that can be accommodated under the forefoot while the heel remains on the floor. Self-tests provide evidence of progress and success to the exerciser. Therefore, the test chosen should show meaningful improvement. For example, a program to increase walking endurance could include a choice of "measures of success" such as a greater distance walked, less exertion, or less time required to walk the original distance.

PAIN AND EXERCISE

Pain can be assessed in several ways: 1) as a general experience; 2) with respect to performance of a specific physical activity; or 3) by the impact of pain on performance of daily activities. The apparent effect of exercise on arthritis-related pain depends on the questions used to assess pain. Research in exercise and arthritis has shown inconsistent results when general pain is measured. Conversely, exercise studies that assessed pain related to specific activities reported significant reductions in pain. A study of exercise in RA compared outcomes for persons instructed to use pain as an exercise guide and others who were instructed to set exercise goals and not consider pain. This study found that the goal-setting group increased exercise performance and reported less pain than the group who used pain as an exercise guide (19). A consistent finding in exercise research is the improvement in function and physical activity levels without increased pain or arthritis symptoms. Thus, it is not necessary to include pain reduction as an exercise objective or expectation; however, it is often an added benefit.

Of all the physical modalities, exercise appears to be the most consistently effective in reducing arthritis-related pain (23). Pain may indicate tissue damage and should be respected and investigated in the process of prescribing and implementing rest and exercise. However, persons who have previously experienced severe pain or who are depressed or inactive may have a lower threshold for stimuli that are interpreted as pain. In the presence of pain, exercise should be assessed for the pain generated by specific motions or by a musculoskeletal examination for activity-induced injury.

At the beginning of an exercise program, the most common pain reports arise from delayed-onset muscle soreness and overstretching. Fortunately, both situations can be avoided by modifying subsequent exercise sessions. Overuse of a joint may be accompanied by swelling, heat, and pain. Immediate treatment consists of ice, elevation, and rest to reduce the swelling; modification of the exercise regimen to avoid re-injury; and implementation of appropriate exercises to condition the joint. Increased joint pain in weight-bearing joints most often follows prolonged standing, fast walking, or walking on uneven ground. Planned periods of non–weight bearing, slower walking speeds, use of shock absorbing footwear, and walking on level surfaces can minimize or eliminate this type of pain.

JOINT PROTECTION AND EXERCISE

Exercise plays an important role in joint protection. Joints can be injured by inflammatory activity, biomechanical stress, pathologic joint loading, immobilization, increased intraarticular pressure, and diminished blood flow. Regular dynamic exercise is associated with improved blood flow (12) and cartilage health, as well as improved range of motion and increased strength and endurance of surrounding muscles. Strong and fatigue-resistant muscle can provide shock attenuation of impact forces crossing a joint. Weak, easily fatigued muscle cannot provide joint stability or control. An intact neuromuscular mechanism is the most important component of shock attenuation and is vital to adequate proprioception. Exercise can protect joints by conditioning muscles surrounding the joint to improve stability, strength, endurance, and power during functional activities. In addition, exercise helps maintain adequate flexibility to allow pain-free, active range of motion and joint alignment.

Joint protection principles must be followed while exercising. For example, joint loading should be alternated with periods of unloading; and activities and equipment should be

Table 4. Guidelines for minimizing biomechanical stresses during exercise.*

- Determine the minimal joint ROM values needed to safely and correctly perform the activity.
- Select activities that involve only a single plane of motion when joint instability is present.
- Change planes of motion (direction) in a slow or controlled manner or ensure the individual has adequate joint stability (static and dynamic), proprioception, and muscular strength to reduce the risk of injury.
- Select activities with minimal joint compression, rotary, and shearing forces.
- Avoid activities that load or generate resistance rapidly (e.g., running, skipping rope).
- Ensure equipment can be adjusted to accommodate individual's limb lengths and joint restrictions.
- Use joint protection principles while exercising (positioning, alternating activities).
- Use orthoses, splints, and other external devices as prescribed.
- Select activities with a low risk of injury.

*ROM = range of motion.

chosen with knowledge of individual needs and biomechanical factors (Table 4). Biomechanics of the joint are discussed in Chapter 1, Musculoskeletal Systems.

ROLE OF THE HEALTH CARE PROFESSIONAL

Self-efficacy is the degree of confidence a person feels in his or her ability to perform a particular behavior. Higher self-efficacy is associated with willingness to adopt and maintain a behavior. Strategies that foster self-efficacy include successful experience with the behavior, reinterpretation of signs and symptoms associated with the behavior, encounters with others who have been successful with the behavior, and encouragement and persuasion.

Strategies to enhance self-efficacy can be embedded in an

Table 5. Guidelines for evaluating community-based exercise settings.

Physical accessibility
  Proximity to parking or public transportation
  Ability to move easily and safely about within the facility, especially bathrooms and changing areas
Social accessibility
  Attitude and friendliness of staff and members
  Willingness of instructors to listen and respond to members about special needs or modifications
  Ongoing classes of appropriate size, intensity, and activities
Cost
  Possibility of paying only for classes or times attended rather than a prepaid membership fee
  Flexibility in membership policy to allow for times when participation is medically inadvisable
  Able to observe and participate before making a financial commitment
Qualifications of staff/instructors
  Current certification by a professional organization and CPR certification
  Training or experience in teaching exercise for people with arthritis or other special needs
  Demonstrated interest in learning about arthritis and exercise
Equipment
  Adequate choice of aerobic and strengthening equipment
  Strengthening equipment of suitable low resistance/weights
  Able to easily adjust and modify devices
  Able to use recommended joint protection techniques
  Equipment is clean and in good condition

exercise recommendation by prescribing exercise that can be successfully performed and that produces a desired result. In addition, the health care provider should help the exerciser recognize sensations such as faster breathing, warmth, or muscular tension as normal and desirable effects of exercise. Referral to an exercise class in which other persons with arthritis are successful exercisers, and providing an encouraging and supportive environment are additional strategies. Referral to self-management classes is also an effective way to promote skill acquisition. Courses developed by the Stanford University Patient Education Research Center (Arthritis Self-Management Program, Chronic Disease Self-Management Program) are effective in increasing participants' exercise behaviors, function, and quality of life and in decreasing pain, fatigue, and medical costs (24). The Arthritis Foundation and other health care providers offer these programs.

With knowledge and support from health care providers, the person with arthritis can use community-based resources for exercise and physical activity. The advantages of community-based exercise include economy, socialization, self-management, wellness focus, and variety in activities and equipment, participants, and locations. Communication between community-based providers and health care professionals provides positive, successful exercise experiences and continuity for the client. Exercise programs are available through local YMCA organizations, health clubs, hospital-sponsored fitness facilities, community colleges, parks and recreation departments, senior centers, and cooperative programs between the Arthritis Foundation and local groups. Not all community-based programs are appropriate for persons with arthritis. Both the health care provider and the person with arthritis should keep in mind guidelines for evaluating a facility or program in addition to the usual requirements of safety (Table 5).

REFERENCES

1. Van den Ende CHM, Vliet Vlieland TPM, Munneke M, Hazes JMW. Dynamic exercise therapy for rheumatoid arthritis (Cochrane Review). In: The Cochrane Library. Issue 2. Oxford: Update Software; 1999.
2. Minor MA. Exercise in the treatment of osteoarthritis. Rheum Dis Clin North Am 1999;25:387–415.
3. ACSM's guidelines for exercise testing and prescription. 6th ed. Philadephia: Lippincott Williams & Wilkins; 2000.
4. Ettinger WH Jr, Burns R, Messier SP, Applegate W, Rejeski WJ, Morgan T, et al. A randomized trial comparing aerobic exercise and resistance exercise with a health education program in older adults with knee osteoarthritis. JAMA 1997;277:25–31.
5. Minor MA, Hewett JE, Webel RR, Anderson SK, Kay DR. Efficacy of physical conditioning exercise in patients with rheumatoid arthritis and osteoarthritis. Arthritis Rheum 1989;32:1396–405.
6. Noreau L, Martineau H, Roy L, Belzile M. Effects of modified dance-based exercise on cardiorespiratory fitness, psychological state and health status of persons with rheumatoid arthritis. Am J Phys Med Rehabil 1995;74:19–27.
7. Westby MD, Wade JP, Rangno KK, Berkowitz J. A randomized controlled trial to evaluate the effectiveness of an exercise program in women with rheumatoid arthritis taking low dose prednisone. J Rheumatol 2000;27:1674–80.
8. Sanford-Smith M, MacKay-Lyons M, Nunes-Clement S. Therapeutic benefit of aquaerobics for individuals with rheumatoid arthritis. Physiother Can 1998;50:40–6.
9. Hurley MV, Scott DL. Improvements in quadriceps sensorimotor function and disability of patients with knee osteoarthritis following a clinically practicable exercise regime. Br J Rheumatol 1998;37:1181–7.
10. Rall LC, Meydani SN, Kehayias JJ, Dawson-Hughes B, Roubenoff R. The effect of progressive resistance training in rheumatoid arthritis: increased strength without changes in energy balance or body composition. Arthritis Rheum 1996;39:415–26.
11. Houlbrooke K, Vause K, Merrilees MJ. Effects of movement and weight-bearing on the glycosaminoglycan content of sheep articular cartilage. Aust J Physiother 1990;36:88–91.
12. James MJ, Cleland LG, Gaffney RD, Proudman SM, Chatterton BE. Effect of exercise on 99Tc-DTPA clearance from knees with effusions. J Rheumatol 1994;21:501–4.
13. Krebs DE, Elbaurn L, O'Mey P, Hodge WA, Mann RW. Exercise and gait effects on in vivo hip contact pressures. Phys Ther 1990;71:301–9.
14. Neumann DA. Biomechanical analysis of selected principles of hip joint protection. Arthritis Care Res 1989;2:146–55.
15. Schnitzer TJ, Popovich JM, Andersson GBJ, Andriacchi TP. Effect of piroxicam on gait in patients with osteoarthritis of the knee. Arthritis Rheum 1993;36:1207–13.
16. Byers PH. Effect of exercise on morning stiffness and mobility in patients with rheumatoid arthritis. Res Nurs Health 1985;8:275–81.
17. Van Deusen J, Harlowe D. The efficacy of the ROM dance program for adults with rheumatoid arthritis. Am J Occup Ther 1987;41:90–5.
18. Ekdahl C, Andersson SI, Moritz U, Svensson B. Dynamic versus static training in patients with rheumatoid arthritis. Scand J Rheumatol 1990;19:17–26.
19. Stenström CH. Home exercise in rheumatoid arthritis functional class II goal setting versus pain attention. J Rheumatol 1994;21:627–34.
20. Hall J, Skevington SM, Maddison PJ, Chapman K. A randomized controlled trial of hydrotherapy in rheumatoid arthritis. Arthritis Care Res 1996;9:206–15.
21. McNeal RL. Aquatic therapy for patients with rheumatic disease. Rheum Dis Clin North Am 1990;16:915–29.
22. Melton-Rogers S, Hunter G, Walter J, Harrison P. Cardiorespiratory responses of patients with rheumatoid arthritis during bicycle riding and running in water. Phys Ther 1996;76:1058–65.
23. Minor MA, Sanford MK. The role of physical therapy and physical modalities in pain management. Rheum Dis Clin North Am 1999;25:233–47.
24. Superio-Cabuslay E, Ward MM, Lorig KR. Patient education intervention in osteoarthritis and rheumatoid arthritis: a meta-analytic comparison with nonsteroidal drug treatment. Arthritis Care Res 1996;9:292–301.

Additional Recommended Reading

American College of Sports Medicine. Position stands. Accessed March 13, 2001. URL: http://www.acsm.org/positionstands.htm
Coleman EA, Buchner DM, Cress ME, Chan BKS, de Lateur BJ. The relationship of joint symptoms with exercise performance in older adults. J Am Geriatr Soc 1996;44:14–21.
Exercise and arthritis [special issue]. Arthritis Care Res 1994;7(4).
Feigenbaum MS, Pollock ML. Prescription of resistance training for health and disease. Med Sci Sports Exerc 1999;31:38–45.
Felson DT, Lawrence RC, Hochberg MC, McAlindon T, Dieppe PA, Minor MA, et al. Osteoarthritis: new insight. Part 2. Treatment approaches. Ann Intern Med 2000;133:726–37.
U.S. Department of Health and Human Services. Physical activity and health: a report of the Surgeon General, 1996. Accessed March 13, 2001. URL: http://www.cdc.gov/nccdphp/sgr/sgr.htm
Van Baar ME, Assendelft WJJ, Dekker J, Oostendorp RAB, Bijlsma JWJ. Effectiveness of exercise therapy in patients with osteoarthritis of the hip or knee: a systematic review of randomized clinical trials. Arthritis Rheum 1999;42:1361–9.

Physical Modalities

CHAPTER 27

KAREN W. HAYES, PhD, PT

Physical modalities of heat, cold, and electricity are often used to alleviate the symptoms of rheumatic disease. While no modality is capable of curing arthritis, amelioration of symptoms may lead to improved function. Overall function depends on freedom from impairments such as weakness, limitation of motion, and pain. Specific treatment goals may include decreasing pain, increasing flexibility, and decreasing swelling. Heat, cold, and electrical stimulation are commonly used to produce improvement in these impairments.

SUPERFICIAL AND DEEP HEAT

Superficial and deep heat are used primarily to decrease pain and improve flexibility. Heat contributes to pain relief by increasing the pain threshold, increasing blood flow, and washing out pain-producing metabolites. Heat also decreases muscle guarding through its effects on the muscle spindle and Golgi tendon organs (1). Ultrasound, a deep heat produced by the conversion of sound waves into heat, was once thought to produce preferential slowing of nerve conduction in small sensory fibers. However, more recent evidence has shown that sensory conduction usually increases after heating (2). An effect on nerve conduction is therefore unlikely to explain the action of ultrasound in reducing pain.

Heat may improve flexibility by reducing pain or by increasing the extensibility of connective tissue (3). Thus, the use of heat allows collagen to deform more readily, leading to increased range of motion if combined with low-load, prolonged stretch (4).

Application of Superficial Heat

Superficial heat can be applied by using hot packs, paraffin wax baths, Fluidotherapy (a bath of small solid particles suspended in a stream of warmed air), infrared radiation (heat lamps), or hydrotherapy. Regardless of the source, superficial heat is in the infrared portion of the electromagnetic spectrum; thus, it penetrates the skin only a few millimeters. Superficial heat should be applied for about 20 minutes to elevate skin temperature and activate optimal heat loss responses by the body. Physiologic effects occur through these reflex vascular and neural responses.

Superficial heat is convenient and safe for home use if patients have received proper instruction on its use. Instructions should include the purpose of the treatment; the method of application; the duration, intensity, and frequency of the application; precautions for use; and a telephone number for the patient to contact a professional practitioner with questions and concerns. The practitioner should demonstrate the treatment and watch the patient perform it to ensure proper administration.

Application of Deep Heat

Deep heat is provided through short-wave diathermy and ultrasound. Like superficial heat, deep heat elevates temperature, but it reaches deeper tissues such as muscle and connective tissue. Short-wave diathermy is usually applied for 20 minutes to fairly large areas of the body. Ultrasound, on the other hand, may be focused on very small areas and is applied for shorter periods of time (3–10 minutes). The heat from short-wave diathermy and ultrasound is produced by conversion of electrical or sound energy into heat energy below the level of the skin heat receptors. Consequently, people perceive the heat from deep heat sources to be much milder. Because of the mechanisms of heat production and the milder but deceptive heat perception, deep heat sources can be hazardous. With short-wave diathermy, any condition that concentrates the electric field, such as metal or perspiration, can produce a burn. Ultrasound, if focused too long at a particular site, can also produce burning. Deep heat should be used under the supervision of a physical therapist. Sources for providing deep heat usually are not portable, and they are too expensive and dangerous for home use.

Contraindications and Precautions

Heat applications to large areas of the body, producing systemic heat loss responses, are contraindicated for people with conditions that prevent adequate thermoregulatory responses (such as cardiac insufficiency or impaired peripheral circulation). They are also contraindicated in conditions that could be aggravated or spread, such as swelling, fever, infection, hemorrhage, or malignancy (1). Local heat applications to small areas may be used safely in stable cardiac conditions or when applied to areas of the body at a distance from areas of swelling, infection, hemorrhage, and malignancy. Because the amount of heat applied depends on the patient's perception, it should not be used with people who have impaired sensation, judgment, or cognition.

In addition to these contraindications, there are several precautions associated with the use of heat in persons with acute, inflammatory arthritis. Heat may increase inflammation, thus increasing edema of the synovial membrane (5). Increasing the intraarticular temperature could damage joint surfaces due to increased activity of collagenolytic enzymes (6). It was previously thought that short applications of superficial heat (less than 10 minutes) cooled the joint and that superficial cooling warmed the joint (7). However, new evidence shows that both joint and skin temperature elevate following superficial heating, especially with treatment times more like those used in clinical practice (e.g., 20 minutes) (8,9). Short-wave diathermy also heats the interior of the joint along with the skin, although not as much as superficial heat (8).

There is no clinical evidence that heat affects progression of rheumatoid arthritis (RA) as evidenced by elevations in erythrocyte sedimentation rate (10), white blood cell count and phagocytosis (11), and radiography (12), but the use of heat for people with acute inflammatory arthritis is best avoided. People with RA often have unstable vascular reactions in response to heat. They may vasodilate more slowly, causing them to retain heat (13). People with vasculitis associated with RA also may have impaired vasomotor heat loss responses (14). When heat is used in people with RA, therefore, they should be monitored carefully for susceptibility to heat stress.

Effectiveness

Some investigators have shown that superficial heat can decrease pain and increase range of movement (15–17), but others have found that superficial heat is not effective (10,18). When superficial heat combined with exercises is compared with exercises alone, heat produces no greater effect than produced by the exercises alone (15,19).

Many patients report global improvement following superficial heat treatments, despite lack of clinical evidence for improvement (17). If the appropriate contraindications or precautions are observed, patients who feel better or are more inclined to be active following heat treatments should be encouraged to use them. There is little danger or cost associated with superficial heat and no apparent negative effects.

Deep heat appears to be capable of increasing range, decreasing pain (20), and decreasing functional incapacity, especially in younger patients and those with less severe disease (21). On the other hand, some investigators have found that deep heat is not effective (22,23), and when combined with exercises, deep heat appears to be no more effective than exercise alone (18,24,25). In one study, the only people whose symptoms worsened were those who received short-wave diathermy (25).

Patients who receive deep heat treatment have been shown to perceive a more satisfactory outcome than those who receive placebo treatments, even when they have persistent disability (20). However, deep heat must be applied in a clinical setting. Such treatments are expensive and may be harmful. When exercise or superficial heat can accomplish the same goals, there is little rationale for using deep heat.

COLD

The primary reasons for using cold applications are to decrease pain, swelling, and inflammation. Pain is decreased by slowing or blocking nerve conduction, decreasing activity of the muscle spindle (1), or releasing endorphins (16). Swelling is decreased through vasoconstriction, which decreases blood flow and capillary pressure. Gentle cold also blocks histamine release, decreasing inflammation. The intraarticular temperature decreases as skin temperature decreases (8), perhaps reducing collagenolytic enzyme activity and inflammation in the joint.

Application

Cold is applied to the skin through ice or cold packs, ice massage, cold baths, or vapocoolant sprays. It is usually applied for 10–30 minutes, depending on the intensity of the cold source and the depth of the tissue to be reached. Deeper tissues require longer treatment times. Milder cold sources are more appropriate for swelling; very cold sources, capable of producing skin anesthesia, are more appropriate for pain reduction. Care should be taken not to frost the skin. As when using superficial heat, cold treatments can be used at home with proper instruction.

Contraindications and Precautions

Contraindications are essentially the same as those for heat. People must have sufficient vasoconstriction capabilities to conserve heat. In addition, because cold causes vasoconstriction, its use may delay healing.

As with the use of heat, several precautions must be taken when using cold treatments. Cold produces stiffness in connective tissues in laboratory studies (3), but that stiffness does not necessarily manifest clinically in decreased range of motion. Nonetheless, caution must be exercised to move cooled joints more slowly. Force generation also may be affected by cold treatments. After using a cold treatment that is sufficient to cool the motor neurons and block nerve conduction, entire motor units may temporarily cease to function, with resulting weakness.

Some people are hypersensitive to cold; others actually exhibit cold allergy manifested as urticaria. People with RA have been shown to experience increased pain with cold exposure (26), especially if they smoke (27). Patients with RA have more vasomotor instability and get colder and stiffer in response to cold exposure. They also have been shown to cool and rewarm more slowly (13). Raynaud's phenomenon, a condition aggravated by cold exposure, is associated with a history of joint pain (28) and systemic sclerosis (29).

Effectiveness

Cold treatments can be effective in decreasing pain, improving function, and decreasing stiffness (16,17,30). The effect of cold on swelling in arthritis patients has not been extensively studied, but one study showed that postsurgical hand volume and pain did not change following cold treatments (31). The small sample in this study may have prevented the observed decreased pain and hand volume from being statistically significant.

Heat and cold appear to be about equally effective for managing pain, stiffness, and limitation of motion (16,17). Cold has been shown to produce earlier decreases in pain and stiffness than short-wave diathermy or placebo treatments (30). Heat appears to be better for improving motion, while cold may be better for reducing pain (17).

TRANSCUTANEOUS ELECTRICAL NERVE STIMULATION

Treatment with transcutaneous electrical nerve stimulation (TENS) may decrease pain and inflammation. Stiffness may decrease as well (32,33). The use of TENS was originally based on the gate control theory advanced by Melzack and Wall (34). Stimulation of the large sensory fibers is thought to prevent impulses from the smaller pain fibers from being transmitted in the ascending tracks in the spinal cord. Theoretically, impulses from C fibers are blocked better than impulses from other fiber types. Because C fibers innervate the synovium and joint capsule, TENS could prove useful in the treatment of arthritis (32). In addition, other forms of TENS have been shown to cause the release of endogenous opioids in the midbrain (35).

Use of TENS has been shown to raise intraarticular temperature about 0.5° C in rabbits after a 5-minute treatment, but it also decreased inflammatory exudate and joint pressure and volume (36). The decreased inflammation and joint volume may help relieve pain in inflammatory arthritis.

Application

There are several modes of TENS, but the 3 most common are high frequency TENS, low frequency or acupuncture-like TENS, and burst mode TENS. High frequency TENS stimulates only the sensory nerve endings, using a continuous train of 100 μsec pulses in a frequency range of 70−100 Hz. The usual electrode placement for people with arthritis is around the involved joint (32,37−42). High frequency TENS is often used for several hours, depending on the pain relief achieved. Pain relief, if it occurs, has a rapid onset.

Low frequency TENS stimulates the motor endplates of muscles using wider, 250 μsec pulses at a frequency of 1−3 Hz. This mode causes the release of endorphins, which theoretically produces longer lasting pain relief. Electrodes are placed over motor points of muscles in the myotome related to the painful joint.

Burst mode TENS combines elements of both the high and low frequency modes. In burst mode, the carrier frequency of the current is high (70−100 Hz), but it is delivered in small "bursts" at a low rate (3–4 bursts per second). Burst mode also uses motor level stimulation with electrode placements similar to those used with low frequency TENS. This method produces longer lasting pain relief, apparently through the same mechanisms as low frequency TENS (43). The advantage of burst mode is the greater comfort of the current, as compared with low frequency TENS. Low frequency and burst mode TENS are usually applied for about 30 minutes.

Contraindications and Precautions

People with cardiac pacing problems or who use pacemakers should not use TENS near the heart. Electrodes should not be placed over the carotid sinus or the laryngeal or pharyngeal muscles (43). In addition, TENS should not be used during the first trimester of pregnancy, because the effect on the fetus is unknown.

As with the other modalities, there are precautions associated with the use of TENS. Persons using TENS should use the joint carefully while being treated. Some people receiving TENS treatments find them uncomfortable. Discomfort may arise from skin irritation from the electrode couplant or adhesion system as much as from the electricity itself.

In a case report, one patient with RA reportedly developed paresthesias and increased pain following heat and TENS. These effects were delayed, so patients should be monitored closely by a qualified therapist (44).

Effectiveness

Pain relief from TENS has been found to range from 50–90% (32,38−40,45). In some studies, pain relief is significantly greater than relief achieved from placebo treatments (37,38,41,42), while in others, both placebo and actual treatments produce similar amounts of relief (41,45−47). The usual amount of pain relief attributed to placebo in studies with patients having RA or OA is about 30−40%. Pain relief beyond that may be attributed to the TENS treatment (48).

In people with rheumatic disease, pain relief from high frequency and burst mode TENS has been shown to last from 2.5 hours (38) to 18 hours (39), although patients in 2 studies remained improved for several days (40) or weeks (45) following termination of treatment. The duration of pain relief from low frequency TENS has not been studied extensively, but in one study, pain relief lasted 4 hours (39).

There is little evidence to favor one mode of TENS over another for patients with rheumatic disease. All 3 modes have been shown to be effective in some studies, with no one mode more effective than another (41,47). Other studies have shown that high frequency and burst modes produce more and longer lasting pain relief compared with low frequency TENS (39,41). In a comparison of burst mode TENS with high frequency and placebo TENS in persons with osteoarthritis (OA), neither mode produced more pain relief than placebo, but the burst mode produced longer pain relief than placebo. High frequency TENS decreased stiffness better than placebo, and both modes produced longer stiffness relief than placebo. High frequency TENS reduced knee circumference better than burst mode, and burst mode was better than placebo for increasing range of motion (33).

In comparing TENS with other treatments, pain relief produced by TENS has been shown to be longer lasting than that produced by medications (38). On the other hand, a nonsteroidal antiinflammatory medication was shown to be superior to TENS for patients with OA of the knee (46), although less than optimal electrode placements were used in the study, and it had a very small sample. In people with OA of the hip, electrical stimulation alone decreased pain as well as ultrasound, shortwave diathermy, or ibuprofen did (25). Appropriate use of TENS could decrease the need for pharmacologic interventions and would be superior to deep heat, which requires clinic-based application.

Overall, TENS appears to be useful for decreasing pain and stiffness, and the symptomatic relief may last longer than relief produced by other treatments. The mode should be selected based on the desired goal. Either high frequency or burst mode will provide long lasting relief from pain, but high frequency might be selected if the goal is also to decrease stiffness. Low frequency TENS does not appear to be useful for patients with arthritis. Because TENS is controlled by the patient, it is a good tool for home use when people are properly instructed and monitored.

SUMMARY

The therapeutic goals for people with arthritis include decreased pain, stiffness and swelling. Superficial heat is helpful in achieving these goals, but may not be necessary if patients exercise appropriately. However, if patients who do not have acutely inflamed joints feel better after using superficial heat treatments, there appears to be no reason not to use them. Deep heat is costly, potentially hazardous, and requires clinic visits. Because other, safer means such as exercise can meet these goals without aggravating symptoms (especially in inflammatory arthritis), there is little reason to use deep heat in patients with arthritis.

In addition to the goals of symptomatic relief, it may be desirable to decrease the destructive inflammatory process for patients with inflammatory arthritis by cooling the joint. Cold treatments also promote improvement in pain, motion, and swelling. Cold treatments are not often considered for patients with arthritis, and patients may prefer heat, even when their symptoms are relieved better with cold (16,17). Patients should be encouraged to try cold treatments, especially when joints are acutely inflamed.

Use of TENS is effective for decreasing pain and stiffness without the potential hazard to joint surfaces. The high frequency and burst modes appear to work best for patients with arthritis. Patient improvement may be longer lasting, and patients may be able to decrease medication use.

Appropriate professional supervision and instruction must accompany the use of any of the physical modalities with patients having rheumatic diseases. Any of these modalities can produce harm if improperly applied. Education by a knowledgeable professional is crucial for correct and safe application.

REFERENCES

1. Lehmann JF, DeLateur BJ. Therapeutic heat. In: Lehmann JF, editor. Therapeutic heat and cold. 3rd ed. Baltimore: Williams and Wilkins; 1982. p. 404–562.
2. Currier DP, Kramer JF. Sensory nerve conduction: Heating effects of ultrasound and infrared. Physiother Can 1982;34:241–6.
3. Wright V, Johns RJ. Quantitative and qualitative analysis of joint stiffness in normal subjects and in patients with connective tissue diseases. Ann Rheum Dis 1961;20:36–46.
4. Lentell G, Hetherington T, Eagan J, Morgan M. The use of thermal agents to influence the effectiveness of a low-load prolonged stretch. J Orthop Sports Phys Ther 1992;16:200–7.
5. Weinberger A, Fadilah R, Lev A, Levi A, Pinkhas J. Deep heat in the treatment of inflammatory joint disease. Med Hypotheses 1988;25: 231–3.
6. Harris ED, McCroskery PA: The influence of temperature and fibril stability on degradation of cartilage collagen by rheumatoid synovial collagenase. N Engl J Med 1974;290:1–6.
7. Hollander JL, Horvath SM: The influence of physical therapy procedures on the intraarticular temperature of normal and arthritic subjects. Am J Med Sci 1949;218: 543–8.
8. Oosterveld FG, Rasker JJ, Jacobs JW, Overmars HJ: The effect of local heat and cold therapy on the intraarticular and skin surface temperature of the knee. Arthritis Rheum 1992;35:146–51.
9. Weinberger A, Fadilah R, Lev A, Pinkhas J: Intra-articular temperature measurements after superficial heating. Scand J Rehabil Med 1989;21: 55–7.
10. Harris R, Millard JB. Paraffin-wax baths in the treatment of rheumatoid arthritis. Ann Rheum Dis 1955;14:278–82.
11. Dorwart BB, Hansell JR, Schumacher HR: Effects of cold and heat on urate crystal-induced synovitis in the dog. Arthritis Rheum 1974;17: 563–71.
12. Mainardi CL, Walter JM, Spiegel PK, Goldkamp OG, Harris ED. Rheumatoid arthritis: Failure of daily heat therapy to affect its progression. Arch Phys Med Rehabil 1979;60:390–3.
13. Martin GM, Roth GM, Elkins EC, Krusen FH. Cutaneous temperature of the extremities of normal subjects and of patients with rheumatoid arthritis. Arch Phys Med 1946;27:665–82.
14. Dyck PJ, Conn DL, Okazaki H. Necrotizing angiopathic neuropathy: Three-dimensional morphology of fiber degeneration related to sites of occluded vessels. Mayo Clin Proc 1972;47:461–75.
15. Green J, McKenna F, Redfern EJ, Chamberlain MA. Home exercises are as effective as outpatient hydrotherapy for osteoarthritis of the hip. Br J Rheumatol 1993;32:812–5.
16. Utsinger PD, Bonner F, Hogan N. The efficacy of cryotherapy (CR) and thermotherapy in the management of rheumatoid arthritis (RA) pain: Evidence for an endorphin effect (Abstract). Arthritis Rheum 1982;25:S113.
17. Williams J, Harvey J, Tannenbaum H. Use of superficial heat versus ice for the rheumatoid arthritic shoulder: A pilot study. Physiother Can 1986;38:8–13.
18. Hamilton DE, Bywaters EGL, Please NW. A controlled trial of various forms of physiotherapy in arthritis. Br Med J 1959;1:542–4.
19. Hecht PJ, Bachmann S, Booth RE, Rothman RH. Effects of thermal therapy on rehabilitation after total knee arthroplasty. Clin Orthop 1983;178:198–201.
20. Konrad K. Randomized, double blind, placebo-controlled study of ultrasonic treatment of the hands of rheumatoid arthritis patients. Eur J Phys Med Rehabil 1994;4:155–7.
21. Jan M, Lai J. The effects of physiotherapy on osteoarthritic knees of females. J Formos Med Assoc 1991;90:1008–13.
22. Hashish I, Harvey W, Harris M. Anti-inflammatory effects of ultrasound therapy: Evidence for a major placebo effect. Br J Rheumatol 1986;25:77–81.
23. Mueller EE, Mead S, Schulz BF, Vaden MR. A placebo-controlled study of ultrasound treatment for periarthritis. Am J Phys Med 1954; 33:31–5.
24. Falconer J, Hayes KW, Chang RW. Effect of ultrasound on mobility in osteoarthritis of the knee: A randomized clinical trial. Arthritis Care Res 1992;5:29–35.
25. Svarcová J, Trnavský K, Zvárová J: The influence of ultrasound, galvanic currents and shortwave diathermy on pain intensity in patients with osteoarthritis. Scand J Rheumatol Suppl 1988;67:83–5
26. Jahanshahi M, Pitt P, Williams I. Pain avoidance in rheumatoid arthritis. J Psychosom Res 1989;33:579–89.
27. Helliwell P, Wallace F, Evard F. Smoking and ice therapy in rheumatoid arthritis. Physiotherapy 1989;75:551–2.
28. Leppert J, Åberg H, Ringqvist I, Sörensson S. Raynaud's phenomenon in a female population: Prevalence and association with other conditions. Angiology 1987;38:871–7.
29. Medsger TA, Steen V. Systemic sclerosis and related syndromes: B. Clinical features and treatment. In: Schumacher HR, Klippel JH, Koopman, WJ. editors. Primer on the rheumatic diseases. 10th ed. Atlanta: Arthritis Foundation; 1993. p. 120–7.
30. Clarke GR., Willis LA, Stenner L, Nichols PJR. Evaluation of physiotherapy in the treatment of osteoarthrosis of the knee. Rheumatology and Rehabilitation 1974;13:190–7.
31. Rembe EC. Use of cryotherapy on the postsurgical rheumatoid hand. Phys Ther 1970;50:19–23.
32. Kumar VN, Redford JB. Transcutaneous nerve stimulation in rheumatoid arthritis. Arch Phys Med Rehabil 1982;63:595–6.
33. Grimmer K. A controlled double blind study comparing the effects of strong burst mode TENS and high rate TENS on painful osteoarthritic knees. Australian Journal of Physiotherapy 1992;38:49–56.
34. Melzack R, Wall PD. Pain mechanisms: a new theory. Science 1965; 150:971–9,
35. Sjolund BH, Eriksson MBE. Endorphins and analgesia produced by peripheral conditioning stimulation. In: Bonica JJ, Liebeskind J, Albe-Fessard DG, editors. Advances in pain research and therapy, vol. 3. New York: Raven Press; 1979. p. 587–92,
36. Levy A, Dalith M, Abramovici A, Pinkhas J, Weinberger A. Transcutaneous electrical nerve stimulation in experimental acute arthritis. Arch Phys Med Rehabil 1987;68:75–8.
37. Abelson K, Langley GB, Sheppeard H, Wigley RD. Transcutaneous electrical nerve stimulation in rheumatoid arthritis. N Z Med J 1983; 96:156–8.
38. Lewis D, Lewis B, Sturrock RD. Transcutaneous electrical nerve stimulation in osteoarthrosis: a therapeutic alternative? Ann Rheum Dis 1984;43:47–9.
39. Mannheimer C, Carlsson CA. The analgesic effect of transcutaneous electrical nerve stimulation (TNS) in patients with rheumatoid arthritis. A comparative study of different pulse patterns. Pain 1979;6:329–34.
40. Mannheimer C, Lund S, Carlsson CA. The effect of transcutaneous electrical nerve stimulation (TNS) on joint pain in patients with rheumatoid arthritis. Scand J Rheumatol 1978;7:13–6.

41. Møystad A, Krogstad BS, Larheim TA. Transcutaneous nerve stimulation in a group of patients with rheumatic disease involving the temporomandibular joint. J Prosthet Dent 1990;64:596–600.

42. Zizic TM, Hoffman KC, Holt PA, Hungerford DS, O'Dell JR, Jacobs MA, et al. The treatment of osteoarthritis of the knee with pulsed electrical stimulation. J Rheumatol 1995;22:1757–61.

43. Foley RA. Transcutaneous electrical nerve stimulation. In: Hayes KW, editor. Manual for physical agents. 5th ed. Saddle River, NJ: Prentice Hall; 2000. p. 121–47.

44. Griffin JW, McClure M. Adverse responses to transcutaneous electrical nerve stimulation in a patient with rheumatoid arthritis. Phys Ther 1981;61:354–5.

45. Smith CR, Lewith GT, Machin D. Preliminary study to establish a controlled method of assessing transcutaneous nerve stimulation as a treatment for the pain caused by osteo-arthritis of the knee. Physiotherapy 1983;69:266–8.

46. Lewis B, Lewis D, Cumming G. The comparative analgesic efficacy of transcutaneous electrical nerve stimulation and a non-steroidal anti-inflammatory drug for painful osteoarthritis. Br J Rheumatol 1994;33:455–60.

47. Langley GB, Sheppeard H, Johnson M, Wigley RD. The analgesic effects of transcutaneous electrical nerve stimulation and placebo in chronic pain patients. Rheumatol Int 1984;4:119–23.

48. Fields HL, Levine, JD. Placebo analgesia- A role for endorphins? Trends Neurosci 1984;7:271–3.

Additional Recommended Reading

Aubin M, Marks R. The efficacy of short-term treatment with transcutaneous electrical nerve stimulation for osteo-arthritic knee pain. Physiotherapy 1995;81:669–75.

Amundson H. Thermotherapy and cryotherapy - effects on joint degeneration in rheumatoid arthritis. Physiother Can 1979;31:258–62.

Bruce JR, Riggin CS, Parker JC, Walker SE, Meyer AA, Wellman FE, et al. Pain management in rheumatoid arthritis: Cognitive behavior modification and transcutaneous neural stimulation. Arthritis Care Res 1988;1:78–84.

Hayes KW. Heat and cold in the management of rheumatoid arthritis. Arthritis Care Res 1993;6:156–66.

Marks R, Cantin D. Symptomatic osteo-arthritis of the knee: the efficacy of physiotherapy. Physiotherapy 1997;83:306–12.

Minor MA, Sanford MK. Physical interventions in the management of pain in arthritis: An overview for research and practice. Arthritis Care Res 1993;6: 197–206.

Nicholas JJ. Physical modalities in rheumatological rehabilitation. Arch Phys Med Rehabil 1994;75:994–1001.

Robinson AJ. Transcutaneous electrical nerve stimulation for the control of pain in musculoskeletal disorders. J Orthop Sports Phys Ther 1996;24:208–26.

Shafshak TS, El-Sheshai AM, Soltan HE. Personality traits in the mechanisms of interferential therapy for osteoarthritic knee pain. Arch Phys Med Rehabil 1991;72:579–81.

Simpson CF. Adult arthritis: Heat, cold, or both? Am J Nurs 1983;83:270–73.

CHAPTER 28

Splinting of the Hand

PAMELA B. HARRELL, OTR, CHT

Splints have been used throughout history to protect, immobilize, or mobilize various parts of the body. A splint may be defined as "a rigid or flexible appliance used for the prevention of movement of a joint or for the fixation of displaced or moveable parts." In current practice, splints are used to maintain and enhance motion, as well as to prevent it. Splints serve various purposes in the management of the hand with rheumatic disease; however, controversy exists over the roles and benefits of splinting. Studies have supported the use of splints to reduce pain and inflammation, but further studies are indicated to determine the outcome of splinting to prevent and correct deformity. Although indications for and use of splints vary widely among practitioners, most agree that splinting plays an important role in the overall management of rheumatic disease.

The use of splints should be based on knowledge of rheumatic disease, mechanisms of joint inflammation, and pathomechanics of joint deformity. The type of arthritis and stage of joint involvement should influence the treatment program, which may include splinting. How the joint has been affected by arthritis, and more importantly, how joint involvement has affected the person's ability to function should also be considered.

EVALUATION

A complete evaluation is necessary prior to establishing goals for a splinting program. An evaluation should include the following components.

Interview and Subjective Assessment. Obtain a clear history of the disease, including duration, medical management, functional performance, and effect of the arthritis on a person's lifestyle. Subjective assessment of pain, stiffness, and fatigue should include such information as intensity, duration, and activities that increase or decrease symptoms.

Objective Measurements. Assessment of range of motion, strength, sensation, and functional abilities will also provide input into splint design. Observation skills should be used to aid objective measurements. For example, during grip and pinch strength testing, observe the stability of the metacarpophalangeal (MCP) joints. Is there an increase in ulnar deviation during gripping activities? Observe metacarpal/interphalangeal joint motion during lateral pinch. Is there hyperextension? Is there pain at the carpometacarpal (CMC) joint during pinch activities?

Visual Inspection. Through observation of swelling, joint alignment, and tendon and ligamentous integrity, articular and nonarticular manifestations of disease can be identified. These manifestations should be addressed in the splinting process. For example, a splint may be utilized to provide external support for ligamentous laxity of proximal interphalangeal

(PIP) joints, which may in turn reduce pain and improve function.

ESTABLISHING SPLINTING GOALS

An individualized approach should be used in establishing splinting program goals, based on problems identified through the evaluation. For example, in the case of a patient with rheumatoid arthritis (RA) who has MCP ulnar drift, goals for splinting should be established as follows: 1) the splint will place the fingers in a more functional position for hand use; and 2) the splint will rest the MCP joints to reduce pain and inflammation. Caution should be utilized in the application of splints. They should only be implemented after fully evaluating the patient's functional ability and establishing goals of splinting. Table 1 lists questions that may help define the parameters of a splinting program for the specific problems identified on the hand evaluation.

PURPOSES OF SPLINTING

Reducing Pain

Splints reduce pain by immobilizing or supporting painful joints and periarticular structures (1–4). Immobilization reduces stress on the joint capsule and synovial lining, thereby reducing pain. Supporting a painful joint with a splint allows improved functional use through reduction of pain. By reducing joint pain, reflexive muscle spasm is also reduced, which further reduces joint pain (3). Splints can reduce pain in such periarticular structures as tendons and ligaments by restricting full excursion and overstretching. The benefits of splinting in terms of pain reduction are well documented (2–8). One study found that more than 60% of patients had moderate to great pain relief by using splints (6,9). Another study showed that patients with splints achieved greater relief from pain than relief from morning stiffness (10). The same study also found that patients continued to wear splints because of the benefits of pain reduction.

Decreasing Inflammation

Splints reduce joint and tendon inflammation by restricting motion. Inflammation is also reduced by decreasing external forces on the inflamed tissues. Several studies have demonstrated reduction in joint inflammation through splinting and rest (1,2,4,7,8,10). Consensus has not been reached on how much rest is necessary to reduce inflammation. It has been suggested, however, that splints used for the purpose of reducing inflammation be continued at night for several weeks after

191

Table 1. Questions to aid in establishing the parameters of a splinting program for the hand.

What is the goal of the splint? Is the splint being used to reduce pain and inflammation or to support an unstable joint? Is the splint being used to prevent or possibly correct deformity?

What is the best splint design for this particular person? Which joint or joints need to be supported or immobilized to achieve the goal? Should the splint be dorsal or volar? Which materials will best achieve the goals of the splint?

When should the splint be worn? Is the splint a resting splint for night wear or a functional daytime splint? How long should the splint be worn?

acute inflammation has resolved (6,11,12). Patients can be taught to monitor their inflammation and adjust their use of splints accordingly.

Preventing Deformity

Splints are often used to support joints in an attempt to prevent deformity. Controversy exists in this area, as there is a lack of outcome data supporting the use of splints for this purpose. Despite this, splints are often prescribed for patients with early signs of deformity to hopefully delay progression, and for patients with more advanced deformity to prevent further deterioration. Wrist involvement in juvenile arthritis is common, and wrist splints are often prescribed to prevent deformities of subluxation and ulnar deviation (13,14).

Wrist splints have been shown to improve writing skills in more than 60% of children with arthritis; however, prevention of deformity has not been documented.

Hand deformity, particularly MCP ulnar deviation, is a common finding in RA (5). Resting hand splints and other ulnar deviation supports are commonly used to prevent or delay progression of deformity. Few studies have addressed the role of splinting in preventing or correcting deformity. The use of a resting splint at night for at least 1 year was not found to delay the progression of ulnar deviation in one controlled study (5). However, the study suggested that dynamic splints could reduce ulnar deviation of MCP joints. Splints used for the purpose of preventing a deformity should be monitored closely.

Correcting Deformity

Splints may be used to correct flexion deformities of the fingers and wrist. Splinting for this purpose can be static (using serial, progressive splinting or casting) or dynamic. Whichever method is used, joint inflammation should be under control, because dynamic forces may exacerbate inflammation. Lateral deformities of the fingers and wrist can also benefit from splinting by providing support to unstable or poorly positioned joints, thereby improving function.

Supporting Function

Hand function can be decreased by painful, inflamed, poorly positioned, or unstable joints. Splinting may improve function by reducing pain and inflammation and by supporting joints in a more stable and functional position. Wrist supports, both commercial and custom, reduce forces on the wrist and protect the joint during daily activities, allowing for function of the

distal joints. Finger and thumb splints place the joints in positions of function and support weakened ligaments, allowing for pinching and gripping with improved dexterity and strength.

Postoperative Management

Dynamic and static splints are used in the postoperative rehabilitation of the hand with rheumatic disease. Dynamic splints allow early postoperative motion in controlled ranges and planes, assist weakened muscles, and protect reconstructed joints and periarticular structures. Dynamic splints also assist in scar formation for stability and motion. Static splints immobilize surgical repairs and stabilize joints in proper alignment. In the case of MCP joint arthroplasty, a dorsal dynamic MCP extension outrigger is used continuously for the first 6–8 weeks postoperatively to maintain alignment of the joints and to allow exercise in a controlled range of motion. This type of splint may also be used for the same purposes in an extensor tendon repair or transfer. Postoperative splinting for repair of a boutonniere or swan neck deformity is usually static, maintaining the position of the PIP joint while allowing for removal of the splint for periods of exercise. Proper use of splinting postoperatively requires a preoperative knowledge of the hand, an understanding of operative procedures, established postoperative goals, and a concerted team effort among the surgeon, therapist, and patient.

TYPES OF SPLINTS

Resting Splints

Resting splints are used primarily to reduce joint inflammation and pain. They may be used during the day as well as at night. Resting splints may also be used to reduce symptoms of nerve entrapment or tendon irritation, such as triggering and tenosynovitis. Caution should be used when determining the wearing time for resting splints in order to maintain joint motion and muscle strength. For this reason, resting splints may be worn at night and intermittently during the day during periods of active synovitis or tenosynovitis, alternating with gentle range of motion and functional activities.

Functional Splints

Functional splints are worn to improve hand function by reducing pain, improving joint alignment, or providing stability to weakened ligaments. Functional splints support or immobilize the minimum number of joints, thereby allowing all other joints to move freely. Functional splints may be *static* (to support weakened or painful joints) or *dynamic* (to gently realign joint deformity).

Corrective Splints

After a complete hand evaluation, it may be determined that joint contracture is the result of a shortening of periarticular structures. If the joint space is preserved, inflammation is at a minimum, and a "soft" end feel is present, splinting may be

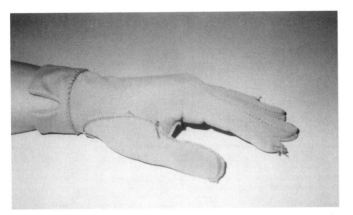

Figure 1. Stretch gloves can be used at night to help decrease morning stiffness and pain.

used to gently correct the contracture. Splints indicated for this purpose may be dynamic or static. Dynamic splinting should be approached cautiously in patients with rheumatic disease. Inflammation and pain may be exacerbated by excessive force on the joint. Static splints that are progressively molded to increase range of motion are often better tolerated due to a lesser amount of force being placed on the joint.

Soft Splints

Support can be provided to joints with gloves, wraps, and soft splints. Soft splints are often more comfortable to patients and may provide as much symptom relief as rigid splints. Using stretch gloves at night has been shown to decrease morning stiffness and pain, allowing for improved hand function (Figure 1) (16). These gloves work by providing gentle compression and neutral warmth to involved joints. Stretch gloves may be contraindicated if carpal tunnel syndrome is present, due to reports of exacerbation of paresthesia. Compressive wraps (such as Coban, Ace, and Tubigrip) also provide support and neutral warmth to joints while allowing joint motion.

Circumferential sleeves and tubes (such as Digisleeve, Digitube, and Compressogrip) can be used as soft splints for joint support. These splints only slightly limit joint mobility. In addition to cushioning and protecting the joint, individual finger wraps and sleeves also act as reminders to protect inflamed finger joints. Soft splints made of neoprene provide joint support and gently assist in realigning joints. Neoprene can be trimmed to fit the patient; however, it does not breathe and may be difficult to put on and wear. Nevertheless, neoprene wraps are often easier to don than tubes, especially when hand weakness is present. Another type of soft splint is fabricated from strapping material to support or realign joints (17). Strapping may be used to reposition ulnar-deviated fingers or to block full motion of interphalangeal joints.

FABRICATED VERSUS PREFABRICATED SPLINTS

A multitude of prefabricated splints, custom-ordered splints, and splinting materials exist. It is often difficult to determine whether it is best to custom fabricate a splint or to use a prefabricated design. There are several advantages to using

custom fabricated splints. The splint is molded to the patient, allowing for conformity to joint surfaces. The materials can be selected according to each individual's needs. In addition, a splint can be designed to support certain joints and allow for movement of others. Finally, modifications in the fit and design are easily made as needed.

The main disadvantage of custom fabricated splints is the cost. Custom fabricated splints are usually the most costly type of splint, due to fabrication time and materials used. Also, making these splints requires a skill that not all therapists possess. The time needed to fabricate the splint is longer than fitting time of a prefabricated splint.

Prefabricated splints also have advantages and disadvantages. They are usually less expensive than custom fabricated splints; however, they may not have the desired fit or provide as much support or immobilization. Prefabricated splints are usually available in only 3 or 4 basic sizes. Achieving a good fit may be problematic due to deformity, size of the forearm in relation to the hand, or general design of the splint. Some prefabricated splints allow for customization by molding of a metal bar or thermoplastic insert, trimming of splint edges, or adjustment of strapping.

PROBLEM IDENTIFICATION AND SPLINT SOLUTION

Identification of the problem through evaluation is the first step toward determining the best type of splint. Some of the more common hand joint problems associated with rheumatic disease are listed in Table 2, along with suggested splinting solutions.

Wrist Splints

A wrist support splint provides support for the wrist while allowing motion of the thumb and fingers (Figure 2). Indications for a wrist splint include wrist pain, synovitis, tenosynovitis, subluxation, nerve entrapment, and epicondylitis. A wrist support splint may be *dorsal*, which allows for sensation on the volar surface of the hand but does not support volar subluxation, or *volar*, which supports volar subluxation but is often difficult to wear with activities that require resting the forearm on a surface. Custom fabricated wrist splints are more likely to restrict motion, while prefabricated wrist supports tend to allow more mid-range motion. One study demonstrated a reduction in finger dexterity with commercially available wrist splints and suggested that when commercial wrist orthoses are used during tasks that require maximum dexterity, this reduction should be weighed against the benefits of splinting (18). A functional position of 20° to 30° of extension is advocated for most conditions; however, in the case of carpal tunnel syndrome 10° of extension maximizes the carpal tunnel. Special care should be taken when fitting a wrist support for a patient with RA. If the MCP joints are involved, restricting the wrist motion may place excess stress on these joints, possibly increasing ulnar deviating or subluxing forces. A position of wrist ulnar deviation is advocated to reduce ulnar deviating forces on the MCP joints.

Table 2. Problem identification and suggested splinting solution in the hand with rheumatic disease.*

Problem identified on evaluation	Splint solution
Wrist joint Synovitis, tenosynovitis Pain Instability, subluxation Nerve entrapment, carpal tunnel syndrome	**Wrist support splint** Dorsal, volar, or combination Worn at rest and/or with activity Removed for range of motion Positioned in neutral to 10° extension
Wrist/thumb Synovitis of wrist and thumb Tenosynovitis of first dorsal compartment Pain in wrist and thumb	**Thumb spica splint** Volar design Radial design to limit thumb motions and allow midrange wrist motion C-bar necessary for CMC joint; thumb IP may/may not be included depending on functional needs
Wrist/hand Synovitis of multiple joints Flexor/extensor tenosynovitis Pain at rest Changes in joint alignment	**Resting hand splint** Full resting splint for immobilization of multiple joints/tendons Modified resting splint for immobilization of wrist/MCPs
MCP joint Synovitis Ulnar deviation Ligamentous laxity	**MCP ulnar deviation support** Built into resting hand splint Hand-based for functional activities May be static or dynamic for function
Finger Boutonniere deformity Swan neck deformity Lateral instability Flexion deformity	**Finger splints** PIP extension with DIP free to stretch oblique retinacular ligament PIP hyperextension block Support for deviation Static progressive or dynamic Serial casts for PIP flexion deformities
Thumb CMC osteoarthritis with pain MCP instability/deformity IP hyperextension IP lateral instability	**Thumb splints** Hand-based CMC support with C-bar Figure-eight MCP support IP hyperextension block Support for deviation

*CMC = carpometacarpal; MCP = metacarpophalangeal; PIP = proximal interphalangeal; DIP = distal interphalangeal; IP = interphalangeal.

Combination Wrist/Thumb Splints

Indications for combination wrist/thumb splints include synovitis of the wrist and thumb joints, tenosynovitis of the wrist and thumb tendons, de Quervain's tenosynovitis, wrist and thumb pain, and instability limiting functional use. Types of wrist and thumb supports include a volar wrist support with an added thumb support, a thumb spica with a C-bar for carpometacarpal involvement, a thumb spica without a C-bar, and a radial thumb spica (Figure 3).

Combination Wrist/Hand Splints

Indications for combination wrist/hand splints include pain or synovitis in multiple joints, tenosynovitis in flexor/extensor tendons, pain and/or stiffness at night or in the morning, and reports of waking with the hand in a fist. A full resting hand splint immobilizes the wrist and fingers to promote relief of pain and inflammation. Studies have shown these splints to be cumbersome to wear, leading to varying rates of use (19). An alternative to a full resting hand splint is the modified resting hand splint, which supports the wrist and MCP joints while allowing interphalangeal movement (Figure 4). The modified resting splint often results in better patient adherence and comfort with less pain and stiffness related to splint wear. If a

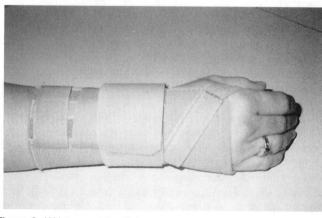

Figure 2. Wrist support splint.

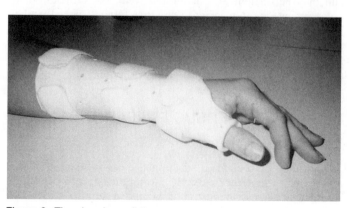

Figure 3. Thumb spica splint.

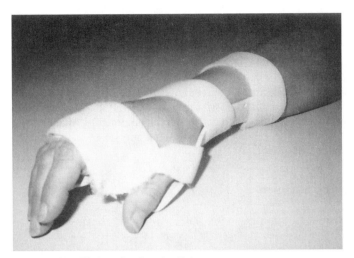

Figure 4. Modified resting hand splint.

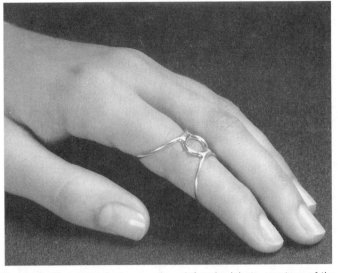

Figure 6. Ring splint for boutonniere deformity (photo courtesy of the Silver Ring Splint Company).

patient requires bilateral resting hand splints, an alternating schedule of night wear may improve adherence.

Finger Splints

Splints for ulnar deviation of the MCP joints may be used to place the fingers in a more functional position or to possibly delay progression of deformity (Figure 5). Ulnar deviation splints may also lessen joint pain by supporting weakened ligaments and by resting the joint. Dynamic ulnar deviation splints apply a gentle force to realign the joints in a more radial direction. Static splints hold the MCP joint in a more radial direction. These splints must be fitted carefully so that they do not interfere with function.

Proximal and Distal Interphalangeal Joint Splints

Splints for the proximal and distal interphalangeal joints are used for synovitis, deformity, instability, pain, and tendon/ligament involvement. A volar or dorsal resting splint may reduce pain and inflammation. For the distal joint, a volar splint is often more supportive, but it may limit functional use

by restricting sensation on the pad of the fingertip. A boutonniere splint (Figure 6) places the PIP joint in extension while allowing flexion of the DIP joint. A swan neck splint (Figure 7) supports the volar surface of the PIP joint from hyperextension, but allows flexion of the joint. Lateral instability of the proximal and distal interphalangeal joint limits functional abilities of pinch and fine precision activities. A splint to address lateral instability should provide support in the direction of the instability while allowing motions needed to perform daily hand tasks.

Thumb Splints

The thumb accounts for 60% of hand function. When thumb use is limited by pain, instability, or deformity, hand function is greatly reduced. Osteoarthritis of the CMC joint of the thumb is a common problem. A hand- or forearm-based thumb support can improve function by reducing pain and supporting

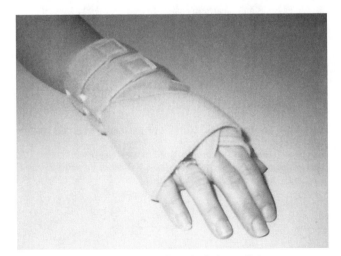

Figure 5. Metacarpophalangeal ulnar deviation splint.

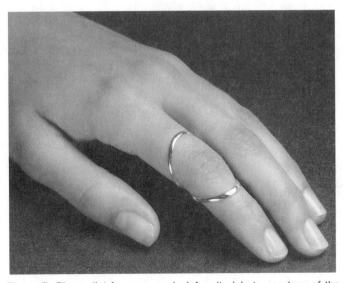

Figure 7. Ring splint for swan neck deformity (photo courtesy of the Silver Ring Splint Company).

ligamentous laxity and joint subluxation (20). Patients may prefer a short hand-based splint over a forearm-based splint, and both types have been found effective in decreasing pain and reducing subluxation of the CMC joint (21). The splint should be fitted carefully to address an adequate C-bar for maintenance of the web space (22). The thumb should be placed in a functional position of opposition to the index finger. In addition, wrist and thumb interphalangeal joint motion should not be restricted.

An unstable, painful, or poorly positioned MCP joint of the thumb can also have a negative influence on hand function. Splints to support the MCP joint of the thumb can improve pinching abilities by providing support and relieving pain. A simple "figure 8" splint for this joint allows movement of the CMC and interphalangeal joints while providing lateral support and positioning the MCP joint for function. Splints for hyperextension and lateral instability of the interphalangeal joint of the thumb follow the same guidelines as for the PIP joints of the fingers.

SPECIAL CONSIDERATIONS

There are several special considerations in splinting the hand with rheumatic disease to ensure that goals of the splinting program and patient satisfaction are achieved. Patients who become involved in a splinting program should be willing to participate and should be educated as to the benefits of wearing the splint. Those who are not interested in wearing splints and who do not understand the purposes of splinting are less likely to adhere to this type of intervention.

Materials used to fabricate splints range from rigid to soft and should be selected according to the type of splint and the purpose of its use. Strapping materials can be integral in fitting the splint, ensuring proper support and joint alignment. Different strapping materials, ranging from elastic to cushioned, may help in achieving the best fit. Precautions for joint position, skin integrity, effect on other joints, and wearing times should be communicated clearly to patients. Persons with arthritis may have more fragile skin due to their disease or to medications used to treat the disease. Splint fitting, padding, and lining can address this issue. Effects of immobilization on the targeted joint, as well as on adjacent joints, should be addressed when developing a schedule for splint wear. Splints should be removed periodically for range of motion exercise and to allow for skin care.

PATIENT EDUCATION

Principles of patient education should be applied in teaching patients about their splinting program (see Chapter 23, Patient Education for Arthritis Self-Management). Patients who learn the purposes of splint use, expectations of splint use, and precautions for splint wear have improved adherence to splint regimes (23). Use of a positive affective tone and encouragement were shown in one study to positively influence splint

wearing (23). Results from studies assessing adherence to splinting programs vary widely, ranging from 25% to 82.5% (21). When patients are better educated about their splinting program, adherence rates should increase. Contracting, written directions, and daily reports are some of the methods used to teach patients about their splints. Regular followup visits to ensure proper fit and wearing of the splints are crucial in meeting treatment goals. Partnership among team members, including the patient, therapist, and physician, is crucial in managing arthritis.

REFERENCES

1. Partridge REH, Duthie JJR. Controlled trial of the effect of complete immobilization of the joints in rheumatoid arthritis. Ann Rheum Dis 1963;22:91.
2. Gault SS, Spyker JM. Beneficial effects of immobilization of joints in rheumatoid arthritis and related arthritides: a splint study using sequential analysis. Arthritis Rheum 1969;12:34–44.
3. Melvin JL. Rheumatic disease in the adult and child: occupational therapy and rehabilitation 3rd ed. Philadelphia PA: FA Davis; 1982.
4. Feinberg J, Brandt KD. Use of resting splints by patients with rheumatoid arthritis. Am J Occup Ther 1981;35:173–8.
5. Malcus Johnson P, Sandkvist G. The usefulness of nocturnal resting splints in the treatment of ulnar deviation of the rheumatoid hand. Clin Rheumatol 1992;11:72–5.
6. Philips CA. Management of the patient with rheumatoid arthritis. The role of the hand therapist. Hand Clinics 1989;5:291–309.
7. Ellis M. Splinting the rheumatoid hand. Clin Rheum Dis 1984;10:673–96.
8. Fred DM. Rest versus activity in arthritis and physical medicine. In: Licht E, editor. Arthritis and physical medicine. Baltimore: Waverly Press; 1969.
9. Zoeckler AA. Prenyl hand splints for rheumatoid arthritis. Phys Ther 1969;49:377–9.
10. Nicholas JJ, Gruen H. Splinting in rheumatoid arthritis: I. Factors affecting patient compliance. Arch Phys Med Rehab 1982;63:92–4.
11. Philips CA. Rehabilitation of the patient with rheumatoid hand involvement. Phys Ther 1989;69:1091–8.
12. Flatt AE. Care of the rheumatoid hand. 3rd ed. St. Louis MO: CV Mosby; 1974.
13. Eberhard BA, Sylvester KL. A comparative study of orthoplast cock-up splints versus ready-made Droitwich work splints in juvenile chronic arthritis. Disabil Rehab 1993;15:41–3.
14. Findlay TW, Halper ND. Wrist subluxation in juvenile rheumatoid arthritis: pathophysiology and management. Arch Phys Med Rehab 1983;64:69–74.
15. Overton EJ, Walcott LE. The role of splints in preventing deformity in the rheumatoid hand and wrist. Missouri Medicine 1966;6:423–7.
16. Erlich GE, DiPiero AM. Stretch gloves: nocturnal use to ameliorate morning stiffness in arthritic hands. Arch Phys Med Rehab 1971;51:479–80.
17. Byron P. Splinting the arthritis hand. J Hand Ther 1994;7:29–30.
18. Stern EB, Ytterberg SR. Finger dexterity and hand function: effect of three commercial wrist extensor orthoses on patients with rheumatoid arthritis. Arthritis Care Res 1996;9:197–205.
19. King JW. Splinting the arthritic hand. J Hand Ther 1993;6:46–8.
20. Wolock BS, Moore JR. Arthritis of the basal joint of the thumb. J Arthroplasty 1989;4:65–78.
21. Weiss S, LaStayo P. Prospective analysis of splinting the first carpometacarpal joint: an objective, subjective, and radiographic assessment. J Hand Ther 2000;13:218–26.
22. Poole JU, Pellegrini VD Jr. Arthritis of the thumb basal joint complex. J Hand Ther 2000;13:91–107.
23. Feinberg J. Effect of the arthritis health professional on compliance with use of resting hand splints by patients with rheumatoid arthritis. Arthritis Care Res 1992;5:17–23.

CHAPTER 29

Enhancing Functional Ability

JILL NOAKER LUCK, OTR/L

Rheumatic diseases have a profound, and often debilitating, effect on an individual's ability to perform normal life activities or occupations. These diseases are now recognized as the leading cause of disability in the United States (1). It is estimated that "over 7 million Americans are limited in their ability to participate in daily activities . . . simply because of arthritis" (2). As the prevalence of arthritis grows to affect an estimated 60 million citizens, those limited in ability to participate in daily activities is projected to increase to 11.6 million people.

In addition to well-documented evidence of the impact of arthritis on such daily living tasks as dressing, bathing, eating, and walking, work (paid and unpaid) and leisure activities are frequently disrupted as well. Work disability estimates range from 25% to 50% for persons with rheumatoid arthritis (RA) (3). Labor force participation among individuals with RA and some work experience was reported to be 50% in those with disease duration of 10 years; 60% had stopped working within 15 years of diagnosis, and 90% within 30 years (4). Ability to participate in leisure activities is an often overlooked area of assessment and intervention, yet one study found that disruption of leisure activities occurred in 33% of community-dwelling elderly persons with arthritis (5). In another study, loss of valued activities (including leisure) was identified in nearly 80% of RA respondents (6). Activities disrupted most often and/or missed most were gardening, crafts, walking/shopping, socializing, participating in sports, and housework (5–7).

This chapter will focus on enhancing functions in self-care, work, and leisure activities within the context of disability as defined by the World Health Organization (8) (Table 1). Combinations of these vital activities are recognized to form the basis of life roles; therefore, addressing disability in these 3 domains can subsequently impact handicap as well. Interventions to minimize disability (and enhance ability) discussed in this chapter include: 1) *alternative techniques* (also known as alternate work methods), including joint protection and energy conservation; 2) *assistive devices* to improve ease and safety of activity performance; and 3) *environmental modification* to promote accessibility.

ASSESSMENT

In general, arthritis-related impairments may include, but are not limited to 1) pain of varying location, intensity, and duration; 2) intra- and extraarticular swelling; 3) stiffness; 4) loss of motion; 5) muscle weakness or loss of strength; 6) fatigue; 7) joint instability or deformity; and 8) skin, nail, or systemic involvement. In light of the variable nature of many rheumatic diseases and their impact on the whole person, health professionals should also be aware of such psychological issues as frustration, anxiety, depression, perceived helplessness, and

Table 1. International classification of impairment, disability, and handicap, World Health Organization, 1980.

Classification	Example
Impairment: Loss or abnormality of an anatomic, physiologic, cognitive or emotional structure or function	Decreased range of motion, strength, pain, stiffness, fatigue, depression
Disability: Difficulty or lack of ability to perform every day activities	Eating, bathing, dressing, household work, school tasks, child care, leisure
Handicap: Limited ability or inability to fulfill roles relevant to age, gender, social and cultural norms	Role of parent, spouse/partner, child, employee, volunteer, student

altered self-image (see Chapter 39, Mood Disorders) and understand their impact on the client's ability to function in their valued activities and normal life roles.

Therapists or other health professionals new to rheumatology should understand, in addition to the fundamentals of assessment, the unique issues posed by individuals with rheumatic disease. The health professional should obtain and understand the individual's specific diagnosis. The rheumatic diseases encompass more than 100 individual conditions and, while many of these conditions share common characteristics, each has its signs, symptoms, findings, and often treatments that define it.

An initial history is essential for gathering helpful background information about the client. In addition to demographic and social information, components of this portion of the assessment might include a medical/surgical history (including use of complementary or alternative therapies); presenting issues such as pain, swelling, or stiffness; impact of disease on global function, including self-care, work, and leisure activities; any treatments or coping strategies that have been used and their effectiveness (e.g., warm showers, ice packs, splints, relaxation techniques); and patient's level of knowledge about the condition.

The assessment of functional activity is best performed within the environment relevant to the activity being addressed (home, work, school, or other location) and at the time of day when those activities occur or are most commonly performed. Often, however, the therapist cannot evaluate the person under such ideal conditions and must rely on the results of the activity assessment performed in the clinical setting. Optimally, the assessment should be performance-based, allowing the health professional to see which activities are difficult for the client and to determine the cause of the difficulty. At this juncture, goal setting should focus on areas of greatest priority and value to the client, engaging him or her in education about treatment options and the problem-solving process (9).

INTERVENTION

After establishing relevant goals, the therapist and the individual with rheumatic disease must collaboratively plan treatment. Treatment recommendations to restore or improve functional abilities include instruction in alternative techniques, provision of assistive devices, and modification of the environment.

Alternative Techniques

If possible, the identified functional limitations should be corrected or minimized by instructing the person in alternative techniques. Individuals with rheumatic diseases most often prefer to do an activity in a modified fashion without the use of a device, rather than with one. Alternative techniques are methods of performing activities that reduce pain, conserve energy, reduce joint stress, and preserve joint structures. The principles of joint protection and energy conservation are practically applied to guide activity performance for persons with arthritis (10,11). Some of these principles are reviewed below.

Respect Pain. Individuals with rheumatic diseases often learn to live with some level of pain in their daily activities. It is important to enable those individuals to recognize the difference between what is a "usual" amount and type of pain versus the pain that is caused by incorrect use or overuse of a joint or muscle. If pain intensity increases or there are overt signs of inflammation, the precipitating activity should be reviewed and strategies to diminish joint stress applied.

Balance Work and Rest. Fatigue can play a significant role in robbing persons with rheumatic diseases of their maximum productivity and ability to accomplish desired activities. Even short rest breaks from activities during the day can help prevent fatigue. Activity scheduling should be paced so that heavy tasks like vacuuming or mowing the lawn are balanced with light ones, such as reading a book.

Conserve Energy. Conservation of energy and reduction of effort in activity can be important for a person with an active inflammatory rheumatic disease who may tire quickly and feel exhausted after a few hours of activity. Fatigue associated with increased disease activity poses a significant challenge to the performance of daily activities as extra time is often required in the course of the day or week to accommodate for this activity-induced fatigue. Minimizing excessive or stressful body movements helps conserve energy. Suggestions for activity modification may include 1) prioritizing tasks that are most important; 2) gathering all necessary supplies before beginning a project; 3) limiting the number of trips needed, especially up and down stairs; 4) sitting to perform tasks when able; and 5) using elongated handles on tools to prevent excessive bending or reaching.

Avoid Positions of Deformity. Positions of comfort are often positions of potential deformity, particularly during acute inflammatory attacks involving the elbows, wrists, fingers, hips, and knees. The resting position of flexion can lead to soft tissue contractures if the joints and soft tissues are not moved through the full range or stretched out. Individuals with arthritis should be educated regarding these positions and instructed to avoid them, especially for prolonged periods.

Use Larger/Stronger Joints. Forces applied to larger joints are more efficiently dispersed than when applied to smaller, more vulnerable joints. Use of mechanical advantage in handling or moving objects can effectively reduce joint stress. Recommendations may include using the forearm to carry packages with handles, using both arms to lift and carry packages close to the body, and when possible, sliding objects with both arms rather than carrying them.

Use Each Joint in its Most Stable Plane. Joint involvement such as synovitis or bony osteophytes can contribute to laxity in the supporting structures and subsequent joint instability and deformity. It is important, therefore, to use each joint in its most stable plane. The individual may be advised to safeguard against rapid and torsional movement of the joints.

Avoid Staying in One Position. Individuals with rheumatic diseases should move and change positions frequently to prevent stiffness and pain. Sitting and standing activities should be alternated to reduce load on the spine and lower extremities. Hand use in activities such as needlework, holding a book, or typing should also be alternated with periods of rest and stretching.

Both joint protection and energy conservation principles are essentially new behaviors to learn. Adoption of these behaviors, at least for the short term, is enhanced by strategies such as identifying and focusing on tasks that individuals view as significant, using experiential teaching and problem solving to reach desired outcomes, practicing goal setting and reflection, and enhancing skill mastery (12–17).

Long-term outcome studies of these techniques are difficult to carry out, but a few short-term studies have provided valuable insights regarding the use and benefits of joint protection and energy conservation. In an observational assessment of joint protection methods used by persons with RA, greater utilization of hand joint protection was noted in those people needing to compensate for hand joint pain and weaker grip strength (13). Outcomes of a 3-week joint protection course in women with RA indicated that 95% of subjects demonstrated a significant increase in ADL ability after the intervention (16).

Another study evaluated a 6-week workbook-based program for teaching energy conservation compared with a program of standard occupational therapy techniques. At 3 months, those in the experimental workbook-based group had a greater level of increased physical activity and a better balance of rest and activity than controls (15). Although these studies provide a basis for evaluating these interventions, future research is needed to further validate their benefits.

ASSISTIVE DEVICES

Assistive devices, which are frequently used by persons with arthritis, are included in the broader term of *assistive technology*. Assistive technology can be defined as "any item, piece of equipment, or product system, whether acquired commercially off the shelf, modified, or customized, that is used to increase, maintain, or improve functional capabilities of individuals with disabilities" (18). Hence, assistive devices can be something as common as enlarged grip kitchen utensils and writing instruments (Figure 1) or a more specialized device, such as a sock aid or motorized scooter.

Availability of assistive devices has grown exponentially. Although not generally covered by insurers, an increasing number and variety of devices are offered commercially in

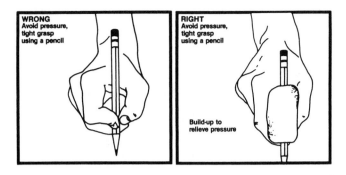

Figure 1. Using enlarged grips for writing relieves pressure on the finger and hand joints.

retail stores and nonmedical specialty shops (see sources in Chapter 44, Links and Organizations). The influence of the aging population and its functional needs, along with the recognition and integration of universal design and ergonomics, has resulted in new features of household items, furniture, computers, and tools.

Assistive devices can be invaluable in preserving or improving functional independence as well as decreasing pain with activity (16). These devices have the potential to compensate for such physical impairments as diminished grip, mobility, strength, manual dexterity, joint stability, and fatigue. Depending on the purpose of the device, use may be long-term or temporary.

Once the need for an assistive device is determined, several factors, including physical, emotional and financial concerns, need to be considered (Table 2). The health care professional should be aware of the impact of these factors on the use—or potential non-use—of assistive devices. Usage of assistive devices as prescribed ranges from an overall 41% among total hip arthroplasty patients at 10 weeks followup (19) to 91% among RA patients after a 3-week arthritis education program (17). A review article on assistive device use identifies factors that have been shown to affect use (20).

Use of assistive devices may be enhanced when the following conditions are met: 1) the device is useful, efficient, durable, dependable, and safe; 2) the user values independence in the activity for which it is intended; 3) the user has confidence in the device and his or her ability to use it; 4) the device is promptly provided and the user is trained to use and maintain it; 5) training occurs in the context of where it will be used

(e.g., home, car, school, work); and 6) the device assists caregivers or partially alleviates some of their work.

Factors that negatively impact prescribed use include incompatibility with the architecture or structures of the home, unreliability or awkwardness of the device, preference for human help, and concern about device use inconveniencing others in the home. User dissatisfaction may be greater when devices are self-recommended or prescribed by non-(occupational) therapy personnel. This is important to note, given the trend of direct-to-consumer marketing of assistive devices and limited access to therapy personnel for collaboration when needed.

Assistive devices can be classified as aids for general daily living; self-care; transfers and mobility; home management; and school, work, and leisure activities. Activities that are commonly difficult within these categories are presented along with assistive devices or adaptations that may increase functional independence.

General Daily Living

Activity	Recommended Device or Adaptation
Turning knobs or faucets	Knob turner, faucet turner
	Single lever faucet
Opening doors	Lever handle
	Automatic garage door opener
Holding/using a key	Key holder (Figure 2)
	Orthotic material built-up handle
Cutting with scissors	Loop or spring-loaded scissors

Self-Care: Personal Hygiene

Personal hygiene is a very important component in maintaining one's appearance and self-esteem. Most often these activities, such as brushing teeth, hair and nail care, shaving, and toileting are limited by diminished hand grasp and arm motion. This is often compounded by the presence of morning stiffness when many of these activities are performed.

Activity	Recommended Device or Adaptation
Comb/brush hair	Enlarged handle brush/comb
	Long-handled brush/comb
Dental hygiene	Cylindrical foam on toothbrush handle
	Denture brush mounted on suction cup base
	Pump toothpaste dispenser or toothpaste key
Shaving	Enlarged handle razor or cylindrical foam
	Electric razor
Nail care	Clippers and emery board mounted on suction cup base
	Electric or battery-operated file/buff
Toileting	Toilet tongs to hold paper and extend reach

Table 2. Factors to consider in prescribing assistive devices.

Physical factors	Does the device reduce pain, stiffness, or joint stress?
	Does the device reduce energy or time expenditure?
	Is the device convenient, easy to use, and if needed, transportable?
	Will the device only be needed at certain times (mornings, bad days)?
	Does the device substitute for an activity that can be done safely without it? Does it promote loss of motion in mobile joint?
Social/emotional factors	Does the person desire or value independence in activities of daily living?
	Does the person have a negative response to the appearance or use of the assistive device?
	Is there a fear of failure or low frustration tolerance that may impede learning to use the device?
	Would the person prefer human help as a device?
Environmental factors	Are the assistive devices or modifications compatible with the architecture and environment of the home/workplace?
	If needed, is there an individual available to install or maintain the equipment?
Financial factors	Can these devices be made less expensively than purchased?
	Are the devices commercially available rather than available only from medical suppliers?

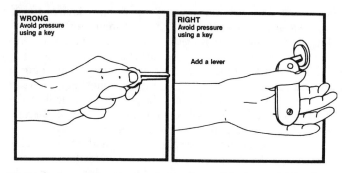

Figure 2. Incorrect and correct ways to avoid pressure to the fingers and hand when using a key.

Self-Care: Bathing

Bathing requires joint mobility, especially in the shoulders, hips, and spine, to reach all body parts. In addition, one needs to be able to grasp and hold a washcloth or sponge and apply soap, as well as manipulate a towel to dry the body after bathing.

Activity	Recommended Device or Adaptation
Washing/drying	Long-handled sponge or brush
	Sponge or wash mitt
	Hand-held shower
	Terry robe after bathing
Using soap or shampoo	Liquid soap in pump or wall-mounted dispenser

Self-Care: Dressing

Dressing can pose a great challenge to a person with rheumatic disease because of its many physical demands. Like grooming, dressing is often performed at times of maximum stiffness. It requires endurance, mobility, strength, and dexterity. Dressing may best be performed after a warm shower to alleviate morning stiffness and in a seated position to reduce energy consumption. In addition to assistive devices for dressing, individuals often benefit from choosing loose-fitting clothing with easier or larger closures and no-wrinkle fabrics.

Activity	Recommended Device or Adaptation
Putting on bra	Choose front closure style
	Replace hooks with Velcro closure
Putting on shirt or jacket	Dressing stick for extended reach
Putting on pants or shorts	Sit to perform task
	Dressing stick to start garment over legs
	Sewn-in loops for easy pull-up
Putting on socks/stockings/ shoes	Sock device and/or long-handled shoehorn
	Slip-on shoes
	Elastic shoelaces or Velcro closure shoes
Fasteners (buttons, snaps, zippers)	Button hook, zipper pull, or zipper ring
	Replace snaps with Velcro

Self-Care: Eating

Eating is not only necessary to health, it is often a highly social and culturally significant activity. The ability to eat independently is of immeasurable value to most individuals. Rheumatic diseases can make it difficult to prepare food for eating and get the food or drink to the mouth. This is frequently due to limitations in strength and mobility of the cervical spine, elbow flexion/extension, forearm rotation, and hand grasp.

Activity	Recommended Device or Adaptation
Holding/using utensils	Utensils with larger handles
	Lightweight utensils
Cutting food	Rocker or angled knife; sharpness decreases cutting pressure
	Nonslip matting under plate
	Dishes with raised edges
Getting food/drink to mouth	Extended-handle utensils, swivel utensils
	Straws
	Lightweight mugs and glasses

Transfers and Mobility

Transfers, or moving from one location to another, are often hampered by limited motion of the hips, knees, ankles, and upper extremities; muscle weakness; joint instability; and pain or stiffness. Independence in transfers is necessary for freedom of normal movement. Safety is of equal importance in preventing falls and reducing the risk of potential injury. Increasing independence and safety in transfers can generally be accomplished by either elevating the seated surface or adding supports for upper extremity assistance.

Activity	Recommended Device or Adaptation
Getting on/off chair	Look for chair with arm supports
	Pillow or elevated cushion on seat
	Lift chair or lift seat insert
Getting into/out of bed	Transfer assist rail
	Use of stool to step up/down
Getting on/off toilet	Elevated toilet seat or frame
	Commode rails
	Higher toilet
Getting in/out of tub or shower	Tub rails and wall-mounted grab bars
	Shower stool or transfer tub bench
Getting in/out of car	Elevated or swivel seat cushion
	"Back" into car seat, turn body, and lift legs in
Driving	Use of wide-angle mirrors
	Power accessories
	Seat cushion or support

Home Management

Home management encompasses the many activities involved in running a household. Persons with rheumatic diseases may benefit from the recent growth in commercially available power, convenience, and ergonomically designed products for these activities. Not all such appliances or products are convenient or easily used by a person with a rheumatic disease, however. Appliance or product use may be difficult due to the weight, force/pressure, or mobility required. Encourage the person to try the product before purchasing to see if it is easily operable. Above all, home management activities are more safely performed by not only using devices, but also by incorporating the principles of joint protection and energy conservation.

Activity	Recommended Device or Adaptation
Opening jars, cans, boxes	Jar openers, electric can opener
	Small kitchen shears, knife, or box top opener
Preparing food	Sit to work when possible
	Utensils with enlarged handles
	Electric food chopper/processor; microwave

Table 3. Guidelines for accessible areas within the home.

Outside entrance	Railings on both sides of stairs (1.5″ diameter) 32–36″ from ground Nonslip surface ramp (portable or permanent) at slope of 1″ rise: 12″ run
Interior halls/doors	Hallways 36″ + width, railings at 32–36″ adults, 18–24″ children Rails 1.5″ diameter mounted on supports 1.5″ from wall Doors 32″ minimum with lever knobs and push-button locks Light switches at 32–36″ from floor
Steps/stairs	Light switches at either end Railings on both sides—extend past last step to help step up/down Recommended 4″ rise to 11″ step (standard 7″ rise to 11″ tread) Stair glide if needed
Bathroom	Toilet at 17–19″ from floor—may add elevated seat to 22″ or install elevated toilet Grab bar or commode rails at both sides of toilet Walk-in shower with built-in seat or wheel-in version Tub with non-slip surface, vertical grab bars at either end, long grab bar mounted at angle on long wall; may use tub mounted rail as well 30″ clearance under sink and 60″ turnaround diameter to accommodate wheelchair
Kitchen	U-shaped or corridor kitchen design with sink between refrigerator and stove and minimum of 18″ counter in between Lazy Susan, pull-out shelves, drawer dividers, and baskets for storage Rolling utility cart for transport; pegboard or wire rack with hooks for storage Movable stool or chair to sit when preparing foods
Bedroom	Bedside organizational table—phone, remote control, touch lighting Book holder or lap desk Power controls for house lighting and security system

Reaching/carrying items	Long-handled reacher to retrieve items Utility cart Lightweight dishes and pans Slide objects rather than carry them
Cleaning	Long-handled non-wringing sponge or mop Long broom with attached dustpan, long-handled duster Lightweight sweeper Terry or sponge wash mitt
Maintenance tasks	Tools with enlarged and cushioned handles Lightweight power tools Spray lubricant or nonslip matting to turn nozzles, valves Easy-to-start self-propelled lawn mower or riding mower Garbage can on wheels

Work/School Activities

The ability to perform and sustain one's occupation, whether as an employee or student, is crucial in maintaining normal life roles. Federal legislation, such as the Americans with Disabilities Act, has established regulations promoting the accessibility of public buildings and transportation, as well as reasonable accommodations to allow an individual to perform his or her job. Possible accommodations depend on the environment, job, or task and the functional level of the individual.

Activity	Recommended Device or Adaptation
Writing	Large diameter pens, markers, or enlarged grips Writing aids Tape recorder for lectures, meetings, dictating notes Laptop computer
Using a computer	Wrist at neutral, cushion in front of keyboard Document holder at eye level Good posture with feet supported on floor Stretch frequently
Using a phone	Large number pad phone or phone holder Speaker phone or headset Lightweight cordless phone
Reading/studying	Book holder with or without page turner Books on tape or CD-ROM

Leisure Activities

Leisure activities and hobbies are an important component of a healthy and balanced lifestyle. Individuals with rheumatic diseases may struggle to perform even routine activities, leaving little energy to participate in leisure pursuits. Depression and pain can also prevent people from enjoying valued activities. Health professionals should assess the leisure interests of individuals with arthritis and any difficulty in the performance of those activities. As desired, modifications may be suggested to enhance ease of participation.

Activity	Recommended Device or Adaptation
Gardening	Tools with cushioned handles Cushioned kneeler with handles to help stand up Window box or raised bed gardening
Playing cards	Card holder Automatic shuffler
Crafts	Table-top clamp to hold work Self-feeding glue gun Enlarged-handle brushes, sponges, or other tools Stretch hands frequently
Woodworking	Lightweight power tools (sander, drill, staple gun) Precut kits to assemble and finish Cushioned foam handles on tools

ENVIRONMENTAL MODIFICATION

Environmental modification is another vital component in the comprehensive care of the person with rheumatic disease. The rapid progression of technology along with the recognition and adoption of ergonomic and universal design concepts potentially provides greater independence in desired activities and roles. Environmental accessibility depends on the nature and extent of the individual's impairment and the limitations posed by his or her specific environment. The clinician must evaluate the individual's ability to function within the relevant environment before suggesting modifications. Psychosocial and economic factors, along with expectations and concerns of others in the environment should also be assessed.

The primary goal of environmental modification is to match the needs of the person with demands of the intended tasks, such as self-care, work, home management, school, or leisure activities (21). Specific guidelines for environmental accessibility can be found in Table 3. Resources such as ABLEDATA, an on-line database of more than 27,000 assistive technology products (sponsored by the National Institute on Disability and Rehabilitation Research) and the Job Accommodation Network, an on-line employment accommodation resource (sponsored by the United States Department of Labor, Office of Disability Employment Policy) can be exceedingly helpful to the health care professional working with individuals in need of modifications and accommodations.

REFERENCES

1. CDC. Prevalence of disability and associated health conditions - United States, 1991-1992. MMWR Morbid Mortal Wkly Rep 1994;43:730-1, 737-9.
2. CDC. Arthritis prevalence and activity limitations - United States, 1990. MMWR Morbid Mortal Wkly Rep 1994;43:433-8.
3. Allaire SH, Anderson JJ, Meenan RF. Reducing work disability associated with rheumatoid arthritis: identification of additional risk factors and persons likely to benefit from intervention. Arthritis Care Res 1996;9:349-57.
4. Yelin E, Henke C, Epstein W: The work dynamics of the person with rheumatoid arthritis. Arthritis Rheum 1987;30:507-12.
5. Jordan, JM, Bernard SL, Callahan LF, Kincade JE, Konrad TR, DeFriese GH. Self-reported arthritis-related disruptions in sleep and daily life and the use of medical, complementary, and self-care strategies for arthritis: the National Survey of Self-care and Aging. Arch Fam Med 2000;9:143-9.
6. Katz P. What is the impact of RA on life activities? Modifications and losses of valued activities attributable to rheumatoid arthritis. Arthritis Care Res 1994;7:S10.
7. Mann WC, Hurren D, Tomiko M. Assistive devices used by home-based elderly persons with arthritis. Am J Occup Ther 1995;49:810-21.
8. World Health Organization. International classification of impairments, disabilities and handicaps. Geneva, Switzerland, 1980.
9. Sotosky JR, Melvin J. Initial interview: a client-centered approach. In: Melvin J, Jensen G, editors. Rheumatologic rehabilitation series, volume 1: assessment and management. Bethesda, MD: American Occupational Therapy Association; 1998.
10. Cordery JC. Joint protection: a responsibility of the occupational therapist. Am J Occupation Ther 1965;19:285-94.
11. Cordery J, Rocchi M. Joint protection and fatigue management. In: Melvin J, Jensen G. Rheumatologic rehabilitation series, volume 1: assessment and management. Bethesda, MD: American Occupational Therapy Association; 1998.
12. Hammond A, Lincoln N, Sutcliffe L. A cross over trial evaluating an educational-behavioral joint protection programme for people with rheumatoid arthritis. Patient Education and Counseling 1999;37:19-32.
13. Hammond A, Lincoln N. Development of the Joint Protection Behavior Assessment. Arthritis Care Res 1999;12:200-7.
14. Gerber LH, Furst GP. Validation of the NIH activity record: a quantitative measure of life activities. Arthritis Care Res 1992;5:81-6.
15. Gerber L, Furst G, Shulman B, Smith C, Thornton B, Liang M, et al. Patient education program to teach energy conservation behaviors to patients with rheumatoid arthritis. Arch Phys Med Rehabil 1987;68:442-5.
16. Nordenskiold U, Grimby G, Hedberg M, Wright B, Linacre JM. The structure of an instrument for assessing the effects of assistive devices and altered working methods in women with rheumatoid arthritis. Arthritis Care Res 1996;9:358-67.
17. Nordenskiold U. Daily activities in women with arthritis. Aspects of patient education, assistive devices and methods for disability and impairment assessment. Scand J Rehabil Med Suppl 1997;37:1-72.
18. Technology-Related Assistance for Individuals with Disabilities Act of 1988 (Public-Law 100-407).
19. Haworth RJ. Use of aids during the first three months after total hip replacement. Br J Rheumatol 1983;22:29-35.
20. Rogers JC, Holm MB. Assistive technology device use in patients with rheumatic disease: a literature review. Am J Occup Ther 1992;46:120-7.
21. Salmen JPS. The doable renewable home. Washington, DC: American Association of Retired Persons, 1991.

Additional Recommended Reading

Backman C. Functional assessment. In: Melvin J, Jensen G, editiros. Rheumatalogic rehabilitation series, volume 1: assessment and management. Bethesda, MD: American Occupational Therapy Association, 1998.

Resources

Title: Job Accommodation Network (A service of the US Dept of Labor Office of Disability Employment Policy)
Copyright: West Virginia University
Write to: West Virginia University
             PO Box 6080
             Morgantown, WV 26506-6080
             800-526-7234
             http://www.jan.wvu.edu

Title: ABLEDATA
             (An online repository of assistive technology products)
             http://www.abledata.com
             8630 Fenton Street, Suite 930
             Silver Spring, MD 20910
             800-227-0216

Note: The World Health Organization recently released the final draft of its new version of the ICIDH (the original version is noted in the chapter introduction), known as the ICIDH-2: International Classification of Functioning, Disability and Health. At press time, the final draft of the new classification system can be found at http://www.who.int/icidh.

CHAPTER 30

Evaluation and Management of the Foot and Ankle

H.J. HILLSTROM, PhD; K. WHITNEY, DPM; J. McGUIRE, DPM, PT;
K.T. MAHAN, DPM, MS; and H. LEMONT, DPM

It has been estimated that 15% of Americans (~40 million) had some form of arthritis as of 1995 (1), a number projected to increase to 18.2% by the year 2020. The Centers for Disease Control and Prevention has estimated that 20.7 million U.S. citizens have osteoarthritis (OA) as of 1990, and rheumatoid arthritis (RA) has been estimated to occur in 2.1 million individuals. Clinically, the involvement of the foot and ankle may be more common in RA than in OA. Gout, pseudogout, Charcot arthropathy, juvenile RA, ankylosing spondylitis, dermatomyositis, scleroderma, systemic lupus erythematosus, polymyalgia rheumatica, and fibromyalgia all may involve the foot and ankle. Paradoxically, little if any rheumatologic data identifies the prevalence of foot and ankle involvement, except for OA.

The National Health Examination Survey reports that 20.8% of individuals aged 25–74 had mild, moderate, or severe radiographic evidence of OA in the feet (2). This estimate dropped to 2.3% when only moderate to severe radiographic evidence was considered. A 1966 study reported a 2% prevalence of symptomatic and radiographic evidence of moderate to severe OA within the metatarsophalangeal (MTP) joints, with women affected twice as often as men (3). When 500 patients with limb joint OA were evaluated, the relative prevalence of joint OA was 41.2% in the knees, 30% in the hands, 19% in the hips, and 4.4% in the ankles (4). Lower extremity malalignment appears to be related to OA of the knee (5).

ANATOMIC CONSIDERATIONS

The foot and ankle comprise 28 bones (including sesamoids), 33 joints, and 112 ligaments. The foot and ankle can be divided into segments that include the hindfoot (ankle and subtalar joints), rearfoot (ankle, subtalar, and midtarsal joints), midfoot (intertarsal and tarsometatarsal joints), and the forefoot (MTP and interphalangeal joints). The subtalar joint is a tri-planar mechanism whose axes of rotation span a large range of positions in the sagittal and transverse planes across individuals (6–9). These studies indicate that there is more than one type of architecture for the human foot.

FOOT AND ANKLE ALIGNMENT

When examining and treating the foot and ankle, it is important to recognize that in a closed chain system, each segment is interrelated and interdependent. No one segment can move independently of the others. Loss of mobility at any one joint

sets in motion a complex series of compensations that may affect many, if not all, the other articulations of the foot.

Anterior ankle joint spurring or contracture of the Achilles tendon restricts dorsiflexion of the ankle and may cause the patient to compensate by one or more mechanisms that include knee flexion or hyperextension, subtalar joint pronation, or midfoot hypermobility. Loss of dorsiflexion of the first MTP joint or hallux limitus places significant constraints on the closed chain system during the transition from mid-stance to propulsion in the gait cycle. If the foot cannot pivot over the MTP joints—and in particular the first MTP joint—the patient must either pick up the foot early (steppage), abduct and roll off the medial aspect of the foot (pronate), or shorten the stride on the involved side (limp). Each of these compensations is associated with a set of correlated and compensatory postures and movements at the knee, hip, and spinal articulations that can place undue stress and promote commensurate injuries elsewhere (10).

Segments of the foot and ankle have a range of available motion that is well tolerated by the system and dependent on the natural architecture of the bones. A certain degree of pronation and supination within the hindfoot is necessary for normal function, such as absorbing shock at heel strike during locomotion. When joints compensate for malalignments or conditions that cause hyper- or hypomobility, pain and disability often result. Small deviations from ideal alignment can impose large changes in stress to pedal structures during locomotion (for example, the effects of pronation on induction and perpetuation of hallux limitus or hallux abductovalgus).

Controlling the alignment of the foot and ankle with orthotic devices and footwear can prevent painful complications by reducing unwanted correlated motions and the need for compensation. In the malaligned state, the foot is likely to have excessive vertical or shear loading on one or more plantar regions, which may result in mechanically induced skin lesions such as corns and calluses. In the severe stages of degenerative joint disease within the foot and ankle, surgical management is an option for treatment.

EVALUATION AND TREATMENT CONSIDERATIONS

The condition of a joint depends on structural (alignment, deformity, flexibility), functional, immunologic, and biochemical factors, as well as a history of trauma. When managing an arthritic condition, it is helpful to categorize the patient's condition as *reactive* or *nonreactive*. This effectively divides treatment strategies into those designed to rest or protect an inflamed structure (*reactive*) and those that accommodate, re-align, or stabilize a *nonreactive* joint. Reactive joints are hot, swollen, and often painful. Examples include RA flares, acute synovitis, and Charcot arthropathy. These joints must be protected and treated with various antiinflammatory medications, physical modalities, or rest until they become nonreactive. The involved joint then can be rehabilitated with appropriate exercises, orthotic devices, and footwear to allow the patient to return to maximum functional capacity.

It is also important to evaluate the biomechanical integrity, including the stability, skeletal alignment, and presence or absence of deformity of a joint or joint complex. *Stability* indicates the quality of a joint's flexibility in both rotational and translational aspects (e.g., excessive anterior drawer at the tibio-talar joint implies an unstable ankle joint). *Skeletal alignment* is the relative osseous positioning of a joint, which may be modifiable by soft tissue contractures or laxity. *Deformity*, often occurring at the extremes of malalignment, refers to a fixed osseous deviation, such as a rigid hammer toe.

Reactive joints should be splinted in a position of rest and treated with physical modalities designed to decrease inflammation and swelling. Various medications and therapeutic modalities can be used to reduce discomfort and allow for early mobilization and return to function. Early mobilization to prevent contracture and reduce muscle wasting can benefit joints that exhibit biomechanical integrity. However, mobilization of reactive joints must often be postponed until the structures involved become nonreactive and can be protected with bracing during strengthening activities.

Nonreactive joints should be evaluated immediately for biomechanical integrity. If biomechanically aberrant, then appropriate support (stabilization), balancing (osseous alignment and muscular forces), and accommodation should be employed. A combination of mobilization, strengthening exercises, orthoses, and footwear are used to restore the patient to maximal function. These interventions may include electrical modalities for muscle strengthening, heating modalities to aid in joint mobilization, open and closed kinetic chain exercises, and various types of orthoses and appropriate footwear to maximize both comfort and function. Joint complexes function best when they are maintained in a range of positions that represent good skeletal alignment, allow the surrounding musculature to work most efficiently, and afford an appropriate level of flexibility.

Osteoarthritis is often accompanied by a loss of joint mobility or flexibility that places excessive demands on the adjacent joints. Joint stability, a requirement for biomechanical integrity, is usually provided by the combination of inherent bony architecture, ligamentous support, and muscle tension. When joints become hypomobile because of protective splinting of surrounding musculature or bony hypertrophy, which develops from years of joint malalignment, the surrounding skeletal system must accommodate the restriction. This may necessitate specifically designed foot orthoses (devices that realign musculoskeletal structures) to transfer demands to other, more flexible articulations. For example, when hallux limitus, rigidus, and abductovalgus occur, loss of motion at the first MTP joint prevents a normal progression from midstance through propulsion in gait referred to as "sagittal plane blocking" (11). The patient may compensate by externally rotating the limb, reducing walking speed, lifting the foot early in the gait cycle, and shortening the stride length.

Limited range of motion at the big toe joint can invoke many different correlated and compensatory motions in posture and locomotion (12). Loss of motion at the first MTP joint places additional demands on the interphalangeal joint. Hallux extensus or hypermobility in extension will develop if the skeletal architecture permits, and a painful interphalangeal joint callus or degenerative joint disease may follow. Treatment strategies include an in-shoe foot orthosis to reduce dorsiflexion demands on the first interphalangeal joint, the addition of a rocker sole to the patient's shoe, or surgical correction of the joint to allow for increased mobility in dorsiflexion.

Hypermobility places a different set of demands on the system and requires increased strength of surrounding musculature and/or an orthosis to add biomechanical integrity. A classic example is hyperpronation, which can place unreasonable demands on the joints of the forefoot, midfoot, and hindfoot. If untreated, hyperpronation can lead to posterior tibial musculotendinous dysfunction or even rupture in the patient with accompanying transient tenosynovitis. Realignment of the pronating foot with a posted in-shoe orthosis can decrease demands placed on the joints of the rear and forefoot and prevent recurrent tenosynovitis caused by repetitive microtrauma.

Once the posterior tibial tendon has been compromised by partial or complete rupture, the foot will quickly decompensate and become very painful, limiting the patient's ability to ambulate. Unless the foot and ankle can be realigned and stabilized with an appropriate ankle-foot orthosis coupled with a rocker-soled shoe, the only relief from pain may be rearfoot surgery. If the midfoot and rearfoot are beyond reconstruction, fusion of the subtalar, talonavicular, and calcaneocuboid joints (triple arthrodesis) may be required to restore stability to the foot and ankle.

Understanding and treating correlated and compensatory patterns associated with mild to severe foot deformity is challenging. A careful lower extremity examination should be performed with the goal of understanding the underlying biomechanics via a comprehensive assessment of the patient at rest and during stance and gait. One must assess the foot in the context of the lower extremity and the whole body if an understanding of the pathology is to be achieved. The remainder of this chapter is concerned with the intricacies of foot and ankle assessment and management. To integrate these techniques with the management of the lower extremity see also Chapter 31, Lower Extremity Conservative Realignment Therapies and Ambulatory Aids.

FOOT TYPE BIOMECHANICS

Planar Dominance

The foot and ankle is a triplanar mechanism that may, at any joint, exhibit a complete 6 degrees of freedom movement: that is, rotations about, and translations along, each of 3 axes. *Triplanar* implies that motions occur in all 3 planes (e.g., ankle rotation is not a purely sagittal plane motion due to the orientation of the trans-malleolar axis). The osseous and soft tissue architecture is a major determinant of foot and ankle function. This architecture is known as the foot type, including pes planus (low arch), rectus (normal arch), and pes cavus (high arch).

Each foot type elicits distinctly different biomechanical function, as demonstrated by Song et al (13). A group of

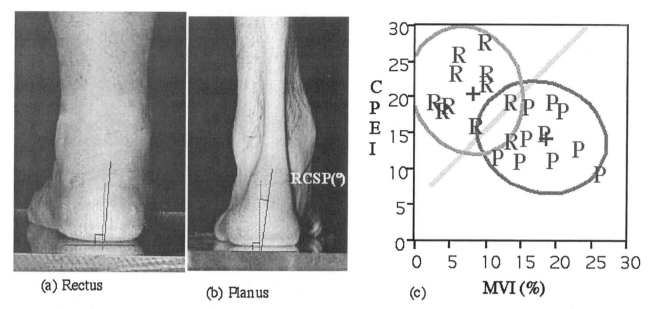

(a) Rectus   (b) Planus   (c)

Figure 1. Foot type biomechanics: The rectus (a), or well-aligned, hindfoot has a nearly perpendicular calcaneal bisection. The pes planus (b), or pronatory, hindfoot has 4° or greater valgus orientation of the calcaneal bisection. As shown in the discriminant analysis (c), rectus and planus feet exhibited different static (MVI) and dynamic (CPEI) function. Adapted from reference 13.

healthy young individuals with hyperpronating (Figure 1b) and well-aligned (Figure 1a) foot types were evaluated. Each subject's foot type was classified *a priori* based on goniometric measures (13,14). As shown in Figure 1c, a scattergram was constructed of static foot function versus dynamic foot function. The rectus and pes planus foot types were clearly separable, indicating that anatomically distinct structures yielded biomechanically distinct functions.

The term *planal dominance* refers to the concept that triplanar joints usually exhibit a greater proportion of motion in one plane than in the other two (15). For example, if a pes planus foot has a lower, more sagittally oriented, subtalar joint axis compared with the rectus foot type, the resulting motion will be dominant in the frontal plane.

Triplanar Assessment

The comprehensive biomechanical examination should include the patient at rest, during posture, and during locomotion. The patient assessment at rest must include a morphologic and arthrometric examination to note the location and degree of malalignment, deformity, or motion limitation. A palpation examination should also be performed to determine any areas of tenderness or pain and the presence of abnormal fluid, masses, or muscle tone.

Failure to properly identify triplanar deformity in the foot may prevent successful management of secondary postural aberrations at more proximal joints. Careful assessment will help the practitioner identify malalignments of the foot in all 3 planes. If these deformities are recognized early, prophylactic measures, including appropriate footwear and orthoses, may be employed to reduce much of the negative sequelae associated with rheumatologic conditions. Anatomic, foot-referenced borderlines can serve as a basic evaluation of pedal structure in each of 3 planes with the patient prone (Figure 2).

At Rest. *Sagittal* plane assessment is performed by viewing the foot from the medial and lateral aspects. The examiner

should visualize the medial and lateral surfaces, noting any variation of normal contours. Increased convexity of dorsal contours and increased concavity of plantar contours will generally indicate cavus foot types (16). In the *transverse* plane, the examiner views the plantar aspect of the foot, noting any variation from the normally straight medial and lateral borderlines. Lateral deviations of these reference borderlines are indicative of abductus foot types, and medial deviations are associated with adductus foot conditions. Finally, the examiner should perform the *frontal* plane assessment by viewing from the toes to the heel. Ideally, the forefoot reference line (lying below the five metatarsal heads) should be parallel with the posterior reference line (which lies below the plantar aspect of the heel). When the forefoot line is inverted relative to the heel line, a forefoot varus attitude is present; conversely, an everted relationship is indicative of a forefoot valgus posture.

With the patient prone on the examination table, an *arthrometric* (joint alignment, range of motion, and deformity) examination of the lower extremities should be performed. Ankle equinus, or insufficient dorsiflexion, is one of the most common lower extremity conditions and may be of neurologic (spasticity), soft tissue (contracture), or osseous origin. As a result, functional or pathologic compensation via foot pronation will occur during posture and locomotion.

To determine if an ankle equinus exists, the examiner should

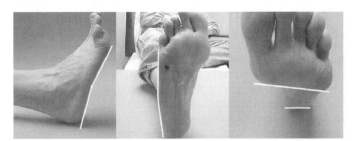

Figure 2. Example of sagittal, transverse, and frontal plane reference lines.

perform the Silfverskiold test (17). With the patient prone, the foot is maintained in a subtalar neutral position (neither pronated nor supinated) and forcibly dorsiflexed upon the ankle to the end range of motion. The Silfverskiold test is performed with the knee both extended and flexed to determine gastrocnemius versus gastrocnemius-soleal musculotendinous involvement. If less than 10° of dorsiflexion is observed with the knee extended (gastrocnemius contracture) or flexed (gastrosoleal contracture), an ankle equinus condition exists.

Osseous restrictions should be ruled out with lateral and antero-posterior radiographs. Neurologic assessment (e.g., reflexes, clonus, etc) must be performed, while an instrumented gait analysis may be used to confirm the diagnosis and define the patients' functional limitations or disabilities (18,19).

To measure the subtalar joint range of motion and neutral subtalar joint position, the examiner draws a vertical bisection line on the posterior aspect of the heel (calcaneus) and the posterior leg. When the foot is maximally supinated and pronated, the degree of calcaneal inversion and eversion is measured with a goniometer on the posterior heel and leg reference lines. Ideally, the subtalar joint neutral position will demonstrate co-linear heel and leg lines. Patients commonly have a neutral position in which the heel bisection is inverted relative to the leg bisection, termed *subtalar varus*. This position may compensate during posture and locomotion via pronation of the subtalar joint to an extent similar to the varus deformity.

Forefoot position can be observed by noting the relationship of the forefoot to rearfoot reference lines. Inverted (varus) and everted (valgus) forefoot positions reflect the structural relationship of the midtarsal joint orientation to the ankle/subtalar joint complex (hindfoot). Forefoot varus deformities can compensate via foot pronation, and rigid forefoot valgus deformities may compensate via a supinatory foot function during posture and locomotion.

Deformities and conditions affecting the first ray are often associated with the first ray position. Elevation deformities of the first ray (metatarsus primus elevatus) generally lead to increased stress on the first MTP joint, which may promote accelerated OA changes. Plantarflexion deformities of the first ray (metatarsus primus equinus) may produce increased pressure or stress beneath the first metatarsal head, which can result in painful submetatarsal head pathology.

Another arthrometric measurement that should be performed is the first MTP joint range of motion. Utilizing a goniometer, the hinge is placed at the medial center of the first MTP joint with each arm centered along the long axes of the hallux and first metatarsal. The end range of available dorsiflexion is then measured with the patient prone and the subtalar joint in neutral position. When dorsiflexion ranges are 60° or less, the patient may be at risk of developing OA due to jamming of the joint during the propulsive phase of gait.

Standing. A weight-bearing postural appraisal of the patient is performed in the frontal, sagittal, and transverse planes. The patient's foot alignment and balance should be carefully assessed. With the patient in quiet standing, the base of support, transverse plane foot angle, and posterior leg to rearfoot alignment should be evaluated. The *base of support* is measured as the distance between the medial malleoli, and normally spans 2–5 cm. Larger values are associated with genu valgum deformities or postural instability. The *transverse plane foot angle* is normally 5° to 10° abducted, as measured by the arc between the foot (second toe axis) and the midline of the body. Measured or observed angles of greater than 10° may be associated

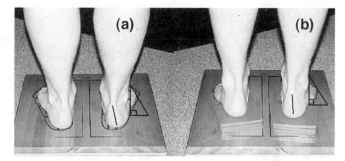

Figure 3. Lateral malleolar index (LMI) and block balance testing: LMI is the deviation from a right triangle to the lateral malleolus (a). With the patient in a comfortable base of support and transverse plane foot angle, note the excessive LMI and valgus resting calcaneal stance position (RCSP). With appropriate wedges of material inserted plantarly (b), note the improvement in LMI and RCSP.

with externally rotated femoral or tibial torsion deformities and with hyperpronated (abducted) foot positions. Pronation of the subtalar joint is clinically observed with calcaneal eversion angles greater than 4° as measured from a posterior calcaneal reference line (bisection) relative to the supporting surface (transverse plane). This closed kinetic chain goniometric measurement, known as resting calcaneal stance position, is one of the few clinical foot alignment measures with good intrarater (0.92) and interrater (0.75) reliability (20).

The degree and severity of pronation also can be determined by the measured amount of medial drift of the lateral malleolus relative to the lateral heel border. This measurement, referred to as the *lateral malleolar index,* allows the practitioner to obtain the optimal rearfoot balance position when prescribing foot orthoses by aligning the lateral malleolus with the lateral heel fat pad so that a colinear relationship exists (21) (Figure 3). As the subtalar joint is manually placed in the optimal "neutral" balance position, alignment changes of the legs, as well as changes in knee position should be observed. Based on exam findings performed with the patient at rest, the practitioner can also place firm material wedges under the forefoot, midfoot, or rearfoot until the ideal foot and limb posture is obtained. This technique allows the practitioner to observe the corrected balance position that orthosis management will attain (22).

To help determine if the patient has hallux limitus, and is at risk of developing the more painful and debilitating condition, hallux rigidus, the *hubscher maneuver* is performed. With the patient in quiet standing, the examiner dorsiflexes the hallux to its end range of motion. Ideally the patient will demonstrate 65° or greater dorsiflexion with an increase in arch height (via the Windlass mechanism). A patient with functional hallux limitus will not achieve 65° of dorsiflexion in weight-bearing, yet may have normal range of motion in the open kinetic chain. After realignment with foot orthoses, the patient may have improved hallux dorsiflexion in weight-bearing, indicating that the big toe joint may be better protected from degenerative joint disease.

Gait. To help the practitioner appreciate the dynamic interrelationships of the ankle and foot joints during walking, an observational gait evaluation of the lower extremities should be performed. The examiner should note limping, antalgic, rigid, apropulsive, or guarded gait patterns. The knee, ankle, and rearfoot positions and the angle and base of gait should also be assessed. Finally, the ankle and foot motions should be care-

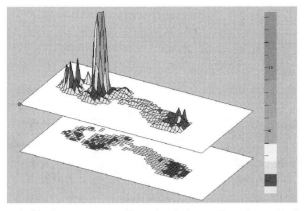

Figure 4. Maximum pressure throughout stance phase in a patient with hammer toe deformities on the second and third digits. Pressures ≥10 kg/cm² in gait are considered pathologic.

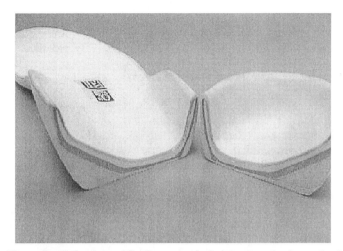

Figure 5. Orthosis modifications may include a deep heel cup, heel elevation, and medial skive technique for enhanced balance and foot alignment.
- Neutral subtalar frontal plane posting (when possible)
- Extended flanges for greater transverse plane stability
- Modest heel elevation to reduce ankle equinus stress
- First metatarsal head cut-out with kinetic wedge to improve first ray function associated with functional hallux limitus
- Deep heel cup with medial (Kirby) heel skive technique for cases with hyperpronation (23)

fully scrutinized. As the patient's foot first strikes the ground, is the heel inverted, perpendicular, or everted? Does the heel remain in a fixed everted position, indicating maximally pronated foot function during gait? When viewing in the sagittal plane, does the patient exhibit early heel off, indicative of an ankle equinus? Does the arch height remain unchanged or does it lower significantly in midstance? Can the patient obtain 65° of first MTP joint dorsiflexion during propulsion?

Patients with a severe or complex rheumatic disease may benefit from a computerized gait analysis, which can provide valuable information contributing to a differential diagnosis, treatment plan, prognosis, and treatment efficacy determination. Figure 4 depicts the maximum pressure throughout stance phase in the barefoot condition for a patient with rigid hammer toes, as measured with a pedobarograph. Pressures in excess of 10 kg/cm² during comfortable cadence locomotion are considered pathologic. Mechanically induced metatarsalgia, a common condition associated with RA, can cause significant pain in the patient.

CONSERVATIVE THERAPIES

Orthosis Management

Many posture and gait patterns associated with osseous and soft tissue malalignments of the foot may be eliminated or minimized with correctly balanced *orthoses*, devices that correct maladjustments of the body. By modifying foot alignment and gait, orthoses can relieve symptomatic stress on the lower extremities through control of excessive or inadequate motion at specific joints.

Foot orthoses can be categorized as rigid, semi-rigid, or flexible and are selected based on the patient's needs. Rigid orthoses should be considered for patients requiring greater biomechanical control, as they reduce unwanted motion and help maintain the desired alignment. For patients who require improved foot alignment but want to maintain some degree of motion, the use of a semi-rigid device may be warranted. Patients who need protective accommodation for osseous deformity or lesions will generally do best with flexible orthoses.

The primary goals of orthosis management should be to reduce pain; limit motion of painful, inflamed, or unstable joints; and slow or arrest progression of deformity. Orthoses

may also help to redistribute forces from high to low pressure areas, reduce shock and shear loading, correct positional (flexible) joint malalignments, accommodate fixed (rigid) deformities, and reduce abnormal shoe wear.

The type and shape of the orthosis and the degree of posting necessary is based on clinical measurements of the foot, postural and gait assessment, and the severity of radiographic changes. Patients with changes in the ankles and feet due to OA will generally demonstrate numerous joint malalignments associated with pathologic pronation. For example, increased stress in the medial column of the foot with pronation may lead to continuous jamming of the first MTP joint during the propulsive phase of gait. For this reason, orthosis management must restore both rearfoot alignment and first ray function. Specific features of orthoses for pronatory patients with OA changes in the feet are illustrated in Figure 5.

For patients with rheumatic disease associated with significant foot deformity, orthoses should provide stability to unstable or inflamed joints and should also address accommodative or protective needs for osseous deformity, nodules, and splayed metatarsals with associated bunion deformities. In addition to the features mentioned in Figure 5, the orthosis prescription should include a cushioned top liner material to protect lesions and inflamed or irritated areas, as well as accommodative submetatarsal head apertures to off-load prominent or plantarflexed metatarsals.

When complete resolution of symptoms may not be possible, the outcome measure should reflect the patient's expectations within the constraints of a realistic prognosis. For example, a realistic goal of orthotic therapy in a patient with chronic OA may be to reduce foot pain by 30–50%.

The extent to which correlated and compensatory motions (supinatory or pronatory) will occur depend on the severity and type of foot or limb deformity and the specific joint axis orientations. Several studies have demonstrated an association between foot and ankle malalignment and lower extremity pathology. For example, excessive foot pronation may be associated the development of patello-femoral syndrome (23). Studies also have demonstrated that excessively pronated or supinated foot types are more susceptible to knee pain than neutral foot types (24). Fewer studies, however, have demonstrated the relationship between improved foot and ankle realignment therapies and reduction of foot or limb pathology. A double-blind, randomized clinical trial of people with recently diagnosed RA found that subjects who used a neutral positioned foot orthosis were 73% less likely to develop hallux valgus deformity than those who used a placebo orthosis (25).

Treatment of hallux abductovalgus deformity should be based on an evaluation of the pattern, degree, and reducibility of deformity. Mild deformities that are minimally deviated with a hallux abductovalgus angle of 15° to 25° and easily reducible should be treated conservatively. Moderate deformities demonstrating a malalignment angle of 25° to 35°, mild subluxation, or mild to moderate tracking of the joint will generally require a combined orthodigital and surgical (soft tissue rebalancing) approach. Advanced to severe hallux abductovalgus deformities of 35° or greater, with a nonreducible trackbound first MTP joint, will usually require soft tissue and osseous reconstructive surgery. Following surgery, orthosis management and retentive orthodigital measures should be employed to maintain correction and prevent future recurrence. When surgical intervention is not an option, accommodative shoe prescription and protective shielding may be used (26).

FOOTWEAR CONSIDERATIONS

Many people with arthritis have some type of foot problem during their lives. RA and the connective tissue diseases affect the forefoot more frequently than the rearfoot. The loss of connective tissue strength produced by repetitive inflammation of the periarticular structures can result in the development of a number of malalignments, deformities, and mechanical problems. Feet affected in this manner need a wide, high toe box with soft compliant material that does not irritate the toes and can accommodate deformities such as bunions or splayed feet. A loss of plantar fat, which protects the metatarsal heads, requires the use of soft protective inserts or orthotics specifically designed to shift weight from the forefoot to the midfoot. Proper shoe sizing, including adequate heel width, instep height, toe box depth, and forefoot width, is essential for a good clinical outcome. Orthotics or inserts take up significant space in the shoe and should always be worn when trying on new shoes to ensure a proper fit.

Osteoarthritis affects the first MTP joint and rearfoot more often. Inherent skeletal malalignments or secondary OA in the presence of repetitive microtrauma produce joint restriction, periarticular hypertrophy, and destruction of articular cartilage. This tends to restrict motion at the involved joint or produce pain with range of motion that will require foot orthoses, sole modifications to alter gait, or restrictive bracing to prevent motion and the resultant pain. Shoes must accommodate orthoses and have the appropriate sole design to facilitate a smooth, pain-free gait.

When considering footwear for patients with arthritis, one typically chooses boxy, in-depth shoes. However, a number of choices exist depending on the degree of foot deformity and the specific goals of the therapy. Shoe choices are also restricted

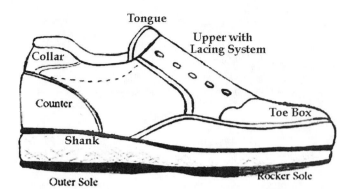

Figure 6. Foot segments and shoe design.

by nonmedical considerations such as style, color, and feel of the shoe. Men's shoes are roomier and closer in style to the shoes commonly prescribed for moderate to severe foot deformity. Women often have to sacrifice a great deal of style to have a shoe with a firm supportive heel counter, reinforced midfoot, and wide roomy toe box (Figure 6). If a prescription orthotic or a cushioned inner sole is added to a narrow, high-heeled woman's shoe such as a pump, it will often make the toe box tight and the shoe so bulky that the patient is unable to wear it. Women with wide or splayed feet, or those who are developing bunions or "hammer toes" have a difficult time finding shoes that will accommodate their condition.

The key to foot comfort is preventing the development of stress or irritation. Shoes need to support areas of instability and protect areas of deformity. The back or heel of the shoe is often reinforced by stiff leather or cardboard-like materials and is referred to as the *counter*. The counter helps keep the heel bone vertical and resist the tendency to roll inward with weight bearing. The *collar* of the shoe extends forward along the top of the counter to the laces and is often padded to help protect the ankle bone from irritation. The sole of the shoe should be reinforced in the back by a stiff piece of plastic or metal referred to as the *shank*. This keeps the shoe from bending in the middle and provides most of the shoe's midfoot or arch support.

The remaining support for the midfoot comes from the lacing or fastening system of the shoe. Laces are the best way to adjust the shoe to allow for swelling and achieve a snug fit. Velcro closure or elastic laces are acceptable alternatives if the patient has hand involvement that prevents lacing. These features are important because they help the shoe contain or restrain a foot that often wants to deform and produce pain.

The front of the shoe is called the *toe box* and must be sufficiently flexible to allow for toe movement. It should be roomy enough to prevent crowding of the digits. Insufficient toe box room can not only affect circulation but lead to nail pathology and hard callus or corns forming on the toes.

The shoe should be constructed of good quality leather or soft breathable material to allow it to stretch easily around digital deformities. Patients with arthritis need extra padding or cushioning for the ball or widest part of the foot. It is often best to purchase a shoe with a removable innersole, so that a softer or more supportive orthosis may be easily incorporated.

Patients should be provided with all the information necessary to make an informed choice about their shoes. The individual is usually the best judge of whether something hurts or not. Every patient with developing arthritis should be seen by

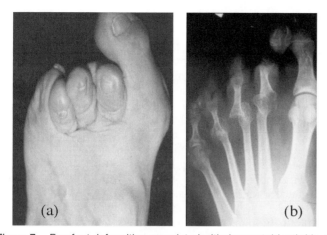

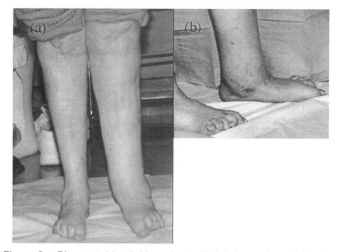

Figure 7. Forefoot deformities associated with rheumatoid arthritis. **a,** Clinical photo demonstrating dorsal contracture of toes 2, 3, and 4 and hallux valgus. **b,** Antero-posterior radiograph demonstrating dislocation of the 2nd, 3rd, and 4th metatarsal proximal phalangeal joints.

Figure 8. Rheumatoid arthritis patient with left foot valgus deformity. **a,** Note valgus malalignment at the knee as well. **b,** Medial view demonstrates medial column collapse.

a podiatrist or other foot health professional to determine their foot type and advise them on any potential problems facing them in the future. People with existing foot pain may also benefit from a discussion about footwear options to help them function with less discomfort. If a clinician is not comfortable recommending shoes for patients, it is appropriate to refer them to a podiatric physician or pedorthist specially trained to help with the decision.

SURGICAL TREATMENT

Rheumatoid Arthritis

RA is the most common inflammatory arthropathy that leads to foot and ankle problems. In one study, 93 of 99 patients had foot and ankle involvement at some time since their diagnosis, and over 50% of the patients had foot and ankle problems at any given time (27). The most common problematic areas for patients with RA are the forefoot, ankle, and rearfoot. In the forefoot, subluxation of the MTP joints with prominence of the metatarsal heads is the primary problem (Figure 7). Surgical treatment involves resection arthroplasty with excision of metatarsal heads 2–5. The base of the proximal phalanx is maintained, and severe digital deformities should be corrected (28). For the first MTP joint, the options are arthrodesis, implant arthroplasty, or resection of the first metatarsal head. The choice of procedure depends on the overall foot structure, location of the pain, and extent of deformity. Improvement with respect to shoe wear, pain, and the ability to stand and walk are typical goals for this surgery. Because loss of the MTP joints is accomplished with this surgery, the procedure is limited to patients who have significant, advanced disease and are already apropulsive.

Valgus foot deformities can occur in the rearfoot, often in conjunction with failure of the tibialis posterior tendon, resulting in severe abduction of the midtarsal joint and severe calcaneal eversion (Figure 8). Patients with RA are best treated with some combination of fusion procedures, such as double arthrodesis of the midtarsal joint or triple arthrodesis (29).

The ankle is frequently a site of severe pain in patients with RA. Surgical stabilization by means of fusion can restore alignment and significantly reduce pain. Frequently, because of the deterioration of the rearfoot joints, a pantalar (i.e., ankle, subtalar, and midtarsal joints) fusion may be necessary.

People with RA require specific surgical considerations. Because bone density may be decreased from a lack of use or prior corticosteroid therapy, purchase of screws may be inadequate. Stabilization by means of Steinmann pins or staples may be preferable in the midfoot. A locking intramedulary nail may be used to stabilize the subtalar and ankle joints (Figure 9). Immobilization support may be necessary for a longer period of time in RA patients until adequate structural stability is obtained.

Osteoarthritis

For OA, a broader array of options is available. The first MTP joint is frequently involved, resulting in hallux limitus. Treat-

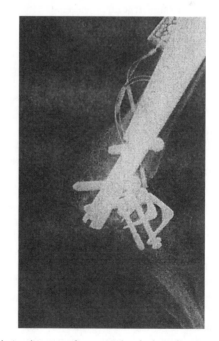

Figure 9. Lateral x-ray after pantalar fusion demonstrating staple, screw, and intramedullary nail fixation.

ment choices include simple resection of hypertrophic bone, reconstruction by means of shortening or plantar flexor osteotomy, resection arthroplasty such as the Keller procedure for resection of the base of the proximal phalanx, single- or double-sided implant arthroplasty, or arthrodesis. Single-sided silicone implant arthroplasty is no longer recommended. Although a number of dual component implants are now available, the long-term efficacy remains to be seen. For OA in other areas of the foot, such as the tarsometatarsal joints or the midtarsal or subtalar joints, fusion is the usual procedure if there is significant loss of cartilage. Debridement of hypertrophic bone formation may occasionally be adequate.

The ankle may be surgically treated by resection arthroplasty of the hypertrophic bone, mosaic plasty for replacement of deteriorated cartilage with autologous cartilage grafts, and arthrodesis. Recently, implant arthroplasty has become popular again. Although these implants have been used in Europe for some time, the long-term efficacy remains to be seen (30).

MECHANICALLY INDUCED SKIN AND SOFT TISSUE CHANGES

Patients with RA, partially as a result of interosseous muscle atrophy, lose their ability to plantar flex the proximal phalanges of the toes, allowing the long extensors to dominate and causing hammered digits. As a sequela of this deformity, the metatarsal fat pad frequently becomes displaced distally under the toes, allowing the metatarsals and interdigital nerves to be subjected to increased contact stress during locomotion. Interdigital neuralgia or Morton's neuroma and metatarsalgia frequently develop as a consequence.

As a protective mechanism to diminish the loading on skin, soft tissue, and bone, adventitial bursae may develop as a soft tissue replacement for the loss of the metatarsal fat pad. Most bursae develop around the head of the first metatarsal medially to protect the soft tissue structures associated with rheumatoid bunion deformity. These lesions also develop beneath the heads of the lesser metatarsals.

In addition, as a consequence of retrograde metatarsal loading to the plantar skin, the patient may develop painful corns and calluses over the ball of the foot. *Corns* are characterized by a sharply circumscribed keratinous funnel shaped plug, which extends through most of the underlying dermis. *Calluses*, in contrast, lack a central plug and have a more even appearance. Corns are usually the more painful, because the plug pressure induces the formation of fibrous scarring within the dermis, dermal nerve thickening, and at times mild inflammation within the dermis. The latter occurs when the plug ruptures and evokes a foreign body tissue response. Calluses, while painful, do not exhibit the severity of dermal changes and therefore tend to be less symptomatic. The presence of dried blood or old hemorrhage within callus is seen on occasion in patients with RA. These collections of dried blood usually suggest the presence of associated angiitis seen in late-stage RA. Precipitated by increased metatarsal pressure on an underlying fragile inflamed vasculature (angiitis), these vessels rupture and extravasate blood within the overlying callus. These patients frequently exhibit associated vasculitic skin change around the digits called *Bywaters lesions*.

Treatment

Conservative treatment options of these structural alterations consist of the use of accommodative foot orthoses. Because 90% of these alterations affect the forefoot, biomechanical off-loading to this area is the focus. Orthoses are modified to provide a substitute for loss of the plantar fat pad by using a combination of materials that exhibit shock attenuation and energy return. Decreasing interdigital nerve contact stress, metatarsal callus, and adventitial metatarsal bursa formation is accomplished by prescribing in-shoe build-ups or orthoses that include a longitudinal arch with a metatarsal bar. Metatarsal bars attached to the soles of shoes redistribute the load from the ball of the foot toward the toes. They are also used to relieve symptoms in more severe cases, but a rocker sole is preferred when cosmetically acceptable to the patient. Painful callus caused by hammer toe and bunion deformities requires shoes with a large toe box. A shoe that has a super wide shank with depth inlay, a depth inlay (contour last), or a custom-molded shoe should be prescribed to accommodate severely deformed feet. Use of latex or silicone toe shields is helpful in reducing pain from severe deformities. Inter-metatarsal joint corticosteroid injections using a combination of soluble and insoluble steroids should be used judiciously when dealing with inflammatory metatarsal joint synovitis, bursitis, or interdigital neuralgia. These injections are best given dorsally, parallel to the metatarsal heads at approximately a 45° angle, with the needle gradually inserted plantar and distally. Triamcinolone acetonide (5–10 mg) and dexamethasone phosphate (2 mg) mixed with lidocaine 2% (30 mg) per interspace helps relieve these symptoms. In advanced recalcitrant deformity, surgery may provide dramatic relief.

REFERENCES

1. Lawrence RC, Helmick CG, Arnett FC, Dayo RA, Felson DT, Giannini EH, et al. Estimates of the prevalence of arthritis and selected musculoskeletal disorders in the United States. Arthritis Rheum 1998;41:778–99.
2. Engle A. Osteoarthritis in adults by selected demographic characteristics, United States-1960-1962. Vital Health Stat 1966;11:20.
3. Lawrence JS, Bremner JM, Bier F. Osteo-arthrosis. Prevalence in the population and relationship between symptoms and x-ray changes. Ann Rheum Dis 1966;25:1–24.
4. Cushnaghan J, Dieppe P. Study of 500 patients with limb joint osteoarthritis. I. Analysis by age, sex, and distribution of symptomatic joint sites. Ann Rheum Dis 1991;50:8–13.
5. Brower DJ, Hillstrom HJ, Song J, Kahler MA, Zonay LJ, Schumacher HR. Lower extremity malalignment incidence in knee osteoarthritis. Arthritis Rheum 1997;40(9Suppl);S174.
6. Inman VT. The joints of the ankle. Baltimore: Williams & Wilkins; 1976, pp xii, 117.
7. Lundberg A, Goldie I, Kalin B, Selvik G. Kinematics of the ankle/foot complex: plantarflexion and dorsiflexion. Foot Ankle 1989;9:194–200.
8. Lundberg A, Svensson OK, Bylund C, Goldie I, Selvik G. Kinematics of the ankle/foot complex. Part 2: Pronation and supination. Foot Ankle 1989;9:248–53.
9. Lundberg A, Svensson OK, Bylund C, Slevik G. Kinematics of the ankle/foot complex. Part 3: Influence of leg rotation. Foot Ankle 1989;9:304–9.
10. Riegger-Krugh C, Keysor JJ. Skeletal malalignments of the lower quarter: correlated and compensatory motions and postures. J Orthop Sports Phys Ther 1996;23:164–70.
11. Dananberg HJ. Gait style as an etiology to chronic postural pain. Part I. Functional hallux limitus. J Am Podiatr Med Assoc 1993;83:433–41.
12. Dananberg HJ. Gait style as an etiology to chronic postural pain. Part II. Postural compensatory process. J Am Podiatr Med Assoc 1993;83:615–24.
13. Song J, Hillstrom HJ, Secord D, Levitt J. Foot type biomechanics. Comparison of planus and rectus foot types. J Am Podiatr Med Assoc 1996;86:16–23.

14. Root ML, Orien W, Weed JH. Normal and abnormal function of the foot. Vol. 2. Los Angeles: Clinical Biomechanics Corporation; 1977.
15. Green DR, Carol A. Planal dominance. J Am Podiatry Assoc 1984;74: 98–103.
16. Whitney A, Whitney K. Anterior cavus foot problems. In: Jay RM, editor. Current therapy in podiatric surgery. Philadelphia: B.C. Decker; 1989, pp. 230–41.
17. Silfverskiold N. Reduction of the uncrossed two-joint muscles of the leg to one-joint muscles in spastic condition. Acta Orthopaedica Scandinavica 1924;56:315–30.
18. Maurer BT, Siegler S, Hillstrom HJ, et al. Quantitative identification of ankle equinus with applications for treatment assessment. Gait & Posture 1995;3:19–28.
19. Hillstrom HJ, Perlberg G, Siegler S, Sanner WH, Hice GA, Downey M, et al. Objective identification of ankle equinus deformity and resulting contracture. J Am Podiatr Med Assoc 1991;81:519–24.
20. Diamond J, Mueller MJ, Delitto A, Sinacore DR. Reliability of a diabetic foot evaluation. Phys Ther 1989;69:797–802.
21. Sanner W. The functional foot orthosis prescription. In: Jay RM, editor. Current therapy in podiatric surgery. Philadelphia: B.C. Decker; 1989, pp. 302–7.
22. Whitney A, Whitney K. Orthodigita techniques. In: Principles and practice of podiatric medicine. New York: Churchill Livingstone; 1990, pp. 693–707.
23. Bennett P. A randomised clinical assessment of foot pronation and its relationship to patello-femoral syndrome. Aust Pod 1988;6–9.
24. Dahle L, Mueller M, Delitto A, Diamond J. Visual assessment of foot type and lower extremity injury. J Orthop Sports Phys Ther 1991;14:70–4.
25. Budiman-Mak E, Conrad K, Roach K, et al. Can orthoses prevent hallux valgus deformity in rheumatoid arthritis? A randomized clinical trial. J Clin Rheumatol 1995;1:313–21.
26. Whitney A, Whitney K. Orthodigital evaluation and therapeutic management of digital deformity. In: Hallux valgus surgery. New York: Churchill Livingstone; 1993.
27. Michelson J, Easley M, Wigley FM, et al. Foot and ankle problems in rheumatoid arthritis. Foot Ankle Int 1994;15:608–13.
28. Coughlin MJ. Rheumatoid forefoot reconstruction. A long-term follow-up study. J Bone Joint Surg Am 2000;82:322–41.
29. Schuberth JM. Pedal fusions in the rheumatoid patient. Clin Podiatr Med Surg 1988;5:227–47.
30. Kofoed H, Sorensen TS. Ankle arthroplasty for rheumatoid arthritis and osteoarthritis: prospective long-term study of cemented replacements. J Bone Joint Surg Br 1998;80:328–32.

CHAPTER 31

Lower Extremity Conservative Realignment Therapies and Ambulatory Aids

H.J. HILLSTROM, PhD; K. WHITNEY, DPM; J. McGUIRE, DPM, PT;
D.J. BROWER, BA; C. RIEGGER-KRUGH, ScD, PT;
and H. RALPH SCHUMACHER, MD

When treating patients with rheumatic disease that involves the load-bearing joints, a thorough assessment of lower extremity alignment is an important component of the clinical exam. Before selecting a conservative therapy or ambulatory aid for the patient, determining the biomechanical integrity of the lower extremity, including stability, malalignments, deformities, and movement performance, is imperative for successful treatment. A thorough understanding of these biomechanical concepts is just as important as making the physical assessments in achieving this goal.

SKELETAL ALIGNMENT

When alignment is normal, the force of weight bearing is transmitted from the center of the femoral head and neck through the center of the knee and ankle as a kinetic chain (1). The lower extremity can exhibit a spectrum of alignments within which an ideal or neutral position exists. Malalignment is defined by the degree of deviation from this neutral position. Irreversible osseous or soft-tissue deformity does not generally occur until the skeletal structures approach significant levels of malalignment. In various malalignments of the lower extremity, the forces passing through the joints may be directed away from the ideal position and concentrated in other regions of the joint that are ill-equipped to handle the stress. For example, in varus knee osteoarthritis (OA), the joint reaction force is more medially directed, resulting in excessive wear across the medial tibio-femoral joint (1,2). Frontal, transverse, and sagittal plane malalignments in OA patients are common (3–10).

Malalignment can be assessed with visual observations of gait and with static measurements taken from radiographs and clinical examinations, all of which are largely subjective. Static measurements such as radiographs may not correlate with dynamic lower extremity function (11).

CORRELATED AND COMPENSATORY MOTIONS AND POSTURES

Correlated motions and postures occur in direct response to changes in dynamic and static skeletal alignment (12). They are linked motions in adjacent or distant joints from the site of original alignment change. Compensatory motions and postures develop in response to this skeletal malpositioning and correlated movements as an attempt to optimize neuromuscu-

loskeletal function. Neuromuscular disorders often result in compensatory motions and postures at multiple locations along the kinetic chain (12,13). Lower extremity malalignments at regions other than the site of primary pathology have been observed at the tibio-femoral (14) and patello-femoral (15) joints.

GENERAL EVALUATION AND TREATMENT CONSIDERATIONS

The condition of a joint depends upon structural (alignment, deformity, flexibility), functional (limitations in posture, locomotion, and activities of daily living), immunologic, and biochemical factors as well as a history of trauma. The biomechanical integrity of a joint includes assessment of stability, alignment, deformity, and movement performance. *Stability* refers to the quality of a joint's flexibility in rotation and translation (e.g., excessive anterior drawer indicative of anterior cruciate ligament pathology). *Alignment* refers to the relative osseous positioning of a joint, which may be modifiable by soft-tissue contracture or laxity (e.g., genu varum). *Deformity*, often occurring at the extremes of malalignment, refers to a fixed osseous malposition (e.g., coxa vara).

To ensure proper treatment for the patient with arthritis involving the lower extremities, a comprehensive clinical exam that includes these concepts is highly recommended. Close attention to the lower extremity alignment in the context of the whole body is essential. Distinguishing between osseous malpositioning and soft-tissue contracture or laxity is important. In the unstable joint, an aberrant instant joint center over the range of motion may compromise cartilage function, such as squeeze film lubrication. Important coupled motions within a given joint may also be altered, which may increase stress at other sites within the kinetic chain (lower extremity).

JOINT BIOMECHANICS

Instant Joint Center

As 2 congruent bones move, at each instant in time there is a theoretical point between the bones of zero motion referred to as the *instant center* (axis of rotation). A joint's instant center of rotation depends largely upon the osseous geometries. The healthy knee has an instant joint center of rotation that describes a "C"-shaped pattern (analogous to a moving hinge) over the range of sagittal plane motion. Injuries to one or more structures, such as a ligament, will significantly affect this instant center and compromise joint stability. A deranged instant center may promote excessive compression or distraction motions within the joint, as opposed to the normally gliding movements that are desired (16).

The Diarthrodial Joint, Cartilage, and Squeeze Film Lubrication

The diarthrodial joint is the essential component that allows humans to exhibit large ranges of motion between limb segments and hence perform purposeful movements. It comprises the subchondral bone of 2 opposing osseous structures, a 1–5 mm layer of articular cartilage on the load-bearing surfaces of each bone, synovial fluid (primarily a high molecular weight hyaluronic acid), and a capsule that encases these structures.

Articular cartilage contains no blood vessels, nerves, or lymph elements, yet it may withstand the repetitive stresses imposed within a joint over the average person's lifetime. It is structurally composed of chondrocytes and an organic matrix, which includes primarily type II collagen, proteoglycans, water, and to a lesser extent, inorganic salts, lipids, and matrix and glycoproteins.

Articular cartilage has 2 important tasks: 1) to distribute the load across the joint surfaces to minimize stress, and 2) to allow relative movement of the opposing joint surface with minimal friction and wear. As the joint is loaded, articular cartilage is compressed and self-lubricating. While undergoing a joint movement, synovial fluid is exuded from the region of joint contact to elsewhere within the joint space. As the region of joint contact becomes unloaded and contact is abandoned, synovial fluid is imbibed back into the articular cartilage. This transient response to deformation is often referred to as "squeeze film" lubrication. For normal rates of loading, this mechanism may actually help attenuate shock to underlying structures, but when the rate of loading exceeds flow response (e.g., repetitive impact), damage to cartilage is likely (16,17).

LOWER EXTREMITY BIOMECHANICS

Planar Dominance

Planar dominance is the plane of greatest motion for a given joint and is determined by the orientation of the joint rotation axis. The osseous and soft-tissue architecture, or foot type, is a major determinant of foot and ankle function. When the axis orientation of the subtalar joint tends to vertical, an increase in transverse plane motion results. A more horizontal (i.e., anterior–posterior) axis orientation produces increased frontal plane motion.

Eccentrically Loaded Columns

Patients with knee OA often exhibit either genu varum or genu valgum. These patients may present with several correlated and compensatory lower extremity malalignments, such as hip abduction, limb length discrepancy, or varus forefoot, that are associated with the primary pathology (12). A lower extremity

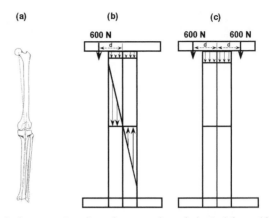

Figure 1. Lower extremity column analogy (adapted from 18): **a,** an osseous schematic of the tibiofemoral joint; **b,** an eccentrically loaded column that imposes both vertical and bending moment stresses; and **c,** if the vertical load is doubled but symmetrically distributed, then no bending moment and reduced total compressive stress results.

malalignment can increase or reduce stress, as well as alter the location of stress, within the knee.

Consider the analogy of a column as a lower extremity (18), (Figure 1). Figure 1a is a schematic of the lower extremity osseous structures without the foot and ankle. As shown in Figure 1b, a column is eccentrically loaded in an architecturally similar manner to the lower extremity. The vertical load divided by the column cross-sectional area imposes a compressive stress. Because the load is eccentrically located with respect to the midline of the lower extremity, an additional bending moment is generated. By definition, a compressive stress on the loaded side of the column is counterbalanced with a tensile stress on the opposite side (indicated by arrows). The bending moment stress is proportional in magnitude to the moment arm about which the eccentric load is applied. Varus knee deformity exacerbates this phenomenon by increasing the bending moment arm. The net compressive stress experienced on the medial aspect of the column (lower extremity) is the sum of the vertical and bending moment compressive stresses. As shown in Figure 1c, if the vertical load is doubled but symmetrically distributed, then no bending moment stress results. Even though the compressive stress due to vertical loading is twice that of Figure 1b, the net compressive stress is much lower because no bending moment is generated.

Figure 2 represents a static equilibrium diagram based on a frontal plane knee radiograph of a patient with varus knee OA. The typical medial joint space narrowing of the tibio-femoral joint is illustrated for this patient's left knee. The force from the mass of the body supported by the knee (Fm) and the force from the lateral musculotendinous and ligamentous tension band components (Ft) form the resultant force (Fr). That resultant force is directed at the medial compartment. The external varus knee moment (Fm * y) must be counterbalanced by an internal valgus knee moment (Ft * x) to maintain static equilibrium. Healthy individuals with well-aligned knee joints have no medial joint space narrowing, and the resultant force (Fr) is more centrally located within the tibio-femoral joint.

The foot and ankle contain 28 bones, 33 joints, and 112 ligaments (19). The large number of degrees of freedom within the foot and ankle permit a wide variety of architectural alignments or foot types. As described by Song et al, pes planus (low arch) foot types have significantly different static and

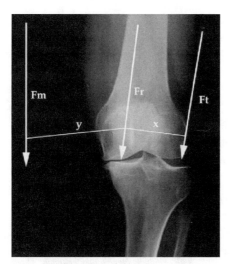

Figure 2. Static equilibrium representation of the varus knee in the frontal plane. Fm = force from the mass of the body supported by the knee; Ft = force from the lateral musculotendinous and ligamentous tension band components; Fr = resultant force; x = moment arm of Ft; and y = moment arm of Fm. Note the excessively medial position of the resultant force in the varus knee.

Table 1. Normative values of passive joint range of motion.

Joints	Planes of motion		
	Sagittal Ext(+):Flx(−)	Frontal Var(+):Valg(−)	Transverse Int(+):Ext(−)
Hip	+15°:−140°	+30°:−25°	+70°:−90°
Knee	+0°:−140°	+2°:−2°	+30°:−45°
Ankle	+20°:−35°		
Subtalar		+20°:−5°	
First MTPJ*	+90°:−30°		

* MTPJ = metatarsophalangeal joint

dynamic function compared with rectus (ideally aligned) foot types (20). Most of the literature examining the relationship between lower extremity malalignment and OA does not include the foot and ankle in free body diagrams (21–27). Since foot and ankle alignment affects the distal tibia, it is unlikely that tibio-femoral alignment is functionally independent of the foot and ankle.

Coupled Motions

Motions within a joint or a family of joints may be coupled across anatomic planes. *Coupling* refers to motions that are imposed in one plane as a result of motion in another plane (i.e., a correlated motion within a joint). An example of this phenomenon is the screw home mechanism. In healthy knees, the medial femoral condyle is 1.7 cm longer than the lateral, which forces the tibia to externally rotate during knee extension in the open kinetic chain. The Helfet test for screw home integrity requires drawing one vertical bisecting line on the patellar and the other on the tibial tuberosity. As the knee extends, the tibial tuberosity bisection should rotate laterally indicating that the tibia externally rotated (16).

BIOMECHANICAL INTEGRITY ASSESSMENT

One of the keys to successful treatment of OA and other rheumatic diseases is a comprehensive assessment of the biomechanical integrity of the lower extremity. This includes determining joint stability, lower extremity alignment, deformity, and movement performance.

Joint Stability

If one or more ligamentous structures are partially or completely ruptured, joint instability will result. These passive restraints to the joint system comprise much of what clinicians perceive as flexibility or stiffness when examining a patient's passive range of motion. Additional stability may be offered in both the passive and active contractile states by the musculotendinous structures. For these reasons, every lower extremity biomechanical exam should include manual muscle testing, passive joint range of motion, and manual ligament stress tests. Manual muscle testing is conducted by resisting each muscle's primary action during a concentric contraction and grading the strength (28).

Passive joint range of motion assessment is conducted with the patient in the supine position in each plane that a joint is expected to have movement. Only a 1° resolution goniometer should be used. During this exam, one should note joint crepitus and effusion. Table 1 shows normative values (16).

Stress tests must be performed to determine ligamentous instability. Strong ligaments acting about the anterior, posterior, medial, and lateral compartments stabilize the knee. In the frontal plane, the collateral ligaments provide resistance to excessive motion. A valgus stress test may be conducted with the patient supine and the knee slightly flexed to unlock from full extension. The examiner secures the ankle with one hand while placing the other hand on the fibular head and pushes medially against the knee and laterally against the ankle (i.e., implementing a 3-point bending). The varus stress test is literally the reverse; that is, pushing the knee laterally. Medial or lateral "gapping" in the direction of applied stress indicates frontal plane instability.

Joint stability in the sagittal plane is maintained by the anterior (ACL) and posterior (PCL) cruciate ligaments. The anterior drawer sign is evaluated with the patient supine, knee flexed to 90°, and feet flat on the table. The examiner stabilizes the foot by sitting on it; then cupping the hands around posterior knee with thumbs placed on the joint lines, draws the tibia towards him or her. The posterior drawer test is the reverse, whereby the tibia is pushed away from the examiner. When 1 cm or greater displacement is elicited, a ligament laxity is suspected.

The Ortolani click test can be used to evaluate the patient for congenital hip dislocation. While the patient is supine, the flexed thigh is abducted and externally rotated. The femoral head can sublux or dislocate with an audible click during this maneuver.

Tibio-femoral OA is differentiated from patello-femoral OA to aid in the selection of appropriate treatment (15). The patella femoral grinding test requires the examiner to push the patella distally in the trochlear groove while the patient contracts the quadriceps. The patella is then palpated with slight resistance through motion; any roughness in articular surfaces will cause palpable crepitation and possible pain as the patella moves. The apprehension test for dislocation/subluxation of the patello-femoral joint requires the patient to be supine with the quadriceps relaxed and knee extended. The examiner presses against the medial aspect of the patella and attempts to dislocate the joint laterally. During this maneuver, the examiner watches the patient's facial expression for apprehension, indicating pain and pathology.

Malalignments and Deformity

A common, but often overlooked, aspect of the patient with rheumatic disease is limb length discrepancy. To assess for this problem, one should first form a clinical impression. Mark each medial malleolus with a marker. Then observe the medial malleoli from above and note whether one malleolus appears higher than the other. A true limb length discrepancy is measured with the patient supine. A 1-mm resolution tape measure is used to determine the distance from the anterior-superior iliac spine to the medial malleolus on each side. An apparent limb length discrepancy is assessed from the umbilicus to each medial malleolus. A functional limb length discrepancy is assessed in quiet standing. The distance from the anterior-superior iliac spine to floor (fifth metatarsal head) is measured bilaterally. The limb length discrepancy may be altered in the closed kinetic chain due to correlated and compensatory postures or segment length differences.

Postural hip alignment and function is assessed in several ways. In the frontal plane, it is important to rule out coxa vara and coxa valga (radiographic neck-to-shaft angle). The normal neck-to-shaft angle is approximately 125°. *Coxa vara* is present when the neck-to-shaft angle is <125°, and *coxa valga* is the opposite (i.e. >125°). The Ober test for iliotibial band contracture is conducted with the patient lying on his or her side and the leg maximally abducted with the knee at 90°. While keeping the hip in neutral position to relax the iliotibial tract, the examiner releases support of the abducted leg. If it does not return to the adducted position, a contracture is present. In the transverse plane, anteversion or antetorsion (femoral in-toeing) and retroversion or retrotorsion (femoral out-toeing) can be assessed by viewing the femur axially. The femoral head to greater trochanter line should be approximately 12° anterior to the lateral and medial condyle line for ideal alignment. In the sagittal plane, a flexion contracture can be detected by performing the Thomas test. The patient is supine, with the pelvis level and the anterior-superior iliac spine perpendicular to the long axis of the body. The examiner places a hand under the lumbar spine and flexes the hip, stopping when the lumbar spine flattens and the pelvis is stabilized. Further flexion will occur only at the hip. If the limb does not return to flat when gradually released from this position, a flexion contracture is present.

Postural knee alignment and function is first assessed in the frontal plane. *Genu varum* or bow-legged stance is more prevalent in knee OA (Figure 3). The tibia may independently be in a varus malalignment as well. Normally the tibia is in slight valgus with respect to the femur. If this posture becomes exaggerated, a *genu valgum* or knock-kneed malalignment is present. Radiographic confirmation of the tibio-femoral angle and concomitant joint space narrowing (Figure 2) is important to assess disease severity.

In the transverse plane, it is important to distinguish between femoral torsion, tibial torsion, and pedal torsion when your patient stands out-toed or in-toed. Tibial torsion is assessed with the patient supine, knees flexed, and legs hanging down

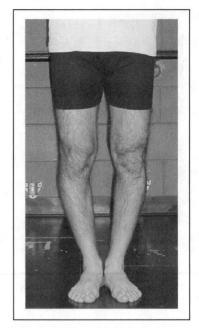

Figure 3. A patient with tibial varum and genu varum.

over the edge of the exam table. The examiner views the patient axially from above the knee and measures the angle between the femoral epicondyles and the transmalleolar axis (where 18–23° external is within normal limits). Femoral torsion is more apparent in quiet standing. If the greater trochanter and head of the femur are positioned parallel to the frontal plane, then each patella should be positioned approximately straight ahead. In the sagittal plane it is possible for the patient to hyperextend the knees or exhibit recurvatum, where the tibio-femoral segments appear slightly "C"-shaped.

Triplanar assessment of the foot and ankle is discussed in Chapter 30, Evaluation and Management of the Foot and Ankle. It is strongly recommended that the biomechanical integrity of the entire lower extremity be assessed when evaluating patients with rheumatic disease that affects the hip, knee, ankle, or foot.

Movement Performance

Observational gait analysis (29) and activities of daily living such as stair ascent and descent are important clinical assessments of movement performance. Computerized gait analysis (posture and locomotion) can provide additional assistance in objectively defining a patient's functional limitations and/or disability (30–32). Assessment of specific parameters can be especially useful for developing a treatment strategy and tracking disease progression (21). Pre- and post-treatment gait analysis can provide objective data for determining the efficacy of therapy.

CONSERVATIVE THERAPIES

Neoprene Sleeves

Neoprene sleeves have provided some pain relief for mild knee OA (33). When used alone they provide warmth and mild

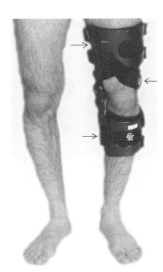

Figure 4. Valgus knee brace.

compression to control edema. Neoprene sleeves may also reinforce joint proprioception by providing constant external stimulation to the skin. They do not provide structural support or realignment of the lower extremity. Many knee braces include a neoprene sleeve as an undergarment for their devices, which can provide realignment.

Knee Braces

Two forms of conservative realignment therapy, knee bracing and foot orthoses, are biomechanically consistent with the aforementioned theoretical concepts. The valgus knee brace should minimize the eccentric loading (Figure 1b) of the varus knee malaligned lower extremity, by reducing the moment arm "y" (Figure 2), shifting the resultant force "Fr" laterally, and reducing the maximum compressive joint stress. Some knee braces use 3-point bending, in which a custom-molded carbon graphite thigh and calf shell supply the laterally directed forces to the proximal and distal knee in the frontal plane, while a Velcro strap that wraps around the lateral aspect of the knee supplies the corrective medially directed load (Figure 4). This configuration results in a valgus correction moment that increases as a function of the hinge adjustment. Outcome studies for a limited number of OA knee brace designs have demonstrated reduced pain (33–42) and improved function (33,35, 37,39,41,42).

Knee braces are available in both over-the-counter and custom-molded (or custom fit) designs. The advantage to over-the-counter designs is primarily in cost savings. The key disadvantage is the lack of a full range of sizes. Custom-molded or custom-fit braces have several advantages: 1) the device is fabricated either from a plaster cylinder cast of the patient's lower extremity or a set of pertinent anthropometric measurements obtained from the patient, 2) the materials employed within the shell and hinges are often of higher quality, and 3) in some custom braces it is possible to adjust the amount of correction. The primary disadvantage is the additional cost, compared with the cost of over-the-counter designs. The treatment goals, hinge designs, shell designs, materials employed, and fabrication techniques vary considerably from one manufacturer to another. Because few of the braces have clinical

outcome studies to support their efficacy, it is difficult to determine the relative effectiveness of each design.

Currently available braces meet 4 basic treatment goals: ligament protection, tibio-femoral realignment, patello-femoral realignment, and bicompartmental realignment. Ligament protection braces have the primary goal of increasing sagittal plane stability (43,44). They are designed to augment or replace the role of the ACL and PCL. Many of the patients who benefit from this therapy are between 20–50 years of age and have injured a ligament as a result of overuse or trauma during sports activities.

Tibio-femoral OA braces have the primary goals of stabilizing and realigning the knee in the frontal plane. The mechanism of action for each brace varies according to design features, but the general aim is to reduce the load to the narrowed region of the joint space via a corrective moment.

Most braces have flat hinges that are constrained to planar function. These planar hinges may be uniaxial, biaxial, or exhibit a coupled planar motion about 2 axes. Two of the commercially available braces have single upright hinges that move in a triplanar manner, which could be an advantage for preserving coupled motions, such as the screw home mechanism. The majority of knee braces have double upright hinges that are parallel to one another, which may be beneficial for enhanced stability but causes constraint in the transverse plane.

Also of interest is the amount of realignment. Some braces offer no realignment (only a restraint for further dynamic malalignment), some offer a fixed amount of realignment, and other braces offer adjustable correction. At this point, there has not been enough investigation into the subtleties of knee brace design to know which ones are preferred or perform best for a specific type of patient.

OA knee braces can have a variety of hinge designs (e.g., adjustable or fixed alignment, single or double upright, polyaxial or uniaxial), shell designs (carbon graphite fibers or polypropylene), and fitting methods (custom-molded or off-the-shelf) which few of the existing knee brace studies completely delineate. As clinical outcome may be affected by these design elements, it is important to specify these features when reporting data. Only 2 abstracts to date have studied varus knee OA pain and function at different knee brace alignments (39,42).

Patello-femoral braces have the primary goal of improving patellar tracking about the femoral condyles. Malpositioning or dysfunctional tracking of the patella has been suspected to be at least a component of patello-femoral OA pathogenesis. Devices for conservative therapy range from simple neoprene sleeves with a cutout for the patella to more complex bracing systems affording adjustable amounts of corrective load. Clinical outcome studies with objective biomechanical data are scarce. One company has recently announced a bicompartmental brace that is designed to treat medial or lateral knee OA and patello-femoral OA; however, it has not been objectively studied.

Caution is necessary when prescribing and fitting knee braces for patients with rheumatic disease. If the prescribing physician's experience with these technologies is limited, it may be best to refer to a professional such as a certified orthotist who has the training and experience needed. In addition, followup care is necessary in order to check the patient's sensation, local swelling, and proper use of the brace. Finally, it is important to become familiar with the literature in order to assimilate the evidence-based medicine from new clinical outcome studies in this rapidly changing area of conservative care.

Site-Specific Stability Orthoses

Lower extremity site-specific stability orthoses are often utilized in the management of malalignments and weakness of the leg in patients with rheumatic disease. Contrary to the perception that "braces" are only used to manage weakness or paralysis caused by neuromuscular disease, these devices are used to unload painful joints, stabilize joints with poor ligamentous or muscular support, and prevent deformity when extreme weakness has developed from disuse atrophy in the presence of marked dyskinesia.

Ankle-Foot Orthoses. Several different orthoses have been developed for either temporary or permanent control of the foot and ankle (45). When patients experience a simple drop foot due to pain or weakness of the anterior muscles and do not require medial or lateral support, a relatively inexpensive, easily dispensed, custom-fitted or off-the-shelf molded plastic orthosis may suffice.

The classic double-upright ankle-foot orthosis with fixed or moveable ankle joints has long been considered the workhorse of lower extremity bracing. Two metal uprights attached to a calf cuff are joined to the patient's shoe. The brace uses these uprights to establish medial/lateral support for the ankle and subtalar joints and relies on fixed or mobile articulations at the ankle to control pedal motions in the sagittal plane. Several types of ankle joints are available (e.g., solid, simple hinge, Klenzak, and double-action). These joints use adjustable stops or pins, or a posterior spring insert to provide a dorsiflexion assist.

The most common use of the ankle-foot orthosis in patients with arthritis is for control of hyperpronating feet resulting from a partial or complete rupture of the tibialis posterior tendon. The patient's ankle motion is restricted, and the valgus attitude of the rear foot is realigned with the use of a leather T-strap attached to the lateral upright. Additional support is provided by an in-shoe foot orthosis posted in varus. Another use for the ankle-foot orthosis is to provide knee control for the patient with weak or absent quadriceps. Alteration of the ankle joint stop to lock the brace in 5–10° of plantar-flexion tends to cause the knee to hyperextend slightly during mid-stance, preventing buckling and falls. Setting the brace in 5–10° of dorsiflexion induces slight flexion in midstance and can be used to prevent genu recurvatum or back knee in gait (45).

Plastic or Molded Ankle-Foot Orthosis. The plastic or molded ankle-foot orthosis is rapidly replacing the double-upright brace as the modality of choice in lower extremity bracing (45). Comfort, reduced weight, low cost, and ease of application are only some of the reasons for its rise in popularity. Because the device uses a molded foot section as its base, the patient has the freedom to change shoe styles without having to modify each one. The close contact of the polypropylene allows for excellent medial-lateral stability. Innovations in ankle joint and spring-assist technology allow versatility in application. One can use a molded, posted insert in the foot section of a polypropylene ankle-foot orthosis for added control and pedal realignment. It is possible to utilize the offset-varus heel seat in the Kirby-Skive orthosis to manage posterior tibial tendon dysfunction (45). However, cuneo-navicular pressure and breakdown can occur, where the foot collapses against the medial longitudinal arch of the brace.

Two types of molded ankle-foot orthoses are commonly utilized: the inexpensive, readily available custom-fitted or off-the-shelf device, and the custom-made or custom-molded device. Whenever fixed-ankle braces are used, the clinician should consider the addition of a rounded heel and rocker sole to promote a more fluid gait. Custom-molded devices are more expensive but can provide greater stability via their more precise fit. Customized padding, positioning, or angulation can be incorporated during the casting and fabrication of the device. Components such as ankle joints, stops, or spring assists can be easily incorporated as well.

Patellar Tendon Bearing Braces. The patellar tendon bearing brace consists of a standard double-upright or molded orthosis construction. It incorporates a molded leg section designed to provide cylindrical support for the limb, thus reducing weight on the foot and ankle. The leg section is constructed in 2 parts, either hinged or secured with Velcro, and designed to resemble the below-knee patellar tendon bearing prosthetic socket. With this modification, the physician can expect a 10–40% reduction in stress applied to the foot and ankle. Patellar tendon bearing braces are most commonly used for severely painful joints with collapse of the articular surfaces from OA, trauma, or rheumatoid arthritis. Although bulky, the patellar tendon bearing brace is sometimes the only way to unload a painful joint in a patient with a complicated medical history who cannot undergo joint fusion or replacement surgery.

Knee-Ankle-Foot Orthoses. Knee orthoses, in combination with ankle-foot orthoses, are occasionally used in the management of more involved lower extremity neurologic or muscular conditions. The knee joint provides stability in the sagittal and frontal planes, preventing buckling in the weak limb. This stability is largely dependent on the integrity of the hip joint and the strength of the thigh, hip, and pelvic girdle musculature. When hip stability is compromised, use of a hip-knee-ankle-foot orthosis with a pelvic band and articulating hip joint may be required.

Foot Orthoses. Foot orthoses can realign and protect the arthritic foot as well as incorporate a correction for limb length discrepancy as described in Chapter 30, Evaluation and Management of the Foot and Ankle.

Ambulatory Aids

Ambulatory aids can be divided into those that increase stability by increasing the patient's base of support, or those that serve to unload painful or unstable joints. No ambulatory aid should be dispensed to a patient without a consultation with a physical therapist for proper fitting and, if needed, pre-ambulatory conditioning to make sure the patient is capable of safely using the device. The physical therapist is specially trained to evaluate patients for balance and coordination and is best suited to decide which of the various devices is most appropriate for a given patient.

Canes. In the arthritic hip, joint loading may be reduced by using a cane in the hand opposite to the involved hip. Canes come in many designs ranging from the simple wooden cane (adjusted by sawing off a portion of the base to achieve the proper height) to the aluminum adjustable cane that can be fit to the patient immediately by choosing one of several predetermined built-in heights.

Wider, flatter handgrips, compared with the standard narrow cane handle, provide a more comfortable resting surface for the hand while allowing the patient to produce greater grip strength. These improved grips can have a cone shape, narrower at the thenar border and wider at the ulnar side of the hand, which aids in improving grip strength of the ulnar digits and resists the tendency toward ulnar drift seen with the rheumatoid arthritis hand. When greater stability is needed due to a lack of wrist strength, a Canadian or forearm crutch with or without a platform addition can be substituted for a cane. Although these devices are technically considered crutches, when used singly they provide no weight reduction for an involved extremity and function as a cane.

The last feature of a cane is its base. Most canes use a simple wide rubber tip to provide stability on a variety of surfaces. Metal spiked tips can be used for ice or when walking off paved surfaces. When a patient's balance is severely compromised, a tripod or quad base can be added to the cane to increase the base of support. However, this adds more weight to the cane—a factor that must be considered when ordering for your patients.

Crutches. Crutches come in a variety of designs and can utilize the wider handgrips described previously. The standard axillary crutch comes with sponge rubber pads over the tops to protect the patient's ribs and upper arms from irritation during use. The hand pieces are also padded to increase the grip size and protect the hands from irritation during ambulation. The tips of the crutches are covered with a wide rubber base and may be ordered with metal tips for ice or unpaved surfaces.

Crutches both increase the base of support and significantly reduce the weight carried by an involved extremity depending on the type of crutch gait used. Weight can be borne on a single uninvolved extremity utilizing a non–weight-bearing 3-point gait, or distributed between the 2 extremities using a partial weight-bearing 3-point or 4-point gait.

Crutches are measured to allow the patient's weight to be borne on the hands and wrists and should never touch the skin under the axilla. Weight bearing through the axilla may result in serious damage to the nerves of the arm and hand. Crutch tops should be 2–3 inches below the axilla when the crutch tips are 6 inches in front of and 6 inches lateral to the ends of the toes. The hand pieces should be positioned with the elbow bent at a 15–20° angle when standing. When a patient needs crutches for an extended period of time and has excellent hand, arm, and shoulder strength, forearm crutches should be considered. These crutches increase the base of support and reduce loading without putting pressure on the upper arm and chest wall and are therefore more comfortable to use. If the patient has a painful hand, wrist, or elbow and limited arm strength, a platform crutch may be a better choice.

Walkers. Walkers provide the greatest stability of all the ambulatory aids but are the most cumbersome to use and provide the most storage problems when traveling in a car or on public transportation. It is impossible to climb stairs with a walker, and negotiating curbs is a difficult and often dangerous task. Walkers are well suited for patients who need to ambulate limited distances and have significant balance or muscle control problems that make them highly unstable.

The standard walker has 4 legs, each fitted with a large rubber tip for stability on smooth surfaces. The patient has to lift the walker, move it forward, and step up to it in order to ambulate. Wheeled walkers have wheels on the front 2 legs to make it easier for patients who find it difficult to lift the walker to move. Patients who have pain or weakness of the hands, wrists, or elbows can have their walkers fitted with a platform attachment that allows them to bear weight on their forearms and use their shoulders to move the walker. Bags or baskets can be attached to the walker to allow patients to carry things when both their hands are occupied manipulating the walker. Some walkers have brakes and a seat for rest periods.

REFERENCES

1. Bradley J. Nonsurgical options for managing osteoarthritis of the knee. J Musculoskel Med 1994;11:14–26.
2. Swanson S. Biomechanics. In: Freeman MAR, Aubriot JH, editors. Arthritis of the knee: clinical features and surgical management.New York: Springer-Verlag; 1980. p. 1–30.
3. Sasaki T, Yasuda K. Clinical evaluation of the treatment of osteoarthritic knees using a newly designed wedged insole. Clin Orthop 1987;221:181–187.
4. Yagi T, Sasaki T. Tibial torsion in patients with medial-type osteoarthritic knee. Clin Orthop 1986;213:177–182.
5. Yagi T. Tibial torsion in patients with medial-type osteoarthrotic knees. Clin Orthop 1994;302:52–56.
6. Yasuda K, Sasaki T. The mechanics of treatment of the osteoarthritic knee with a wedged insole. Clin Orthop 1987;215:162–172.
7. Moussa A, Bridges-Webb C. Quality of care in general practice. A delphi study of indicators and methods. Aust Fam Physician 1994;23:465–8, 472–3.
8. Goh JC, Bose K, Khoo BC. Gait analysis study on patients with varus osteoarthrosis of the knee. Clin Orthop 1993;294:223–31.
9. Brower DJ, Hillstrom HJ, Song J, Kahler MA, Zonay LJ, Schumacher HR, et al. Lower extremity malalignment incidence in knee osteoarthritis (OA). Arthritis Rheum 1997;40(9Suppl):S174.
10. Sharma L, Hurwitz DE, Thonar EJ, Sum JA, Lenz ME, Dunlop DD, et al. Knee adduction moment, serum hyaluronan level, and disease severity in medial tibiofemoral osteoarthritis. Arthritis Rheum 1998;41:1233–1240.
11. Wang H, Olney S. Relationship between alignment, kinematic and kinetic measures of the knee of normal elderly subjects in level walking. Clin Biomech 1994;9:245–252.
12. Riegger-Krugh C, Keysor JJ. Skeletal malalignments of the lower quarter: correlated and compensatory motions and postures. J Orthop Sports Phys Ther 1996;23:164–170.
13. Vlahovic TC, Ribeiro CE, Lamm BM, Denmark JA, Walters RG, Talbert T, et al. A case of peroneal neuropathy-induced footdrop. Correlated and compensatory lower-extremity function. J Am Podiatr Med Assoc 2000; 90:411–420.
14. Brower D, Song J, Hillstrom HJ, Kahler MA, Zonay L, Schumacher HR. Lower extremity malaignments associated with knee osteoarthritis. Paper presented at: Annual Meeting of the Podiatric Research Society; 1998; Orlando, FL.
15. Elahi S, Cahue S, Felson DT, Engleman L, Sharma L. The association between varus-valgus alignment and patellofemoral osteoarthritis. Arthritis Rheum 2000;43: 1874–1880.
16. Nordin M, Frankel VH. Basic biomechanics of the musculoskeletal system. 2nd ed. Philadelphia: Lea & Febiger; 1989. p. xxiii, 323.
17. Mow VC, Ateshian GA, Spilker RL. Biomechanics of diarthrodial joints: a review of twenty years of progress. J Biomech Eng 1993;115:460–467.
18. Maquet PGJ. Biomechanics of the knee: with application to the pathogenesis and the surgical treatment of osteoarthritis. New York: Springer-Verlag; 1983. p. xviii, 306.
19. Hirsch B, Minugh-Purvis N. Anatomy of the lower extremity. Philadelphia: Temple University School of Podiatric Medicine; 1999.
20. Song J, Hillstrom HJ, Secord D, Levitt J. Foot type biomechanics. comparison of planus and rectus foot types. J Am Podiatr Med Assoc 1996; 86:16–23.
21. Andriacchi TP. Dynamics of knee malalignment. Orthop Clin North Am 1994;25:395–403.
22. Chao EY, Neluheni EV, Hsu RW, Paley D. Biomechanics of malalignment. Orthop Clin North Am 1994;25:379–386.
23. Paley D, Herzenberg JE, Tetsworth K, McKie J, Bhave A. Deformity planning for frontal and sagittal plane corrective osteotomies. Orthop Clin North Am 1994;25:425–465.

24. Paley D, Maar DC, Herzenberg JE. New concepts in high tibial osteotomy for medial compartment osteoarthritis. Orthop Clin North Am 1994;25:483–498.

25. Murphy SB. Tibial osteotomy for genu varum. Indications, preoperative planning, and technique. Orthop Clin North Am 1994;25:477–482.

26. Tetsworth K, Paley D. Malalignment and degenerative arthropathy. Orthop Clin North Am 1994;25:367–377.

27. Catagni MA, Guerreschi F, Ahmad TS, Cattaneo R. Treatment of genu varum in medial compartment osteoarthritis of the knee using the Ilizarov method. Orthop Clin North Am 1994;25:509–514.

28. Kendall FP, McCreary EK, Kendall HO. Muscles, testing and function. 3rd ed. Baltimore: Williams & Wilkins; 1983. p. xix, 326.

29. Perry J. Gait analysis: normal and pathological function. Englewood Cliffs, NJ: SLACK; 1992. p. xxxii, 524.

30. Horak FB, Nashner LM, Diener HC. Postural strategies associated with somatosensory and vestibular loss. Exp Brain Res 1990;82:167–177.

31. Woollacott MH, Shumway-Cook A, Nashner LM. Aging and posture control: changes in sensory organization and muscular coordination. Int J Aging Hum Dev; 1986;23:97–114.

32. Winter DA. The biomechanics and motor control of human gait: normal, elderly and pathological. 2nd ed. Waterloo, Ontario: University of Waterloo Press; 1991,. p. x, 143.

33. Kirkley A, Webster-Bogaert S, Litchfield R, Amendola A, MacDonald S, McCalden R, et al. The effect of bracing on varus gonarthrosis. J Bone Joint Surg Am 1999;81:539–548.

34. Pollo FE, Otis JC, Wickiewicz TL, Warren RF. Biomechanical analysis of valgus bracing for the osteoarthritic knee. Paper presented at: North American Clinical Gait Laboratory Conference; April 9, 1994. Portland, OR.

35. Pollo FE, Otis JC, Wickiewicz TL, Warren RF. Biomechanical analysis of valgus bracing for the osteoarthritic knee. Arthritis Rheum 1995;38: S241.

36. Horlick SG, Loomer RL. Valgus knee bracing for medical gonarthrosis. Clinical Journal of Sports Medicine 1993;3:251-255.

37. Matsuno H, Kadowaki KM, Tsuji H, Generation II knee bracing for severe medial compartment osteoarthritis of the knee. Arch Phys Med Rehabil 1997;78:745–749.

38. Hillstrom H, Brower DJ, Bhimji S, McGuire J, Whitney K, Snyder H, et al. Assessment of conservative realignment therapies for the treatment of varus knee osteoarthritis: biomechanics and joint pathophysiology. Gait Posture 2000;11:170–1.

39. Otis JC, Backus SI, Polle FE, Wickiewicz TL, Warren RF and et al. Load sharing at the knee during valgus bracing for medial compartment osteoarthritis. Gait Posture 1996;4:189.

40. Hewett TE, Noyes FR, Barber-Westin SD, Heckmann TP. Decrease in knee joint pain and increase in function in patients with medial compartment arthrosis: a prospective analysis of valgus bracing. Orthopedics 1998;21:131–138.

41. Lindenfeld TN, Hewett TE, Andriacchi TP. Joint loading with valgus bracing in patients with varus gonarthrosis. Clin Orthop 1997;344:290–297.

42. Otis J, Backus SI, Campbell DA, Furman GL, Montalvo E, Warren RF, et al. Valgus knee bracing for knee osteoarthritis: a biomechanical and clinical outcome study. Gait Posture 2000;11:116.

43. Liu SH, Mirzayan R. Current review. Functional knee bracing. Clin Orthop 1995;317:273–281.

44. Beynnon BD, Johnson RJ, Fleming BC, Peura GD, Renstrom PA, Nichols CE, et al. The effect of functional knee bracing on the anterior cruciate ligament in the weightbearing and nonweightbearing knee. Am J Sports Med; 1997;25:353–359.

45. Braddom RL. Physical Medicine and Rehabilitation. Philadelphia: WB Saunders; 1996.

Pre- and Post-Surgical Management of the Hip and Knee

SANDY B. GANZ, PT, MS, GCS; and GIGI VIELLION, RN, ONC

Total joint arthroplasty (TJA) of the lower extremity is a highly successful surgical procedure that has revolutionized the outlook of patients with arthritis. Over 450,000 total hip and total knee arthroplasties are performed annually in the United States (1). While the majority of TJAs are performed for osteoarthritis, other rheumatic diseases also cause joint destruction and may result in the need for surgery. In the early years of TJA, incapacitating pain was the sole indication for surgery. Today, relief of pain is still the primary indication for most arthroplasties; however, other considerations include quality of life issues such as limited function, deformity, and joint instability that limit activities of daily living (ADLs) (2).

Members of the surgical health care team should work closely with those responsible for the medical management of the patients' disease. Total joint arthroplasty of the lower extremity is a highly successful surgical procedure with an excellent outcome. As with any major surgery, there are inherent risks that must be carefully weighed. The patient must be willing to prepare for the surgery and be an active participant in rehabilitation.

PREOPERATIVE EVALUATION

Total joint arthroplasty is an elective procedure and therefore allows for preoperative education and evaluation of the patient. Once it is decided that the patient will benefit from a TJA, the health care team begins the evaluation process. It is important to determine the patient's expectations. Because some outcomes of surgery are more predictable than others, the health care team can assist patients in determining if their goals are realistic.

Disease management issues must be considered for all patients, but are especially critical for persons with one of the more complex rheumatic diseases (3). Assessment of the patient's disease activity and the systems involved, as well as any physical and psychosocial limitations, is essential to developing a plan of care. Special consideration should be given to the routines, medications, and modalities utilized by patients to manage their disease. Patients are advised to stop taking aspirin and nonsteroidal antiinflammatory drugs (NSAIDs)—including cyclooxygenase-2 (COX-2) inhibitors—approximately 1 week before surgery to avoid the risk of increased bleeding (4). The time frame for stopping these drugs varies according to drug half-life.

Most patients will be placed on anticoagulant therapy for several weeks postoperatively. During this time, methods other than aspirin or NSAIDs (except in low doses and with close monitoring of prothrombin times) should be used to manage pain. Analgesics that can be used in place of NSAIDs include acetaminophen, nonacetylated salicylates, tramadol, and mild narcotics. Increased disease activity in individuals with inflammatory rheumatic disease may be managed using larger doses of NSAIDs if necessary, with very careful titration based on the prothrombin time. Patients with ankylosing spondylitis, rheumatoid arthritis (RA), and juvenile rheumatoid arthritis must be evaluated for cervical spine involvement to avoid potentially dangerous manipulation of the neck during anesthesia (2). Preoperative cervical spine x-rays should include a lateral flexion view.

Patients should be made aware of factors that could increase their risk of postoperative complications. Smoking, a history of heart or lung disease, use of steroids and/or other immunosuppressive drugs, diabetes, RA, and obesity are factors that can affect rehabilitation and delay wound healing (2). Sources of infection must be eliminated preoperatively to prevent hematogenous seeding at the site of the joint replacement. The most common sources of infection are the teeth, the genitourinary tract, and open areas on the skin (2). A dental checkup is recommended within 6 months before surgery is scheduled. A preoperative urine culture is necessary as asymptomatic bacteriuria is common in women and prostatic hypertrophy can present increased risk of infection in men. Known medical problems should be treated prior to TJA.

A preoperative physical therapy evaluation should be performed to identify and address areas that may be problematic postoperatively. Early identification of potential problems will expedite rehabilitation and enable the team to plan for appropriate home care. The evaluation should include assessment of gait, range of motion of all joints, strength of all extremities, respiratory status, and a functional assessment. This evaluation is especially important in patients with multiple joint involvement or one of the more complex rheumatic diseases (5). An observational gait analysis is performed to determine the patient's weight-bearing ability and any abnormal loading on the affected/unaffected limbs. Measurement of range of motion of joints and gross manual muscle testing of the upper extremities and uninvolved lower extremity are performed to determine the type of ambulatory aids that may be needed during the postoperative period. A respiratory evaluation should include auscultation and a measurement of the number of cubic centimeters a patient inspires and expires utilizing an incentive spirometer (6). Pain assessment, using a visual analog scale or pain disability index scale, should be performed. Finally, each patient should be assessed preoperatively using a functional rating scale in order to determine if there is a change in functional status following surgery (7). Indices that may be utilized in both the pre- and postoperative evaluation include the Medical Outcomes Survey Short Form-36 (SF-36) (8), Western Ontario and MacMaster University Osteoarthritis Index (WOMAC) (9), Harris Hip Score (10), Functional Status Index (9), and the Knee Society Clinical Rating System Score

(11). Additional functional assessments are described in Chapter 9, Functional Ability, Health Status, and Quality of Life.

Consideration must be given to the support that will be available to the patient after discharge from the hospital. The home environment should be assessed to ensure patient safety and ability to function. Upon discharge from the hospital, most arthroplasty patients can expect to perform self-care and manage at home with minimal assistance and decreased pain. Patients should be informed prior to surgery of their expected length of hospitalization and their postoperative abilities and limitations. This will allow the social worker or discharge planner, patient, and family the opportunity to make appropriate arrangements for managing at home. Preoperative preparation of the home should include removal of scatter rugs, provision of clear pathways for ambulation, and advance meal preparation. Arranging for someone to assist with errands and transportation should be done prior to hospitalization.

PREADMISSION EDUCATION

Preoperative patient education is crucial in the management of the TJA patient (10,12). Studies have shown that preoperative interventions, in the form of patient education classes, enhance the postoperative course. Education may be provided individually or in a group session and should include the patient's family and/or significant other. For every surgical procedure, there are routine events that occur. A *clinical pathway* is a multidisciplinary timetable that depicts these events. This allows the patient and the health care providers to be aware of what should occur on each postoperative day. Reviewing a clinical pathway that outlines the course of treatment can help the patient to prepare preoperatively for surgery, hospitalization, and recuperation. The expected length of stay should be made clear. Realistic goals should be set, including appropriate time frames.

Explain to patients that their active participation is necessary for an optimal recovery. Description of hospital routines, stressing what will be expected of the patient, gives people a sense of control over their recovery (3). Patients and their families may benefit from a visit to the inpatient unit and the opportunity to meet the staff. It is helpful to have an anesthesiologist discuss with the patient the type of anesthesia to be used and the impact of anesthesia on recovery. Instruction and demonstration of postoperative exercises and any precautions the patient will be required to follow should be included. Additionally, if time allows, patients should be taught and encouraged to do exercises to improve muscle strength and tone. This will accelerate the recovery process (12).

The greatest concern of most patients is how they will manage after surgery. Patients who cannot manage at home alone, or with home care, may need to be discharged to a subacute facility or rehabilitation center. Patients may need reassurance about their postoperative functional abilities and the discharge setting. Attention must be paid to any other comorbid conditions and current medical management of the individual (12,13).

POSTOPERATIVE MANAGEMENT

Patients may be given general or regional anesthesia. Patients who are given epidural anesthesia will be alert but insensate below the level of the epidural when they arrive in the postanesthesia care unit. Regardless of the type of anesthesia used, special care must be taken when moving the patient who has had a total hip arthroplasty to avoid dislocating the hip. In most cases, patients having TJA of the lower extremity will have a Foley catheter to prevent urinary retention or incontinence while the epidural is in effect.

As the effects of the anesthesia wear off, the pain experience will vary. Pain control can be managed by use of epidural analgesia or intravenous patient-controlled analgesia (IV-PCA). With IV-PCA, the patient is able to control the frequency of their pain medication. However, patients must understand the importance of using enough medication to promote bed mobility, early ambulation, and deep breathing (to avoid pulmonary complications). Patients with ankylosing spondylitis may be more susceptible to pulmonary problems due to diminished chest expansion.

Anesthesia—especially epidural anesthesia—and pain medication can slow down the gastrointestinal tract. The patient's abdomen must be auscultated for missing or hyperactive bowel sounds and observed for distention. Waiting until the patient reports being hungry and bowel sounds are present before starting oral intake may prevent an ileus from occurring. The stress of surgery may cause other gastrointestinal problems such as ulcers. Patients who have been taking aspirin or NSAIDs are at increased risk for gastrointestinal bleeding, which may have serious consequences for patients who are already anemic secondary to their chronic disease.

Other known complications of TJA are deep vein thrombosis and subsequent pulmonary embolus. One of the available methods of prophylaxis to prevent deep vein thrombosis should be used for patients following total hip or total knee arthroplasty. Mechanical devices such as the pneumatic sequential compression device or a venous foot pump are often used in conjunction with a pharmacologic method such as warfarin or low molecular weight heparin (14). While this approach is important in the postoperative period, it may present problems for patients who depend on aspirin or NSAIDs to manage their rheumatic disease, because these drugs cannot be used without careful monitoring of the patients' prothrombin time. In addition to these methods of preventing deep vein thrombosis, active ankle pump exercises and early ambulation are essential.

Infection is a potential complication of TJA. Measures to protect the patient from infection include laminar flow in the operating room, prophylactic antibiotics, and educating the patient about the importance of constant vigilance in preventing and recognizing signs of infection (15). Most TJA surgeons support the use of prophylactic antibiotics before any dental work, including cleaning, and before any invasive medical procedures. Immediate attention to early infection can protect the joint and avoid a long and costly hospitalization. Patients with inflammatory arthritis who have been treated with immunosuppressive therapy tend to be at increased risk for intraoperative and postoperative complications (2). In the postoperative period, patients who are treated with corticosteroids are at increased risk for many complications including friable skin, delayed wound healing, and infection. The risk of infection is also increased in patients with enteropathic arthritis through hematogenous seeding from the bowel and in patients with psoriatic arthritis (2).

REHABILITATION

In the 4 decades since the first TJA was performed, methods and philosophies of rehabilitation have changed, but the goals of rehabilitation have remained the same. The primary goals following TJA are to restore function, decrease pain, and gain muscle control so that individuals can return to previous levels of functioning (6,16).

Total Hip Arthroplasty

Rehabilitation following cemented and cementless total hip arthroplasty is influenced by many factors, including surgical technique and approach. The most common approach used is the posterior/posterior lateral. When this approach is used, precautions during rehabilitation must be taken to avoid extremes of hip flexion, adduction, and internal rotation. When an anterior approach is used, extremes of external rotation, extension, and abduction must be avoided. Dislocation occurs in approximately 1–4% of total hip arthroplasty patients and may occur during any one or a combination of these movements (16). If hip arthroplasty is performed in conjunction with a trochanteric osteotomy, weight-bearing must be protected and active hip abduction must be avoided for 8–12 weeks postoperatively or until the osteotomy site is well healed. The most common maneuvers in which dislocations occur following a posterior lateral approach are: 1) rising off a low surface such as a toilet or recliner; 2) twisting the trunk toward the operated side in either a standing or seated position with feet planted on the floor; and 3) bending down to tie shoes from a seated position. There is controversy regarding the length of time patients should adhere to postoperative TJA precautions. Opinions range from 4 weeks to life. Positions to avoid are listed in Table 1.

Regardless of the institution, the postoperative rehabilitation routine will consist of therapeutic exercise, transfer training, gait training, and instruction in ADLs (17). Therapeutic exercises are performed in order to increase muscle strength and gain control of the limb for various necessary activities. Lower extremity exercises consist of supine ankle circles, quadriceps sets, gluteal sets, hip internal rotation to neutral, and hip and knee flexion to 45° supine and 90° sitting. Transfer training consists of bed to standing, sitting posture, and toilet transfers. The type of prosthesis fixation used will determine whether the patient will be non–weight-bearing, toe-touch weight-bearing, partial weight-bearing, or full weight-bearing during gait training. Prior to discharge, patients should be instructed in managing stairs and curbs. In the early postoperative period, patients often have the sensation that their operated limb is longer, because temporary abduction contractures can result from enforced abduction in bed or from distal advancement of the trochanter. Unless there is a true leg-length discrepancy, shoe lifts should not be applied for at least 4–6 weeks when the temporary hip abduction contracture resolves (16,17).

Following discharge from the hospital, the long-term goal is to improve ambulation to a normal gait without abductor weakness or lurch. It is important to include abductor strengthening in patients' home exercise program. Prolonged weakness in the hip abductors causes abnormal stress on the hip joint. Over time, these abnormal forces can lead to implant loosening (16). A cane should be used until abductor weakness is resolved. Patients should be advised to carry loads on the side

Table 1. Positions to avoid following total hip arthroplasty.

- Knees higher than hips, such as sitting in a low chair or on a low toilet
- Crossing legs while sitting, standing, or lying down
- Bending down to tie shoes or pick up an object from the floor
- Twisting from the trunk while seated or standing with the operative leg planted on the floor
- Leaning forward from the waist while seated
- Any other activity in which hip flexion is greater than 90°, hip is adducted past neutral, and/or hip is internally rotated past neutral

that underwent arthroplasty. Research has shown that loads carried on the contralateral side significantly increase force demands placed on the side of the arthroplasty, while loads as large as 20% of body weight carried on the operative side produce no more hip abductor muscle activity, as measured by electromyogram, than that produced while walking without a load (18). Patients must be cognizant of the fact that although the artificial joint causes little or no pain, it is in fact not a normal joint.

There is no consensus regarding which sporting activities a person with a hip replacement can safely participate in following surgery. Non-impact loading activities such as bicycle riding, swimming, dancing, golf, and doubles tennis are usually encouraged. Impact loading activities, such as running, jogging, and contact sports, can result in increased stress on the bone-cement interface and may lead to loosening of the prosthesis. Studies have shown that intelligent participation in activities such as walking, golf, bowling, and swimming—where there is no excess load (>20 lbs) placed on the hip—has no influence on the outcome of the total hip arthroplasty (19). In general, high activity levels are associated with increased failure rates in conventional cemented hip arthroplasty.

Patients must be warned that no type of hip replacement can withstand the forces of strenuous loads on the hip without possible loosening (20). Patients may resume sexual activity as soon as they feel comfortable doing so, as long as they adhere to the precautions to avoid hip dislocation. Studies have shown that patients usually resume sexual activity 4–6 weeks postoperatively (21).

Total Knee Arthroplasty

Rehabilitation following total knee arthroplasty has dramatically changed over the past 3 decades, but the goals remain the same. Whether referring to a unicondylar or bicondylar knee replacement that is constrained, semi-constrained, or unconstrained; cemented or cementless; the primary goal is to provide a stable joint with a functional range of motion. Patients who underwent knee arthroplasty 25 years ago remained in the hospital for 3 weeks and were placed in a cylinder cast for 7–10 days before flexion was initiated. Today, mechanical flexion is initiated immediately after surgery, and the average length of stay for an uncomplicated total knee arthroplasty is 3–5 days after surgery (1).

Continuous passive motion (CPM) is a method of mechanical flexion. A machine is applied to the lower extremity to passively flex the knee at a designated speed and degree of flexion, as programmed by the physical therapist or nurse. The efficacy of CPM is controversial. Some studies indicate that it may be beneficial in counteracting the effect of joint immobilization (22); other studies indicate the opposite (23). Contraindications to the use of CPM are: 1) sensory deficits excluding epidural anesthesia; 2) excessive wound drainage; and 3) postoperative confusion.

Patients who are having difficulty with flexion and who have a concomitant knee flexion contracture should have limited time in the CPM machine. A dynamic knee brace may be indicated in these patients. Factors to consider when placing a knee arthroplasty patient in the CPM machine include the type of anesthesia, type of dressing, pain tolerance, and presence of deformity. Continuous passive motion is usually increased to the patient's tolerance, which should be equal to or more than what is achieved with active flexion.

Initiation of transfer activities, gait training, and range of motion usually occurs on the first postoperative day. Weight-bearing status will be determined by the type of implant fixation used. Patients may be discharged with crutches for protected weight bearing for 4–6 weeks postoperatively or with a cane for full weight bearing. To date, no prospective, controlled, randomized studies have addressed implant loosening in patients who received different weight-bearing instructions in the immediate postoperative period.

Important factors that influence postoperative range of motion in the knee are the type of prosthesis, preoperative deformity, and intraoperative bone resection. An exercise program that incorporates flexibility and strengthening may consist of active range of motion, active assisted range of motion, passive range of motion, isometrics (quadriceps and hamstring), straight leg raising, short arc quadriceps, patellar mobilization, and use of a stationary bicycle. Cryotherapy is often used concomitantly with exercise sessions. Aggressive quadriceps strengthening exercises (e.g., isokinetics or weights) should not be performed until soft tissue healing has occurred and there is adequate active ROM (7). Historically patients have been discharged from the hospital when they achieve 90° of knee flexion, are able to transfer in and out of bed independently, and can ambulate with a cane unassisted on level surfaces and stairs. Currently patients are being discharged 3–5 days after surgery, with varying degrees of flexion. Patients are more frequently managed in their home with home health services or are placed in short-term rehabilitation centers.

The most common type of failure in total knee arthroplasty is mechanical loosening. By placing undue forces on the knee joint, the patient increases the chance of prosthetic loosening and endangers the overall success of the knee replacement. Patients are often instructed prior to and after surgery to avoid sports that place excessive force on the prosthetic knee joint, such as running, jumping, or singles tennis. Most orthopedic surgeons allow patients to play golf. Reports of pain severity during and after golf have been found to be significantly higher in golfers with left knee versus right knee arthroplasty. This may be a direct result of increased torque on the left knee in right-handed golfers (24). The effect of total knee arthroplasty on driving reaction time was studied in 40 patients (25). Results indicated that reaction time returned to normal approximately 8 weeks after surgery for patients with right knee arthroplasty. Thus, driving reaction time, range of motion, and strength should be considered when advising patients to resume driving.

REFERENCES

1. American Academy of Orthopaedic Surgeons. Available at: http://www.aaos.org. Accessed July 6, 2001.
2. Sculco TP, editor. Surgical treatment of rheumatoid arthritis. Chicago: Mosby Year Book; 1992.
3. Mabrey JD, Toohey JS, Armstrong DA, Lavery L, Wammack LA. Clinical pathway management of total knee arthroplasty. Clin Orthop 1997;345:125–133.
4. Connelly CS, Panush RS.: Should nonsteroidal anti-inflammatory drugs be stopped before elective surgery? Arch Intern Med 1991;151:1963–1966.
5. Rodgers JA, Garvin KL, Walker CW, Morford D, Urban J, Bedard J. Preoperative physical therapy in primary total knee arthoplasty. J Arthoplasty 1998;13:414–421.
6. Sculco TP, Ganz SB, Noaker LJ. Knee surgery and rehabilitation. In: Melvin JL, Gall V, editors. Rheumatologic rehabilitation series: surgical rehabilitation. Bethesda: American Occupational Therapy Association; 1999.
7. Ganz SB. Physical therapy of the knee. In: Insall JN, Windsor RE, Scott WN, Kelly MA, Aglietti P, editors. Surgery of the knee. 2nd ed. New York: Churchill Livingstone; 1993. p. 1171–1191.
8. Ware JE Jr, Sherbourne CD. The MOS 36-item short-form health survey (SF-36). Med Care 1992;30:473–483.
9. Jette AM. Health status indicators: their utility in chronic-disease evaluation research. J Chronic Dis 1980;33:567–579.
10. Laupacis A, Bourne R, Rorabeck C, Feeny D, Wong C, Tugwell P, et al. The effect of elective total hip replacement on health-related quality of life. J Bone Joint Surg Am 1993;75:1619–1626.
11. Insall JN, Dorr LD, Scott RD, Scott WN. Rationale of The Knee Society clinical rating system. Clin Orthop 1989;248:13–14.
12. Haines N, Viellion G. A successful combination: preadmission testing and preoperative education. Orthop Nurs 1990;9:53–57.
13. Lichtenstein R, Semaan S, Marmar E. Development and impact of a hospital-based perioperative patient education program in a joint replacement center. Orthop Nurs 1993;12:17–25.
14. Arcelus J, Caprini J, Reyna JJ. Finding the right fit: effective thrombosis risk stratification in orthopaedic patients. Orthopedics 2000;23:S633–638.
15. Total Hip Replacement. NIH Consensus Statement Online 1994 September 12-14;12:1-31. Available at: htpp://text.nlm.nih.gov/nih/ cdc/www/ 98cvr.html.Accessed July 6, 2001.
16. Martin S, Zavadak K, Noaker LJ. Hip surgery and rehabilitation. In: Melvin JL, Gall V, editors. Rheumatologic rehabilitation series: surgical rehabilitation. Bethesda: American Occupational Therapy Association; 1999. p. 82–113.
17. Ganz SB. Physical therapy in rheumatoid arthritis. In: Sculco TP, editor. Surgical treatment of rheumatoid arthritis. Chicago: Mosby Year Book; 1992. p. 379–395.
18. Neumann DA. Hip abductor muscle activity in persons with a hip prosthesis while carrying loads in one hand. Phys Ther 1996;76:1320–1330.
19. Ritter MA, Meding JB.: Total hip arthroplasty: can the patient play sports again? Orthopedics 1987;10:1447–1452.
20. McGrory BJ, Stuart MJ, Sim FH. Participation in sports after hip and knee arthroplasty: review of literature and survey of surgeon preferences. Mayo Clin Proc 1995;70:342–348.
21. Stern SH, Fuchs MD, Ganz SB, Classi P, Sculco TP, Salvati EA. Sexual function after total hip arthroplasty. Clin Orthop 1991;269:228–235.
22. Coutts RD, Kaita J, Barr R, Mason R, Dube R, Amiel D, et al. The role of continuous passive motion in the postoperative rehabilitation of the total knee patient. Orthopaedic Transactions 1982;6:277–278.
23. Ritter MA, Gandolf VS, Holston KS. Continuous passive motion versus physical therapy in total knee arthroplasty. Clin Orhop 1989;244:239–243.
24. Mallon WJ, Callaghan JJ.: Total knee arthroplasty in active golfers. J Arthroplasty 1993;8:299–306.
25. Spalding T, Kiss J, Kyberd P, Turner-Smith A, Simpson AH.: Driver reaction times after total knee replacement. J Bone Joint Surg Br 1994;76:754–756.

Complementary and Alternative Treatments

SHARON L. KOLASINSKI, MD

Since the first edition of this text appeared, continuing patient interest in complementary and alternative medicine (CAM) therapies, a rapidly expanding body of published clinical trials, and a substantially increased research budget at the National Center for Complementary and Alternative Medicine within the National Institutes of Health (NIH) have contributed to an expanded literature on this topic. Furthermore, a recent American College of Rheumatology (ACR) position statement recommends that rheumatologists should be able to knowledgeably discuss CAM therapies with their patients and integrate such therapies that are proven safe and effective as appropriate. However, the ACR also advises caution in the use of therapies that are not validated (1). Because of the breadth of CAM interventions (Table 1), this chapter will focus on those therapies for which well-designed trials provide some evidence-based grounds for discussion.

SCOPE OF USE

In a landmark 1993 article, Eisenberg and colleagues brought the previously unrecognized extent of complementary and alternative medicine use to the attention of the traditional medical community (2). They defined CAM interventions as those not traditionally taught in U.S. medical schools and not traditionally available in U.S. hospitals and reported that 34% of randomly selected telephone interviewees had used such a therapy in the preceding year. A followup study in 1997 documented that use of CAM had increased to more than 42% of those interviewed, with clinical encounters for alternative care exceeding visits to primary care providers (3). These studies suggested that CAM therapies are often used for chronic disease and chronic pain, a finding confirmed in a number of observational studies in the rheumatologic literature in the United States as well as in Europe, Australia, and Canada (4,5). The definition of CAM has expanded to include numerous specific interventions (Table 1), and information regarding them is now taught in more than 40 medical schools. The Cochrane Collaboration currently lists more than 4,000 randomized, controlled CAM trials and PubMed has recently added CAM as a search category (see Appendix).

Subsequent research has clarified what therapies rheumatology patients are using and why. Although earlier studies suggested that CAM users were more likely to be middle-aged and white, and to have a higher level of education and income (2,3), subsequent studies in arthritis patients have shown that CAM is frequently used across racial, ethnic, education, and income groups (4). Studies in Hispanic and rural African

Table 1. Common complementary and alternative therapies.

Acupressure	Meditation
Acupuncture	Naturopathy
Aromatherapy	Nutritional therapy
Ayurveda	Osteopathy
Chiropractic	Reflexology
Herbal medicine	Reiki
Homeopathy	Relaxation and visualization
Hypnosis	Spiritual healing
Kinesiology	Therapeutic touch
Massage	Yoga

Data compiled from Eisenberg (3) and Zollman C, Vickers A. ABC of complementary medicine. What is complementary medicine? BMJ 1999;319: 693–6.

American communities show high rates of use as well, though the spectrum of alternative therapy differs.

Among rheumatology patients, complementary and alternative therapies are often used to supplement standard medical care, rather than replace it. Those who tend to use CAM have inadequately controlled pain. In a survey of rheumatology outpatients, 87% said they used CAM to control pain and 62% had heard it helped someone else (6). The perception that CAM therapies were safe was held by 72%, but only 10% believed that they would cure arthritis. This study also confirmed that physicians asked about CAM use only 30% of the time, but that patients expected their doctors to know about the efficacy of CAM treatments as well as potential interactions with prescription medications.

DIET

The use of dietary interventions is appealing as a readily accessible and seemingly controllable factor in the treatment of arthritis symptoms. While medical history is rich with descriptions of the relationship between food and drink and gout, more recent systematic study has shown that only rarely can clinical symptoms in other arthritis patients be documented to occur in relation to specific foods (7). However, certain findings suggest that this will continue to be an area of active investigation. Some rheumatoid arthritis (RA) patients have been shown to benefit on occasion from the use of fish or plant oil preparations. Eicosapentaenoic acid and docosahexaenoic acid are present in cold-water fish as well as widely available in capsule form. Each has been shown to lead to the suppression of arachidonic acid-derived prostaglandins and leukotrienes. Similar in vitro findings have been demonstrated for plants oils derived from borage (*Borago officinalis*), evening primrose (*Oenothera biennis*), and flaxseed (*Linum usitatissimum*). However, optimal patient selection criteria and appropriate dosing have not been established in controlled clinical trials (8).

Fasting has been demonstrated to have short-term anti-rheumatic efficacy. While not a practical or recommended intervention, fasting for 7–10 days has led to reductions in pain, stiffness, evidence of inflammation on physical examination and laboratory testing, and medication requirements in studies of patients with RA. The mechanisms for this effect remain obscure, but could include the reduction in the antigenic challenge to the immune system provided by food ingestion (9).

VITAMINS

The use of vitamin supplementation is an area of considerable interest for patients, for both health promotion and improvement of arthritis symptoms. Two recent studies have led to new speculation about the role of vitamin D in osteoarthritis (OA). Analysis of Framingham data, including food frequency questionnaires and measurement of serum $25-(OH)_2D$ levels, suggested that those with the lowest intake and serum levels of vitamin D were 3 times more likely to have progression of established OA, although no preventive benefit was noted (10). This contrasted with a subgroup analysis in the Study of Osteoporotic Fractures (11), which found that those with the lowest levels of $25-(OH)_2D$ were 3 times more likely to develop OA of the hip as measured by radiographic joint space narrowing. Despite these intriguing epidemiologic extrapolations, it is not known if taking vitamin D supplements prevents the onset or progression of osteoarthritis.

Analysis of another Framingham population subset, again by food frequency questionnaire, revealed that high vitamin C intake was associated with a 3-fold reduction in OA disease progression. A weaker positive association was found for beta-carotene. No association could be demonstrated for vitamins E, B1, B6, niacin, or folate (12). However, vitamin E was found to be of benefit in one small study of RA patients that showed modest analgesic benefits, though no alterations in swollen or tender joints were noted (13). Finally, vitamin A has been implicated in worsening osteoporosis and increasing osteoporotic fracture risk. In Sweden, where dietary intake of vitamin A is the highest in Europe due to dairy product supplementation, retinol intake >1.5 mg/day led to a 10% reduction in bone density and a doubling of hip fractures (14).

GLUCOSAMINE AND CHONDROITIN

These building blocks of normal connective tissue have been used for osteoarthritis pain relief for decades in Europe. Their increasing use in the United States followed the publication of the popular bestseller, *The Arthritis Cure*, by Dr. Jason Theodosakis in 1997 (15). This book not only brought glucosamine and chondroitin to the attention of the American public, it also forced an examination of the accumulated clinical data available to evaluate these substances.

Glucosamine is an aminomonosaccharide that is a component of glycoproteins, proteoglycans, and glycosaminoglycans. It is involved in a rate-limiting step of proteoglycan synthesis and, when added to chondrocytes *in vitro*, stimulates proteoglycan production. Glucosamine is known to be reduced in osteoarthritic cartilage. Limited laboratory studies have demonstrated glucosamine's effectiveness in reducing cellular production of inflammatory mediators, as well as in reducing inflammation in the rat adjuvant arthritis model. Pharmacokinetic data suggest that oral administration of radio-labeled glucosamine results in detectable serum levels of ^{14}C within hours of administration, but there has been no direct demonstration that the glucosamine is incorporated into cartilage. Nonetheless, rabbit data have suggested a preventive role for glucosamine.

Most clinical trials of glucosamine have been of short duration and small size. However, several randomized, double-blinded, placebo-controlled trials have been carried out (5,16,17). Virtually all published studies suggest benefit in terms of pain relief, and some have shown improvement in tenderness, swelling, and functional status as well. The benefit has been comparable to that of nonsteroidal antiinflammatory drugs (NSAIDs), but the time of onset for symptom relief by glucosamine is delayed over a period of weeks. The effects of glucosamine may also persist weeks after discontinuation. Adverse events have been minimal and comparable to placebo; gastrointestinal upset is most often mentioned. A controversial 3-year trial has suggested that glucosamine use was associated with a slowing in the rate of radiographic progression of OA (18), but has been criticized on the basis of the difficulty in interpreting the radiographic technique used. A large, NIH-funded multicenter trial is underway in the United States to further study the role of glucosamine in treatment of OA.

Chondroitin sulfate is available over-the-counter as an individual preparation, as well as in combination with glucosamine with or without a variety of vitamins, minerals, and other supplements. Less experimental and clinical data are available on the use of chondroitin, and none has been published on the combinations. Meta-analysis of short-duration studies with small numbers of patients has shown positive trends for analgesia in OA of the knee and hip.

A recent meta-analysis was intended to address some of the shortcomings of the published trials on glucosamine and chondroitin (19). The authors identified 6 randomized, double-blind, placebo-controlled trials of glucosamine and 9 of chondroitin. Although the trials showed moderate to large effect of these nutraceuticals, interpretation of the results was limited by inconsistencies in study methods and industry sponsorship. Nonetheless, the authors concluded that glucosamine and chondroitin have some efficacy in treating OA symptoms and that they are safe. Most studies have used a daily dose of 1500 mg of glucosamine sulfate and 1200 mg of chondroitin sulfate.

HERBAL PREPARATIONS

A visit to the local health food store will reveal a large number of preparations devoted to the treatment of arthritis. The array of herbal ingredients present in these preparations can be quite impressive, some coming from folk tradition, others of less clear origin. A small, but growing, body of well-designed trials is beginning to address the role of some of these preparations in the rheumatologic armamentarium.

Willow Bark (*Salix sp.*)

The bark of the willow and poplar trees has been used since antiquity for the treatment of pain, fever, and gout. Willow bark remains a popular ingredient in over-the-counter antirheumatic preparations due to its content of salicin, a source of salicylic acid. A randomized, double-blind, placebo-controlled trial has demonstrated efficacy of willow bark preparations for relieving pain in OA of the knee and hip over a 2-month period. The agent used in this study contained only 20–40 mg of salicylic acid equivalent in a 2-tablet dose (20). Preparations containing willow bark are generally thought to be less effective than nonsteroidal antiinflammatory drugs because of lesser effects on the inflammatory pathways, but no head-to-head comparisons have been made. This may also explain why these preparations have fewer adverse effects. A more recent study looked at over 200 individuals with low back pain recruited from the community (21). After 6 months, patients treated with willow bark extract had a significant increase in pain-free intervals without the need for rescue medications.

Devil's Claw (*Harpagophytum procumbens*)

The medicinal roots of this native African plant have been used in folk medicine for relief of pain due to rheumatism. A handful of small but well-designed studies have shown significant improvement in pain in OA patients using *Harpagophytum procumbens* (devil's claw). Double-blind trials have demonstrated reductions in pain scores and increases in mobility for patients taking devil's claw over a 2-week period. Short-term tolerability was high, but long-term efficacy and side effects have yet to be determined. While the mechanism of action is unknown, those with a history of ulcer should avoid this herb due to its stimulatory effect on gastric secretions.

Feverfew (*Tanacetum parthenium*)

A resident of many suburban backyards in the United States despite its European origins, feverfew is another herb long used to treat rheumatism. As the name implies, feverfew has been used as an antipyretic and antiinflammatory folk remedy. It is known to reduce platelet aggregation, prostaglandin synthesis, and histamine release, although its effects appear to be independent of cyclooxygenase. More recent data suggest that feverfew extract may inhibit cytokine-induced adhesion molecule expression on rheumatoid synovial fibroblasts, although studies of feverfew in patients with RA have shown little or no benefit. In a 6-week trial using a powdered extract of *Tanacetum parthenium*, 41 women with RA had no improvement in pain, stiffness, or the number of swollen or tender joints on physical examination. Feverfew should be avoided by those with allergies to chamomile, ragweed, or yarrow.

Thunder God Vine (*Tripterygium wilfordii*)

Considerable interest has been focused on *Tripterygium wilfordii*, also known as Chinese thunder god vine. Roots, leaves, and flowers of this herb were used in the 16th century as part of traditional Chinese medicine. It fell out of use for centuries, perhaps because of its toxicity, and was later used as an agricultural insecticide. Interest in its medicinal use was revived when Chinese physicians during the Cultural Revolution became more familiar with traditional herbal practices.

Pharmacologic preparations have been developed and numerous Chinese publications have documented the use of *Tripterygium* derivatives for a host of rheumatologic disorders, including rheumatoid arthritis, systemic lupus erythematosus, Henoch-Schönlein purpura, Sweet's syndrome, systemic sclerosis (scleroderma), Behçet's syndrome, and psoriatic arthritis. Pharmacologic, toxicologic, and chemical analyses suggest that the therapeutic activity of *Tripterygium* derives from the diterpenoid components with epoxide structures. T2, a chloroform-methanol extract, and EA, an ethyl acetate extract, have been shown to have a number of antiinflammatory and immunosuppressive effects.

In vitro and in vivo studies have demonstrated inhibition of the production of pro-inflammatory cytokines (interleukin-2, interferon-γ) and inflammatory mediators such as prostaglandin E_2 and nitric oxide. The mechanism may include the suppression of the transcription of genes for inflammatory mediators. Animal studies have shown efficacy in the adjuvant arthritis model that is comparable to immunosuppressive drugs such as azathioprine and corticosteroids.

Most information about the use of *Tripterygium* comes from uncontrolled clinical trials and retrospective reports, but some reports have detailed observations in patients treated for up to a decade. One case report describes a woman with systemic lupus erythematosus and diffuse membranoproliferative glomerulonephritis. After developing *Pneumocystis* pneumonia while on cyclophosphamide, she self-medicated with a combination of steroids and thunder god vine and achieved a resolution of proteinuria and a normalization of serum creatinine. One prospective, randomized, double-blind study of T2 in rheumatoid arthritis patients showed significant improvements in joint tenderness scores, as well as in physician and patient global assessment. Erythrocyte sedimentation rate, C-reactive protein levels, and levels of rheumatoid factor fell in actively treated patients; however, considerable toxicity was documented as well. Up to a third of patients had gastrointestinal side effects and many patients experienced amenorrhea. Other studies have suggested that amenorrhea may be irreversible in perimenopausal women exposed to *Tripterygium* and that exposed men may experience azoospermia. Treatment-related deaths have occurred as a result of myocardial damage, renal failure, and hypotensive episodes related to severe gastrointestinal side effects. Nevertheless, thunder god vine continues to be the subject of continued study due to its impressive array of immunosuppressive effects.

Avocado Soybean Unsaponifiables

A preparation made from the unsaponifiable fractions of avocado and soybean oils remains a popular remedy for osteoarthritis pain in Western Europe. A substantial body of in vitro and animal studies suggests a variety of potentially relevant effects of avocado soybean unsaponifiables (ASU). Laboratory studies have shown that interleukin-1 mediated events may be affected by ASU and that collagen synthesis may be stimulated in articular chondrocyte culture. Additional cytokine levels and prostaglandin production may be altered as well. Reduction in cartilage lesions was seen in a rabbit model of OA. One multicenter randomized double-blind, placebo-controlled trial of 164 patients showed significant reductions in pain, functional disability, and use of nonsteroidal antiinflammatory drugs (22). Side effects were comparable to placebo.

BUYER BEWARE

Patients and physicians interested in taking or prescribing over-the-counter dietary supplements should be aware of the provisions of the Dietary Supplement and Health Education Act passed by Congress in 1994. This legislation permits the over-the-counter sale of numerous herbal and other preparations, exempting them from documentation requirements for efficacy and safety that are required for prescription medications. Unfortunately, under this law, consumers cannot be assured of the purity or dosage of the herb or presumed active ingredient in over-the-counter "natural" products. Nor do manufacturers have any incentive to participate in clinical trials to further evaluate such products, since they may be sold for a variety of indications without demonstration of efficacy. This state of affairs has clearly impeded progress in establishing evidence-based guidelines for the use of herbal medications.

Adverse Effects of Herbal Preparations

The adverse effects of herbal preparations are not well studied, although patients clearly expect their physicians to be aware of and advise patients about potential side effects. Case reports have documented several instances of marked toxicity due to Chinese herbal preparations. These preparations generally contain multiple ingredients, which may vary between different batches. Gastrointestinal bleeding due to the adulteration of Chinese herbs by nonsteroidal antiinflammatory drugs has been well documented. Hepatotoxicity, including fulminant liver failure, has been reported as well. An inadvertent manufacturing error led to contamination of a batch of Chinese herbs used for weight reduction imported to Belgium. The nephrotoxic herb, *Aristolochia fangchi*, was implicated in subsequent development of rapidly progressive renal failure resulting in end-stage renal disease and, more recently, the appearance of urothelial carcinoma in almost half of those patients with renal failure.

Caution should be exercised when herbal preparations are used in combination with prescription medications. In particular, the potential for increased bleeding risk should be appreciated in patients on anti-platelet therapy or anticoagulants who are also taking feverfew, ginseng, garlic, or gingko. It has also been suggested that willow bark could increase plasma levels of methotrexate and that echinacea should not be used in combination with methotrexate due to the risk of increased hepatotoxicity. Theoretically, the use of "immune boosters" such as echinacea, *Astragalus*, licorice root, and alfalfa sprouts could interfere with the action of immunosuppressive medications. A review of selected clinical considerations focusing on known or potential drug-herb interactions has been published (23).

PHYSICAL INTERVENTIONS

Acupuncture

Acupuncture is an ancient Chinese technique traditionally indicated for redressing imbalances of *chi*, or energy. Needles placed along a series of meridians, or pathways, could be used to therapeutically direct the flow of chi in the body. More recent Western explanations of the analgesic efficacy of acupuncture invoke various alterations in the neurochemical microenvironment. Some observations suggest that stimulation of high-threshold small-diameter nerve fibers occurs, which leads to specific blockage of pain messages in higher centers of the brain. However, the absence of a clear understanding of the mechanism of action has led to debate about what the appropriate placebo control should be in clinical trials. Some studies have used no treatment as a control, while others have used needle placement in non-meridian locations. However, it is known that even sham acupuncture can have analgesic effects.

Despite the long history of use and popularity of acupuncture, studies in arthritis patients have been relatively few. In patients with OA awaiting knee replacement, acupuncture led to diminution of pain, while those who did not receive acupuncture reported increasing pain as their time to undergo surgery neared. Pain relief has been demonstrated in a few other small and brief trials of patients with OA as well as in other clinical pain models. A recent meta-analysis of acupuncture used for the treatment of low back pain showed that acupuncture was superior to a variety of control interventions, although not clearly better than placebo (24). Similarly, a recent systematic review of acupuncture for OA of the knee revealed strong evidence to support the use of acupuncture for pain control, although its role in improving function was less clear (25). After a review of the available data, the National Institutes of Health has concluded that results for acupuncture in control of chemotherapy-associated nausea and vomiting and control of postoperative pain have been promising. In addition, they concluded that disorders such as tennis elbow, fibromyalgia, myofascial pain, osteoarthritis, low back pain, and carpal tunnel syndrome may be treated either primarily or adjunctively with acupuncture.

T'ai Chi

T'ai chi is an ancient Chinese practice that incorporates cognitive, cardiovascular, and musculoskeletal responses. This classical conditioning exercise has been performed for centuries to promote health and to be used in self-defense. It has been suggested that t'ai chi might maintain flexibility and mobility in arthritis patients after investigations showed improvements in muscle strength and aerobic efficiency. One recent prospective, randomized, controlled study demonstrated enhanced self-efficacy, quality of life, and functional mobility among older adults with OA who practiced t'ai chi for 12 weeks (26).

ADVISING PATIENTS

The rigors of evidence-based medicine are only beginning to be applied to the vast and diverse practices encompassed by

Table 2. Advising patients about the use of complementary and alternative medicine.

1. Ask all patients about use of herbal therapies and dietary supplements and document their use in the medical record.
2. "Natural" does not necessarily mean safe.
3. Interactions between herbal products and pharmaceutical products do occur; therefore, avoid combined use.
4. Lack of standardization of herbal agents may result in variability in herbal content and efficacy among manufacturers.
5. Lack of quality control and regulation may result in contamination during manufacture and potential misidentification of plant species.
6. Herbal treatments should not be used before or during pregnancy or lactation because of lack of long-term clinical trials proving safety.
7. Herbal treatments should not be used in larger-than-recommended doses.
8. Herbal treatments should not be used for more than several weeks, because of lack of studies proving long-term safety.
9. Herbal treatments with known adverse effects and toxic effects should be avoided.
10. Infants, children, the elderly, or anyone with impaired immune function should not use herbal treatments without professional advice.
11. An accurate diagnosis and discussion of proven treatment options are essential prior to the patient's considering use of herbal treatments.
12. If adverse effects occur, they should be documented in the patient's chart and therapy should be discontinued.

Reprinted with permission from Cirigliano M, Sun A. Advising patients about herbal therapies. JAMA 1998;280:1565–6.

complementary and alternative medicine. However, epidemiologic data suggest that CAM use is increasing. Patients will continue to expect physicians to understand potential medication interactions, as well as other risks and benefits of seeking alternative approaches. As the field of complementary and alternative medicine grows, one of the most useful interventions physicians can make is to ask their patients what alternative therapies they are using and why. A number of authors have suggested guidelines for practitioners that have wide applicability (Table 2) and, as health care providers, we must continue to inform ourselves as research results become available.

In the meantime, patients will continue to gather information from family, friends, and the Internet (see Chapter 44 for web sites of interest).

REFERENCES

1. Panush RS. American College of Rheumatology position statement. Complementary and alternative therapies for rheumatic diseases II. Rheum Dis Clin N Am 2000;26:189–192.
2. Eisenberg DM, Kessler RC, Foster C, Norlock FE, Calkins DR, Delbanco TL. Unconventional medicine in the United States. Prevalence, costs, and patterns of use. N Engl J Med 1993;328:246–52.
3. Eisenberg DM. Advising patients who seek alternative medical therapies. Ann Intern Med 1997;127:61–9.
4. Kolasinski SL. The use of alternative therapies by patients with rheumatic diseases. J Clin Rheum 1999;5:253–4.
5. Kolasinski SL. Complementary and alternative therapies for rheumatic disease. Hosp Pract 2001;36:31–6, 39.
6. Rao JK, Mihaliak K, Kroenke K, Bradley J, Tierney WM, Weinberger M. Use of complementary therapies for arthritis among patients of rheumatologists. Ann Intern Med 1999;131:409–16.
7. Panush RS, Stroud RM, Webster EM. Food-induced (allergic) arthritis. Inflammatory arthritis exacerbated by milk. Arthritis Rheum 1986;29:220–6.
8. Ernst E, Chrubasik S. Phyto-anti-inflammatories. A systematic review of randomized, placebo-controlled, double-blind trials. Rheum Dis Clin North Am 2000;26:13–27, vii.
9. Henderson CJ, Panush RS. Diets, dietary supplements, and nutritional therapies in rheumatic diseases. Rheum Dis Clin North Am 1999;25:937–68.
10. McAlindon TE, Felson DT, Zhang Y, Hannan MT, Aliabadi P, Weissman B, et al. Relation of dietary intake and serum levels of vitamin D to progression of osteoarthritis of the knee among participants in the Framingham Study. Ann Intern Med 1996;125:353–9.
11. Lane NE, Gore LR, Cummings SR, Hochberg MC, Scott JC, Williams EN, et al. Serum vitamin D levels and incident changes of radiographic hip osteoarthritis: a longitudinal study. Study of Osteoporotic Fractures Research Group. Arthritis Rheum 1999;42:854–60.
12. McAlindon TE, Jacques P, Zhang Y, Hannan MT, Aliabadi P, Weissman B, et al. Do antioxidant micronutrients protect against the development and progression of knee osteoarthritis? Arthritis Rheum 1996;39:648–56.
13. Edmonds SE, Winyard PG, Guo R, Kidd B, Merry P, Langrish-Smith A,. Putative analgesic activity of repeated oral doses of vitamin E in the treatment of rheumatoid arthritis. Results of a prospective placebo controlled double blind trial. Ann Rheum Dis 1997;56:649–55.
14. Melhus H, Michaelsson K, Kindmark A, Bergstrom R, Holmberg L, Mallmin H, et al. Excessive dietary intake of vitamin A is associated with reduced bone mineral density and increased risk for hip fracture. Ann Intern Med 1998;129:770–8.
15. Theodosakis J, Adderly B, Fox F. The arthritis cure: the medical miracle that can halt, reverse, and may even cure osteoarthritis. New York: St Martin's Press; 1997.
16. Deal CL, Moskowitz RW. Nutraceuticals as therapeutic agents in osteoarthritis. The role of glucosamine, chondroitin sulfate, and collagen hydrolysate. Rheum Dis Clin North Am 1999;25:379–95.
17. Delafuente JC. Glucosamine in the treatment of osteoarthritis. Rheum Dis Clin North Am 2000;26:1–11, vii.
18. Reginster JY, Deroisy R, Rovati LC, Lee RL, Lejeune E, Bruyere O, et al. Long-term effects of glucosamine sulphate on osteoarthritis progression: a randomised, placebo-controlled clinical trial. Lancet 2001;357:251–6.
19. McAlindon TE, LaValley MP, Gulin JP, Felson DT. Glucosamine and chondroitin for treatment of osteoarthritis: a systematic quality assessment and meta-analysis. JAMA 2000;283:1469–75.
20. Mills SY, Jacoby RK, Chacksfield M, Willoughby M. Effect of a proprietary herbal medicine on the relief of chronic arthritic pain: a double-blind study. Br J Rheumatol 1996;35:874–8.
21. Chrubasik S, Eisenberg E, Balan E, Weinberger T, Luzzati R, Conradt C. Treatment of low back pain exacerbations with willow bark extract: a randomized double-blind study. Am J Med 2000;109:9–14.
22. Maheu E, Mazieres B, Valat JP, Loyau G, Le Loet X, Bourgeois P, et al. Symptomatic efficacy of avocado/soybean unsaponifiables in the treatment of osteoarthritis of the knee and hip: a prospective, randomized, double-blind, placebo-controlled, multicenter clinical trial with a six-month treatment period and a two-month followup demonstrating a persistent effect. Arthritis Rheum 1998;41:81–91.
23. Miller LG. Herbal medicinals: selected clinical considerations focusing on known or potential drug-herb interactions. Arch Intern Med 1998;158:2200–11.
24. Ernst E, White AR. Acupuncture for back pain: a meta-analysis of randomized controlled trials. Arch Intern Med 1998; 58:2235–41.
25. Ezzo J, Hadhazy V, Birch S, Lao L, Kaplan G, Hochberg M, et al. Acupuncture for osteoarthritis of the knee: a systematic review. Arthritis Rheum 2001;44:819–25.
26. Hartman CA, Manos TM, Winter C, Hartman DM, Li B, Smith JC. Effects of T'ai Chi training on function and quality of life indicators in older adults with osteoarthritis. J Am Geriatr Soc 2000;48:1553–9.

Additional Recommended Reading

Panush RS, editor. Complementary and alternative therapies for rheumatic diseases I. Rheum Dis Clin North Am 1999;25.
Panush RS, editor. Complementary and alternative therapies for rheumatic diseases II. Rheum Dis Clin North Am 2000;26.
Eisenberg DM, Kessler, RC, Foster C, Norlock FE, Calkins DR, Delbanco TL. Unconventional medicine in the United States. Prevalence, costs, and patterns. N Engl J Med 1993;328:246–52.
Eisenberg DM. Advising patients who seek alternative medical therapies. Ann Intern Med 1997;127:61–9.
Eisenberg DM, Davis RB, Ettner SL, Appel S, Wilkey S, Van Rompay M, et al. Trends in alternative medicine use in the United States, 1990-1997: results of a follow-up national survey. JAMA 1998;280:1569–75.

Fugh-Berman A. Alternative medicine: what works. A comprehensive, easy-to-read review of the scientific evidence, pro and con. Baltimore: Williams & Wilkins; 1997.

Rao JK, Mihaliak K, Kroenke K, Bradley J, Tierney WM, Weinberger M. Use of complementary therapies for arthritis among patients of rheumatologists. Ann Intern Med 1999;131:409–16.

Appendix

Definition of Complementary and Alternative Medicine by the Cochrane Collaboration

"Complementary and alternative medicine (CAM) is a broad domain of healing resources that encompasses all health systems, modalities and practices and their accompanying theories and beliefs, other than those intrinsic to the politically dominant health system of a particular society or culture in a given historical period. CAM includes all such practices and ideas self-defined by their users as preventing or treating illness or promoting health and well-being. Boundaries within CAM and between the CAM domain and that of the dominant system are not always sharp or fixed."

Shoulder Disorders and Treatments

MAREN LAWSON MAHOWALD, MD

Approximately 20–25% of adults experience shoulder problems that cause pain and impair normal functioning (1,2). Symptoms may begin abruptly or gradually and may be an acute, subacute, or chronic problem. Identification of the specific shoulder disorder requires a thorough knowledge of the anatomy and complex muscle actions that produce motion and stability. Physical examination based on the anatomy and biomechanics of the shoulder permits accurate diagnosis in most but not all patients. Analysis of the biomechanical dysfunctions in shoulder disorders provides the basis of treatment and rehabilitation. The goals of therapy for the painful shoulder are to decrease pain, improve function, and prevent recurrences and disability.

More than 90% of shoulder pain involves rotator cuff tendinitis, tears, or contracture. Limitation of motion due to pain from rotator cuff problems predisposes to adhesive capsulitis as a secondary complication, which further increases pain and loss of motion. Prompt initiation of physical therapy or home exercises to put the arm through its full range of motion passively or actively will decrease the likelihood of developing this contracture and additional disability.

ETIOLOGY

Causes of shoulder disorders are generally distributed by age, work and recreational activities, and trauma. Young people and vigorous athletes are more likely to experience abrupt, severe stress forces causing acute supraspinatus tendinitis, bicipital tendinitis, rotator cuff tear, dislocation, or fracture. Middle-aged adults who engage in intermittent repetitive vigorous activities (weekend jocks and do-it-yourselfers) are susceptible to acute inflammatory supraspinatus and bicipital tendinitis. In elderly patients, normal activity superimposed on chronic degenerative or inflammatory arthritis is associated with tendinitis or a contracted rotator cuff ("frozen shoulder"). The elderly may develop polymyalgia rheumatica or referred shoulder pain from other comorbid conditions.

ANATOMY AND BIOMECHANICS

There are 3 synovial joints (sternoclavicular, acromioclavicular, glenohumeral) and a bone-muscle-bone scapulothoracic articulation in the shoulder. The glenohumeral joint is a diarthrodial joint that is only minimally constrained by the bony components. The joint is supported by the rotator cuff and joint capsule surrounding the bony anatomy (3). The rotator cuff is made up of the tendons of 4 muscles: the subscapularis, supraspinatus, infraspinatus, and the teres minor muscles. Forces generated by contraction of the rotator cuff muscles depress the humeral head and stabilize it in the shallow glenoid, thus permitting abduction of the humerus by the deltoid. The scap-

ula is stabilized by 6 muscles: trapezius, major and minor rhomboids, levator scapulae, serratus anterior, and pectoralis minor (Figure 1).

Understanding biomechanical dysfunctions in shoulder disorders involves kinetics and kinematics. *Kinetics* deals with the motion of a body under the action of given forces. Kinetic analysis involves calculation of loads acting on the shoulder joint complex. *Kinematics* describes the motion of a body without reference to force or mass and defines the range of motion and surface motion of a joint in the frontal (coronal or longitudinal), sagittal, and transverse (horizontal) planes. The uniplanar motions at the glenohumeral joint are given in Table 1. Surface motion describes the relative position of the contact point on the humeral head and the contact point in the glenoid. With rotation of the humerus, the contact point in the glenoid remains constant while the contact point on the humeral head moves. During shoulder elevation (flexion), there is a combination of rolling (contact point on glenoid and contact point on humeral head both change) and gliding (contact point on humeral head is constant while contact point on glenoid changes).

Kinetic analysis of shoulder motion involves calculation of loads or forces acting on the shoulder joint complex. The weight of the arm and load being carried plus the forces generated by the muscles that move the arm must not dislocate the glenohumeral articulation. The glenohumeral joint has both static stabilizers (anterior, middle, and inferior glenohumeral ligaments; posterior capsule; and labrum) and dynamic stabilizers, which are the muscles for each planar movement and the co-contracting stabilizer muscles acting to resist dislocation. A free body diagram is used to calculate the reaction forces acting on the glenohumeral joint through a 3-force system. This system includes the forces from the weight of the arm (approximately 5–9% of body weight) and the deltoid muscle contraction moving the humerus up and out, which may be as much as 8 times the weight of the arm (approximately 70% of body weight). This must be counteracted by the glenohumeral joint reaction force (approximately 10 times the arm weight or 90% of body weight) plus the co-contracting rotator cuff muscles, which generate approximately 9.6 times arm weight (infraspinatus, supraspinatus, teres minor, and subscapularis muscles).

EVALUATION

Disorders of the shoulder joint complex cause pain, stiffness, upper arm weakness or instability, sleep disruption, and impaired activities of daily living, work, and recreation. Pain in the shoulder region may also be referred from pathology in the cervical spine, brachial plexus, peripheral nerve, tumor in the apex of the lung, lesions in or near the diaphragm (pleura, gall bladder, liver), and rarely, angina.

The differential diagnosis of shoulder pain includes rotator cuff tendinitis, rotator cuff tear, bicipital tendinitis, rotator cuff

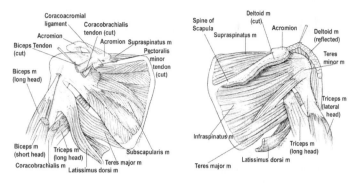

Figure 1. Shoulder anatomy, anterior and posterior views.

contracture ("frozen shoulder"), acromioclavicular arthritis, glenohumeral arthritis, and referred pain from sites extrinsic to the shoulder joint complex. It should be noted that more than one pathology often exists in the painful shoulder (4).

The Nature of Shoulder Pain

Patients often have difficulty localizing pain around the shoulder accurately. The sites causing the pain are so close together that differentiation is difficult. Pain originating from a site in the shoulder may be referred to the lateral mid-humerus or into the neck. The muscles near the lesion often contract to minimize painful movement and become another source of more diffuse pain in the taut muscles.

Pain is more likely to be localizable early in the course of supraspinatus tendinitis, bicipital tendinitis, and acromioclavicular arthritis. For example, the patient with acute supraspinatus tendinitis will localize the pain to the lateral tip of the shoulder or the lateral mid-humerus near the deltoid insertion. Typically the pain begins after the first 30° of abduction of the arm and is increased by resisted abduction of the arm or when rolling onto the painful shoulder during sleep. Interestingly, the pain often abates when abduction exceeds 120°.

History

The key to the diagnosis of shoulder disorders is precise data obtained with a focused interview. Probe for information about the exact onset of pain and its severity, character, location, periodicity, and impact. It is important to identify activities or trauma associated with the onset of shoulder pain. Inquire about prior episodes of shoulder pain, specifically asking about cause, workup, treatment, and time course. Determine pain severity using a 0 to 10 scale (0 = no pain, 10 = worst possible pain), and ask whether the pain is constant or incident to movement. Ask the patient to characterize the pain using descriptors such as sharp, aching, boring, gnawing, deep, burning, or tingling. If possible, have the patient pinpoint the most painful site.

Identify impact factors by asking which positions and movements increase or relieve the pain. Determine functional impairments by asking about activities of daily living (e.g., combing hair, dressing, overhead lifting), work capabilities (how much can be lifted and carried, can the patient work full time, is job security in jeopardy?) and leisure activities that can no longer be enjoyed. Ask whether the pain is worse at night when rolling onto the affected side (a positive response indicates rotator cuff problems).

Painless and full active range of motion strongly suggests referred pain. The patient with referred pain from the cervical spine may associate increased pain with certain neck movements and/or postures. Patients with referred pain from lung or diaphragmatic lesions tend to have persistent gnawing or aching pain not affected by shoulder movements or position.

Physical Examination

The shoulder examination should systematically compare the affected with the unaffected side. Information from all the examination elements is required for an accurate diagnosis. Elements of the examination include observation, range of motion and muscle strength testing, palpation, and special/provocative testing.

Observation. Look for bony prominences and swelling over the acromioclavicular and sternoclavicular joints and the normal sulcus between the humerus and thorax anteriorly (glenohumeral joint). Note any muscle atrophy, ecchymoses, abrasions, or other signs of trauma around the shoulder. Erythema is suggestive of infection.

Range of Motion and Muscle Strength Testing. First observe the arc (degrees) and ease of *active range of motion* during forward flexion (raise hands up above the head), external rotation (place hands behind occiput), internal rotation (place hands behind the back), and abduction (raise arms out from the sides bringing hands together above the head). *Passive range of motion* testing is carried out with the examiner fixing the scapula to the thorax with one hand while using the other hand to put the arm through all the motions. Compare the

Table 1. Uniplanar motions at the glenohumeral joint.

Motion	Description	Primary muscles involved (secondary contributors)
Flexion	Shoulder elevation or forward movement of the arm in the sagittal plane	Anterior deltoid, pectoralis major and minor (medial deltoid, supraspinatus, infraspinatus, subscapularis, clavicular pectoralis)
Extension	Backward movement of the arm in the sagittal plane	Posterior deltoid, latissimus dorsi, teres major, trapezius, rhomboid triceps (long head)
Abduction	Shoulder elevation in the frontal plane or abduction of the arm away from the side of the body	Medial deltoid, supraspinatus (posterior deltoid, infraspinatus, ± teres minor)
Adduction	Holding the arm at the side of the body and moving it across the chest	Anterior and posterior deltoid, clavicular pectoralis, teres major, subscapularis latissimus dorsi, triceps (long head)
Internal rotation	Move hand behind back or across the chest	Subscapularis, anterior deltoid, pectoralis major, latissimus dorsi, teres major
External rotation	Move hand behind head and away from the body while the elbow is close to the side of the body	Posterior deltoid, infraspinatus, teres minor
Shoulder elevation	Shrug	Trapezius, levator scapulae

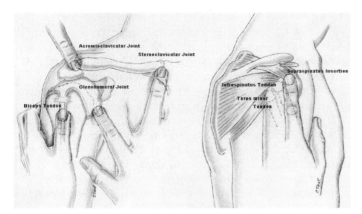

Figure 2. Landmarks for palpation of the shoulder.

arc of passive motion and point of pain near end ranges with the observed arc of active motion and point where pain is produced. Greater pain with active motion compared to passive motion suggests rotator cuff problems, whereas pain with both passive and active motion suggests glenohumeral joint arthritis.

Muscle strength should be tested in the deltoid, supraspinatus, subscapularis, internal rotators, external rotators, and biceps muscles; however, findings may be unreliable when pain is present. Pain with weakness that is described as burning or tingling suggests an underlying neuropathic process such as cervical radiculopathy, plexopathy, or neuropathy that may be further localized by testing deep tendon reflexes and cutaneous sensation.

Palpation. Note areas of warmth. Carefully palpate for tenderness over the sternoclavicular joint, acromioclavicular joint, glenohumeral joint beneath the coracoid process and at the insertions of the supraspinatus tendon, infraspinatus tendon, teres minor tendon, over the anterior aspect of the rotator cuff, and the biceps tendon in the bicipital groove (Figure 2). Identify areas of focal swelling with or without tenderness. Palpation should be done with the fingertip pad (rather than the fingertip) applying firm direct pressure. A grinding rotation of the palpating finger may produce a misleading pain response in the absence of tissue pathology.

Special/Provocative Testing. Special tests and examination maneuvers to reproduce pain with specific actions can be very helpful in identifying the source of pathology in the shoulder joint complex. These provocative tests are designed to isolate an individual muscle action or integrated force as much as possible and deliver a counterforce or strain to reproduce the pain symptom. For example, the impingement test is performed by forward flexing the extended arm with forearm pronation while fixing the scapula to the thorax with the other hand to determine whether anterior shoulder pain is reproduced. This test is fairly sensitive for rotator cuff impingement between the head of the humerus and the acromion, but it is not very specific, as a positive sign may occur with adhesive capsulitis, glenohumeral arthritis or instability, or acromioclavicular arthritis.

Rotator muscles should be tested individually. Supraspinatus is tested by resisted abduction of the arm positioned in slight abduction, flexion, and internal rotation. The infraspinatus is tested by resisted external rotation of the arm with elbow flexed to 90°. The subscapularis is tested with the arm at the side and the elbow flexed to 90° with resisted internal rotation. Additional tests will be described in the sections on individual

shoulder disorders. Shoulder pain with minimal loss of motion, no palpable tenderness, or no increase in pain with provocative tests suggests referred pain to the shoulder, a bone lesion, or a neuropathic process, especially if muscle atrophy is present.

Imaging Studies

Imaging studies are usually required to confirm the clinical diagnosis and to rule out other pathologic conditions. In some cases, diagnostic studies are useful to determine the size and severity of the lesion, which may direct choice of treatment and prognosis.

Plain x-rays should be performed routinely as part of the shoulder evaluation, including the anteroposterior view with internal and external rotation, scapular Y view, and the axillary view. These will reveal dislocation; fracture; arthritic changes characteristic of rheumatoid arthritis, osteoarthritis, and calcium pyrophosphate dihydrate crystal deposition disease; tendon calcifications; and bone cysts and sclerosis in the humeral head due to chronic rotator cuff disease tumors or avascular necrosis. The Y view will show variations in acromion morphology. A decrease in the acromiohumeral space due to upward migration of the humeral head indicates a rotator cuff tear. The axillary view will demonstrate posterior dislocation of the humeral head and calcifications in the tendon of the subscapularis. Additional views are needed to visualize acromioclavicular and sternoclavicular pathology specifically.

Arthrography with computed tomography (CT) or magnetic resonance imaging (MRI) is emerging as a valuable tool to evaluate soft-tissue lesions and intraarticular lesions in the glenohumeral joint. Availability of this technology depends on the experience level of radiology staff. CT scans provide good detail of lesions in the glenohumeral, acromioclavicular, and sternoclavicular joints. MRI scans allow visualization of soft tissue lesions, bone tumors, and ischemic necrosis of bone. MRI is sensitive for rotator cuff problems, but may not differentiate between tendinitis, partial tears, and small complete tears (5).

Ultrasonography provides an inexpensive, noninvasive method of identifying rotator cuff lesions with high sensitivity and specificity when carried out by an experienced technician. Scintigraphy (bone scan) is a very sensitive but nonspecific method to demonstrate increased uptake due to inflammation, arthritis, infection, or bone lesions.

Arthroscopy is becoming the preferred diagnostic study for patients with shoulder pain not responding to initial conservative therapy because it also affords the opportunity for treatment (debridement, removal of loose bodies, cuff repair, labrum repair, excisional decompression, tenodesis and tendon transfers, subacromial decompression, and repair of some chondral lesions).

SPECIFIC SHOULDER DISORDERS

Rotator Cuff Tendinitis

Rotator cuff tendinitis is the most common cause of shoulder pain. Tendinitis rather than bursitis is the underlying pathologic process, which may be acute or chronic. Rotator cuff tendinitis is caused by trauma, repetitive overhead activities, variations in acromion morphology, osteophytes on the undersurface of the acromion, or inflammatory processes such as rheumatoid arthritis or microcrystalline (apatite) deposits. Symptomatic calcific tendinitis occurs when a preexisting calcific deposit begins to resorb and produces intense inflammation (see also Chapter 21, Periarticular Rheumatic Diseases).

About 25 years ago, Neer coined the term "impingement" and reported on 100 anatomic dissections of the shoulder. He described various pathologic changes associated with the impingement of the rotator cuff between the acromion, coracoid, coracoacromial ligament, acromioclavicular joint, and the humeral head (6). He created a staging system for impingement lesions and their characteristic features, as follows:

- *Stage I* (mild tendinitis) with edema and hemorrhage in the rotator cuff is usually seen in those under age 25 who engage in overhead activities.
- *Stage II* (chronic tendinitis) occurs in the third and fourth decade as fibrosis, thickening, and tearing of the cuff following repeated impingement and recurrent attacks of rotator cuff tendinitis.
- *Stage III* (cuff tears) develops after age 40 and includes full thickness rotator cuff tears, biceps tendon rupture, and/or degenerative bone changes.

Acute lesions produce excruciating sharp pain that is exacerbated by overhead activities. Chronic lesions produce a persistent ache over the lateral upper arm that increases with active abduction. Dressing is painful, and sleep is often disrupted by pain. Pain is greater with active and resisted abduction than with passive abduction. Tenderness to palpation is localized to the greater tubercle of the humerus (the insertion of the supraspinatus tendon). Edema and swelling of the supraspinatus tendon (inflamed rotator cuff) results in impingement of the rotator cuff between the greater tuberosity and the acromion during abduction of the arm.

Neer devised an "impingement" test to demonstrate the pathophysiology of rotator cuff impingement (i.e., inflammation in the subacromial space); however, it may also be positive with other periarticular disorders. In Neer's test, the examiner fixes the scapula to the thorax with one hand and forcefully moves the arm into forward flexion with the other hand, reproducing the patient's shoulder pain. Impingement may be confirmed if the pain is eliminated during repeat testing after an injection of lidocaine into the subacromial bursa. Hawkins sign, another "impingement" test, is elicited by internally rotating the arm at 90° of forward flexion while the elbow is flexed at 90°.

External and internal rotation strength and pain response should be tested with the flexed elbow supported by the examiner and rotational force applied to the wrist. Weakness or pain during resisted external rotation from the neutral position (0° adduction) suggests inflammation or tear of the infraspinatus tendon. Weakness or pain with resisted abduction while the arm is at 30° of forward flexion, or resisted abduction while the arm is at 90° of forward flexion and pronation so the thumb is pointing at the floor ("empty can position"), suggests a lesion in the supraspinatus tendon.

In Stage I, plain x-rays are normal but may demonstrate abnormal acromion morphology. With recurrences and progression of rotator cuff tendinitis, sclerosis and cyst formation occurs in the humeral head, and spur formation on the undersurface of the lateral side of the acromioclavicular joint develops. When tears occur, the acromiohumeral distance decreases due to superior subluxation of the humeral head, and erosive changes in the anterior acromion develop. Calcification in the tendon may be seen on plain x-rays. On MRI, tears demonstrate increased signal in both T1- and T2-weighted images.

Treatment depends on staging as well as the age and activity level of the patient. Pendular exercises are basic to all therapy programs because the weight of the arm distracts the subacromial space and permits maintenance of motion, flexibility, and reduction of pain. The earlier that physical therapy is begun, the more likely it is to be successful. Pain must be controlled to permit the patient to exercise daily. Patient education regarding the home exercise program is critical for adherence. Application of heat or ultrasound before exercising reduces pain and facilitates stretching (7).

With Stage I lesions, rest (but not immobilization), nonsteroidal antiinflammatory drugs (NSAIDs), and stretching are followed by progressive internal and external rotation strengthening exercises. Restoration of rotator cuff muscle strength will prevent superior migration of the humeral head, thereby reducing pain and restoring shoulder function (8). Corticosteroid injections often provide dramatic improvement and permit earlier physical therapy (9).

With Stage II lesions, initial corticosteroid with bupivacaine injection plus NSAIDs or analgesics is preferred to permit more extensive passive, active-assisted, and active stretching and strengthening exercises to reduce contracture. Cessation of overhead activities and job modifications are necessary during the treatment period and may have to be continued to prevent recurrence of impingement.

Patients with refractory Stage II or III impingement (failure of 6 months of physical therapy) will usually need surgery. The surgical approach, called anterior acromioplasty, is designed to decompress the subacromial space (subacromial bursectomy, coracoacromial ligament section, and resection of bone at the undersurface of the acromion), repair any full thickness cuff tears if possible, and resect the distal clavicle if it is contributing to the impingement. Surgical sectioning of the coracoacromial ligament with subacromial bursectomy or open anterior acromioplasty may be needed to prevent recurrences and disability.

Prevention of recurrences and disability depends on patient education. Identifying the overuse pattern or cause of repeated trauma permits development of modifications to reduce or eliminate such activities. In a deconditioned or debilitated individual, normal activities of daily living may injure the rotator cuff. Muscle strengthening and general conditioning exercises are key to preventing recurrences in these individuals.

Rotator Cuff Tears

Rotator cuff tears occur with trauma, or they may be spontaneous in later stages of rotator cuff tendinitis, with chronic inflammation due to rheumatoid arthritis, spondylarthropathies, or systemic lupus erythematosus. Fibers of the rotator cuff are intertwined with the glenohumeral joint capsule so that complete tears of the rotator cuff result in communication between the joint and the subacromial bursa. Rotator cuff tears are classified by size and by individual rotator cuff tendon involved.

Traumatic tears are usually the result of a fall directly on the shoulder or an outstretched arm or of lifting a heavy object. The patient often feels a snap, followed by severe pain and inability to abduct the arm. If there is a history of direct trauma, x-rays should be obtained to rule out dislocation or fracture. Many patients do not recall a specific traumatic event, suggesting gradual progressive degeneration of the rotator cuff to a complete tear or cuff attrition such that a trivial stress on the rotator cuff extends a smaller, incomplete tear. Partial tears occur in overhead athletes due to repetitive tensile overload.

Patients have pain and difficulty with upper extremity activities requiring abduction or internal and external rotation (dressing, combing hair, reaching into a back pocket). On exam the patient is unable to maintain the arm in abduction after it is passively raised (the "drop arm test"). Weakness of external rotation with the arm near the side of the body suggests a full thickness tear. Symptoms of rotator cuff tear and tendinitis may be differentiated by repeating the "drop arm test" after injecting a local anesthetic. With tendinitis, the patient is able to maintain abduction after the pain is eliminated; however, abduction cannot be maintained by those with a complete tear.

Imaging studies of rotator cuff tears should include plain x-rays initially to identify humeral head lesions, acromion type and osteophytes, unsuspected fractures and dislocation, and superior subluxation of the humerus. Ultrasonography and MRI are replacing arthrography for definitive diagnosis.

Treatment of acute cuff tears should be conservative initially, including NSAIDs, ultrasound, or local heat before stretching exercises, and ice after overhead activity. If pain precludes physical therapy, local injection of a corticosteroid with local anesthetic can be given. When pain and motion improve, a progressive strengthening program for rotator cuff muscles, deltoid, and scapular stabilizers should be started. A gradual return to overhead activities at work and recreation is implemented when symptoms are minimal and shoulder function is restored. If pain and shoulder impairment persist after 3-6 months of conservative treatment, arthroscopic or open surgical repair is considered. Subacromial decompression and removal of acromion osteophytes usually relieves pain and improves function even if the tear is found to be irreparable at the time of surgery (10). Earlier surgery may be indicated for full thickness tears in a younger person with loss of function.

Bicipital Tendinitis and Rupture

The bicipital tendon has a long head and a short head. The long head of the biceps is in a groove between the lesser and greater tubercle of the humerus and passes through the glenohumeral joint to insert on the superior rim of the glenoid. The biceps is a forward flexor of the arm, a forearm flexor, and a supinator when the elbow is flexed. *Bicipital tendinitis* is caused by acute or chronic impingement of the tendon between the bicipital groove and the acromion causing tenosynovitis of the long head of the biceps. Rupture of the long head of the biceps is rare in the absence of concomitant rotator cuff problems and impingement. Spontaneous rupture may occur with sudden anterior shoulder pain and ecchymosis with a sagging prominence of the biceps belly.

Bicipital tendinitis causes anterior shoulder pain with focal tenderness to palpation in the bicipital groove. Excessive pressure of the palpating finger can readily produce a misleading pain response in the absence of tendon inflammation. The pain can be provoked by several test maneuvers. Pain is increased by resisted supination of the forearm with the elbow flexed (Yergason's supination test) and resisted forward flexion of the arm with the elbow extended (Speed's test).

Treatment of biceps tendinitis includes rest, NSAIDs, local corticosteroid injection, and ultrasound therapy. Tendon rupture repair is controversial, and options include tenodesis of the distal end of the tendon into the bicipital groove or tendon transfer to the coracoid process to maintain biceps power.

Adhesive Capsulitis

Adhesive capsulitis (frozen shoulder syndrome, pericapsulitis, periarthritis) describes the painful or painless loss of active and passive shoulder motion in all planes. The cause may be idiopathic, as seen in patients with diabetes, parkinsonism, or thyroid disorders. X-rays and bone scans are not abnormal in this idiopathic form. Adhesive capsulitis also occurs secondarily to other intrinsic shoulder lesions or extrinsic lesions that cause referred pain to the shoulder, such as cervical radiculopathy or apical lung lesions. A mild inflammatory process results in cytokine and growth factor production leading to capsular fibrosis (11). Four stages of adhesive capsulitis have been described (12).

- *Stage I* is an early hypervascular inflammatory (lymphocytic) phase that lasts approximately 3 months. Shoulder pain is described as a deep aching that is present at rest and may radiate to the upper arm, back, and neck. Pain is exacerbated by any attempts at movement. Night pain is common and prevents sleeping on the affected side. On examination, there is a loss of internal and external rotation of the arm that is improved by injection of lidocaine into the glenohumeral joint. Flexion and extension are fairly well-preserved.
- During *stage 2*, progressive loss of motion with persistent pain occurs over 3–9 months. Injection of lidocaine or scalene block eliminates the pain but does not improve range of motion, reflecting a loss of capsule volume and flexibility. Biopsy reveals a dense proliferative synovitis and hypervascularity, as well as capsular fibroplasias without inflammation. On examination, the practitioner fixes the scapula to the thorax with one hand and is unable to abduct or internally and externally rotate the arm with the other hand.
- In *stage 3*, after 9–14 months of symptoms, patients report mild pain or pain-free stiff shoulder. No increase in range of motion occurs with local anesthetic or general anesthesia. Arthroscopy reveals synovial thickening but no hypervascularity.
- *Stage 4* is called the "thawing stage" during which range of motion is slowly recovered as increased motion begets increased stretching and capsule remodeling.

The primary treatment of adhesive capsulitis is physical therapy with NSAIDs and periodic corticosteroids injected into the glenohumeral joint. Treatment of stages 1 and 2 should include corticosteroid and local anesthetic injection, gentle stretching, and NSAIDs. In stages 3 and 4, analgesics and physical therapy are recommended. Patient education about the natural course and anticipated spontaneous resolution is critical to prevent discouragement and increase adherence to the exercise therapy program. Only rarely are arthroscopy or manipulation under anesthesia to ease the contracture needed (13).

Acromioclavicular Disorders

Acromioclavicular arthritis produces pain at the superior aspect of the shoulder that may radiate to the neck or jaw. The pain is produced or increased by activities involving adduction of the arm such as sleeping on the affected side, golfing, buckling a seatbelt, or doing bench presses and pushups. Acute acromioclavicular joint pain may be caused by infection, crystal-induced inflammation, or direct trauma that injures the distal clavicle or ligaments. Chronic disorders are due to repetitive trauma (e.g., heavy construction work, weightlifting, gymnastics, or swimming), chronic inflammatory disease, or idiopathic osteolysis of the distal clavicle.

On examination, there may be a visible "step-off" between the distal clavicle and medial acromion indicating separation. Examination reveals tenderness to palpation of the acromioclavicular joint, and crepitus may be felt during a shoulder shrug. The pain is reproduced during forced adduction of the arm over the chest. Imaging studies should include specific acromioclavicular views because routine shoulder x-rays do not demonstrate the joint well. X-ray changes include osteophytes, subchondral cystic changes and sclerosis, and osteopenia of the distal clavicle. Later resorption of the distal clavicle produces widening of the joint space.

Treatment includes pain control with local heat, NSAIDs, corticosteroid injections, and shoulder rehabilitation to increase motion and strength of shoulder muscles. In refractory cases, resection of the distal clavicle via arthrotomy or arthroscopy may be required to control pain and preserve function.

Sternoclavicular Arthritis

Sternoclavicular arthritis produces pain with shoulder activities that involve movement of the clavicle or thorax. Causes of acute sternoclavicular arthritis include infection (especially in intravenous drug abusers), seronegative spondylarthropathy, and less commonly, rheumatoid arthritis. There is focal tenderness and swelling at the sternoclavicular joint, and pain may be reproduced by a shoulder shrug or rotation of the upper thorax.

Treatment includes antibiotics and needle or surgical drainage for septic arthritis. Intraarticular corticosteroid injections are beneficial for those with underlying chronic inflammatory arthritis.

Glenohumeral Joint Disorders

Glenohumeral disorders produce variable pain with active and passive motion, often accompanied by locking and clicking. The pain is generalized over the shoulder region and may radiate into the neck, back, and upper arm. Tenderness to palpation is sought by producing direct pressure 1 cm below the coracoid process; care should be taken not to employ a rotatory motion, which will produce pain and involuntary contraction of the pectoral muscle overlying the glenohumeral joint capsule. Joint pathology and pain decrease glenohumeral range of motion, which is compensated by increased scapulothoracic motion that temporarily minimizes functional losses. Periarticular contractures develop and are associated with muscle atrophy and weakness that lead to substantial functional deficits.

Inflammatory Arthritis of the Shoulder

Rheumatoid arthritis and the spondylarthropathies commonly cause mild to severe chronic synovitis in the glenohumeral, acromioclavicular, and sternoclavicular joints. Acute inflammation of the glenohumeral joint is seen with infection, pseudogout, gout (rare), hydroxyapatite deposition in dialysis patients, or recurrent hemarthrosis due to hemophilia or chronic anticoagulation. Synovitis in the glenohumeral joint causes rotator cuff tendinitis and may result in tears with a cystic swelling over the anterior shoulder.

On examination, the acromioclavicular and sternoclavicular joints often have focal tenderness, swelling, and warmth. Effusion in the glenohumeral joint may be discerned by bimanual palpation of the anterior and posterior aspect of the shoulder. X-rays reveal erosions at the greater tuberosity, humeral head osteoporosis, and uniform narrowing of the glenohumeral joint space. At the acromioclavicular joint, erosions and widening of the joint with osteoporosis of the distal clavicle are seen.

The goal of treatment is to control the underlying inflammatory process and reduce pain with NSAIDs, analgesics, and corticosteroid injections. Patients with inflammatory arthritides must develop a habit of daily stretching and strengthening exercises to prevent functional loss and increased pain (see Chapter 26, Rest and Exercise). Patients with refractory disease will usually require total shoulder arthroplasty, which should be done before rotator cuff tendon attenuation and/or contractures are extensive.

Degenerative Disorders of the Shoulder

Osteoarthritis. Primary osteoarthritis of the glenohumeral joint is rare. Degenerative changes increase with age and may be related to recurrent trauma associated with boxing, heavy construction, pneumatic hammer use, neuropathic conditions such as syringomyelia, calcium pyrophosphate dihydrate crystal deposition disease, diabetes (Charcot joints), or other conditions such as hemochromatosis, hemophilia, and chronic dislocation of the shoulder.

The patient usually describes an insidious onset of mild to moderate shoulder pain. On examination, pain and crepitus occur with both active and passive range of motion testing. There is greater loss of external rotation compared to internal rotation. Osteophytes are seen at the anterior and inferior joint margins with sclerosis and subarticular cysts in the humeral head.

Symptomatic treatment is often successful with analgesics and NSAIDs, with or without corticosteroid injections. Because there is no reversible component underlying the symptoms, improvement in range of motion is limited. Vigorous stretching should be avoided, as it is likely to increase pain and further limit motion. When pain is refractory, total shoulder replacement is effective.

Osteonecrosis. Osteonecrosis of the humeral head may follow humeral neck fracture or be associated with lupus, pancreatitis, asthma, corticosteroid therapy, organ transplantation, sickle cell disease, or barotraumas ("the bends"). Necrosis of the humeral head leads to subchondral fracture and collapse with secondary degenerative changes of the articular surface. Pain is described as deep aching or boring, and x-rays are often normal in the early stages. MRI scan is highly sensitive and specific for osteonecrosis.

Treatment is directed at pain control to preserve motion and strength. If symptoms cannot be controlled with analgesics, total shoulder arthroplasty or hemiarthroplasty is indicated.

Shoulder Instability Problems

Tears of the glenoid labrum may be associated with disruption of portions of the glenohumeral ligament causing anterior or posterior instability or internal derangement similar to knee meniscal tears. A fall on an outstretched arm in abduction and slight forward flexion is the most common acute injury producing a SLAP (superior, labral, anterior, posterior) lesion; chronic lesions occur in athletes who throw repetitively. Patients usually describe pain associated with a catching or popping sensation during overhead activities. A SLAP lesion at the anterosuperior labrum involves injury of the long head of the biceps at its insertion to the superior glenoid labrum. Type I SLAP is a frayed superior labrum; Type II is an unstable labral biceps complex anchor to the glenoid; Type III is a bucket handle tear of the labrum; and Type IV is a bucket handle tear of the labrum that extends into the biceps tendon. On examination, pain is reproduced by resisting a downward force on the hand when the arm is in 90° of forward flexion, full internal rotation, and 30° of adduction (O'Brien test).

Glenohumeral instability results in recurrent transient subluxation or even dislocation of the humeral head. Anterior instability is the most common and presents with anterior shoulder pain when the arm is abducted and externally rotated. Pain may be associated with a feeling of slipping and clicking or that the joint is loose. Posterior instability typically follows unusual trauma with the arm flexed forward and internally rotated; on examination, the patient is unable to externally rotate the arm. Instability with recurrent anterior subluxation causes impingement of the rotator cuff between the subluxed humeral head and the acromion.

Glenohumeral instability can follow trauma and may be associated with generalized laxity and hypermobility, capsular tears or avulsions, and lesions in the glenoid labrum. Cuff-tear arthropathy and Milwaukee shoulder are 2 terms that likely refer to the same or similar shoulder disorders. When a large tear in the rotator cuff causes instability and permits proximal migration of the humeral head, destructive erosions and crystal deposition are seen. The primary treatment approach to glenohumeral instability is prolonged rehabilitation designed to strengthen all the muscles of the shoulder girdle.

Extrinsic Causes of Shoulder Pain

Cervical radiculopathy can transmit pain to the shoulder region with altered sensation (numbness or tingling) and/or motor weakness. The pain is initiated or exacerbated by neck motions rather than shoulder movement and is localized to the dermatome distribution. Weakness with decreased deep tendon reflexes localizes to the myotome distribution of C6, C7, and C8 nerves. Diagnosis may be confirmed by imaging studies and electromyography.

Brachial plexopathy (Parsonage Turner syndrome) causes a deep severe shoulder pain and loss of motion due to muscle weakness and atrophy. It may be due to brachial plexus injury, irradiation, or diabetes; occur after viral infection or immunization; or be a paraneoplastic phenomenon (14). The pain is usually abrupt in onset, intense, and described as sharp, throbbing, stabbing, or aching in the shoulder region. The pain may be bilateral and is constant, worsened by arm movements, and associated with paresthesias, numbness, and objective sensory deficits. Pain may remit in a few weeks or last a few years, leaving striking weakness and muscle atrophy that gradually improve over 1–3 years. The diagnosis of plexopathy can be confirmed by electromyography. Treatment includes oral systemic corticosteroids or intraarticular corticosteroid injections for pain relief. During the period of weakness, a regular passive stretching exercise program is used to prevent contractures. Progression to active exercises for stretching and strengthening is recommended as soon as the patient is able.

Suprascapular neuropathy occurs secondary to direct trauma, nerve stretch injury, or compression in the suprascapular or spinoglenoid notch. The suprascapular nerve (C5, C6) innervates the supraspinatus and infraspinatus muscles and is the sensory nerve to the glenohumeral joint capsule and acromioclavicular joint. Neuropathy produces weakness on abduction and external rotation and a burning pain that increases during abduction. Deep tendon reflexes and passive range of motion are normal. Atrophy of the infraspinatus muscle may occur early. The diagnosis can be confirmed by finding prolonged latency and decreased amplitude of the motor response to suprascapular nerve stimulation. Nerve entrapment in the suprascapular notch produces posterolateral shoulder pain that may radiate down the extremity and/or up into the neck, associated with weakness of abduction and external rotation and atrophy of the infraspinatus muscle. The pain is described as deep, burning, or aching and can be elicited by palpation of the suprascapular notch. The suprascapular nerve may be contused by direct trauma, compressed by a mass lesion, tethered by the suprascapular ligament, or recurrently traumatized during competitive overhead sports such as volleyball. The diagnosis is confirmed by electromyography and nerve conduction studies. The initial approach should be to rule out a mass lesion with MRI, reduce overhead activities, and control pain with analgesics and NSAIDs or with a suprascapular nerve block.

Thoracic outlet syndrome is caused by compression of the neurovascular bundle (brachial plexus, subclavian artery, and vein) at the thoracic outlet. Pain, paresthesia, and numbness radiate from the neck and shoulder down the arm and into the ring and little fingers and are worsened by activities. Associated vascular abnormalities include discoloration, temperature change, claudication, and Raynaud's phenomenon. On physical examination, the radial pulse decreases as the arm is raised above the head (hyperabduction maneuver) or when the patient holds a deep breath and turns the head to the affected side (Adson's test). However, both of these tests may be positive in normal individuals and are therefore not conclusive. A chest x-ray may reveal a cervical rib, elongated transverse process of C7, fracture, or exostoses. An angiogram or venogram can demonstrate significant vascular compression.

The mechanisms that lead to *visceral referred pain to the shoulder* are poorly understood. Nociceptive impulses from the diaphragm via the phrenic nerve produce referred pain to the trapezius area. The phrenic nerve may also be irritated by lesions in the upper thorax, mediastinum, and pericardium. Cardiac pain is referred to the axilla and left pectoral region. Gallbladder irritation refers pain to the tip of the shoulder and scapular region. Referred pain may be associated with cutaneous hypersensitivity and muscle spasm. Treatment is directed at the underlying visceral disease.

REFERENCES

1. Croft P, Pope D, Silman A. The clinical course of shoulder pain: prospective cohort study in primary care. BMJ 1996;313:601–2.
2. Sommerich CM, McGlothin JD, Marras WS. Occupational risk factors associated with soft tissue disorders of the shoulder: a review of current investigations in the literature. Ergonomics 1993;36:697–717.
3. Frieman BD, Albert TJ, Fenlin JM. Rotator cuff disease: a review of diagnosis, pathophysiology, and current trends in treatment. Arch Phys Med Rehabil 1994;75:604–9.
4. DeWinter AF, Jans MP, Scholten RJ, Deville W, van Schaardenburg D, Bouter LM. Diagnostic classification of shoulder disorders: interobserver agreement and determinants of disagreement. Ann Rheum Dis 1999;58:272–7.
5. Iannotti JP, Zlatkin MB, Esterhai JL, Kressel HY, Dalinka MK, Spindler KP. Magnetic resonance imaging of the shoulder: sensitivity, specificity, predictive value. J Bone Joint Surg Am 1991;73:17–29.
6. Neer CS II. Anterior acromioplasty for the chronic impingement syndrome in the shoulder. A preliminary report. J Bone Joint Surg Am 1972;54:41–50.
7. Van der Heijden GJ, van der Windt DA, de Winter AF. Physiotherapy for patients with soft tissue shoulder disorders: a systematic review of randomized clinical trials. BMJ 1997;315:25–30.
8. Jobe FW, Moynes DR. Delineation of diagnostic criteria and a rehabilitation program for rotator cuff injuries. Am J Sports Med 1982;10:336–9.
9. Blair B, Rokito AS, Cuomo F, Jarolem K, Zuckerman JD. Efficacy of injections of corticosteroids for subacromial impingement syndrome. J Bone Joint Surg Am 1996;78:1685–9.
10. Gazielly DF, Gleyze P, Montagnon C. Functional and anatomical results after rotator cuff repair. Clin Orthop 1994;304:43–53.
11. Rodeo SA, Hannafin JA, Tom J, Warren RF, Wickiewicz TL. Immunolocalization of cytokines and their receptors in adhesive capsulitis of the shoulder. J Orthop Res 1997;15:427–36.
12. Neviaser TJ. Adhesive capsulitis. Orthop Clin North Am 1987;18:439–43.
13. Warner JJ. Frozen shoulder: diagnosis and management. J Am Acad Orthop Surg 1997;5:130–40.
14. Tsairis P, Dyck PJ, Mulder DW. Natural history of brachial plexus neuropathy. Arch Neurol 1972;27:109–17.

Low Back and Neck Pain

DAVID BORENSTEIN, MD

Low back and neck pain are among the most common symptoms evaluated and treated by primary care providers. The common cold is the only medical illness associated with more lost days from work than spine disorders (1). In any 12-month period in the United States, 15–20% of the population has an episode of lumbosacral pain.

Low back and neck pain are symptoms associated with over 70 disorders including both mechanical and medical illnesses (2,3). Mechanical disorders of the spine cause more than 90% of all episodes of back and neck pain (4). Mechanical spine pain may be defined as pain secondary to overuse of a normal anatomic structure (i.e., muscle strain) or pain secondary to trauma or deformity of an anatomic structure (spinal stenosis). These disorders are characterized by exacerbation (sustained spinal extension) and alleviation (supine position) in direct correlation with particular physical activities. The most common mechanical disorders of the spine include muscle strain, herniated intervertebral disc, and spondylosis.

Medical illnesses of the spine may include infections, neoplasms, spondylarthropathies, and metabolic disorders. These systemic illnesses are treated specifically for the associated medical disorder; for example, antibiotics are prescribed for vertebral osteomyelitis, or parathyroidectomy for hyperparathyroidism.

A wide range of therapies, including rest, medications, physical modalities, and surgery, are available to treat mechanical spine pain. The variety of therapies has resulted in confusion for primary care providers concerning appropriate use of therapy for specific forms of mechanical spine pain. This absence of consensus was documented in a study of 2,897 physicians who responded to a questionnaire concerning the prescribing of therapy for patients with acute muscle strain, sciatica, and chronic low back pain (5). Treatment recommendations chosen by the respondents followed a pattern consistent with the specialty of the physician—that is, surgery was chosen by orthopedic surgeons, rehabilitation by physiatrists, and so on. These choices often conflicted with published guideline recommendations for diagnosis and management of low back pain (6).

The practicing physician must be able to determine a cost-effective choice of therapy for the spinal pain patient. Except in the rare circumstance of individuals with a surgical emergency such as cauda equina syndrome, ruptured abdominal aneurysm, or cervical myelopathy with cord compression, nonsurgical treatment is effective for most patients with acute spine pain. At 2 weeks, 50% of patients show improvement, while 90% return to their baseline state by 2 months (7). Acute spine pain is defined by a duration of less than 12 weeks, while chronic spine pain has a duration of 12 weeks or longer.

MECHANICAL DISORDERS OF THE AXIAL SKELETON

Common mechanical disorders of the lumbar and cervical spine include muscle strain, whiplash, intervertebral disc herniation, spondylosis, and spinal stenosis. The clinical characteristics of these disorders are listed in Table 1.

Muscle Strain

Muscle strain is preceded by a physical event, such as lifting a weight greater than the forces that can be supported by the muscular and ligamentous structures of the spine. Back or neck pain associated with muscle injury radiates up and across the paraspinous muscles, with radiation limited to the buttocks or the shoulders, respectively. Physical examination reveals limited range of motion of the lumbar or cervical area with muscle contraction and a normal neurologic examination. Radiographic evaluation of the spine may be normal or may demonstrate a loss of lordosis.

Whiplash

Cervical hyperextension injuries of the neck are associated with rear-collision motor vehicle accidents (8). Impact from the rear causes acceleration–deceleration injury to the soft tissue structures in the neck. Paracervical muscles (sternocleidomastoid, longus coli) are stretched or torn, and the sympathetic ganglia contiguous to these muscles may be damaged, resulting in Horner's syndrome (ptosis, meiosis, anhydrosis), nausea, or dizziness. Cervical intervertebral disc injuries may occur.

The symptoms of stiffness and pain with neck motion are first noticed 12–24 hours after the accident. Headache is commonly reported. Patients may have difficulty swallowing or chewing and may have paresthesias in the arms. Physical examination reveals decreased range of neck motion and persistent paracervical muscle contraction. Neurologic examination is unremarkable, and radiographs do not show soft tissue abnormalities other than loss of cervical lordosis.

Intervertebral Disc Herniation

Intervertebral disc herniation occurs with a sudden physical event, such as lifting a heavy object or sneezing. Herniation of the disc causes nerve impingement and inflammation resulting in radiating pain in the leg (sciatica) or arm (brachialgia). Back or neck pain may be present, but it is not universally noted by individuals with a disc herniation. Physical examination reveals radicular pain with tension on the affected nerve with a

Table 1. Mechanical disorders of the axial skeleton.

	Muscle strain	Herniated nucleus pulposus	Spinal stenosis	Whiplash	Spondylosis	Myelopathy
Typical age at onset	20–40	30–50	>60	30–40	>50	>60
Pain pattern						
Location	Back/neck	Back/leg	Neck/arm/leg	Neck	Back/neck	Arm/leg
Onset	Acute	Acute	Insidious	Acute	Insidious	Insidious
Extension	Increase	Decrease	Increase	Increase	Decrease	Increase
Flexion	Decrease	Increase	Decrease	Decrease	Increase	Decrease
Straight leg raising	−	+	+ with stress	−	−	+ with stress
Plain x-ray	−	−	+	−	+	+
Computed tomography	−	Disc herniation	Canal narrowing	−	Joint arthritis	Canal narrowing
Magnetic resonance	−	Disc herniation	Canal narrowing	−	Joint arthritis	Canal narrowing

straight leg raising test or Spurling's sign. Neurologic examination may reveal sensory deficit, reflex asymmetry, or motor weakness corresponding to the location of the damaged spinal nerve root and degree of impingement. Radiographic evaluation with magnetic resonance scan is obtained to confirm the level of disc herniation that corresponds to physical findings in patients who do not improve in an 8–12 week period.

Spondylosis

Osteoarthritis (OA) of the spinal zygapophyseal joints may cause localized low back or neck pain. As the intervertebral disc degenerates, intersegmental instability and approximation of the vertebral bodies shift the compressive forces across the zygapophyseal joints. The transition of these facet joints from non–weight-bearing to weight-bearing joints leads to zygapophyseal OA. As a result, patients develop lumbar or cervical pain that increases at the end of the day and radiates across the low back or shoulders. Physical examination reveals that pain worsens with extension of the spine, and no neurologic deficits are present. Pain radiates into the surrounding muscles and is exacerbated by ipsilateral bending to the side with the osteoarthritic joints. Oblique views of the spine demonstrate zygapophyseal joint narrowing, periarticular sclerosis, and osteophytes. These radiographic findings are significant only so far as they correlate with clinical history and physical factors consistent with OA (9).

Myelopathy/Spinal Stenosis

The most serious form of spinal stenosis is cervical myelopathy, which occurs as a consequence of spinal cord compression by osteophytes, ligamentum flavum, or intervertebral disc. Cervical spondylotic myelopathy is the most common cause of spinal cord dysfunction in individuals older than 55 years of age (10). With disc degeneration, osteophytes develop posteriorly and project into the spinal canal, compressing the cord and its vascular supply. Clinical symptoms include a history of peculiar sensations in the hands, associated with weakness and lack of coordination. Neck pain is mentioned by only one-third of patients with myelopathy. In the lower extremities, this disorder can cause gait disturbances, spasticity, leg weakness, and spontaneous leg movements. Older patients may describe leg stiffness, foot shuffling, and a fear of falling. Incontinence is a late manifestation. Physical examination reveals weakness of the appendages in association with spasticity and fasciculations. Sensory deficits include decreased dermatomal sensation

and loss of proprioception. Hyperreflexia, clonus, and positive Babinski's sign are present in the lower extremities. Plain radiographs reveal advanced degenerative disease with narrowed disc spaces, osteophytes, facet joint sclerosis, and cervical instability. Magnetic resonance imaging (MRI) is useful in detecting the extent of spinal cord compression and the effects of compression on the integrity of the cord. Combined computed tomography/myelogram imaging is useful for distinguishing protruding discs from osteophytes.

Lumbar spinal stenosis causes chronic low back pain, frequently lasting longer than 12 weeks. Progression of the disorder causes increased narrowing of the spinal canal, resulting in stenosis and compression of neural elements. The clinical manifestation of spinal stenosis is neurogenic claudication. Narrowing of the spinal canal, which may occur at single or multiple levels, causes radiating lower extremity pain when walking or standing. Neurologic examination may reveal sensory, motor, or reflex abnormalities when the patient is exercised to the point of developing neurogenic claudication. Radiographic evaluation with MRI demonstrates narrowing of the spinal canal resulting from a combination of protruding degenerative intervertebral disc, hypertrophied ligamentum flavum, and apophyseal joint osteophytes. The correlation between radiographic abnormalities and clinical symptoms and signs is more direct with herniated nucleus pulposus than with lumbar spinal stenosis.

THERAPEUTIC INTERVENTIONS

Treatment of acute low back pain differs from treatment of chronic low back pain. Therapies that are appropriate for individuals with chronic pain may not be indicated for patients with acute symptoms. A reasonable goal for therapy of acute spine pain is 100% pain relief and return to normal function, while the goal for therapy of chronic spine pain is maximizing function. Total relief of pain may not be achieved when pain has been present for an extended period of time. Many therapies have been proposed for low back pain without clinical investigation to determine their efficacy. Scientifically proven therapies for acute low back pain are few compared to other common medical disorders.

Review of AHCPR Guidelines for Low Back Pain

In December 1994, the Agency for Health Care Policy and Research (AHCPR) published a 160-page *Clinical Practice*

Table 2. Agency for Health Care Policy and Research (AHCPR) guidelines for management of acute low back pain.

I. Patient education
Patients with acute low back problems should be given accurate information about the following (strength of evidence = B):
- A. Expectations for both rapid recovery and recurrence of symptoms based on natural history of low back symptoms.
- B. Safe and effective methods of symptom control.
- C. Safe and reasonable activity modifications.
- D. Best means of limiting recurrent low back problems.
- E. The lack of need for special investigations unless red flags are present.
- F. Effectiveness and risks of commonly available diagnostic and further treatment measures to be considered should symptoms persist.

II. Medications
Acetaminophen and nonsteroidal antiinflammatory drugs (NSAIDs):
- A. Acetaminophen is reasonably safe and is acceptable for treating patients with acute low back problems (strength of evidence = C).
- B. NSAIDs, including aspirin, are acceptable for treating patients with acute low back problems (strength of evidence = B).
- C. NSAIDs have a number of potential side effects. The most frequent complication is gastrointestinal irritation. The decision to use these medications can be guided by comorbidity, side effects, cost, and patient and provider preference (strength of evidence = C).

III. Physical treatments
Spinal manipulation:
- A. Manipulation can be helpful for patients with acute low back problems without radiculopathy when used within the first month of symptoms (strength of evidence = B).
- B. A trial of manipulation in patients without radiculopathy with symptoms longer than 1 month is probably safe, but efficacy is unproven (strength of evidence = C).

IV. Activity modification
Activity recommendations for bed rest and exercise:
- A. A gradual return to normal activities is more effective than prolonged bed rest for treating acute low back problems (strength of evidence = B).
- B. Prolonged bed rest for more than 4 days may lead to debilitation and is not recommended for acute low back problems (strength of evidence = B).
- C. Low-stress aerobic exercise can prevent debilitation due to inactivity during the first month of symptoms and thereafter may help to return patients to the highest level of functioning appropriate to their circumstances (strength of evidence = C).

Guideline booklet on the diagnosis and management of acute low back pain, based on recommendations of a multidisciplinary panel of practitioners who reviewed 3,918 published scientific articles (11). The panel made recommendations concerning initial assessment, clinical care, and special studies and diagnostic considerations, including surgery. The articles for diagnosis and therapy were rated from A (studies with strong research-based evidence) to D (those with published articles that did not meet inclusion criteria for study design). Greatest support was given to randomized, controlled trials. In the absence of such trials, evidence was described as weak or indirect. In these circumstances, the potential benefit of an intervention had to outweigh its potential risks to be considered cost effective.

Therapeutic interventions recommended by the panel are listed in Table 2. The recommendations are to be implemented after an evaluation, including history and physical examination, that excludes medical disorders that require expedited therapy in the form of surgery or antibiotics. Imaging techniques during initial evaluation are unnecessary as they will not influence treatment choices.

The members of the advisory group agreed that the recommendations are best considered options, and not the sole method, for treating acute low back pain. Most recommendations are based on a small number of articles, although thousands were reviewed. In addition, certain therapies may not be recommended because of the absence of scientific studies demonstrating efficacy, not because of the absence of possible benefit. For example, muscle relaxants are not recommended. A recommendation would not be forthcoming, as no new study of muscle relaxants has been reported in a number of years. The exclusion of this class of agents is based on the absence of information, not the lack of efficacy. Study design may also limit the potential to demonstrate efficacy. For example, investigations of epidural corticosteroid injections that measure benefit at 1 week and at 6 months will miss the beneficial effects of the therapy that occur in the second to twelfth weeks

(12). The relationship between specific disorders and treatment recommendations is lacking. It is also important to remember that the guidelines do not apply to disorders associated with chronic low back pain.

Despite these limitations, the guidelines for acute low back pain provide important clinical recommendations for the primary care providers. Patients should be advised to limit bed rest and encouraged to maintain activity. The guidelines on bed rest, spinal manipulation, and exercise may all be seen as methods to motivate patients to regain normal motion of the lumbosacral spine. Recommendations for medications maximize the use of agents with mild toxicities and little abuse potential. In general, invasive therapies are limited to those low back pain patients who fail to improve over a 4–12 week period. Only a small minority of patients require surgical intervention.

Therapy for Acute Mechanical Spine Pain

The therapy for acute mechanical low back and neck pain should incorporate some of the AHCPR guidelines along with practical recommendations that patients can follow. Many of the recommendations for treatment of mechanical disorders of the low back are also applicable to the neck.

Muscle Strain. Therapy for muscle strain of the spine includes controlled physical activity, nonsteroidal antiinflammatory drugs (NSAIDs), muscle relaxants, and physical therapy. Muscle strain improves with gradually increasing physical activity. However, there are upper limits on the extent of exercises. Individuals who believe that an early return to usual exercise programs is appropriate are at risk for re-injury. Patients should be encouraged to remain in bed only for limited periods of time. A period as short as 2 days has been shown to be effective at relieving acute back and neck pain (13). Limiting physical activity initially allows the injured tissues to rest, permitting a greater opportunity for healing without re-injury;

however, prolonged bed rest results in deconditioning that is detrimental to muscle function. As soon as acute pain diminishes, encourage patients to increase physical activity. This might include walking for increasing periods of time each day. Increasing evidence supports resumption of normal activity early in the course of muscle strain to maximize the return to full function. Research in Finland showed the efficacy of bed rest for 2 days, back-mobilizing exercises, and ordinary activity as tolerated for low back pain therapy (14). Better recovery, improved function, and fewer missed work days were associated with ordinary physical activity.

Non-narcotic analgesics such as NSAIDs relieve pain and allow patients to be more mobile. Nonsteroidal drugs with a rapid onset of action and analgesic properties are most helpful in patients with acute pain. Cyclooxygenase-2 (COX-2) inhibitors are effective for patients with a history of NSAID-associated gastrointestinal injuries. Muscle relaxants may be helpful for patients who have palpable, paraspinous muscular spasm on physical examination or difficulty sleeping at night because of muscle pain. The muscle relaxant may be given 2–3 hours before sleep to limit somnolence the following morning. The combination of an NSAID with a muscle relaxant is better than an NSAID alone at improving pain relief in acute low back pain patients with muscle spasm (15,16). Physical modalities, in the form of ice massage initially, or warm baths subsequently, may also decrease pain and diminish spasm.

Local areas of muscle spasm in the lumbar or cervical spine may be resistant to oral medications. On physical exam, the areas of spasm are identified to be firm to palpation, with radiation of pain to surrounding muscles. This "trigger point" may be injected with a combination of a local anesthetic and semi-soluble corticosteroid preparation. These injections are effective in breaking the pain–spasm cycle that results in muscle tightness. If injections are contraindicated (for example, in patients with sensitivity to local anesthetics), acupressure over the trigger point may also offer symptomatic relief.

Many health care professionals play important roles in the recovery of patients with low back or neck pain. Physical therapists offer pain-relieving modalities early in the course of back or neck strain. Subsequently, range of motion and strengthening exercises restore function to baseline levels. Manipulation by a chiropractor may be helpful early in the course of back pain that is unassociated with leg pain. Massage therapy improves the range of motion of contracted muscles. Although these therapeutic modalities are frequently prescribed, the clinical evidence that proves the efficacy of these interventions is sparse (17).

Whiplash. Treatment of whiplash includes the use of cervical collars for minimal periods of time in addition to therapies effective for muscle strain (8). A cervical collar increases muscle stiffness and slows recovery; therefore, whiplash patients are encouraged to discontinue the use of a cervical collar within a few days of the injury. Mild analgesics, NSAIDs, and muscle relaxants are prescribed to encourage motion of the neck. Most patients improve after about 4 weeks of therapy. Patients with symptoms that persist longer than 6 months rarely experience significant improvement. The mechanism of chronic pain in whiplash patients remains to be determined.

Acute Herniated Nucleus Pulposus. The treatment for most patients with a herniated disc is nonoperative; 80% will respond to conservative medical therapy. The outcome for individuals treated medically or surgically is similar over a 10-year period (18). However, surgical patients obtain earlier relief of leg pain than individuals treated nonsurgically. Patient education is essential for a successful outcome, as the patient must understand the natural history of resolution of disc herniation. The initial component of therapy is controlled physical activity with the patient in a semi-Fowler's position in bed. Once back and leg pain lessen, encourage the patient to walk. Bed rest does not hasten improvement compared to activity as tolerated and causes muscle deconditioning (19).

Drug therapy in the form of NSAIDs, analgesics, and muscle relaxants decreases pain and inflammation. NSAIDs are important for the control of leg and arm pain, because inflammation of the nerve root is the source of sciatica and brachialgia in disc patients. NSAIDs with prolonged action may be better able to control symptoms. Analgesic medications, including narcotics, may be used for severe pain; however, other analgesics should be substituted for narcotics as soon as pain diminishes. Epidural corticosteroid injections are indicated for patients whose continued sciatica does not respond to 2–4 weeks of conservative therapy.

Surgical intervention is reserved for patients in whom all forms of conservative therapy fail. Patients with sciatica, abnormal physical findings, and confirmatory radiographic tests are candidates for discectomy. The success rate for lumbar discectomy ranges from 70% to 95% (20). Surgical intervention for cervical herniated discs is also reported to be successful in a majority of patients with brachialgia and corresponding anatomic abnormalities. Opinion is divided on the need for cervical fusion in addition to discectomy. Fusion requires a bone graft harvested from another surgical site (iliac bone), which may become an additional area of pain. However, patients with cervical fusions have a return to function and more rapid pain relief.

Therapy for Chronic Mechanical Spine Pain

Myelopathy. Nonsurgical therapy should be attempted for cervical myelopathy patients without severe neurologic compromise or for those who are poor surgical risks. Conservative therapy includes immobilization with a firm cervical orthosis, NSAIDs, epidural corticosteroid injections, and cervical traction. However, in general, myelopathy is a surgical disease. The goal of surgery is to decompress the spinal cord to prevent further spinal cord compression and vascular compromise. Surgical intervention has the best opportunity for improvement before irreversible damage is sustained by the cervical spinal cord (21).

Spinal Stenosis. Patients with lumbar spinal stenosis have pain that progresses over an extended period of time. The majority of individuals with spinal stenosis can be treated nonsurgically. Education about appropriate spinal biomechanics used in activities of daily living, and those positions of the spine that exacerbate back and leg pain, is a key component. Inflammation of the soft tissues in the spinal canal and neural foramina result in compression of neural elements.

NSAIDs are useful in decreasing inflammation, soft tissue swelling, and neural compression, and they may be used for an extended period of time while improvement of function continues. Due to the increased age in many patients with spinal stenosis, increased sensitivity to NSAID toxicities—particularly those of the gastrointestinal tract—must be considered. The utility of epidural corticosteroid injections for spinal stenosis is questionable, as they tend to be more effective for radicular pain associated with herniated intervertebral discs than for spinal stenosis. Injections are given once a week for 3 weeks. If a good response is achieved, the injections may be repeated in 4–6 months.

Surgical decompression should be considered for patients with neurogenic claudication that severely limits function. These patients are unable to walk one block or have radicular pain when standing. The first operation has the greatest opportunity for relief of symptoms. In a study of 251 patients with spinal stenosis who underwent decompression surgery, 67% had an excellent or good outcome (22). Good operative outcome was reduced to only 46% of 66 patients with repeat decompressive operations.

Chronic Pain Therapy

A small but significant proportion of spine patients do not respond to acute therapy and require prolonged conservative management. In chronic pain management, the patient must be convinced that the goal of therapy is to maximize physical function. A combination of therapies is necessary to reach this goal. Exercise programs that improve aerobic conditioning and range of motion are helpful. Patients may benefit from increased NSAID dosage or switching to a different chemical class of NSAID. Tricyclic antidepressants offer additional pain relief mediated through the central nervous system. Use of narcotic analgesics is generally discouraged, but they may be used at a specific dose to facilitate function. Long-acting narcotics may decrease pain to allow a return to work without the waxing and waning effect of short-acting agents. Once a regular work schedule is established, a gradual decrease of dose is attempted while function is maintained. Some individuals are unable to reduce their narcotic requirement without a deterioration in physical function and require sustained narcotic medications for extended periods. The benefits and detriments of this form of therapy must be constantly reviewed by the physician and patient.

Return to employment or other productive pursuit is an important goal of therapy. Movement of the back or neck improves function and counters the inactivity that can exacerbate pain. The appearance of new symptoms or marked exacerbation of preexisting problems are indications for reevaluation.

REFERENCES

1. Frymoyer JW. Back pain and sciatica. N Engl J Med 1988;318:291–300.
2. Borenstein DG, Wiesel SW, Boden SD. Low back pain: medical diagnosis and comprehensive management. 2nd ed. Philadelphia: WB Saunders; 1995.
3. Borenstein DG, Wiesel SW, Boden SD. Neck pain: medical diagnosis and comprehensive management. Philadelphia: WB Saunders; 1996.
4. Nachemson A. The lumbar spine: an orthopedic challenge. Spine 1976;1: 59–71.
5. Cherkin DC, Deyo RA, Wheeler K, Ciol MA. Physician views about treating low back pain: the results of a national survey. Spine 1995;20:1–20.
6. Spitzer WO, LeBlanc FE, Dupuis M, Abenhaim L, Belanger AY, Bloch R, et al. Scientific approach to the assessment and management of activity-related spinal disorders: report of the Quebec Task Force on spinal disorders. Spine 1987;12 Suppl:S1–59.
7. Dillance JB, Fry J, Kalton G. Acute back syndrome: a study from general practice. Br Med J 1966;3:82–4.
8. Spitzer WO, Skovron ML, Salmi LR, Cassidy JD, Duranceau J, Suissa S, et al. Scientific monograph of the Quebec Task Force on whiplash-associated disorders: redefining "whiplash" and its management. Spine 1995;20 Suppl 8:1S–73S.
9. Boden SD. The use of radiographic imaging studies in the evaluation of patients who have degenerative disorders of the lumbar spine. J Bone Joint Surg Am 1996;78:114–24.
10. Bernhardt M, Hynes RA, Blume HW, White AA III. Cervical spondylotic myelopathy. J Bone Joint Surg Am 1993;75:119–28.
11. Bigos S, Bowyer O, Braen G, Brown KC, Deyo RA, Haldeman S, et al. Acute low back problems in adults. Rockville (MD): Agency for Health Care Policy and Research, Public Health Service, U.S. Department of Health and Human Services. December 1994. Clinical Practice Guideline No. 14. AHCPR Publication No.95-0642.
12. Spaccarelli KC. Lumbar and caudal epidural corticosteroid injections. Mayo Clin Proc 1996;71:169–78.
13. Deyo RA, Diehl AK, Rosenthal M. How many days of bed rest for acute low back pain? N Engl J Med 1986;315:1064–70.
14. Malmivaara A, Hakkinen U, Aro T, Heinrichs M, Koskenniemi L, Kuosma E, et al. The treatment of acute low back pain: bed rest, exercises, or ordinary activity? N Engl J Med 1995;332:351–5.
15. Borenstein DG, Lacks SL, Wiesel SW. Cyclobenzaprine and naproxen versus naproxen alone in the treatment of acute low back pain and muscle spasm. Clin Ther 1990;12:125–31.
16. Cherkin DC, Wheeler KJ, Barlow W, Deyo RA. Medication use for low back pain in primary care. Spine 1998;23:607–14.
17. Cherkin DC, Deyo RA, Battie M, Street J, Barlow W. A comparison of physical therapy, chiropractic manipulation, and provision of an educational booklet for the treatment of patients with low back pain. N Engl J Med 1998;339:1021–9.
18. Weber H. Lumbar disc herniation: a controlled prospective study with 10 years of observation. Spine 1992;8:983–91.
19. Vroomen PCAJ, de Krom MCTFM, Wilmink JT, Kester ADM, Knottnerus JA. Lack of effectiveness of bed rest for sciatica. N Engl J Med 1999;340:418–23.
20. McCullogh JA. Focus issue on lumbar disc herniation: macro and microdiscectomy. Spine 1996;21 (Suppl 24):45S–56S.
21. Ebersold MJ, Pare MC, Quast LM. Surgical treatment for cervical spondylitic myelopathy. J Neurosurg 1995;82:745–51.
22. Herno A, Airaksinen O, Saari T, Silhoven T. Surgical results of lumbar spinal stenosis: a comparison of patients with or without previous back surgery. Spine 1995;20:964–9.

Additional Recommended Reading

Borenstein DG. Disorders of the low back and neck. In: Klippel JH, editor. Primer on the rheumatic diseases. 11th ed. Atlanta: Arthritis Foundation; 1997. p. 130–6.
Nordin M, Cedraschi C, Vischer TL. New approaches to the low back pain patient. Clin Rheumatol 1998;12:1–180.
Deyo RA, Weinstein JN. Low back pain. N Engl J Med 2001;344:363–70.

Pain Management

CAROL BURCKHARDT, RN, PhD

Patients with rheumatic diseases regard pain as a major challenge and one of the most important consequences of their illness (1). Although acute pain is a universal experience that serves vital life-preserving functions, chronic pain is a significant stressor that promotes neuroendocrine dysregulation, impairs physical and mental performance, and predicts loss of productive work and future disability (2). Uncontrolled chronic pain is destructive to the individual's sense of self and quality of life. Moreover, despite the advances that have been made in the management of the rheumatic diseases, patients seldom experience complete pain relief in response to their medications and other treatment regimens. Thus, comprehensive pain management is an ongoing challenge for both patients and health care providers.

Variations in the chronic pain experience cannot be explained solely by the underlying disease process. Patients with similar disease severity often differ in their pain levels. A biopsychosocial model provides one way of understanding an individual's response to pain (2–4). Pain is influenced by biologic factors, such as inflammation and joint destruction, and by psychosocial factors, such as depression, fear, lack of social support, and difficult work environments (1).

PAIN ASSESSMENT

Accurate pain measurement is critical to both clinical assessment and conclusions regarding treatment outcomes. Because pain is a complex sensory and emotional experience that cannot be measured directly, investigators and clinicians must measure events that are thought to represent various dimensions of the pain experience. Health care providers must make inferences regarding patients' subjective pain experiences on the basis of verbal reports, overt motor behaviors such as grimacing, or responses to various rating scales that measure intensity and coping responses. Several comprehensive reviews of pain measurement are available (5–7).

Pain Rating Scales

Pain ratings are subjective estimates of pain intensity or unpleasantness. Intensity refers to the severity of the pain experience, whereas unpleasantness refers to the emotional arousal produced by this experience. The strategies used most frequently to measure these dimensions of pain are numeric and verbal rating scales, visual analog scales, and pain questionnaires, such as the McGill Pain Questionnaire (8,9), the Brief Pain Inventory (10), and the West Haven-Yale Multidimensional Pain Inventory (11).

Numeric rating scales consist of a series of numbers placed on a horizontal or vertical line in ascending order of intensity (e.g., 0–10). These scales usually are anchored by verbal descriptors at the endpoints such as "No pain at all" and "Unbearable pain." Verbal rating scales are similar to numeric scales, except that they consist of a series of words aligned in ascending order of intensity (Table 1). Both the numbers and the words represent rank-ordered categories that form *ordinal scales*. Although individuals generally find it easy to understand and respond to these scales, the meanings of the intervals between the scale categories are unknown.

There are both strengths and weaknesses associated with the use of numeric and verbal rating scales. Such scales are simple to administer and reliable for use in low literacy populations (12). However, the structure of verbal scales may force patients to choose categories that do not actually represent their pain experiences. For example, patients may not have a good understanding of the English language and, thus, may have difficulty matching their pain experiences with any of the available categories. This problem highlights the need to develop reliable and valid pain measurements for persons from non-English speaking cultures (13).

The *visual analog scale* (VAS) is an alternative to ordinal rating scales (Table 1). The VAS consists of a 100-mm horizontal line with endpoints that are anchored by such verbal descriptors as "No Pain" and "Unbearable Pain." Patients respond to the VAS by placing a mark at the point along the scale that best represents the intensity or unpleasantness of their pain experience. Responses are scored by measuring the distance from the left endpoint to the individual's mark. This distance represents a quantitative measure of the patient's subjective pain experience.

Compared to numeric and verbal category scales, the VAS has several advantages. First, the VAS has a large number of possible response points, which makes it sensitive to treatment-induced changes. Second, the intervals between the response points of the VAS are equal. Finally, children as well as adults can use the VAS to describe their pain experiences. A formidable disadvantage, however, is that VAS scales may be less reliable and valid in low literacy populations and among some cultural groups (12). Additionally, many patients must be provided with detailed instructions and practice to reliably respond to a VAS.

Table 1. Numeric and verbal rating scales of pain intensity and a visual analog scale.

Numeric Rating Scale					
0 No pain at all	1	2	3	4	5 Unbearable pain

Verbal Rating Scale
No pain at all Extremely weak Weak Mild Moderate Strong Intense Extremely intense

Visual Analog Scale
No pain ⌊_____⌋ Unbearable pain

The McGill Pain Questionnaire consists of 20 verbal category rating scales that evaluate the sensory, emotional, and intensity dimensions of the pain experience. The verbal descriptors within each scale are rank ordered by pain intensity. Patients choose 1 descriptor from each relevant scale that best represents their pain experience. The questionnaire is scored by summing the number of words from among the 20 category scales, or by summing the rank values of these words to form a Pain Rating Index. The short form of this questionnaire includes only 15 verbal descriptors; it may be used with patients who are easily tired due to their illnesses. Persons without a good understanding of English are not able to fill out the questionnaire reliably.

The Brief Pain Inventory Short Form contains a body diagram for marking painful areas, and 11 numeric rating scales for measuring intensity and interference with physical, mental, and social activities. The West Haven-Yale Multidimensional Pain Inventory is a 52-item inventory that contains 3 parts: effects of pain on the patient's life; responses of others to the patient's pain; and extent of participation in functional activities. Both of these scales have simple numeric formats that meet the needs of diverse populations of patients and have been used in osteoporosis and fibromyalgia (FM) populations. They also contain valuable information for clinicians regarding the ways in which chronic pain interferes with normal functioning.

Pain Behaviors

Investigators have developed observation methods for recording overt motor behaviors that communicate the subjective experience of pain among patients with osteoarthritis (OA) (14), and adults and children with rheumatoid arthritis (RA) (15,16). These observation methods require patients to perform a standardized, 10-minute sequence of physical maneuvers for video recording, including sitting, standing, walking, and reclining. Trained observers then view the video recordings and count the frequencies of specific, operationally defined pain behaviors (Table 2). Pain behavior can be observed in a reliable manner and counts of these behaviors are characterized by good construct and discriminant validity.

There are benefits associated with the measurement of pain behavior. First, it provides quantifiable observational data regarding patients' functional limitations in activities that are directly related to vocational, social, and leisure endeavors. Second, in contrast to the significant relationships that are found between patients' pain ratings and their emotional distress levels, measures of pain behavior in the laboratory generally are independent of patients' affective states. Finally, measurement of pain behavior, in addition to pain ratings, allows one to determine whether there are differences between patients' reports of subjective pain experiences and their behaviors (1). The major disadvantage to the observation of pain behavior is that it entails a large amount of training, professional time, and expense.

Physiologic Measures

Physiologic assessment is gaining credibility as a way to understand and evaluate chronic pain. Measurement of substance P, a major neurotransmitter of pain (17); evoked potentials (18); abnormal sensory processing (19); cerebral blood flow (20); and positron emission tomography (21) all have potential for increasing the ability to describe and evaluate chronic pain. At present none of these are ready to be used in clinical work, as applicability to individual patients has not yet been determined.

Pain Coping Assessment

Understanding the ways in which patients cope with chronic pain can be useful in helping them develop better coping strategies. The Coping Strategies Questionnaire (CSQ) is a

Table 2. Pain behaviors associated with osteoarthritis, rheumatoid arthritis, and juvenile arthritis.

Osteoarthritis	Adult Rheumatoid Arthritis	Juvenile Rheumatoid Arthritis
Guarding	Guarding	Guarding
Active rubbing	Bracing	Bracing
Unloading joint	Grimacing	Rigidity
Rigidity	Sighing	Active rubbing
Joint flexing	Rigidity	Single flexing
	Passive rubbing	Multiple flexing
	Active rubbing	

reliable and valid instrument that has been used extensively with rheumatic disease patients (22–24). The CSQ consists of 7 subscales containing statements that measure cognitive and behavioral ways of coping with chronic pain, 1 scale that measures the amount of catastrophizing patients do in response to pain, and 2 items that measure perceived ability to control and decrease pain.

Pain Measurement Outcomes

Establishing a clinically significant change in pain is difficult. Using more than one method of measurement can be helpful so that, for example, consistency between verbal report and pain behaviors is seen. Correlating the results of pain measurement with the number of pain medications patients take, activities in which they participate, or use of health care resources can also provide evidence of the efficacy of pain treatment (1,25). Clinicians who use numeric rating scales or VAS generally agree that a score of 4 or lower on a 10-point scale indicates good chronic pain control.

COMPREHENSIVE PAIN MANAGEMENT

Effective treatment of chronic pain usually requires professionals from multiple disciplines to provide appropriate interventions in a coordinated fashion. Goals in both adults and children are to reduce inflammation, pain, and the physical or emotional impairments that accompany unrelieved pain. Most patients with rheumatic disease will require education and pharmacologic, cognitive-behavioral, and physical interventions. There are unresolved issues regarding which combinations of treatment work best for specific individuals during the early and later stages of disease (13). However, group data from well-controlled studies now indicate clearly that multidisciplinary, multicomponent treatment is superior to single focused interventions or usual treatment (26–28).

Education

The Arthritis Self-Management Program (ASMP) is a standardized intervention that has been evaluated primarily with OA and RA patients. It focuses on enhancing patients' self-efficacy, that is, their beliefs that they can perform specific behaviors to achieve their health-related goals. The ASMP produces significant increases in self-efficacy for pain and other symptoms, as well as significant reductions in pain ratings and arthritis-related physician visits among patients with OA and RA that persist for up to 4 years (29).

Telephone-based counseling interventions represent a newer, inexpensive method for improving patients' health status. The first of these interventions, developed for patients with OA, reviewed educational information, medications, and clinical problems with patients and taught them strategies for increasing their involvement in encounters with physicians (30). This intervention produced significant improvements in patients' reports of pain and functional ability and did not substantially increase health care costs. Use of telephone interventions in other rheumatic diseases has yielded mixed results (31). Whether more directive interventions, such as telephone-based coping skills training, would produce similar effects remains to be determined. (See also Chapter 23, Patient Education for Arthritis Self-Management.)

Pharmacologic Treatment

A comprehensive pain management program for any patient must include attention to the optimal drug strategy for controlling inflammation in RA and chronic pain in OA and other rheumatic conditions, such as FM. (See also Chapter 25, Pharmacologic Interventions in the 21st Century.) Drug therapy for pain management in the rheumatic diseases is most effective when combined with nonpharmacologic strategies. For example, a meta-analysis of patient education interventions compared with nonsteroidal antiinflammatory drug treatment concluded that patient education interventions provided 20–30% additional pain relief compared with the use of drugs alone (32).

Nonopioid Analgesics. For many patients, the mild to moderate joint pain of OA can be controlled with acetaminophen in daily doses not exceeding 4 grams. For patients whose pain is not controlled, tramadol, a synthetic opioid agonist not associated with significant abuse, can be considered in dosages of between 200–300 mg daily (33). Studies of tramadol in patients with FM indicate efficacy for pain relief, possibly because of its stimulation of the descending inhibitory systems (opioid effect) and antinociceptive effect through inhibition of serotonin and norepinephrine at the level of the dorsal horn neurons (34). Tramadol should be used with caution in patients with seizure disorders or in those taking high doses of drugs, such as some antidepressants, that are known to reduce the seizure threshold.

Nonsteroidal Antiinflammatory Drugs (NSAIDs). Although acetaminophen is now recommended as the first-line drug for pain control, NSAIDs have historically been the mainstay of pain treatment in the rheumatic diseases. Both nonselective NSAIDs and cyclooxygenase-2 (COX-2) specific inhibitors are well-documented suppressors of pain in patients with OA (33). They should be considered for patients who do not obtain adequate pain relief from acetaminophen. Risks and benefits of nonselective NSAID treatment in populations such as the elderly or those with a history of peptic ulcers disease should be carefully considered. For these patients, as well as for any patient on long-term NSAID therapy, a COX-2 specific inhibitor is likely a better choice because of the significantly lower risk of gastrointestinal adverse events. There is little evidence that NSAIDs significantly decrease pain in patients with FM (34).

Topical Analgesics. Patients with OA of the hands or knees and patients with FM may benefit from such topical analgesics as capsaicin cream and topical salicylates or other NSAIDs. Higher drug concentrations can be achieved at specific sites using this method. A number of controlled trials in the OA population suggest that decreases in pain in specific areas are significant (33,35,36).

Opioid Analgesics. The use of opioid analgesics for chronic pain remains controversial. Some clinicians argue strongly that rheumatic disease patients whose pain is uncontrolled are as deserving of opioid trials as those patients living with chronic cancer pain (37). Others feel that opioids are inappropriate or that the potential for dependence and adverse effects outweighs the benefits.

Data from recent randomized clinical trials of controlled release codeine in OA patients suggest that the drug significantly decreased pain severity and pain interference with functioning (38,39). There are no well-controlled trials of opioid drug treatment in either RA or FM populations. Such studies are needed if a larger percentage of rheumatic disease patients are to get the state-of-the-science pain management they need.

Glucosamine and Chondroitin. The use of these compounds by patients with OA and FM has become common, notwithstanding the lack of well-controlled clinical trials. A meta-analysis of trials in the treatment of OA concluded that although the results were uniformly positive for decreasing pain and increasing function, most of the trials had methodologic deficiencies that could have inflated the results (40).

Cognitive Behavioral Strategies

The psychological and behavioral therapies for rheumatic disease pain share similar treatment components: education, relaxation training, self-efficacy enhancement, coping skills development, cognitive restructuring techniques to decrease helplessness and catastrophizing, and rehearsal of newly learned skills. Cognitive behavioral therapies (CBT) are well-established treatments for OA and RA (See Chapter 24, Cognitive Behavioral Interventions). A number of clinical trials have produced significant improvements in pain rating, reductions in pain behaviors, and increases in self-efficacy for pain (1,3). Some have indicated that spouse participation in the treatment enhanced the outcomes and that gains persisted for more than one year (1). Clinical trials of CBT are beginning to accumulate in the FM population as well. Although most have compared CBT to no treatment rather than attention controls, overall they point to significant changes in pain coping, control, self-efficacy, severity, and interference with functioning, some of which are sustained for 6 months or more (26,41).

Physical Interventions

A number of physical interventions are effective for reducing pain in OA, RA, and FM. These include heat therapy such as paraffin baths; cold therapies using cold packs, ice massage, vapocoolant sprays, or cold laser; and transcutaneous electrical nerve stimulation (TENS) (35). For more detailed information on these interventions, see Chapter 27, Physical Modalities. Exercise therapies have been successful in reducing pain levels in OA, RA, and FM patients (See also Chapter 26, Rest and Exercise). Cardiovascular fitness training programs, as well as combined programs of education, exercise, pool therapy, and fitness training, can produce significant improvements in patients' ratings of pain, disease activity, and physical function (27,35,41,42).

Complementary Therapies

Rheumatic disease patients frequently use complementary and alternative medical (CAM) therapies for relief of pain. Of the many types of CAM available, acupuncture is the leading therapy used by patients. Evidence for the efficacy of real acupuncture when compared to sham acupuncture is strong for both OA and FM (43). For further discussion of these therapies, see also Chapter 33, Complementary and Alternative Treatments.

PREVENTION OF CHRONIC PAIN

The recent development of behavioral interventions for the secondary prevention of chronic musculoskeletal pain among injured workers represents an important advance that may have a positive impact on the high health care costs of treating this condition (44). A controlled study of a cognitive behavioral intervention for people in the community who had experienced 4 or more episodes of relatively intense spinal pain during the past year found that, at the 1-year followup, the cognitive behavioral group had significantly fewer pain-free days and more positive fear-avoidance beliefs. The group also reduced the risk of long-term sick leave threefold—a finding that translates into considerable savings to employers and the social welfare system (45).

A small number of independent studies of secondary prevention programs have produced positive effects similar to those noted above. Although the development of these programs is a recent phenomenon, successful programs seem to share 3 features. First, these programs emphasize increasing patient activity levels soon after injury (preferably 4–12 weeks after pain onset). Second, the programs elicit patients' participation as active partners with the treatment providers. Finally, effective prevention programs emphasize relapse prevention and good adherence to newly learned strategies for managing pain.

SUMMARY

There is consistent evidence that pharmacologic, psychologic, and behavioral therapies produce significant reductions in ratings of pain among patients with rheumatic disease. Several issues concerning pain management therapies need greater attention from clinicians and investigators. First, greater emphasis should be devoted to the prevention of patient relapse following treatment. Second, the role of pain management strategies should be documented when evaluating reductions in health care utilization as well as in the direct and indirect costs of pain. Third, special attention should be devoted to the development and evaluation of "minimal" interventions, such as telephone-based counseling, that may contribute to substantial cost savings. Fourth, secondary prevention of chronic pain should become of increasing interest to providers who care for patients with recent musculoskeletal injuries. Finally, clinicians and investigators should begin to develop and evaluate early intervention therapies for managing pain in patients with newly diagnosed RA, OA, and FM so that the long-term negative consequences of chronic pain can be minimized.

The author of this chapter would like to acknowledge the contributions of Laurence A. Bradley, PhD, who wrote this chapter in the first edition and whose perspective continues to be reflected here.

REFERENCES

1. Bradley LA, Alberts KR. Pain management in the rheumatic diseases. Rheum Dis North Am 1999;25:215–32.

2. Chapman CR, Gavrin J. Suffering: the contribution of persistent pain. Lancet 1999;353:2233–7.
3. Keefe FJ, Caldwell DS. Cognitive behavioral control of arthritis pain. Med Clin North Am 1997;81:277–90.
4. Rapoff MA, Lindsley CB. The pain puzzle: a visual and conceptual metaphor for understanding and treating pain in pediatric rheumatic disease. J Rheumatol 2000;27(suppl 58):29–33.
5. Katz J, Melzack R. Measurement of pain. Surg Clin North Am 1999;79: 231–52.
6. Kuis W, Heijnen CJ, Sinnema G, Kavelaars A, van der Net J, Helders PJ. Pain in childhood rheumatic arthritis. Baillieres Clin Rheumatol 1998;12: 229–44.
7. Bradley LA. Pain measurement in arthritis. Arthritis Care Res 1993;6: 178–86.
8. Melzack R. The McGill Pain Questionnaire: major properties and scoring methods. Pain 1975;1:277–99.
9. Melzack R. The short-form McGill Pain Questionnaire. Pain 1987;30: 191–7.
10. Daut RL, Cleeland CS, Flanery RC. Development of the Wisconsin Brief Pain Questionnaire to assess pain in cancer and other diseases. Pain 1983;17:197–210.
11. Kerns RD, Turk DC, Rudy TE. The West Haven-Yale Multidimensional Pain Inventory (WHYMPI). Pain 1985;23:345–56.
12. Ferraz MB, Quaresma MR, Aquino LRL, Atra E, Tugwell P, Goldsmith CH. Reliability of pain scales in the assessment of literate and illiterate patients with rheumatoid arthritis. J Rheumatol 1990;17:1022–4.
13. Bellamy N, Bradley LA. Workshop on chronic pain, pain control, patient outcomes in rheumatoid arthritis and osteoarthritis. Arthritis Rheum 1996; 39:357–62.
14. Keefe FJ, Caldwell DS, Queen K, Gill KM. Martinez S, Crisson JE, et al. Osteoarthritic knee pain: a behavioral analysis. Pain 1987;28:309–21.
15. McDaniel LK, Anderson KO, Bradley LA, Young LD, Turner RA, Agudelo CA, et al. Development of an observation method for assessing pain behavior in rheumatoid arthritis patients. Pain 1986;24:165–84.
16. Jaworski TM, Bradley LA, Heck LW, Roca A, Alarcon GS. Development of an observation method for assessing pain behaviors in children with juvenile rheumatoid arthritis. Arthritis Rheum 1995;38:1142–51.
17. Russell IJ, Orr MD, Littman B, Vipraio GA, Alboukrek D, Michalek JE, et al. Elevated cerebrospinal fluid levels of substance P in patients with the fibromyalgia syndrome. Arthritis Rheum 1994;37:1593–601.
18. Lorenz J, Grasedyck K, Bromm B. Middle and long latency somatosensory evoked potentials and stimulation in patients with fibromyalgia syndrome. Electroencephalogr Clin Neurophysiol 1996;100:165–8.
19. Kosek E, Ordeberg G. Abnormalities of somatosensory perception in patients with painful osteoarthritis normalize following successful treatment. Eur J Pain 2000;4:229–38.
20. Mountz JM, Bradley LA, Modell JG, Alexander RW, Triana-Alexander M, Aaron LA, et al. Fibromyalgia in women. Abnormalities of regional cerebral blood flow in the thalamus and the caudate nucleus are associated with low pain threshold levels. Arthritis Rheum 1995;38:926–38.
21. Iadarola MJ, Max MB, Berman KF, Byas-Smith MG, Coghill RC, Gracely RH, et al. Unilateral decrease in thalamic activity observed with positron emission tomography in patients with chronic neuropathic pain. Pain 1995;63:55–64.
22. Rosenthiel AK, Keefe FJ. The use of coping strategies in chronic low back pain patients: relationship to patient characteristics and current adjustment. Pain 1983;17:33–44.
23. Burckhardt CS, Clark SR, O'Reilly CA, Bennett RM. Pain-coping strategies of women with fibromyalgia: relationship to pain, fatigue and quality of life. J Musculoskel Pain 1997;5(3):5–18.
24. Keefe FJ, Caldwell DS, Martinez S, Nunley J, Beckham J, Williams DA. Analyzing pain in rheumatoid arthritis patients. Pain coping strategies in patients who have had knee replacement surgery. Pain 1991;46:153–60.
25. Farrar JT. What is clinically meaningful: outcome measures in pain clinical trials. Clin J Pain 2000;16(suppl):S106–12.
26. Buckelew SP, Conway R, Parker J, Deuser WE, Read J, Witty TE, et al.

27. Mannerkorpi K, Nyberg B, Ahlmén M, Ekdahl C. Pool exercise combined with an education program for patients with fibromyalgia syndrome. A prospective, randomized study. J Rheumatol 2000;27:2473–81.
28. Scholten C, Brodwicz T, Graninger W, Gardavsky I, Pils K, Pesau B, et al. Persistent functional and social benefit 5 years after a multidisciplinary arthritis training program. Arch Phys Med Rehabil 1999;80:1282–7.
29. Lorig KR, Mazonson PD, Holman HR. Evidence suggesting that health education for self-management in patients with chronic arthritis has sustained health benefits while reducing health care costs. Arthritis Rheum 1993;36:439–46.
30. Weinberger M, Tierney WM, Cowper PA, Katz BP, Booher PA. Cost-effectiveness of increased telephone contact for patients with osteoarthritis. A randomized, controlled trial. Arthritis Rheum 1993;36:243–6.
31. Maisiak R, Austin JS, West SG, Heck L. The effect of person-centered counseling on the psychological status of persons with systemic lupus erythematosus or rheumatoid arthritis: a randomized, controlled trial. Arthritis Care Res 1996;9:60–6.
32. Superio-Cabuslay E, Ward MM, Lorig KR. Patient education interventions in osteoarthritis and rheumatoid arthritis: a meta-analytic comparison with nonsteroidal antiinflammatory drug treatment. Arthritis Care Res 1996;9:292–301.
33. Felson DT, Lawrence R, Hochberg MC, McAlindon T, Dieppe PA, Minor M, et al. Osteoarthritis: new insights. Part 2: treatment approaches. Ann Intern Med 2000;133:726–37.
34. Bennett RM. Pharmacological treatment of fibromyalgia. J Functional Syndromes 2001;1:79–92.
35. Minor MA, Sanford MK. Physical interventions in the management of pain in arthritis: an overview for research and practice. Arthritis Care Res 1993;6:197–206.
36. Rosenstein ED. Topical agents in the treatment of rheumatic disorders. Rheum Dis Clin North Am 1999;25:899–918.
37. Gonzales GR, Portenoy RK. Selection of analgesic therapies in rheumatoid arthritis: the role of opioid medications. Arthritis Care Res 1993;6: 223–8.
38. Peloso PM, Bellamy N, Bensen W, Thomson GT, Harsanyi Z, Babul N, et al. Double blind randomized placebo control trial of controlled release codeine in the treatment of osteoarthritis of the hip or knee. J Rheumatol 2000;27:764–71.
39. Roth SH, Fleischmann RM, Burch FX, Dietz F, Bockow B, Rapoport Rj, et al. Around-the-clock, controlled-release oxycodone therapy for osteoarthritis-related pain: placebo-controlled trial and long-term evaluation. Arch Intern Med 2000;160:853–60.
40. McAlindon TE, LaValley MP, Gulin JP, Felson DT. Glucosamine and chondroitin for treatment of osteoarthritis: a systematic quality assessment and meta-analysis. JAMA 2000;283:1469–75.
41. Burckhardt CS. Nonpharmacological treatment of fibromyalgia syndrome. J Functional Syndromes 2001;1:103–5.
42. Sim J, Adams N. Physical and other non-pharmacological interventions for fibromyalgia. Bailliere's Clin Rheumatol 1999;13:507–23.
43. Berman BM, Swyers JP, Ezzo J. The evidence for acupuncture as a treatment for rheumatologic conditions. Rheum Dis Clin North Am 2000; 26:103–15.
44. Linton SJ, Bradley LA. Strategies for the prevention of chronic pain. In: Gatchel RJ, Turk DC, editors. Psychological treatments for pain: a practitioner's handbook. New York: Guilford; 1996.
45. Linton SJ, Ryberg M. A cognitive-behavioral group intervention as prevention for persistent neck and back pain in a non-patient population: a randomized controlled trial. Pain 2001;90:83–90.

Resources

American Chronic Pain Association: www.theacpa.org
American Pain Society: www.ampainsoc.org
International Myopain Society: www.myopain.org

Fatigue

BASIA BELZA, PhD, RN

Fatigue is a frequent and bothersome problem for individuals with rheumatic disease. This chapter examines the impact and prevalence of fatigue, causes of fatigue, measurement instruments, and management strategies for fatigue reduction in rheumatic diseases. Researchers in the rheumatic diseases have only recently begun to conduct studies in this area. Fatigue has important implications for overall disease management because it contributes to a sedentary life style. It may be a factor in discontinuing or not fully participating in rehabilitation, reducing quality of life, and impairing functional status.

Health professionals share responsibility for addressing fatigue. Whereas physicians' expertise lies in managing the medical aspects of illness, symptom management is shared by all health professionals. Pain, fatigue, depressed mood, and disability are consequences of the illness. Health professionals are trained to help patients better understand and adjust to the consequences of disease. Collaborative efforts can lead to better utilization of the expertise of our colleagues. Disciplines such as nursing, physical therapy, occupational therapy, and mental health play pivotal roles in the management of fatigue.

DEFINITION AND IMPACT

Fatigue is a perception arising from the complex interplay of biologic processes, psychosocial phenomena, and behavioral manifestations (1). To some, fatigue is the end result of excessive energy consumption, depleted hormones or neurotransmitters, or the diminished ability of muscle cells to contract (2). To others, fatigue is the subjective state of weariness related to reduced motivation, prolonged mental activity, or boredom. Fatigue can also be the awareness of a decreased capacity for physical and/or mental activity due to an imbalance in the availability, utilization, and/or restoration of resources needed to perform activity (1). The impact of fatigue is associated with moderate impairment in functional capacity and reduced productivity. One patient with rheumatoid arthritis (RA) describes the impact as follows: "When I am fatigued everything is too great an effort. Ordinary tasks loom as overwhelming. Feelings of helplessness and hopelessness dominate." The presence of fatigue also makes the management of associated symptoms more challenging. It may also be related to increased human error and associated with increased falls (3).

PREVALENCE

The prevalence and severity of fatigue vary by type of rheumatic disease. Although the diagnostic criteria for RA do not include fatigue, one criterion for clinical remission is the absence of fatigue (4). In patients with RA fatigue has been found to range from 88–100% (4–6). The American College of Rheumatology 1990 Multicenter Study for Fibromyalgia,

which defined fatigue as "usually or always being too tired to do what you want," found that 81% of persons with fibromyalgia reported fatigue (7). Fatigue is also present in 80–100% of patients with systemic lupus erythematosus and is one of the most disabling symptoms for patients (8–10). Levels of fatigue are higher in patients with active lupus than in patients with inactive disease (10). Fatigue has been found in at least 50% of patients with ankylosing spondylitis (11). The occurrence of fatigue across diagnostic categories at all phases of life underscores the need for empirically based interventions.

ETIOLOGY

Fatigue is a complex phenomenon with multiple causes and contributors that include physiologic, psychological, and environmental factors. Components of the inflammatory process may contribute to fatigue. The level of fatigue in RA is strongly associated with pain, sleep disturbance, inactivity, comorbid conditions, poorer functional status, and newly diagnosed disease (5,12). Other factors associated with fatigue are depressive symptoms, female gender, and self-efficacy towards coping with RA (12,13). When in pain, people expend more energy to complete even the simplest tasks. Disturbed sleep leads to daytime fatigue. Inactivity leads to deconditioning and muscle atrophy.

As a result of disuse or reduced use, changes in the cardiorespiratory system reduce the body's energy producing capacity and mechanical efficiency, contributing to decreased endurance. Muscle function may be impaired due to accumulation of metabolic products, which in turn leads to impaired muscle contractility. Functional impairment is associated with less efficient use of the musculoskeletal system or use of less developed muscle groups to minimize pain. Potential psychological causes of fatigue, such as depression and anxiety, have been noted in patients with rheumatic disease. The diagnostic criteria for depression include the presence of fatigue. Impairment in cognitive function, including decreased attention and impaired perception and thinking, has been associated with fatigue. Individuals with rheumatic diseases have reported cognitive changes such as difficulty in thinking and inability to concentrate (9).

MEASUREMENT

Accurate measurement of fatigue is important for several reasons: 1) to understand the relationship of fatigue with other symptoms such as pain and depression, 2) to monitor its natural history over time, 3) to screen or classify, 4) to assess individual health status, 5) to distinguish between disease conditions, 6) to guide management decisions, and 7) to evaluate the magnitude of change in response to treatment. In addition to

Table 1. Selected instruments that measure fatigue in the rheumatic diseases and other chronic conditions.

Instrument	Description	Number and type of items	Comments
Multidimensional Assessment of Fatigue (5,6,17)	Measures 5 dimensions of fatigue: degree, severity, distress, impact on daily activities, and frequency	16-item instrument that uses numerical rating scales with endpoints of 1 (not at all) to 10 (a great deal)	Developed in rheumatoid arthritis and healthy adults; tested in other chronic conditions
Fatigue Severity Scale (9)	Measures symptoms associated with fatigue and its impact on work, family, and social life	9-item instrument that uses numerical rating scales with endpoints of 1 (low) to 7 (high)	Based on the characteristics of fatigue in systemic lupus erythematosus and multiple sclerosis
Fatigue Subscale; Profile of Mood States (POMS) (18)	Measures fatigue severity; the Fatigue Subscale is 1 of the 6 POMS subscales	7-item subscale that uses numerical rating scales with endpoints of 1 (not at all) to 5 (all the time)	Tested in a variety of clinical populations and healthy adults
Fatigue Scale (19)	Measures physical and mental symptoms associated with the presentation of fatigue	14-item instrument that uses numerical rating scales on a continuum with 1 (better than usual) to 4 (much worse than usual)	Developed in chronic fatigue syndrome and patients attending a medical clinic
Activity Record (20)	Captures activities in a day in a person's life: activities are quantified and specific abilities are rated in terms of the presence and amount of associated symptoms	Daily log format in which the individual identifies completed physical activities and amount of associated fatigue	
Profile of Fatigue-Related Symptoms (21)	Assesses the severity and pattern of illness and evaluates the effects of treatment	96-item multidimensional illness-specific instrument	Developed for use in chronic fatigue syndrome

assessing degree, duration, and severity of fatigue, several related areas need to be determined. Key questions to ask patients presenting with fatigue are: What is the status of your rheumatic disease? Do you have any associated disorder(s) such as hypothyroidism? How well do you sleep? Other factors to be assessed include minor or major mood disturbance, psychosocial stressors, and exercise and activity levels (14).

Familiarity with the several different fatigue measures allows clinicians and researchers to select the scale that best meets their and their patients' needs. Many instruments are available that measure fatigue. One website contains multiple instruments purported to measure fatigue (http://www.qlmed.org/) (15). Resources are also available to guide the evaluation of patient education, health promotion, and other health services interventions (16).

Traditionally, single-item measures have been used to assess fatigue in rheumatic diseases. One question frequently used to evaluate outcomes in clinical trials is how many hours elapse from the time of arising to the time of fatigue onset. Various scales have been used to measure fatigue or energy, such as determining energy level on a 10-point scale ranging from "not at all" to "a lot," or determining fatigue intensity on a 4-point scale from "none" to "severe." Although these approaches require minimal patient time and are simple to score, most have not been subjected to stringent psychometric evaluation. While this type of questioning allows for the measurement of a single dimension of fatigue, such as severity, it fails to capture other dimensions such as intensity or timing. Recently there has been a move toward measuring fatigue from a multidimensional perspective. Table 1 includes published instruments used to measure fatigue that have been developed and tested in the rheumatic diseases.

MANAGEMENT STRATEGIES

Treatment goals for the management of fatigue include resolving the underlying problem(s), helping the patient better understand fatigue, and reducing or alleviating the fatigue. If there is a single underlying problem causing fatigue, such as hypothyroidism or anemia, it should be diagnosed and treated. If there is a component of depression, the patient should receive counseling and, if appropriate, antidepressant medication. The clinician and patient need to develop mutually agreed-upon treatment strategies to reduce or alleviate fatigue with the goal of maintaining or improving quality of life.

Self-Appraisal. Monitoring changes in one's own body is a basic activity of self-care (22). Completing a fatigue care wheel (Appendix A) may help a person see the relationship between specific causes and solutions to fatigue. Using standardized measures to assess fatigue or maintaining a log may help identify patterns of, variations of, and contributors to fatigue. Suggesting that patients read the story "A Bowl of Marbles" (Appendix B) may serve as a starting point for discussion about their own energy level.

Optimal Control of Inflammation. Although the mechanism is unknown, it is speculated that the release of interleukin-1, associated with the body's immune response, contributes to fatigue. Whatever the contributing factors, inflammation has been associated with fatigue. Appropriate type and amount of medications must be taken to control the inflammatory process.

Symptom Reinterpretation. One strategy for improving self-efficacy—the belief in one's capability to exercise control over motivation and environmental demands—is reinterpretation of symptoms. This allows an individual to reconceptualize what he or she thinks about fatigue and redefine physiologic symptoms and signs. For example, fatigue may be a warning sign of an impending increase in disease activity, and that warning should stimulate a patient to seek earlier medical treatment. People with high self-efficacy approach difficult tasks as challenges, set challenging goals, increase effort in face of difficulties, and experience low stress and depression. Improving self-efficacy is critical because studies show it is strongly related to fatigue (13).

Increasing Activity Levels. Individuals with rheumatic disease who are involved in aerobic exercise of moderate intensity note improvements in pain and fatigue. Additionally, improvements have been noted in muscle strength and functional status. Providers should encourage patients with arthritis to safely increase their activity level. The level of aerobic conditioning also has a significant influence on performance capability. Individuals with limited aerobic capacity due to pathologic state or a sedentary lifestyle can increase their endurance through training. After evaluation of the cardio-respiratory and musculoskeletal systems, and with consultation from an exercise specialist, patients can start a training program. Training produces improved heart rate, ventilation, and oxygen transport and utilization. Specific improvements in coordination and functional efficiency also occur, depending on type of activity and muscle groups trained. Endurance training thus allows a lower energy expenditure for a given effort, resulting in reduced fatigue and enhanced performance.

Energy Conservation. Energy conservation is the process of saving energy and improving the distribution of energy over time. Proper body positioning conserves energy. Energy is used when the body is in poor posture such as with the use of incorrect work height, poor posture, or hunched shoulders. Rest breaks reduce pain and stress to damaged joints (see Chapter 26, Rest and Exercise). Activity analysis allows the examination of activities that might drain excessive time and energy. Strategies to alter work patterns include pacing, planning ahead, prioritizing, using adaptive equipment, and job simplification.

Sleep and Rest Behaviors. Obtaining adequate rest and sleep is an intuitively logical approach to managing fatigue. Principles of sleep hygiene are discussed in Chapter 38, Sleep Disturbance. For fatigue resulting from sleep apnea, myoclonus, or other suspected sleep disturbances, refer to a sleep clinic for evaluation and treatment.

SUMMARY

Effective management of fatigue is possible. Consideration should be given to the multiple causes of fatigue and varied management strategies. More research is needed on factors that contribute to fatigue, and interventions must be tested to determine those most effective in alleviating or reducing fatigue. Treating fatigue requires an understanding of the inflammatory process, the impact of the rheumatic disease on the psychological system, and the personal attributes and motivations of the individual with arthritis.

REFERENCES

1. Aaronson JS, Teel CS, Cassmeyer V, Neuberger GB, Pallikkathayil L, Pierce J, et al. Defining and managing fatigue. Image J Nurs Sch 1999; 31:45–50.
2. Poteliakhoff, A. Adrenocortical activity and some clinical findings in acute and chronic fatigue. J Psychosom Res 1981;25:91–5.
3. Fessel KD. Fear of falling and activity limitation among persons with rheumatoid arthritis [abstract]. Arthritis Rheum 1995;38 Suppl 9:S305.
4. Pinals RS, Masi AT, Larsen RA, The Subcommittee for Criteria of Remission in Rheumatoid Arthritis of the American Rheumatism Association Diagnostic and Therapeutic Criteria Committee. Preliminary criteria for clinical remission in rheumatoid arthritis. Arthritis Rheum 1981;24:1308–15.
5. Belza B, Henke C, Yelin E, Epstein W, Gilliss C. Correlates of fatigue in older adults with rheumatoid arthritis. Nurs Res 1993;42:93–9.
6. Neuberger G, Press, A, Lindsley H, Hinton R, Cagle P, Carlson K, et al. Effects of exercise on fatigue, aerobic fitness, and disease activity measures in persons with rheumatoid arthritis. Res Nurs Health 1997;20:195–204.
7. Wolfe F, Smythe HA, Yunus MB, Bennett RM, Bombardier C, Goldenberg DL, et al. The American College of Rheumatology 1990 criteria for the classification of fibromyalgia: report of the Multicenter Criteria Committee. Arthritis Rheum 1990;33:160–72.
8. Shur, P. Clinical features of systemic lupus erythematosus. In: Ruddy S, Harris ED Jr., Sledge CB, editors. Kelley's textbook of rheumatology. Philadelphia: WB Saunders; 2001.
9. Krupp L, LaRocca N, Muir-Nash J, Steinberg A. A study of fatigue in systemic lupus erythematosus. J Rheumatol 1990;17:1450–2.
10. Tench CM, McCordie I, White PD, D'Cruz DP. The prevalence and associations of fatigue in SLE. Rheumatology (Oxford) 2000;39:1249–54.
11. Calin A, Edmunds L, Kennedy L. Fatigue in ankylosing spondylitis–why is it ignored? J Rheumatol 1993;20:991–5.
12. Riemsma RP, Rasker JJ, Taal E, Griep EN, Wouters JM, Wiegman O. Fatigue in rheumatoid arthritis: the role of self-efficacy and problematic social support. Br J Rheumatol 1998;37:1042–6.
13. Huyser BA, Parker JC, Thoreson R, Smarr KL, Johnson JC, Hoffman, R. Predictors of subjective fatigue among individuals with rheumatoid arthritis. Arthritis Rheum 1998;41:2230–7.
14. Goldenberg D. Fatigue in rheumatic disease. Bull Rheum Dis 1995;44: 4–8.
15. Researcher's guide to the choice of instruments for quality of life assessment in medicine. Accessed June 21, 2001. URL: www.qlmed.org/
16. Lorig K, Stewart, A, Ritter P, Gonzales V, Laurent D, Lynch J. Outcome measures for health education and other health care interventions. Thousand Oaks (CA): Sage Publications; 1996.
17. Belza, B. Comparison of self-reported fatigue in rheumatoid arthritis and controls. J Rheumatol 1995;22:639–43.
18. McNair D, Lorr R, Dropplemen L. EdITS manual for the profile of mood states. San Diego: Education and Industrial Testing Service; 1992.
19. Chalder T, Berelowitz G, Pawlikowska T, Watts L, Wessely S, Wright D, et al. Development of a fatigue scale. J Psychosom Res 1993;37: 147–53.
20. Gerber LH, Furst GP. Validation of the NIH Activity Record: a quantitative measure of life activities. Arthritis Care Res 1992;5:81–6.
21. Ray C, Weir W, Phillips S, Cullen S. Development of a measure of symptoms in chronic fatigue syndrome: the Profile of Fatigue Related Symptoms (PFRS). Psychol Health 1992;7:27–43.
22. Keller M, Ward S, Baumann L. Processes of self-care: monitoring sensations and symptoms. Adv Nurs Sci 1989;12:54–66.

APPENDIX A

Example of Fatigue Care Wheel

Fatigue is a frequent and bothersome symptom associated with many of the systemic rheumatic diseases. Patients can learn new self-management skills by identifying the causes of fatigue and using effective fatigue management strategies. Using a Fatigue Care Wheel, instruct patients in identifying factors that bring on fatigue (inner circle) and strategies that decrease fatigue (outer circle). Encourage patients to post the Fatigue Care Wheel in a prominent place at home or work to serve as a reminder.

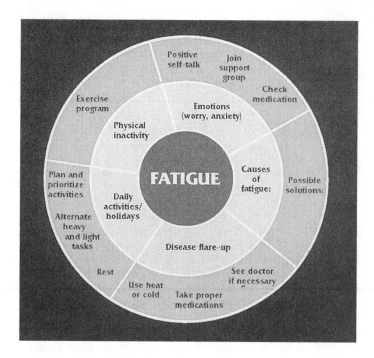

Reproduced, with permission, from Arthritis Foundation. Coping with fatigue. Atlanta: Arthritis Foundation; 1991.

APPENDIX B

My Bowl of Marbles
By Linda Jean Frame

I begin by thinking of energy as marbles. Each small, expendable amount of energy becomes a marble. I have a limited number of marbles to use each day and while the number of marbles may vary from day to day, I can pretty well judge each morning just how many marbles I will have to use that day. I then place my day's supply in an imaginary fish bowl and begin my day.

With each activity such as washing my face or combing my hair I use energy. When I expend one marble's worth of energy, I extract one marble from the bowl. I value each marble at a certain amount and can judge when I use that amount of energy. You might give a different value to each of your marbles, but it will all work out the same way in the end. Bigger projects require more marbles; however, on bad days you will find that even small activities will demand the use of more marbles than those same activities will require on good days. There are times when it is very frustrating to have so little energy and to have to use so much of it to do even simple things, but that's the way it is.

Starting each day with an awareness of your energy supply will enable you to choose what is really important to you, and you can plan accordingly. Try to avoid frustration by accepting your limitations. Frustration is a form of stress and stress is a marble user. Comfort yourself with the thought that you won't always have so few marbles to use. Tomorrow may be a better day. Remember to remove marbles during the day for any type of stress. Remove marbles for anything that causes tension or fear. I throw out a couple of marbles every time I have to drive in rush-hour traffic; not because the traffic bothers me, but because I know that I must be a little more alert and stressed than when I drive at other times of the day. If something really big happens, and I am *really* stressed or shocked, I may throw away the whole bowl and give myself the rest of the day off.

If you should see me or phone me at one of those times, when I have resigned from the human race, you might say, "Linda has lost her marbles," and you would be exactly right!

Arthritis Foundation. SLE self-help course leader's manual. Atlanta: Arthritis Foundation; 1994. p.58. Reprinted with permission from TALS, the San Diego Chapter Newsletter.

Sleep Problems

STEPHEN T. WEGENER, PhD

Sleep problems are common in persons with painful chronic disease, and certain sleep disruptions are associated with specific rheumatic diseases. Clinicians working with rheumatic disease patients will encounter a range of sleep problems requiring a basic knowledge of sleep physiology, cycles, and disturbances as well as fundamental assessment and intervention techniques. Management of these sleep problems has the potential to improve functioning and quality of life.

SLEEP PHYSIOLOGY

Sleep Architecture and Cycles

Human sleep is not a static or unidimensional experience; rather, it is a dynamic process of rest. Healthy adults move through a series of stages during the sleep period. These stages are characterized by distinct patterns of behavioral and physiologic states measured by electroencephalography (EEG), electro-oculography (EOG), and electromyography (EMG). A usual night's sleep is divided into the broad categories of rapid eye movement (REM) and non-REM sleep. Non-REM sleep is further subdivided into 4 stages. Stage 1 is characterized initially by alpha wave pattern (8–13 Hz, low amplitude, high frequency EEG activity), moving to slow activity (2–3 Hz) as the individual moves from wakefulness to sleep. Stage 1 ranges from 30 seconds to 7 minutes in duration and is marked by decreased EEG and EMG activity. The individual may report being awake and is easily aroused by environmental stimuli. During stage 2 there is a further decrease in EEG activity and both researchers and subjects report that true sleep begins. After 15–30 minutes most adults enter stage 3 and 4 sleep. These stages are grouped together as deep or delta sleep, due to the predominance of delta wave patterns (high amplitude, low frequency EEG activity). There is little movement and the person may be very difficult to arouse. Adults typically pass briefly through stages 1 and 2 followed by a period of 30–60 minutes in stage 3/4 sleep.

The typical sleeper returns briefly to stage 2 sleep and then enters the first REM period. REM or dream sleep is characterized by mixed EEG patterns similar to stage 1; however, EMG-measured muscle tension is at its lowest level. Early work on REM sleep seemed to indicate that REM sleep was essential for psychological health; however, recent data do not support this contention (1). The 4 sleep stages and REM occur in cycles each night. Early in the night, stage 3/4 sleep is dominant. As sleep progresses, REM periods increase in length and frequency. The average adult has 4–6 cycles per night depending on age, previous sleep history, and medications. Typical adult sleep is allocated as follows: 2–5% stage 1 sleep, 40–50% stage 2, 12–25% stages 3 and 4, and 20–25% REM (1).

Sleep Requirements

In the U.S., adults average 7–8 hours of sleep per night; however, individual sleep requirements vary greatly. Our society has a significant sleep debt due to the lack of adequate sleep, particularly among school-age children and working adults (2). The typical sleep–wake cycle is approximately 24 hours and is related to the presence of sunlight. The body's Circadian clock controls the sleep cycle, promoting sleeping during the dark hours and peak alertness during daylight hours.

Sleep Across the Life Span

As people age, there is a growing variability in their quality and quantity of sleep. Babies and young children have a higher percentage of stage 3/4 sleep and there is less variation in sleep patterns. As the individual ages, there is an increasing tendency to spend less time in deep sleep and to sleep for shorter periods. The adolescent experiences a dramatic drop in the amount of time asleep to the adult range of 7–8 hours. Throughout middle age there is a decrease in *sleep efficiency*—the amount of time sleeping divided by the amount of time in bed. Older people have greater variability in their sleep patterns, but they often maintain their usual amount of sleep through daytime napping. The elderly also experience more frequent midsleep awakenings. It is not known whether older people need less sleep or are simply less able to achieve the same amount and quality of sleep as before. Factors contributing to changes in sleep quantity and quality include degeneration of the nervous system, increasing prevalence of physical illness, alteration of sleep patterns, reduced level of physical activity, and continued expectation of previous sleep patterns (1).

SLEEP PROBLEMS

Clinicians observe a wide variety of sleep problems that may or may not be related to the rheumatic diseases. The 4 main categories of sleep disturbances are listed in Table 1 (3). Different types of sleep disorders are often seen in various age groups. In children, the most common problems are night terrors, enuresis, and fears related to separation at bedtime. Adolescents experience sleep deprivation with the related problems of difficulty rising and daytime sleepiness. In adults, there is increasing prevalence of sleep apnea, periodic leg movements (PLM) syndrome, disorders of excessive sleepiness, as well as problems initiating and maintaining sleep.

Epidemiology

Insomnia includes difficulty initiating sleep, frequent midsleep awakenings, and nonrestorative sleep. Due to the various def-

Table 1. The 4 main categories of sleep disturbances based on the International Classification of Sleep Disorders (ref. 2).

I. Dyssomnias—including disorders of initiating and maintaining sleep (DIMS) and disorders of excessive sleepiness (DOES)

II. Parasomnias—disorders that are not primarily associated with insomnia or excessive sleepiness such as sleepwalking, rhythmic movement disorder, nightmares, or sleep bruxism

III. Sleep disorders associated with medical or psychiatric disorders—such as alcoholism, mood disorders, Parkinsonism, sleep-related asthma, or gastroesophageal reflux

IV. Proposed sleep disorders—those disorders without sufficient data to include in the classification at this time

initions used in epidemiologic studies, the true incidence and prevalence of insomnia are not known. In sleep disorder centers, approximately 15% of individuals presenting with sleep disturbance have true psychophysiologic insomnia (1). Transient insomnia is common, as is the use of hypnotic medication. Approximately 40 million Americans have chronic sleep disorders, and most cases go undiagnosed (2). Individuals with serious sleep problems have an almost 50% comorbidity rate of psychological distress, anxiety, depression, and medical illness (2). Insomnia is best conceptualized as a symptom, and effective management of the sleep problem begins with accurate diagnosis of the underlying causes or illness.

Sleep Problems and Rheumatic Disease

Individuals with rheumatic disease are at risk for sleep problems due to chronic pain and increased incidence of depression. Patients cite pain as the most common cause of sleep problems (4). Certain sleep disruptions have been linked with specific rheumatic diseases.

Fibromyalgia. Fibromyalgia has the most consistent and well-documented association with sleep disruptions. However, current data do not establish whether sleep disruptions are a cause or effect of fibromyalgia. A pattern of increased nocturnal vigilance, light nonrestorative sleep, insomnia, poor sleep quality, and a high frequency of subjective sleep disruptions is experienced by many persons with fibromyalgia (5). A night of poor sleep is followed by a day of higher pain intensity, which in turn is followed by another night of poor sleep. These sleep patterns are associated with stiffness, fatigue, and cognitive disturbances (6,7).

Sleep studies have repeatedly documented the intrusion of alpha waves during non-REM sleep (alpha EEG non-REM sleep anomaly) in persons with fibromyalgia (5). Alpha waves are indicative of wakefulness seen in early stage 1 sleep. The intrusion of this pattern on other sleep stages is related to poor sleep quality and may be related to the development of fibromyalgia (5). This anomaly is associated with increased pain reports in persons with fibromyalgia (5), and inducing deep pain during sleep is associated with an increase in this anomaly in normal controls (8). However, the alpha EEG non-REM sleep anomaly is not found in all patients with fibromyalgia (9,10). A recent study identified 3 distinct patterns of alpha sleep activity in persons with fibromyalgia, only one of which was related to clinical manifestations of fibromyalgia (11). This suggests that the relationship between the sleep disturbance and clinical symptoms is more complex than originally thought.

Additional sleep anomalies associated with fibromyalgia include delayed sleep onset (12), reduced stage 3 and 4 (deep sleep) time (13), greater number of arousals (13,14), reduced REM sleep (13), greater sleep fragmentation (10), and greater wake time after sleep onset (13). While present in a subset of persons with fibromyalgia, neither sleep apnea nor periodic limb movements are consistently associated with the musculoskeletal symptoms of fibromyalgia and do not appear to be responsible for the development of the disorder (15). Sleep disruptions such as motor agitation, nocturnal awakening, and nonrefreshing sleep seem to be prominent in children with fibromyalgia but may be different than those seen in adults (16).

Studies have not observed reduced sleep time or sleep efficiency in persons with fibromyalgia, suggesting that changes in the quality of sleep, rather than absolute sleep time, may be critical. The mechanisms by which sleep anomalies develop and are related to the etiology and/or maintenance of fibromyalgia remain unclear. One possibility is that low levels of serotonin are related to decreased deep sleep, which may lead to development of this syndrome (9). Alternatively, low levels of the growth hormone somatomedin C have been identified in some patients with fibromyalgia and may serve as a potential link between disturbed sleep and muscle pain (17). Finally, observed reductions in the regional cerebral blood flow to the thalamus and caudate nucleus may be related to disruption of the neuroendocrine system and sleep architecture (18). These abnormalities remain to be confirmed.

Rheumatoid Arthritis. Sleep fragmentation—light, easily disrupted sleep with multiple midsleep awakenings—has been observed by EEG and by self-report in adults and children with rheumatoid arthritis (RA) (19–21). In adults, sleep fragmentation has been associated with higher pain reports and morning stiffness (22); however, these specific findings remain to be replicated. Clinicians should be aware that persons with RA who have cervical instability may be at increased risk for sleep apnea (23).

Other Rheumatic Diseases. Sleep quantity and sleep quality (more stage 1 and less stage 2 sleep) disruptions have been observed in persons with osteoarthritis (24,25). Persons with primary Sjögren's syndrome report a variety of sleep problems including midsleep awakenings and less efficient sleep (26). Poor sleep has been reported as a quality of life concern in a sample of persons with ankylosing spondylitis (27). The importance of these observations for the etiology, prognosis, and treatment of these rheumatic diseases is unknown. The incidence and prevalence of sleep problems in other forms of rheumatic diseases such as systemic lupus erythematosus remain to be determined.

ASSESSMENT

A review of sleep parameters should be included in the initial patient history. Sleep patterns may be affected by pain, respiratory problems, psychiatric or neurologic conditions, medications, or environmental stimuli. Critical information for the diagnosis and treatment of sleep problems is provided by the individual's medical, psychiatric, and family history; medication usage; and environmental assessment. Behavior in terms of eating, substance use/abuse, exercise habits, sleep schedule, and presleep activities should be included in the assessment, as well as an interview with the patient's bed partner. An assessment of the individual's sleep environment with regard to sleep hygiene principles may be indicated.

It is essential for clinicians to determine the type of sleep disturbance experienced by the patient. If the problem involves initiating and maintaining sleep, then it must be determined whether the problem is sleep onset delay, midsleep awakening, or early morning awakening. Short-term complaints and difficulties should be distinguished from chronic problems. Inquiry regarding what steps the patient has taken to address the sleep problem will indicate the chronicity and severity of the symptom. Careful review of medications, including over-the-counter drugs, is necessary to identify pharmacologic agents that may disrupt sleep patterns. Some medications disrupt sleep during active use and others during the withdrawal period.

Sleep diaries are useful in assessing sleep problems. A daily record of the individual's sleep patterns including bedtime, rising time, midsleep awakenings, pain, mood, and medication use, kept for at least a week, is essential. Review of the diary with the patient can provide data for diagnosis and treatment. Subsequent weekly diaries are critical for evaluating treatment response. A full physical and neurologic examination with emphasis on detecting disorders that can affect the nervous system is indicated for those with severe sleep problems. Evaluation of anxiety and depression is critical, because psychiatric illness is common in persons with sleep problems (2). If a severe mood disturbance is identified, referral for psychiatric evaluation and medication is indicated.

Several self-report functional measures for monitoring outcomes in rheumatic diseases can be used to assess sleep quality, including the Multidimensional Health Assessment Questionnaire (MDHAQ; ref. 28) and Nottingham Health Profile (29). Routine use of a functional assessment measure that includes assessment of sleep parameters will aid in identifying sleep problems and determining the effectiveness of any subsequent treatment. (See also Chapter 9, Functional Ability, Health Status, and Quality of Life.)

The need for sleep laboratory evaluation depends on factors such as the individual's presenting complaint, response to initial sleep hygiene, and behavioral and pharmacologic interventions. Excessive daytime sleepiness is often related to an underlying sleep disorder, particularly sleep apnea and narcolepsy. Due to the close association between excessive daytime sleepiness and potentially serious organic pathology, individuals with this presenting problem should be referred to a sleep medicine specialist. Primary symptoms of delayed sleep onset and midsleep awakenings may be initially treated with sleep hygiene education or behavioral therapy if sleep apnea, movement disorders, or disorders of excessive sleepiness such as narcolepsy can be ruled out. The clinician should develop a list of potential causes for the sleep disruption and seek to understand and treat each in turn.

TREATMENT

Treatment is dictated by the underlying cause or causes of the sleep problem. Optimizing the treatment of the underlying rheumatic disease is the first step. Special attention should be given to achieving pain control at night through altering the timing of pain medication or considering alternative medications. Review of medications that may disrupt sleep (e.g.,

Table 2. Once rheumatic disease management is maximized these additional steps should be taken to address sleep problems.*

Sleep hygiene
    Avoid over-the-counter sleep aids
    Avoid late meals
    Reduce caffeine and alcohol intake
    Exercise regularly
    Develop a regular sleep schedule
    Maintain cool, well-ventilated, quiet room
Behavior therapy
    Relaxation therapy
    Sleep habit training
Pharmacotherapy
    Sedative/hypnotic agents
    Low-dose antidepressants

* Adapted from *Assessment and Management of the Rheumatic Diseases: The Teaching Slide Collection for Clinicians and Educators.* Copyright 1997 by the American College of Rheumatology.

clonidine, beta blockers) is indicated. Treatments of other medical, psychiatric, or primary sleep problems such as sleep apnea are part of initial efforts to improve sleep parameters. A hierarchical approach to the treatment of residual sleep problems builds on good sleep hygiene, adds behavioral therapy, and progresses to pharmacologic intervention (Table 2). Treatments can be combined to capitalize on the faster results obtained from pharmacologic intervention and the more prolonged benefits of behavioral treatment. The following treatment recommendations are based primarily on studies in nonrheumatic disease populations; when available, specific data are presented on rheumatic disease patients.

Sleep Hygiene Education

Poor sleep hygiene may be thought of as a primary cause of sleep disruption or as a risk factor for developing this problem. Education regarding principles of good sleep hygiene is the foundation for treating sleep problems. Recommendations provided in brief oral or written form are unlikely to change behavior or have any impact on the sleep problem. Effective sleep hygiene intervention requires ongoing counseling and contact with the patient to translate the advice into behavior change. Sleep hygiene principles are listed in Table 3. Because it is difficult to modify several habits at once, the clinician and patient should target one or two initial habits, establish those new behaviors, and then address additional behaviors.

Exercise

Exercise may be an effective intervention in the short term for improving sleep parameters in persons with fibromyalgia, but problems with adherence undermine long-term benefits (30). The potential for improving sleep quality and quantity is one of many reasons for including exercise in a self-management program for persons with rheumatic disease.

Behavioral Interventions

In adult populations, behavioral treatments may be effective in reducing sleep latency and improving subjective sleep quality (31). In addition, behavioral therapy can improve sleep prob-

Table 3. Sleep hygiene principles.

Regular sleep patterns
    Go to bed and arise the same time each day
    Avoid naps, except for brief 10–15-minute period 8 hours after rising
    Take a hot bath to raise temperature 2°C within 2 hours of bedtime
    A hot drink may also help
    Avoid bright light if you have to arise during the sleep period
Environmental factors
    Avoid large meals 2–3 hours before bedtime
    Establish a bedtime ritual
    Keep clock face turned away
    Make sure sleep environment is dark, quiet, and comfortable
Exercise
    Exercise regularly each day
    Avoid vigorous exercise 2 hours prior to bedtime
Drug effects
    Give up smoking entirely or avoid smoking several hours before bedtime
    Do not smoke if you have a midsleep awakening
    Limit use of alcoholic beverages
    Discontinue caffeine use
    Avoid use of over-the-counter sleep medications
    Use prescribed sleep medication only occasionally
Aging
    Educate patients regarding changes in sleep parameters that occur with age to reduce unrealistic expectations and anxiety

lems associated with chronic pain (32). Behavioral therapy generally employs sleep habit reconditioning known as stimulus control, relaxation training, and cognitive therapy to change negative thoughts about sleep. Specialized training is necessary to teach patients these techniques, and referral to a specialist in behavioral medicine is warranted. The use of self-management techniques may have the additional benefit of promoting self-efficacy, thus leading to positive effects on other aspects of the rheumatic disease.

Pharmacologic Interventions

Optimal medical management of the rheumatic disease is the initial intervention for patients whose sleep problem is related to their primary disease process. Adequate doses and optimal timing of nonsteroidal antiinflammatory drugs or analgesic medications to reduce pain and inflammation may facilitate restful sleep.

The most appropriate use of hypnotic medication is in individuals with sleep problems of recent onset. The role of hypnotics in chronic insomnia is less clear, and they should only be used as part of a coordinated clinical management strategy to address the underlying problems. If chronic use is anticipated and the sleep disturbance is related to pain or fibromyalgia, consider the use of a tricyclic antidepressant (33). Duration of action is the primary consideration in choosing a hypnotic agent. This duration is determined by rates of absorption, distribution, and elimination. Special care must be taken in the elderly due to the slowing of metabolism, which may result in higher plasma levels and greater sensitivity of the central nervous system (1).

The choice of hypnotic is based on whether the intended effect is to reduce time to sleep onset, midsleep awakenings, or anxiety related to sleep disturbance. If the main difficulty is falling asleep, rapidly eliminated agents such as zolpidem or midazolam should be considered. Zolpidem has been shown to improve sleep quality and quantity in persons with fibromyalgia (34). Clinicians need to avoid the tendency to use a larger

dose of these medications to sustain sleep as this practice may lead to respiratory depression or rebound insomnia when withdrawn.

When frequent midsleep awakenings are the problem, hypnotics with moderate duration of action but rapid elimination may be helpful (e.g., brotizolam, zopiclone). In persons with RA, short-term zopiclone was effective in improving subjective sleep problems (35). Residual effects and inevitable accumulation can occur with some longer-acting hypnotics such as flurazepam and nitrazepam (1).

When both insomnia and residual anxiety are present, agents with long duration of action such as clorazepate may be useful. Use the smallest dose possible and avoid chronic use of hypnotic agents. If sleep disturbance persists, further diagnostic evaluation and treatment of underlying causes is indicated.

Sedating tricyclic and tetracyclic antidepressants in less than antidepressant doses at bedtime can be effective in reducing sleep disturbances, particularly in persons with fibromyalgia (36). As a group, both tricyclics and selective serotonin reuptake inhibitors (SSRIs) appear to improve self-reported sleep quality, pain, fatigue, and well-being, but not trigger points. However, it is not clear if these improvements are independent of depression (33). In fibromyalgia, the effectiveness of amitriptyline or fluoxetine alone to improve sleep quality may diminish over time (37–39). One study indicated that a combination of fluoxetine and amitriptyline may be more effective than either agent alone (39).

The effect of tricyclic antidepressants on alpha EEG non-REM sleep anomaly is unclear (9). The positive effects of these agents need to weighed against the side effects related to their anticholinergic activity, particularly in the elderly. Also, tricyclic antidepressants depress REM sleep. For a significant minority of patients SSRIs have a negative effect on sleep (40). For individuals with sleep disturbances and concomitant depression, agents that block the serotonin type 2 (5-HT2) receptor (e.g., nefazodone) may be beneficial (40).

Cyclobenzaprine has also demonstrated improvement in total sleep time in persons with fibromyalgia (37). Alternative therapies such as melatonin have been used to treat sleep problems associated with fibromyalgia and deserve further consideration (41).

REFERENCES

1. Kryger MH, Roth T, Dement WC, editors. Principles and practice of sleep medicine. 3rd ed. Philadelphia: WB Saunders; 2000.
2. National Commission on Sleep Disorders Research. Wake up America: a national sleep alert. Washington (DC): U.S. Department of Health and Human Services; Jan 1993. Program 470-M.
3. American Sleep Disorders Association, Diagnostic Classification Steering Committee Thorpy MJ, chair). International classification of sleep disorders: diagnostic and coding manual. Rochester (MN): American Sleep Disorders Association; 1990.
4. Leigh TJ, Bird HA, Hindmarch I, Wright V. A comparison of sleep in rheumatic and non-rheumatic patients. Clin Exp Rheumatol 1987;5:363–5.
5. Moldofsky H. Sleep and fibrositis syndrome. Rheum Dis Clin North Am 1980;15:91–103.
6. Jennum P, Drewes AM, Andreasen A, Nielson KD. Sleep and other symptoms in primary fibromyalgia and in healthy controls. J Rheumatol 1993;20:1756–9.
7. Affleck G, Urrows S, Tennen H, Higgens P, Abeles M. Sequential daily relations of sleep, pain intensity, and attention to pain among women with fibromyalgia. Pain 1996;68:363–8.
8. Drews AM, Nielson KD, Arendt-Nielsen L, Birket-Smith L, Hansen LM. The effect of cutaneous and deep pain on the electroencephalogram during sleep: an experimental study. Sleep 1997;20:632–40.

9. Carette S, Oakson G, Guimont C, Steriade M. Sleep electroencephalography and the clinical response to amitriptyline in patients with fibromyalgia. Arthritis Rheum 1995;38:1211–7.

10. Shaver JL, Landis CA, Heitkemper MM, Buchwald DS, Woods NF. Sleep, psychosocial distress and stress arousal in women with fibromyalgia. Res Nurs Health 1997;220:247–57.

11. Roizenblatt S, Moldofsky H, Benedito-Silva AA, Tufik S. Alpha sleep characteristics in fibromyalgia. Arthritis Rheum 2001;44:222–30.

12. Horne JA, Shackell BS. Alpha-like EEG activity in non-REM sleep and the fibromyalgia (fibrositis) syndrome. Electroencephalogr Clin Neurophysiol 1991;79:271–6.

13. Branco J, Atalaia A, Paiva T. Sleep cycles and alpha-delta sleep in fibromyalgia syndrome. J Rheumatol 1994;21:1113–7.

14. Jennum P, Drewes AM, Andreasen A, Nielsen KD. Sleep and other symptoms in primary fibromyalgia and in healthy controls. J Rheumatol 1993;20:1756–9.

15. Lario BA, Teran J, Alonso J, Arroyo I, Viejo JL. Lack of association between fibromyalgia and sleep apnea syndrome. Ann Rheum Dis 1992; 51:108–11.

16. Kashikar-Zuck S, Graham TB, Huenefeld MD, Powers SW. A review of biobehavioral research in juvenile primary fibromyalgia syndrome. Arthritis Care Res 2000;13:388–97.

17. Bennett RM, Clark SR, Campbell SM, Burckhardt CS. Low levels of somatomedin C in patients with the fibromyalgia syndrome: a possible link between sleep and muscle pain. Arthritis Rheum 1992;35:1113–6.

18. Mountz JM, Bradley LA, Modell JG, Alexander RW, Triana-Alexander M, Aaron LA, et al. Fibromyalgia in women: abnormalities of regional cerebral blood flow in the thalamus and caudate nucleus are associated with low pain threshold levels. Arthritis Rheum 1995;38:926–38.

19. Mahowald MW, Mahowald ML, Bundlie SR, Ytterberg SR. Sleep fragmentation in rheumatoid arthritis. Arthritis Rheum 1989;32:974–83.

20. Hirsch M, Carlander B, Vergé M, Tafti M, Anaya J-M, Billiard M, et al. Objective and subjective sleep disturbances in patients with rheumatoid arthritis: a reappraisal. Arthritis Rheum 1994;37:41–9.

21. Zamir G, Press J, Tal A, Tarasiuk A. Sleep fragmentation in children with juvenile rheumatoid arthritis. J Rheumatol 1998;25:1191–7.

22. Drewes AM, Svendsen L, Taagholt SJ, Bjerregard K, Nielson KD, Hansen B. Sleep in rheumatoid arthritis: a comparison with healthy subjects and studies of sleep/wake interactions. Br J Rheumatol 1998;37:71–81.

23. Drossaers-Bakker KW, Hamburger HL, Bongartz EB, Dijkmans BA, van Soesbergen RM. Sleep apnea caused by rheumatoid arthritis. Br J Rheumatol 1998;37:889–94.

24. Leigh TJ, Hindmarch I, Bird HA, Wright V. Comparison of sleep in osteoarthritic patients and age and sex matched healthy controls. Ann Rheum Dis 1988;47:40–2.

25. Wilcox S, Brenes GA, Levine D, Sevick MA, Shumaker SA, Craven T. Factors related to sleep disturbances in older adults experiencing knee pain or knee pain with radiographic evidence of knee osteoarthritis. J Am Geriatr Soc 2000;48:1241–51.

26. Tishler M, Barak Y, Paran D, Yaron M. Sleep disturbances, fibromyalgia and primary Sjogren's syndrome. Clin Exp Rheumatol 1997;15:71–4.

27. Ward MM. Health-related quality of life in ankylosing spondylitis: a survey of 175 patients. Arthritis Care Res 1999;12:247–55.

28. Pincus T, Swearingen C, Wolfe F. Toward a multidimensional Health Assessment Questionnaire (MDHAQ): assessment of advanced activities of daily living and psychological status in the patient-friendly Health Assessment Questionnaire format. Arthritis Rheum 1999;42:2220–30.

29. Houssien DA, McKenna SP, Scott DL. The Nottingham Health Profile as a measure of disease activity and outcome in rheumatoid arthritis. Br J Rheumatol 1997;36:69–73.

30. Wigers SH, Stiles TC, Vogel PA. Effects of aerobic exercise versus stress management in fibromyalgia: a 4.5 year prospective study. Scand J Rheumatol 1996;225:77–86.

31. Lacks P. Behavioral treatment for persistent insomnia. New York: Pergamon Press; 1987.

32. Currie SR, Wilson KG, Pontefract AJ, deLaplante L. Cognitive-behavioral treatment of insomnia secondary to chronic pain. J Consult Clin Psychol 2000;68:407–16.

33. O'Malley PG, Balden E, Tomkins G, Santoro J, Kroenke K, Jackson JL. Treatment of fibromyalgia with antidepressants: a meta-analysis. J Gen Intern Med 2000;15:659–66.

34. Moldofsky H, Lue FA, Mously C, Roth-Schechter B, Reynolds WJ. The effect of zolpidem in patients with fibromyalgia: a dose ranging, double-blind, placebo controlled, modified crossover study. J Rheumatol 1996; 23:529–33.

35. Drewes AM, Bjerregard K, Taagholt SJ, Nielsen KD. Zopiclone as night medication in rheumatoid arthritis. Scand J Rheumatol 1998;27:180–7.

36. Arnold LM, Keck PE, Welge JA. Antidepressant treatment of fibromyalgia: a meta-analysis and review. Psychosomatics 2000;41:104–13.

37. Carette S, Bell MJ, Reynolds WJ, Haraoui B, McCain GA, Bykerk VP, et al. Comparison of amitriptyline, cyclobenzaprine, and placebo in the treatment of fibromyalgia: a randomized, double-blind clinical trial. Arthritis Rheum 1994;37:32–40.

38. Wolfe F, Anderson J, Harkness D, Bennett RM, Caro XJ, Goldenberg DL, et al. A double-blind, placebo controlled trial of fluoxetine in fibromyalgia. Scand J Rheumatol 1994;23:255–9.

39. Goldenberg D, Mayskiy M, Mossey C, Ruthazer R, Schmid C. A randomized, double-blind crossover trial of fluoxetine and amitriptyline in the treatment of fibromyalgia. Arthritis Rheum 1996;39:1852–9.

40. Thase ME. Treatment issues related to sleep and depression. J Clin Psychiatry 2000;61 Suppl 11:46–50.

41. Citera G, Arias, MA, Maldonado-Cocco JA, Lazaro MA, Rosemffet MG, Brusco LI, et al. The effect of melatonin in patients with fibromyalgia: a pilot study. Clin Rheumatol 2000;19:9–13.

Resources

American Academy of Sleep Medicine. Accessed September 7, 2001. URL: http://www.aasmnet.org

National Sleep Foundation. Accessed September 7, 2001. URL: http://www.sleepfoundation.org

CHAPTER 39

Mood Disorders

KRISTOFER J. HAGGLUND, PhD; and ROBERT G. FRANK, PhD

Mood disorders are commonly experienced by persons with chronic illness, including those with rheumatic disease. Depression is, arguably, the mood disorder with the greatest personal and societal impact. In fact, depression is a major health problem associated with excessive mortality and morbidity. Impairment and disability associated with depression are equal to that associated with cardiovascular disease and are greater than that due to other chronic disorders such as hypertension or diabetes mellitus (1). Depressed and anxious individuals utilize higher levels of health care services (2). Despite the high personal and fiscal costs associated with depression, it may go undetected and untreated in as many as 50% of depressed individuals seen in medical settings.

Research indicates that patients with undetected depression tend to be only slightly less depressed than those treated for this disorder (3). Furthermore, individuals who are treated for their depression by general medical providers are less likely to receive appropriate, high-quality care (4). Recent emphasis on cost-effective care for both primary care and chronic illness demands careful examination of comorbid conditions and aggressive, high-quality treatment of conditions like depression that can be detected and treated effectively.

Depression or depressive symptoms are common in individuals with all types of rheumatic disease, but they are most clearly documented among individuals with rheumatoid arthritis (RA) (5,6), systemic lupus erythematosus (SLE) (7), and fibromyalgia (8). Research indicates that regardless of the type of rheumatic disease, mood disturbance is associated with increased pain, functional impairment, and poorer outcomes (8,9).

CHARACTERISTICS

The common usage of the term *depression* has necessitated the establishment of clear criteria for depressive illness. The frequently utilized appellate "clinical depression" has no true descriptive value. In general usage, depression describes transient mood changes in response to life's vagaries. The clinical syndrome of depression with persistent impairment of mood and the presentation of associated symptoms is markedly different from normal mood variations and grief. As shown in Table 1, clinical features include impairment in mood, cognition behavior, and somatic functioning (10).

Epidemiology of Depression

Research data suggest that there are increasing rates of depressive disorders among successive birth cohorts throughout this century. These data also indicate an earlier age of onset for the most recent birth cohorts and a persistence of higher prevalence among women, although a less pronounced gender dif-

Table 1. Clinical features of depression.

Feature	Description
Mood (affect)	Sad, blue, depressed, unhappy, down in the dumps, empty, worried, irritable
Cognition	Loss of interest, difficulty concentrating, low self-esteem, negative thoughts, suicide ideation, and less commonly, hallucinations and delusions
Behavior	Psychomotor retardation or agitation, crying, social withdrawal, dependency, suicide
Somatic (physical)	Sleep disturbance, fatigue, appetite disturbance, weight change, pain, gastrointestinal upset, decreased libido

ference is apparent in recent cohorts (11). In family studies, cohorts under 40 years of age have been found to have rates 3 times as high as the oldest cohort (11). In addition, it appears that the lifetime rate of any disorder declines with age, with the lowest rates being found among elderly people. This pattern of decreased lifetime rate with age is particularly pronounced for affective disorders. For men and women, the lifetime rates for affective disorders are 6% and 11%, respectively. In the 18–19 year-old age group, 7% and 15% had affective disorders; in the 45–64 age group, only 4% and 9%; and in the 65 and older age group, 2% and 3% had affective disorders (12).

Depression is a disabling syndrome. Depressed individuals are less able to perform the activities of daily living than patients with medical conditions such as diabetes and rheumatic disorders alone (1). In one study, patients with dysthymia were significantly more limited in physical and social role functioning 2 years after diagnosis than patients with hypertension, despite significant deterioration of function for those with hypertension. Individuals who recover from depressive disorders tend to be employed, have a lower alcohol intake, use active coping strategies, and have a higher level of physical activity and social support in comparison with those who do not recover over time (1).

Depression is a potentially lethal disorder; about 15% of individuals with primary affective disorder eventually kill themselves. Approximately 50% of persons who commit suicide have a primary diagnosis of depression (10). Long-term risk factors for suicide include hopelessness, suicidal ideation, and prior suicide attempts.

Anxiety has received less empirical attention than depression in persons with rheumatic diseases, despite evidence that anxiety disorders can be significantly disabling. Clinically noteworthy levels of anxiety have been reported among large samples of people with rheumatic diseases. A longitudinal investigation involving 400 persons with RA found that initial anxiety scores were related to pain and predicted subsequent physician utilization (13). High lifetime rates of anxiety have also been noted in individuals with fibromyalgia (14). More research is needed to address the prevalence of anxiety, its comorbidity with mood disorders, and its relationship to disease status.

Major Depressive Episode

Major depressive episode (MDE) is the most common mood disorder. Diagnosis of MDE is based on operational criteria including the presence of either a depressed mood or the loss of pleasure/interest and at least 4 other major symptoms of depression over a 2-week period. The symptoms must also cause significant impairment in social, occupational, or other roles, and they must not be due to a "general" medical condition such as hypothyroidism, to bereavement, or to the physical effects of a mood-altering substance (15).

Based on a survey of over 18,000 adults in 5 U.S. communities, epidemiologic studies found a 1-month prevalence of 1.6% and a lifetime prevalence of 4.4% for MDE (12). The mean age at onset of MDE was 27 years with little difference between men and women. The prevalence of depression in women was found to be uniformly higher than in men, with twice as many women having major depression. An average untreated episode lasts 6 or more months, although 21% of patients studied still experienced depression 2 years later.

Major depressive episode is a recurrent disorder; the likelihood of experiencing a single episode is less than 50%, but the risk of further episodes increases with each subsequent episode. Frequently, MDE occurs with other conditions. For example, patients with dysthymic disorder may have MDE superimposed (double depression). Anxiety disorders also coexist with MDE.

Dysthymic Disorder

Dysthymic disorder is characterized by a chronic disturbance involving depressed mood for most of the day, more days than not, for at least 2 years. In addition to depression, 2 or more of the following symptoms are necessary: decreased appetite or overeating, hypersomnia or insomnia, fatigue, poor self-esteem, impaired concentration or difficulty with decision-making, and feelings of hopelessness. Dysthymic disorder differs from MDE in the number and intensity of the symptoms.

A distinction is made between early onset (before age 21) and late onset (age 21 or older) dysthymia (15), although the value of this distinction is unclear. A 3% lifetime prevalence of dysthymia was found in the adult population, with women affected 1.5 to 3 times more often than men. Dysthymia was more common in women under 65, unmarried persons, and young persons with low income. Dysthymia also was associated with greater use of general health and psychiatric services, and with psychotropic drug use. Dysthymic disorders are often accompanied by other psychiatric disorders. Up to 75% of persons with dysthymia may have other conditions, including MDE, panic and other anxiety disorders, and substance abuse (12).

Adjustment Disorder with Depressed Mood

Adjustment disorder with depressed mood refers to a maladaptive reaction to an identified psychosocial stressor or stressors, which occurs within 3 months after the onset of the stressor and has persisted no longer than 6 months. The depressive reaction must either impair the person's occupational or social function or be overreactive in light of the nature of the stressor. Symptoms include depressed mood, tearfulness, and feelings of hopelessness. The distinction between adjustment disorder with depressed mood and MDE is often unclear; stressors play an important role in the onset of both conditions. If the full criteria for MDE are met, that diagnosis takes precedence (15).

Uncomplicated Bereavement

Uncomplicated bereavement is considered a normal reaction to a major loss, such as the death of a family member. It is not classified as a mental disorder, although some symptoms may be identical to those of MDE. In general, uncomplicated bereavement is not associated with a pervasive sense of guilt and worthlessness, marked functional impairment, or thoughts of suicide (15). Guilt is sometimes associated with things done or not done at the time of death of a loved one (15). Marked or prolonged functional impairment is uncommon. Bereavement usually begins shortly after the loss and improves over several months.

Organic and Psychoactive Substance-Induced Mood Disorders

Organic mood syndromes are characterized by mood disturbance created by medical conditions. The clinical presentation mimics functional depression and may range from mild to severe. A common example of organic mood syndrome in rheumatic disease is a depressive effect associated with high doses of corticosteroids in individuals with RA (6). A variety of nonpsychiatric medical conditions are thought to be accompanied by depression, for example, endocrine disorders (including those of the pituitary, adrenal, and thyroid) and collagen-type disorders such as systemic lupus erythematosus.

PREVALENCE

Assessment

Estimates of depression among persons with rheumatic disease vary widely, depending on the assessment methodology. Most studies have relied on self-report questionnaires, which tend to produce higher estimates of the prevalence of depression compared to structural interviews. Self-report approaches to the assessment of depression are flawed in several ways (16). First, the administration of a single questionnaire, even at multiple times, is insufficient to measure depression validly and reliably, even as a syndrome (i.e., signs and symptoms that cluster together). Structured and semi-structured interviews like the Diagnostic Interview Schedule (DIS) are more sensitive and specific (5). The DIS can be used by lay interviewers, provides a lifetime as well as a current diagnosis, and helps investigators differentiate mood changes associated with alcohol and other substance abuse.

Another problem with the use of depression questionnaires is the lack of valid cut-off scores. Most questionnaires have a range of cut-off scores for the designation of depression, depending on the population studied. In addition, designations such as nondepressed, mildly depressed, moderately depressed, severely depressed, or dysphoric are used to describe test results. Comparison between self-report questionnaires and structured interviews becomes almost impossible given the lack of research examining the validity of these diagnostic designations. Moreover, scores in the mild or moderately depressed ranges can be obtained without endorsement of key symptoms, including depressed mood, hopelessness, or feelings of worthlessness. Research has indicated that common self-report measures of depression and anxiety may be measuring global emotional distress rather than specific emotional states. Among patients with RA, common measures of depression demonstrated good convergent validity, but poor discriminant validity.

The symptoms of depression and other mood disorders overlap with symptoms from rheumatic diseases such as RA, fibromyalgia, ankylosing spondylitis, and systemic lupus erythematosus. Most self-report questionnaires of mood disturbance were initially developed and validated among individuals without chronic illness, resulting in possible criterion contamination (13).

Rheumatoid Arthritis

Most examinations of depression and anxiety among individuals with rheumatic disease have focused on RA (13,17,18). The rate of depression among people with RA approximates the rate found in other types of serious chronic illness, but differs substantially from community samples, the latter having a prevalence of about 5.6%. A comprehensive review of the research on depression among people with RA suggested that the point prevalence ranges from 17% to 27% (19). In one of the larger studies involving 137 patients with RA, 42% met criteria for some form of depression, using a structured interview (DIS) (5). Forty-one percent met criteria for dysthymic disorder, and 17% met criteria for MDE.

Using the Arthritis Impact Measurement Scale (AIMS) depression scale in a sample of 6,153 consecutive patients with rheumatic disease (including 1,152 with RA), 25% of the RA patients self-reported depressive symptoms at a level analogous to possible depression, and 20.4% reported depressive symptoms analogous to probable depression (20).

The prevalence rate may be influenced by the age of the participants in most studies, however. As noted above, the incidence of depression appears to decline with age in the general population. Among people with rheumatoid arthritis, Wright and colleagues found that those aged 45 years or younger reported significantly higher levels of self-reported depressive symptoms than those older than 45 years, even after controlling for other demographic and medical variables. The rate of depression appears to decline steadily after age 45 (18).

Osteoarthritis

Few studies have specifically examined mood disorders among people with osteoarthritis (OA). One study found rates of anxiety and depression among people with OA that were higher than would be expected from a community sample (13). Others have found that depression scores for individuals with OA vary according to the area of the body affected, although all exceed the percentage reported in community samples.

Only 14% of individuals with OA reported levels of depression on the AIMS analogous to probable depression, while 17% and 23% respectively, of individuals with OA of the knee/hip and neck indicated levels analogous to probable depression (21). Mild to moderate depressive symptoms were reported by 40% of patients interviewed in a clinic using a self-report depression scale. Another 6% reported severely depressed mood (22). These patients had an average age of 71 years and an average duration of OA of 19 years.

Fibromyalgia

Almost 1 of every 3 patients with fibromyalgia reports symptoms of depression analogous to probable depression (23), although other studies have demonstrated a wide range of prevalence rates of depression. In one study, a lifetime prevalence of depression was found to be approximately 43% (24). A recent study using a structured clinical interview with patients treated in tertiary care centers found a lifetime prevalence of 68% and current prevalence of 22%. Another 10% of the sample currently had dysthymia, 7% had panic disorder, and 12% had simple phobia (14). Differences in methodology are likely to account for these discrepancies. Just as with other rheumatic diseases, scores on common self-reported measures of depression among people with fibromyalgia are likely to be contaminated by disease-related symptoms. For example, when contamination by fibromyalgia symptoms was controlled, researchers found lower rates of MDE using the Beck Depression Inventory (25). Caution should be used when generalizing results from studies not accounting for symptoms such as fatigue. Furthermore, depression and other psychological impairment has been found to be more common among fibromyalgia patients presenting for treatment than among the larger population of people with fibromyalgia (26). The high rate of psychological disorders and coexisting functional disability among those with fibromyalgia seeking treatment indicates that attention to these features of the disorder is critical to effective treatment (27).

Ankylosing Spondylitis

In a sample of 177 individuals with ankylosing spondylitis, rates of depression comparable to other types of rheumatic disease and chronic illness were observed, despite the possibly widespread belief that individuals with ankylosing spondylitis are better adjusted than others with chronic illness (28). Using the Center for Epidemiological Studies-Depression Scale, 31% of the subjects exceeded criteria for depression, with women reporting higher levels of depressive symptoms. There have been few high-quality published studies about psychological functioning among people with ankylosing spondylitis, but further research is warranted.

Systemic Lupus Erythematosus

Psychiatric symptoms among patients with SLE may result from generalized or localized involvement of the central nervous system, secondary phenomena caused by other manifestations of the disease, therapy, or emotional reactions to the chronicity, uncertainty, and severity of the disease. A recent review noted that depression was the most common symptom reported in nearly half of the 19 studies reviewed (29). Depression rates ranged from 20% to 55% of the patients with systemic lupus erythematosus. Anxiety has also been found at a higher rate among patients with SLE compared to individuals in good health (7), but further research is needed before firm conclusions can be made about mood disorders among people with SLE.

PSYCHOLOGICAL FACTORS

Function and Depression

It is widely speculated that the more disabling the disease, the higher the prevalence of depression. Among individuals with RA, those with depressive symptoms have poorer function and are more likely to have a major physical limitation, spend more days in bed, and report more joints with pain as well as higher levels of pain (30). Depression and anxiety predict pain and functional impairment in RA, even after disease activity is considered (9). Conversely, disability has been found to be one of the strongest predictors of depression (31).

The component of functional impairment most often associated with risk for depressive symptoms is loss of valued activities. Patients with higher levels of depressive symptoms perform 12% fewer valued activities than those with lower levels of depressive symptoms (32). A decline in basic activities of daily living appears to be a risk factor for the development of depressive symptoms in women with RA; the most critical risk factor is loss of the ability to perform valued activities (32). Similar patterns may exist among populations with other forms of rheumatic disease, but further research is needed.

Sleep

There is a widely recognized link between sleep pathology and depression, but the causal direction of the relationship is poorly understood. A recently proposed model of fatigue in SLE suggests that depression and sleep problems, precipitated or exacerbated by disease activity, act as mediators that worsen fatigue (33). Similar relationships have been found among people with RA (34). Sleep problems, including sleep disruption and anxiety about sleep, are the proximal link to fatigue. An affective component, characterized by depression and anxiety, can become linked to sleep disruption in a cyclic process. In SLE, disease manifestations appear to have a more proximal effect on depression, sleep disruption, and/or sleep anxiety, which then act on more proximal causes of fatigue. This model may have applications to other types of rheumatic disorders (see also Chapter 38, Sleep Disturbance).

Depression, Cognition, and Pain

In addition to disease-related factors such as pain or disability, numerous other psychological, social, and environmental factors may elicit or result from depression, including learned helplessness and interactions with spouses (35). One recent study suggests that psychological and social variables are better than disease variables at predicting depression and anxiety (36). Depression has been implicated as an independent contributor to pain when both are assessed concurrently among individuals with arthritis (5,9,27). Pain has been found to make an independent contribution to predicting depression when both are assessed concurrently, but its effects on subsequent depression appear to be mediated by coping strategies (37).

Cognitive theory suggests that individuals in pain displaying high levels of cognitive distortion are more likely to develop depressed mood. Individuals with RA who have high levels of depressed mood may exhibit increased concurrent levels of cognitive distortion. Similarly, perceptions of helplessness are associated with higher levels of depression. Patients with a tendency toward cognitive distortion, such as inaccurate overgeneralization, selective abstraction, personalization, and catastrophizing, are more prone to symptoms of depression (38). The tendency toward cognitive distortion increasing the likelihood of depressive symptoms appears to be independent of illness-related disability. Conversely, belief in one's ability to cope (31) and the use of active, problem-solving coping strategies lead to improvements in depression (37). A recent study among people with RA found that those with depressive symptoms reported greater negative impact of disease-related stressors and poorer coping (39).

Similarly, the types of interactions with spouses appear to affect depression levels, but the nature of the relationship is not simple. Patients who perceived their disease as challenging became more depressed over time when spouses offered more positive support (40). Among people with fibromyalgia, depression appears to be related to negative cognitive appraisals regarding the effects of fibromyalgia on daily functioning (41).

PSYCHOBIOLOGY OF DEPRESSION

Advances in the pharmacotherapy of affective disorders over the last 4 decades have illuminated the psychobiology of depressive disorders. Evidence indicates that depression involves dysregulation of 2 major neurobiologic systems: the hypothalamic–pituitary–adrenal axis and the sympathetic–adrenal–medullary axis (6).

Beginning in the 1950s, tricyclic antidepressants replaced monoamine oxidase inhibitors as the treatment of choice for unipolar depression. The tricyclic antidepressants have relatively high affinity for muscarinic, histaminergic, and adrenergic receptors, causing the side effects and toxicity associated with this class of drug. More recently, the selective serotonin reuptake inhibitors and the dual-action serotonin-norepinephrine reuptake inhibitors were introduced. These drugs are widely accepted by patients because they lack the side effects associated with tricyclic antidepressants, and they are simpler to administer. Despite these advantages, as many as 30–40% of patients fail to respond satisfactorily to pharmacologic therapy, and a significant number of patients fail to achieve long-term remission.

The development of antidepressant medications has underscored the role of neurotransmitters in the pathophysiology of depression. It is now accepted that serotonin neuronal systems are involved in many episodes of depression. It is unlikely that only this single neurotransmitter underlies the neurochemical basis of all depressions; other neurotransmitters thought to be involved in depression include norepinephrine, dopamine, and a variety of neuropeptides, most prominently corticotropin releasing factor.

Although most current research on the psychobiology of depression focuses on the roles of serotonin and norepinephrine, there is substantial interdependence among neurotransmitter systems. Currently, no theory adequately describes the role of neurotransmitters in depression. Abnormalities in the hypothalamic–pituitary–adrenal axis have been commonly observed in depression, but possible links with rheumatic disease remain unknown (6).

TREATMENT

Psychological Therapy

Several forms of psychotherapy, including interpersonal psychotherapy, cognitive therapy, behavior therapy, and cognitive behavioral therapy, have been found to be effective in the treatment of mild to moderate major depressive episodes. The goal of interpersonal psychotherapy is to relieve depression by reducing interpersonal conflicts. Treatment length is relatively brief, typically lasting several months. The focus is on current relationships, although historic relationships may be addressed. Interpersonal psychotherapy has been found to be effective in the treatment of major depression and similar to tricyclic antidepressants in overall effectiveness.

Both cognitive therapy and behavior therapy have been shown to be effective in treating depression. Cognitive therapy emphasizes identification and reduction of negative thoughts and beliefs. Behavior therapy focuses on developing new or augmenting existing behavioral patterns to increase positive reinforcement and on "activating" the individuals. Cognitive behavioral therapy uses methods from both of these 2 treatments. In several studies, psychotherapy and pharmacotherapy have been found to be equally effective in the treatment of depressed outpatients.

Over the last decade, a number of studies have investigated psychotherapeutic interventions in patients with rheumatic disease, most often RA. These studies focused on improving symptoms of rheumatic disease globally, with outcome measures including daily functioning, psychological status, and pain. In general, these interventions utilized cognitive and behavioral interventions in groups of patients with RA (42). Reports have consistently indicated improved coping, reduction of pain and mood disturbance, and increased daily functioning. A recent meta-analysis of treatment for patients with fibromyalgia examined both pharmacologic and nonpharmacologic treatments (including exercise programs and cognitive-behavioral treatment) (43). The nonpharmacologic interventions produced, almost without exception, improvements in physical status, report of symptoms, daily functioning, and psychological status. These interventions tended to be more effective than pharmacologic treatment when used alone (43).

Pharmacologic Therapy

All antidepressants marketed in the U.S. have established efficacy for major depression in placebo-controlled studies. When compared to each other, none has proved superior. Outcome studies typically report that 60–80% of subjects improve, compared with 30–40% improvement in those taking placebo (10). As the severity of depression increases, active drug/placebo differences become more apparent. As yet there is no method to identify those who will respond to specific regimens. Little guidance is available to help clinicians determine appropriate antidepressant medication for individuals with rheumatic disorders.

Because there is no evidence to suggest relative advantage of any antidepressant, choice of drug should be determined by factors such as: 1) previous positive response; 2) similar pharmacogenetics to a drug that has been helpful; 3) depressive subtype; 4) side effects and toxicity of the drug; and 5) cost. Selective serotonin reuptake inhibitors (fluoxetine, paroxetine, sertraline) tend to have fewer side effects and can be started at what is usually an effective dose, but maintenance on the medication for at least 4 months after full remission is important.

Several studies have examined analgesic effects of antidepressant medication in patients with RA who may also meet criteria for depression. These studies have used doses of antidepressants that are lower than prescribed for the treatment of depression. Fifty-seven percent of depressed patients with RA who were treated with a combination of imipramine and supportive psychotherapy significantly improved (44). In contrast, another study found no significant difference in depression between RA patients receiving psychotherapy and age-matched controls (45). A randomized, double-blind trial to examine the effects of low-dose trimipramine (25–75 mg) in 36 depressed patients with RA found that joint pain and tenderness were reduced, but depression did not improve (46). Further research is needed to study the effectiveness of the new antidepressant medications for people with OA and RA and other rheumatic diseases.

For older individuals with rheumatic disorders, medications must be used with caution and adjusted appropriately. Side effects are more common due to increased age and the complicated medical regimen common to the treatment of rheumatic disorders.

REFERENCES

1. Hays RD, Wells KB, Sherbourne CD, Rogers W, Spritzer K. Functioning and well-being outcomes of patients with depression compared with chronic general medical illnesses. Arch Gen Psychiatry 1995;52:11–19.
2. Simon G, Ormel J, VonKorff M, Barlow W. Health care costs associated with depressive and anxiety disorders in primary care. Am J Psychiatry 1995;152:352–357.
3. Wells KB, Burnam AM, Camp P. Severity of depression in prepaid and fee-for-service general medical and mental specialty practices. Med Care 1995;33:350–364.
4. Wells KB, Sturm R. Care for depression in a changing environment. Health Aff 1995;14:78–89.
5. Frank RG, Beck NC, Parker JC, Kashani JH, Elliott TR, Haut AE, et al. Depression in rheumatoid arthritis. J Rheumatol 1988;15:920–925.
6. Morrow KA, Parker JC, Russell JL. Clinical implications of depression in rheumatoid arthritis. Arthritis Care Res 1994;7:58–63.
7. Omdal R, Husby G, Mellgren SI. Mental health status in systemic lupus erythematosus. Scand J Rheumatol 1995;24:142–145.
8. Turk DC, Okifuji A, Sinclair JD, Starz TW. Pain, disability, and physical functioning in subgroups of patients with fibromyalgia. J Rheumatol 1996;23:1255–1262.
9. Hagglund KJ, Haley WE, Reveille JD, Alarcón GS. Predicting individual differences in pain and functional impairment among patients with rheumatoid arthritis. Arthritis Rheum 1989;32:851–858.
10. Jefferson JW, Greist JH. Mood disorders. In: Hales RE, Yudofsky SC, Talbott JA, editors. The American Psychiatric Press textbook of psychiatry. 2nd ed. Washington, DC: American Psychiatric Press; 1994. p. 465–495.
11. Fombonne E. Increased rates of depression: update of epidemiological findings and analytical problems. Acta Psychiatr Scand 1994;90:145–156.

12. Weissman MM, Livingston BM, Leaf PJ, Florio LP, Holzer C III. Affective disorders. In: Robins LN, Regier DA, editors. Psychiatric disorders in America: the epidemiologic catchment area study. New York: Free Press; 1991. p. 328–366.
13. Hawley DJ, Wolfe F. Anxiety and depression in patients with rheumatoid arthritis: a prospective study of 400 patients. J Rheumatol 1988;15:932–941.
14. Epstein SA, Kay G, Clauw D, Heaton R, Klein D, Krupp L, et al. Psychiatric disorders in patients with fibromyalgia. A multicenter investigation. Psychosomatics 1999;40:57–63.
15. American Psychiatric Association. Diagnostic and statistical manual of mental disorders. 4th ed. Washington, DC: American Psychiatric Association; 1994.
16. Tennen H, Hall JA, Affleck G. Depression research methodologies in the Journal of Personality and Social Psychology: a review and critique. J Pers Soc Psychol 1995;68:870–884.
17. Callahan LF, Kaplan MR, Pincus T. The Beck Depression Inventory, Center for Epidemiological Studies Depression scale (CES-D), and General Well-Being Schedule depression subscale in rheumatoid arthritis. Arthritis Care Res 1991;4:3–11.
18. Wright GE, Parker JC, Smarr KL, Johnson JC, Hewett JE, Walker SE. Age, depressive symptoms, and rheumatoid arthritis. Arthritis Rheum 1998;41:298–305.
19. Creed F, Ash G. Depression in rheumatoid arthritis: aetiology and treatment. Int Rev Psychiatry 1992;4:23–34.
20. Hawley DJ, Wolfe F. Depression is not more common in rheumatoid arthritis: a 10-year longitudinal study of 6,153 patients with rheumatic disease. J Rheumatol 1993;20:2025–2031.
21. Dexter P, Brandt K. Distribution and predictors of depressive symptoms in osteoarthritis. J Rheumatol 1994;21:279–286.
22. Blixen CE, Kippes C. Depression, social support, and quality of life in older adults with osteoarthritis. Image J Nurs Sch 1999;31:221–226.
23. Hudson JI, Hudson MS, Pliner LF, Goldenberg DL, Pope HG. Fibromyalgia and major affective disorder: a controlled phenomenology and family history study. Am J Psychiatry 1985;142:441–446.
24. Ahles TA, Khan SA, Yunus MB, Spiegel DA, Masi AT. Psychiatric status with patients with primary fibromyalgia, patients with rheumatoid arthritis, and subjects without a pain: a blind comparison of DSM-III diagnoses. Am J Psychiatry 1991;148:1721–1726.
25. Burckhardt CS, O'Reilly CA, Wiens AN, Clark SR, Campbell SM, Bennett RM. Assessing depression in fibromyalgia patients. Arthritis Care Res 1994;7:35–39.
26. Aaron LA, Bradley LA, Alarcon GS, Alexander RW, Triana-Alexander M, Martin MY, et al. Psychiatric diagnoses in patients with fibromyalgia are related to health care-seeking behavior rather than to illness. Arthritis Rheum 1996;39:436–445.
27. Walker EA, Keegan D, Gardner G, Sullivan M, Katon WJ, Bernstein D. Psychosocial factors in fibromyalgia compared with rheumatoid arthritis: I. Psychiatric diagnoses and functional disability. Psychosom Medicine 1997;59:565–571.
28. Barlow JH, Macey SJ, Struthers GR. Gender, depression and ankylosing spondylitis. Arthritis Care Res 1993;6:45–51.
29. Wekking EM. Psychiatric symptoms in systemic erythematosus: an update. Psychosom Med 1993;55:219–228.
30. Katz PP, Yelin EH. Prevalence and correlates of depressive symptoms among persons with rheumatoid arthritis. J Rheumatol 1993;20:790–796.
31. Wright GE, Parker JC, Smarr KL, Schoenfeld-Smith K, Buckelew SP, Slaughter JR, et al. Risk factors for depression in rheumatoid arthritis. Arthritis Care Res 1996;9:264–272.
32. Katz PP, Yelin EH. Life activities of persons with rheumatoid arthritis with and without depressive symptoms. Arthritis Care Res 1994;7:69–77.
33. McKinley PS, Ouellette SC, Winkel GH. The contributions of disease activity, sleep patterns, and depression to fatigue in systemic lupus erythematosus. A proposed model. Arthritis Rheum 1995;38:826–834.
34. Fifield J, Tennen H, Reisine S, McQuillan J. Depression and the long-term risk of pain, fatigue, and disability in patients with rheumatoid arthritis. Arthritis Rheum 1998;41:1851–1857.
35. Bradley LA, Alberts KR. Psychological and behavioral approaches to pain management for patients with rheumatic disease. Rheum Dis Clin North Am 1999;25:215–232.
36. Evers AW, Kraaimaat FW, Geenen R, Bijlsma JW. Determinant of psychological distress and its course in the first year after diagnosis in rheumatoid arthritis patients. J Behav Med 1997;20:489–504.
37. Young LD. Psychological factors in rheumatoid arthritis. J Consult Clin Psychol 1992;60:619–627.
38. Smith TW, Christensen AJ, Peck JR, Ward JR. Cognitive distortion, helplessness, and depressed mood in rheumatoid arthritis: a four-year longitudinal analysis. Health Psychol 1994;13:213–217.
39. Katz PP. The stresses of rheumatoid arthritis: appraisals of perceived impact and coping efficacy. Arthritis Care Res 1998;11:9–22.
40. Schiaffino KM, Revenson TA. Relative contributions of spousal support and illness appraisals to depressed mood in arthritis patients. Arthritis Care Res 1995;8:80–87.
41. Okifuji A, Turk DC, Sherman JJ. Evaluation of the relationship between depression and fibromyalgia syndrome: Why aren't all patients depressed? J Rheumatol 2000;27:212–219.
42. Parker JC, Smarr KL, Buckelew SP, Stucky-Ropp RC, Hewett JE, Johnson JC, et al. Effects of stress management on clinical outcomes in rheumatoid arthritis. Arthritis Rheum 1995;38:1807–1818.
43. Rossy LA, Buckelew SP, Dorr N, Hagglund KJ, Thayer JF, McIntosh MJ, et al. A meta-analysis of fibromyalgia treatment interventions. Ann Behav Med 1999;21:180–191.
44. Fowler PD, MacNeill A, Spencer D, Robinson ET, Dick WC. Imipramine, rheumatoid arthritis and rheumatoid factor. Curr Med Res Opin 1977;5:241–246.
45. Kaplan S, Kozin F. A controlled study of group counseling in rheumatoid arthritis. J Rheumatol 1981;8:91–99.
46. Macfarlane JG, Jalai S, Grace EM. Trimipramine in rheumatoid arthritis: a randomized double-blind trial in relieving pain and joint tenderness. Curr Med Res Opin 1986;10:89–93.

Additional Recommended Reading

Parker JC, Wright GE. The implications of depression for pain and disability in rheumatoid arthritis. Arthritis Care Res 1995;8:279–283.

Rossy LA, Buckelew SP, Hagglund KJ, Thayer JF, McIntosh MJ, Hewett JE, et al. A meta-analysis of fibromyalgia treatment interventions. Ann Behav Med 1999;21:180–191.

Deconditioning

JUDITH A. FALCONER, PhD, MPH, OTR/L

Deconditioning is a generalized physical debilitation that occurs in response to disease and/or to diminishing or habitually low levels of physical (muscular) activity. The hallmarks of physical deconditioning include diminished cardiorespiratory efficiency (increased resting heart rate, decreased VO_2 max), decreased muscle and connective tissue function, bone loss, increased percent body fat, and low endurance.

Stimuli from muscular activity and postural (gravitational) stress with daily activities regulate musculoskeletal and cardiorespiratory function. When muscular activity is reduced or is below threshold levels for prolonged periods of time, Type II (fast twitch, force production) muscle fibers atrophy, especially in the weight-bearing muscles, with a corresponding loss of muscle mass and function. Loss of aerobic enzymes, mitochondrial density (cellular energy), and capillary density render the muscles less able to use oxygen efficiently. When the muscular demand for oxygen and blood flow is diminished by immobilization or disuse, cardiac stroke volume, cardiac output, and plasma volume decrease, with a proportionate increase in resting heart rate. These changes interfere with the capacity of the cardiorespiratory system to deliver oxygen and nutrition to working muscle.

In addition to regulating cardiorespiratory and musculoskeletal function, physical activity (muscular contraction) regulates bone and joint integrity. Physical activity provides the mechanical loading essential to bone formation and maintenance of joint flexibility. Inadequate bone loading decreases bone mass and the supporting matrix, thus increasing the risk for injury and fracture. Immobility of joints causes contracture of the joint capsule and periarticular muscles (stiffness) and interferes with cartilage nutrition.

Deconditioning or poor physical fitness contributes to excess fatigue, low functional status, injury risk (impairments in neuromuscular protective responses), incoordination, low pain threshold, sleep disturbances, and selected diseases such as obesity, coronary heart disease, osteoporosis, and depression. Deconditioning may also impair immune system functioning, including the response to illness and injury.

Deconditioning and rheumatic disease activity are related, but the nature of this relationship is unclear. Deconditioning may increase the products of inflammation, such as cytokines and tumor necrosis factor, or it may be a product of the inflammatory process. Deconditioning is generally worse in inflammatory diseases, suggesting a role for inflammation in the deconditioning process. The role of physical activity in deconditioning has also been shown. Increased physical fitness in persons with inflammatory and noninflammatory rheumatic disease is associated with improved physical performance, elevated mood, and possibly a slower rate of joint destruction (1,2).

Deconditioning in the chronic inflammatory diseases may be confounded by associated comorbidities such as cardiopulmonary involvement and gastrointestinal complications that alter nutritional state. Medications used to manage inflammatory disease and associated comorbidities, such as corticosteroids (steroid myopathy), beta blockers, or chemotherapy may themselves be factors in the deconditioning process.

Although research findings on deconditioning in the rheumatic disease literature are limited, available evidence and clinical observations suggest that it is more prevalent and serious than commonly acknowledged. Low levels of physical fitness have been reported in all of the rheumatic disease groups studied including rheumatoid arthritis, osteoarthritis (OA), juvenile rheumatoid arthritis, juvenile dermatomyositis, fibromyalgia, and systemic lupus erythematosus.

Prevention and management of deconditioning are deceptively simple: daily physical activity of sufficient intensity, duration, frequency, and mode to improve or maintain physical fitness. Patient directives to "be more active" or "get more exercise" are necessary, but they provide limited guidance in terms of therapeutic intervention. Key issues to examine include the patient's reasons for inactivity and possible methods to become more active.

FACTORS LIMITING PHYSICAL ACTIVITY

Disease-specific factors; psychological, social, and environmental factors; and aging influence the level of habitual physical activity. The relative importance of each factor in a particular individual suggests the course of action.

Rheumatic disease alters the energy supply-and-demand balance required to support muscular (physical) activity and prevent fatigue. Lean body mass, a primary energy supply source, is often diminished with rheumatic disease. Loss of muscle mass and muscle strength may be caused by primary inflammation (elevated cytokine production, reduced growth hormone production, increased resting energy expenditure, or increased whole-body protein breakdown rates), reflex inhibition due to pain, changes in muscle metabolism (e.g., polymyositis), neuropathic complications of disease such as entrapment neuropathies, medications (e.g., steroid myopathy), or muscle wasting due to disuse atrophy. Smaller muscles have a lower cross-sectional area to generate force as well as fewer mitochondria for muscle respiration, which contributes to muscle weakness and fatigue.

Caloric intake, especially for proteins, is another important source of energy that may be diminished with rheumatic disease, due to appetite loss or protein malnutrition. *Cachexia*, a general lack of nutrition and wasting associated with excess disability and increased mortality risk, may be common and severe with chronic inflammatory disease (3). In the presence of adequate caloric and protein intake, rheumatoid cachexia may be related to the inflammatory process in addition to the effects of medication and decreased physical activity.

Excess body weight may lower physical activity, increase risk for many diseases (such as OA of the knee), worsen joint symptoms, and increase energy expenditure per unit of force; it is probably both a contributing factor and a consequence of deconditioning. Rheumatic disease and physical inactivity may increase the percentage of body fat with or without a change in body weight. The average body fat content is about 25% for young women and 15% for young men; these percentages increase with age (4).

In addition to low energy supply, energy demand with physical activity is increased by rheumatic disease. Symptoms such as pain, stiffness, and weakness alter joint biomechanics, particularly in the spine and lower extremities, and significantly add to the energy costs of movement. For example, limping or other abnormal gaits may double the energy needed to ambulate.

Chronic inflammation may also cause a hypermetabolism, a primary metabolic abnormality that increases energy expenditure in the resting state (elevated resting heart rate) (3). The elevated resting energy expenditure rate plus the increased energy demand with activity result in an energy deficit, early onset or excess fatigue, and diminished physical activity. Physical training decreases resting heart rate and may help to re-set the basal metabolic thermostat in chronic inflammation.

Psychological, social, and environmental factors propel the deconditioning process by their influence on physical activity. The pain and fatigue accompanying rheumatic disease limit the drive for physical activity. The natural response to pain and fatigue is to rest or curtail physical activity. Ironically, physical inactivity contributes to pain and low endurance, yet the deconditioned individual often feels too bad or too tired to exercise.

Few individuals know intuitively the appropriate level of physical activity for their disease state. Anxiety or fear of damaging the joints or increasing pain often restricts physical activity in an otherwise motivated person. Painful or exhausting experiences following activity, such as delayed-onset exercise-induced pain, further discourages this behavior.

Attitudes and beliefs about physical activity influence habitual activity behaviors and the willingness to change these behaviors. Persons who believe that their activity level can be improved and that increasing physical activity improves their health are likely to initiate a fitness program. Continued involvement in physical activities depends on many factors including the level of enjoyment, convenience, social support, and symptom relief or feeling of well-being that accompanies the activity (see also Chapter 41, Adherence).

Social and environmental factors act as stimuli or constraints to physical activity. For example, physical activity level correlates with weather, occupational requirements, amount and type of leisure pursuits, and social characteristics such as gender, education, and cultural expectations.

Aging may compound the deconditioning effects of rheumatic disease and physical inactivity. Age-correlated losses in cardiorespiratory and musculoskeletal function may include decline in aerobic capacity, muscle weakness, joint stiffness, and bone demineralization. These losses are similar to physiologic deconditioning and are, at least in part, also thought to be caused by diminishing physical activity with age. Age-related decline in physical activity is partially explained by attitudes towards physical activity; perceptions of health, fitness, and activity needs; anxiety and emotional health; and level of encouragement and social support (5).

Table 1. Clinical indications of deconditioning.

Fatigue, daytime tiredness, lack of energy for usual activities
Prolonged bed rest or joint immobilization
Less than 30 minutes per day of moderate physical activity
Decreased daily physical activity
Decreased physical fitness

ASSESSMENT

Prolonged immobilization, self-reports of fatigue or low or diminishing physical activity, and physical activity and physical fitness assessments are used clinically to determine the presence and severity of deconditioning (Table 1).

Some level of deconditioning can be assumed following any prolonged period of bed rest or joint immobilization that is volitional or enforced by acute inflammation, comorbid illness, splinting, or surgery (6). Although the illness or condition dictating the immobilization contributes to the deconditioning effects (and at one time was thought to explain deconditioning), we now know that immobility is an independent cause of deconditioning. Bed rest experiments conducted by the National Aeronautics and Space Administration to study the effects of immobilization and weightlessness during space travel demonstrated the severe physiologic deconditioning inherent in inactivity even in young, healthy adult volunteers (7). Primarily because of the risk of deconditioning, prolonged bed rest in the management of rheumatic disease is rarely recommended.

In the ambulatory adult or child, initial indications of deconditioning may not be readily apparent by physical appearance or from a clinical examination. General self-reports of daytime tiredness, lack of energy for usual daytime activities, prolonged exercise recovery, shortness of breath with minimal exertion, or excessive fatigue with physical exertion may signal deconditioning in the otherwise healthy person.

Because deconditioning is common and preventable, routine monitoring for physical activity is recommended as part of all health care for individuals with rheumatic disease. Simple screening questions about the level of habitual physical activity and regular exercise behaviors help determine the need for assessment or intervention and alert the patient to the importance of physical activity.

Physical Activity Assessment

Physical activity may be assessed by diary or activity logs, activity questionnaires, behavioral observations, and mechanical or electronic monitors (8). Diaries and activity logs involve self-reporting of daily behaviors. One activity log designed for use in rheumatic disease is the Activity Record (ACTRE) (9). The ACTRE is a 24-hour record of pain and fatigue (amount, intensity, time of day, and associated activity); perceptions of daily activities; frequency and duration of rest; and frequency, intensity, duration, and patterns of physical activity (see Figure 1). Instructions, data collection forms, and a computer-based scoring program are available from the developers of this assessment (10).

Activity questionnaires can be used to measure intensity of physical activity in various leisure, occupational, self-care, and home activities (11). Questionnaire data yield estimates of the time spent in various types of activities or the time weighted by

Day 1		Afternoon		During this time I felt pain 1 = Not at all 2 = Very little 3 = Some 4 = A lot	At the beginning of this half-hour I felt fatigue 1 = Not at all 2 = Very little 3 = Some 4 = A lot	I think that I do this 1 = Very poorly 2 = Poorly 3 = Average 4 = Well	I find this activity to be 1 = Very difficult 2 = Difficult 3 = Slightly difficult 4 = Not difficult	For me this activity is 1 = Not meaningful 2 = Slightly meaningful 3 = Meaningful 4 = Very meaningful	This activity causes fatigue 1 = Not at all 2 = Very little 3 = Some 4 = A lot	I enjoy this activity 1 = Not at all 2 = Very little 3 = Some 4 = A lot	I stopped to rest during the activity 1 = yes 2 = no
Key # *	Half-hour beginning at	Category†	Activity								
3	12:30 pm	HA	Prepare lunch	1 2 3 (4)	1 (2) 3 4	1 (2) 3 4	1 (2) 3 4	1 (2) 3 4	1 2 (3) 4	1 2 (3) 4	(1) 2
2	1:00 pm	SC	Eat lunch	1 2 (3) 4	1 (2) 3 4	1 2 (3) 4	1 2 (3) 4	1 2 (3) 4	1 2 (3) 4	1 (2) 3 4	1 (2)
3	1:30 pm	HA	Clean kitchen	1 2 3 (4)	1 (2) 3 4	1 2 (3) 4	1 2 (3) 4	1 2 (3) 4	1 2 (3) 4	1 (2) 3 4	1 (2)

Figure 1. Example of an activity record. * 1 = Mostly lying down; 2 = Mostly sitting (at work, reading, computer, TV, etc.); 3 = Mostly standing, walking, lifting, or moving around. † RE = rest; SC = self care; PP = preparation or planning; HA = household activities; WK = work; RL = recreation or leisure; TR = transportation; RX = treatment; SL = sleep.

an estimate of the intensity of that activity derived from average energy expenditure associated with the specific activity.

Mechanical and electronic monitoring involve the use of motion detectors to quantify physical movement in real time. For example, pedometers are lightweight instruments worn on the body that are useful for counting steps or estimating distance walked; portable accelerometers are small devices attached to the trunk or limbs which enable quantification in various planes of motion.

Physical activity assessments in children usually involve parent or self-report activity measures, heart rate monitors, motion detectors, or behavioral observations (12). Direct observation methods typically include recording and coding the physical activity type and intensity observed in the home, school, or recreational setting during a time-sampling interval.

Physical Fitness Assessment

Physical fitness evaluation is necessary to quantify deconditioning and to determine appropriate and safe exercise recommendations. Cardiorespiratory fitness can be assessed by heart rate (measured either by a heart rate monitor strapped to the chest or by counting beats at the radial or carotid pulse) and by maximum oxygen uptake (VO_2 max, measured directly in the laboratory or estimated from submaximal graded exercise tests or field tests). Graded exercise tests use treadmills, cycle ergometers, or step tests, and involve the assessment of heart rate response to one or more levels of effort. Field tests are time/distance walk/run tests, such as the 1-mile walk test or 5-minute walk test. With minor modifications, these tests appear to be safe, valid, and reliable for use with adults (13,14) and children (15) with rheumatic disease. Due to the importance of physical activity and physical fitness to growth and development, regular clinic or school-based physical fitness testing with normative or criterion-referenced standards are useful for the evaluation of children.

Muscular strength is commonly assessed by dynamometry or the 1-repetition maximum test (the heaviest weight that can be lifted only once using good form); muscular endurance by the total count of push ups and/or curl ups; and flexibility by goniometry or the "sit and reach" test. Hydrostatic weighing, body mass index (body weight in kilograms divided by height in meters squared), waist to hip ratio, and skinfold measure-

ments with calipers are helpful in evaluating healthful body weight and percent body fat.

MANAGEMENT STRATEGIES

In the absence of evidence to the contrary, it is reasonable to assume clinically that individuals with rheumatic disease are either at risk for deconditioning or that they would benefit from improved physical activity level. Some individuals unavoidably lose physical performance capacities and the ability to run or participate in strenuous physical activities. Although the disease process itself imposes a physical fitness ceiling, few individuals with rheumatic disease accumulate sufficient levels of physical activity to maintain maximal physical fitness capacity.

Newly diagnosed patients are usually anxious to retain or regain their previous physical activity capacity. Early intervention prevents excess deconditioning and safely rebuilds exercise tolerance and confidence. Patients with established disease tend to adapt to low levels of physical activity, unnecessarily relinquishing valued activities and functional ability. In this group, intervention to restore activity initiative and motivation may be a prerequisite to improving physical fitness, health, and function.

The physical activity and physical fitness assessments discussed earlier are used to set the goals of intervention, to mark progress towards goals, and to guide the choice of interventions. An accurate understanding of current physical fitness, physical activity level, and activity interests and needs promotes awareness and insight into daily routines and suggests ideas and directions for specific changes.

Deconditioning interventions are targeted to the factors contributing to physical inactivity. A combination of methods is used to alleviate obstacles to physical activity, such as disease factors and psychological, social, or environmental issues, and to motivate and counsel patients towards healthful overall physical activity levels.

Therapies that relieve disease symptoms and restore joint function address some of the disease-specific factors inhibiting physical activity. For example, pain management, joint replacement surgery, or functional activity and gait training increase overall activity level indirectly by reducing pain and energy expenditure and improving joint mechanics and motor skills.

Energy conservation training refers to education in and practice of the efficient use of available energy. Integrating principles of energy conservation such as pacing, delegating, prioritizing, and balancing activity and rest into daily routines does not directly improve performance capacities, but it may minimize functional limitations, delay the onset of fatigue, and encourage higher levels of physical activity.

Social and environmental factors can set the stage for realistic therapeutic recommendations. For example, the approval of peers or partners, guidance from an instructor, or camaraderie among exercise group members all promote exercise adherence. Parental, peer, and school support reinforce appropriate physical activities in an able child. Whereas the weather is frequently cited as a major obstacle to exercise, access to well-maintained and safe parks and walkways, scenic routes, swimming pools, and indoor exercise facilities and equipment facilitate physical activity. The challenge is to help the individual find and participate in activities that are enjoyable, practical, safe, and sufficiently intense and varied to increase physical fitness without aggravating the symptoms of rheumatic disease.

Becoming more physically active involves learning and practicing new behaviors. Learning begins when the problem is personally experienced and meaningful to the individual. Experiential or problem-based learning promotes the development and mastery of the attitudes, skills, and behaviors required to incorporate new physical activity patterns. Physical activities that can be integrated into daily routines are more likely to be rewarding and sustained. Sometimes one small change in a daily routine, such as climbing a flight of stairs or walking around the block, provides the impetus and motivation for meaningful change.

Physical Activity and Exercise

Physical activity and exercise are necessary to overcome deconditioning. The recommended public health guidelines for physical activity in healthy adults provide a benchmark for interpreting low physical activity in individuals with rheumatic disease. All adults should accumulate 30 minutes or more of moderate-intensity physical activity (3.0 to 6.0 metabolic equivalents of task [METs]) on most, preferably all, days of the week (16,17). Examples of moderate-intensity physical activities include walking briskly, bicycling, dancing, and home care or repair. Guidelines for healthy children (18) and adolescents (19) are higher and include vigorous and continuous physical activities.

Regardless of physical status, individuals with controlled rheumatic disease can minimize deconditioning with sufficient amounts of aerobic, resistance, and flexibility exercises. As with anyone else, individuals should be medically screened before beginning an exercise program or significantly increasing activity levels. Coaching by a health professional who is knowledgeable about exercise prescription in rheumatic disease is also recommended. In addition to the specific exercise prescription and progression, individuals may need "permission" to exercise and reassurance that a good exercise program will not worsen symptoms. However, learning to self-regulate physical activity and exercise builds confidence and habit and is essential to safe and effective training.

The specific types, intensity, duration, frequency, and progression of exercise depend on the initial fitness level, rheumatic disease status, general health, exercise goals, preferences, and resources of the individual. Aerobic exercise is the most important type of exercise to improve cardiorespiratory fitness and, in combination with dietary regulation, to lower the percent of body fat. Deconditioned adults (20) and children (15) with rheumatic disease are encouraged to initiate an aerobic exercise program slowly, beginning with a few 5-minute bouts of low-intensity exercise with rest periods between bouts and gradually increasing to 20–40 minutes of continuous or intermittent (minimum of 10-minute bouts) aerobic exercise, 3–4 days per week, at moderate intensity. Intensity of aerobic exercise in adults is determined by exercise heart rate, which can be self-assessed by a heart rate monitor or by counting immediately post-exercise the beats at the radial or carotid pulse for 10 seconds. Alternatively, Borg's scale for rating of perceived exertion (RPE), a subjective rating of exercise intensity, may be the preferred method of determining exercise intensity for individuals who have difficulty palpating heart rate, very low levels of fitness, cardiovascular or pulmonary disease, or medications such as beta blockers that affect the heart rate response to exercise (21).

Intensity, duration, and frequency of aerobic exercise interact to produce the exercise effect. For example, a lower intensity of exercise done for a longer duration may be as effective and preferable to a higher intensity exercise for a shorter duration, particularly for individuals at risk of joint injury. Alternating the mode of aerobic exercise (i.e., alternating low impact aerobic dance with stationary cycling) to vary joint stress and weight-bearing minimizes risk of injury and promotes adherence. Varying the intensity of exercise within a session builds exercise tolerance. The rate of exercise progression depends on many factors such as initial fitness, the exercise stimulus, and the individual's response to exercise, but may reasonably be expected to take several months to reach a maintenance phase.

Dynamic resistance and flexibility exercises complement aerobic exercise and are necessary to improve muscle strength and endurance and joint flexibility. Persons with rheumatic disease should build towards a resistance exercise program 2–3 days per week of 10–12 lifts per major muscle group of a load that can be lifted safely and correctly, and 1–2 sessions per day of stretching exercises (22). Persons who are extremely deconditioned or physically impaired may require an initial program of light flexibility and strength training prior to the onset of aerobic training (see also Chapter 26, Rest and Exercise).

GUIDELINES FOR REFERRAL

Routine office-based management of deconditioning by a physician or nurse-clinician who is trained in exercise prescription may be sufficient to prevent deconditioning or to treat mild to moderate deconditioning. Referral to other health care specialists or programs may be warranted when expertise or resources are not available in the office setting, deconditioning is moderate to severe and requires immediate and intensive training with supervision, the patient appears overwhelmed by disease management and requires specialized assessment and management, or the patient's fitness status declines or fails to improve after a trial of 3 months.

Although there is overlapping expertise among arthritis health care professionals, physical therapists generally focus on disorders of movement and possess expertise in physical fitness assessment, exercise prescription, and physiologic issues underlying deconditioning. Occupational therapists focus on disorders of human performance and offer expertise in physical activity analyses, functional training, and behavioral issues underlying deconditioning. Video and community-based programs may be cost-efficient, safe, and effective when properly instructed and supervised. Because these programs may be conducted by many different disciplines and providers, specific programs should be evaluated for their appeal to consumers and competence in exercise and physical activity prescription in rheumatic disease.

REFERENCES

1. Minor MA, Hewett JE, Webel RR, Anderson SK, Kay DR. Efficacy of physical conditioning exercise in patients with rheumatoid arthritis and osteoarthritis. Arthritis Rheum 1989;32:1396–405.
2. Kovar PA, Allegrante JP, MacKenzie CR, Peterson MG, Gutin B, Charlson ME. Supervised fitness walking in patients with osteoarthritis of the knee. Ann Intern Med 1992;116:529–33.
3. Rall LC, Roubenoff R. Body composition, metabolism, and resistance exercise in patients with rheumatoid arthritis. Arthritis Care Res 1996;9:151–6.
4. McArdle WD, Katch FI, Katch VL. Essentials of exercise physiology. 2nd ed. Philadelphia: Lippincott Williams & Wilkins; 2000.
5. Shephard RJ. Aging, physical activity and health. Champaign, IL: Human Kinetics; 1997.
6. Steinberg FU. The immobilized patient: functional pathology and management. New York: Plenum Publishing; 1980.
7. Sandler H, Vernikos J. Inactivity: physiological effects. Orlando FL: Academic Press; 1986.
8. Montoye HJ, Kemper HC, Saris WH, Washburn RA. Measuring physical activity and energy expenditure. Champaign IL: Human Kinetics; 1996.
9. Gerber LH, Furst GP. Scoring methods and application of the activity record (ACTRE) for patients with musculoskeletal disorders. Arthritis Care Res 1992;5:151–6.
10. Furst G. National Institutes of Health, Building 10, Room 6S235, 10 Center Drive, MSC 1604, Bethesda, MD, 20892-1604.
11. Pereira MA, FitzGerald SJ, Gregg EW, Joswiak ML, Ryan WJ, Suminski RR, et al. A collection of physical activity questionnaires for health-related research. Med Sci Sports Exerc 1997;29(suppl):S1–S205.
12. Pate RR. Physical activity assessment in children and adolescents. Crit Rev Food Sci Nutr 1993;33:321–6.
13. Minor MA, Johnson JC. Reliability and validity of a submaximal treadmill test to estimate aerobic capacity in women with rheumatic disease. J Rheumatol 1996;23:1517–23.
14. Burckhardt CS, Clark SR, Nelson DL. Assessing physical fitness of women with rheumatic disease. Arthritis Care Res 1988;1:38–44.
15. Klepper SE, Giannini MJ. Physical conditioning in children with arthritis: Assessment and guidelines for exercise prescription. Arthritis Care Res 1994;7:226–36.
16. Pate RR, Pratt M, Blair SN, Haskell WL, Macera CA, Bouchard C, et al. Physical activity and public health. JAMA 1995;273:402–7.
17. National Center for Chronic Disease Prevention and Health Promotion. Physical activity and health. Available at: http://www.cdc.gov/nccdphp/sgr/sgr.htm. Accessed August 3, 2001.
18. Corbin CB, Pangrazi RP. Physical activity for children: a statement of guidelines. Reston, VA: National Association for Sport and Physical Education; 1998.
19. Sallis JF, Patrick K. Physical activity guidelines for adolescents: consensus statement. Pediatr Exerc Sci 1994;6:302–14.
20. Minor MA. Cardiovascular health and physical fitness for the client with multiple joint involvement. In: Walker JM, Helewa A, editors. Physical therapy in arthritis. Philadelphia: WB Saunders; 1996.
21. Borg G. Psychophysical scaling with applications in physical work and the perception of exertion. Scand J Work Environ Health 1990;16(suppl 1):55–8.
22. Minor MA, Kay DR. Arthritis. In: American College of Sports Medicine. Exercise management for persons with chronic diseases and disabilities. Champaign, IL: Human Kinetics; 1997.

Additional Recommended Reading

American College of Sports Medicine. The recommended quantity and quality of exercise for developing and maintaining cardiorespiratory and muscular fitness, and flexibility in healthy adults. Med Sci Sports Exerc 1998;30:975–991.

Bouchard C, Shephard RJ, Stephens T, editors. Physical activity, fitness, and health: international proceedings and consensus statement. Champaign, IL: Human Kinetics; 1994.

Moncur C, guest editor. Exercise and arthritis. Arthritis Care Res 1994; 7(theme issue):167–236.

Adherence

MICHAEL A. RAPOFF, PhD

Treatment regimens for adult and pediatric rheumatic diseases are complex, demanding, costly, and the benefits are often delayed (1–3). These factors characterize regimens that are likely to produce nonadherence (4–6).

Adherence has been defined as ". . . the extent to which a person's behavior (in terms of medications, following diets, or executing lifestyle changes) coincides with medical or health advice" (7). This definition has heuristic value because it: 1) specifies the range of adherence behaviors required for various regimens (such as medications, therapeutic exercises, and splinting in rheumatic diseases); 2) requires an evaluation of the "extent" of adherence, emphasizing that adherence is relative and can vary within persons over time, between persons, and across different regimen requirements; and 3) implies there is a standard (that which coincides with medical advice) for determining acceptable adherence.

ADHERENCE MEASURES

A variety of methods have been used to measure adherence, including drug assays, behavioral observations, electronic monitoring, pill counts, treatment outcome, provider estimates, and patient report (6,8,9). As shown in Table 1, each of these methods has both assets and liabilities.

Drug Assays. The detection of drug levels, metabolites, or pharmacologically inert substances added to drugs as tracers can be detected in blood, urine, and, in rare cases, saliva (6). They are quantifiable, useful for dosing adjustments, and do not rely on patient or provider estimates. However, assays can be expensive, invasive (particularly relevant for children), and intermittently obtained, thereby reflecting more recent ingestion. In addition, drug levels may reflect factors other than patient adherence, such as inadequate dosing, non–steady state concentrations in patients taking medications with long half-lives over a short period of time, pharmacokinetics variations due to the type of medication preparations (e.g., enteric coating), physiologic factors such as gastric pH, interactions with other medications, patient age, or patient behaviors such as smoking (10,11).

Behavioral Observations. Direct observations are preferable for nonpharmacologic regimens (such as therapeutic exercises), because the provider can evaluate how patients are carrying out treatments and provide corrective feedback as needed (2,6). A major drawback of observations is the limited access providers have to observe patients. However, family members can provide reliable observations of adherence if they are provided with a specific and relatively simple observational strategy and are adequately trained (12).

Electronic Monitoring. Technological advances in microprocessors have led to the development of electronic monitoring of adherence. Microelectronic monitors are now available for recording, storing, and downloading information on medication removal (13). Electronic monitoring allows for continuous (real-time) and long-term assessments of medication adherence. Monitors can also reveal a spectrum of adherence problems, including underdosing, overdosing, delayed dosing, drug "holidays" (omitting doses for several days in succession without provider authorization), and "white-coat" adherence (giving the appearance of adequate adherence by dumping medications or taking medications consistently several days before clinic visits) (14).

These devices present an exciting new avenue for adherence assessment but opening vials does not guarantee ingestion and their current costs are prohibitively expensive for routine clinical use. However, when supplemented by periodic assays, these measures are likely to become the "gold standard" in adherence research (6).

Pill Counts. Pill counts or volume measurements have been used extensively in adherence research. They are simple and can be routinely done during clinic visits or by phone. As with automated measures, the major liability is that medications removed are not necessarily ingested (6).

Treatment Outcome. Outcomes such as active joint counts, duration of morning stiffness, and functional status measures have been viewed as indirect measures of adherence (6,15). These measures are well integrated into clinical practice and research. However, there is not necessarily a close correspondence between patient adherence and treatment outcome (16). Poorly adherent patients may have acceptable outcomes and fully adherent patients may have bad ones. Adherence and treatment outcome are separate phenomena and need to be assessed separately to determine the level of adherence necessary to achieve desired therapeutic effects (6).

Provider Estimates. Provider estimates generally involve a global rating of the degree to which patients are adherent to a regimen (6). Busy providers may find this the most feasible way to assess adherence. However, provider estimates consistently underestimate levels of nonadherence (6). This may be due to reliance on treatment outcomes for estimating adherence and positive bias or expectancies, such as wanting to believe patients are adhering to recommendations.

Patient Report. Consistent with the emphasis on history-taking in clinical practice, it is not surprising that patient and family reports are often relied on to assess adherence (6). These reports are often obtained by structured interviews or questionnaires (17). However, patient ratings tend to overestimate the degree of adherence (2,6). This may be due to social desirability effects whereby patients and families may want to preserve their relationships with their providers by reporting that they are behaving in socially approved ways.

How patients or family members are questioned about adherence may be critical in the quality of data obtained by reports. Questions that are nonjudgmental, specific, and time-limited are likely to yield more accurate information about adherence, as they are less likely to generate evasive and

Table 1. Assets and liabilities of adherence measures.

Measure	Assets	Liabilities
Assays	1. Can adjust drug dosage 2. Gold standard in adherence measurement	1. Pharmacokinetics may affect absorption and excretion rates 2. Short-term, invasive, and expensive
Observation	1. Direct measure of nonpharmacologic regimen adherence 2. Can measure adherence on repeated occasions	1. Obtrusive and reactive 2. Clinically impractical
Electronic monitoring	1. Precise dosing and interdose interval data obtained 2. Continuous and long-term measurement is possible	1. Medication removal does not guarantee consumption 2. Reactive and mechanical failures
Pill counts	1. Easily obtained 2. Inexpensive	1. Pill removal does not guarantee ingestion 2. Overestimates adherence
Treatment outcomes	1. Evaluate regimen efficacy 2. Clinically feasible	1. Inexact or unknown relationship to adherence 2. Factors other than patient adherence can affect outcome
Physican estimates	1. Clinically feasible 2. Generally more accurate than global patient estimates	1. Overestimates adherence 2. Physician experience or familiarity with patient unrelated to accuracy
Patient report	1. Clinically feasible 2. Generally accurate for nonadherence	1. Overestimates adherence 2. Subject to reporting bias—"faking good"

defensive reactions and are less subject to recall errors or misunderstanding (18). For example, questions about medication adherence can be prefaced by stating that "most people—including the interviewer—miss doses of their medication for one reason or another" (19). In contrast, a judgmental and/or global approach without time referents can be useless or actually induce deception.

An alternative is to have patients or family members monitor and record specific adherence behaviors. This can even be done using computerized diaries (8). The accuracy of such records can be improved by clearly specifying target behaviors, using simple monitoring strategies, emphasizing the importance of accuracy and honesty, demonstrating and having patients practice using the monitoring strategy, and periodic and independent checks on accuracy (6).

ADHERENCE RATES

Adherence rates vary depending on how adherence is assessed and what regimen has been prescribed. Medication adherence rates range from 16% to 84% in the treatment of rheumatoid arthritis (RA), and from 38% to 59% in the treatment of juvenile rheumatoid arthritis (JRA) (1,2,6,20,21). Adherence rates for nonpharmacologic regimens (e.g., for therapeutic exercises) range from 25% to 65% in the treatment of RA and from 47% to 86% in the treatment of JRA (1,15,21).

CONSEQUENCES OF NONADHERENCE

The consequences of nonadherence include compromised efficacy, increased health care costs and utilization, and compromised clinical trials (6). Increased morbidity and possibly mortality (such as with abrupt discontinuation of corticosteroids) can be attributed to nonadherence (22). The cost-effectiveness of health care can also be adversely affected. Money may be wasted on treatments that are not followed, or families may incur the costs of additional but unnecessary diagnostic and treatment procedures (23). These unnecessary costs may further burden society in the form of increased insurance premiums and taxes. Treatment nonadherence can also interfere with clinical trials of therapeutic regimens by complicating judgments of efficacy and adding to the sample sizes needed to detect clinical effects (6).

FACTORS RELATED TO ADHERENCE

Much of the adherence literature has focused on identifying factors that promote or impede adherence (4–6). Typically this is done by correlating various factors with adherence or contrasting adherent and nonadherent patients along factorial dimensions (2). As shown in Table 2, patient/family, disease, and regimen factors have been most frequently studied as correlates of adherence. These studies can help determine risk profiles for adherence problems. Additionally, they can assist in formulating or augmenting theoretical models and suggest potentially modifiable variables for adherence intervention trials (6).

Patient/Family Factors. Adherence is likely to be compromised when patients and their families are not well informed, are dissatisfied with care, lack financial and social resources, and experience adjustment problems such as low self-esteem, decreased self-efficacy, and family disharmony. The search for a "typical" nonadherent patient has not been particularly fruitful (5); therefore, providers are cautioned to examine these potential patient/family factors in terms of their relevance for specific patients.

Table 2. Patient/family, disease, and regimen factors associated with nonadherence to medical regimens.

Patient/family factors
    Dissatisfaction with medical care
    Limited financial and social resources
    Lack of knowledge
    Low self-esteem
    Learned helplessness and pessimism
    Negative overall adjustment
    Poor coping strategies
    Family dysfunction
Disease factors
    Decrements in compliance over time
    Patient asymptomatic or in remission
    Increased number of symptoms
    Younger age at disease onset
    Disease not perceived as severe by patient and/or family
Regimen factors
    Complex and demanding regimens
    Costly regimens
    Questionable efficacy
    Lack of continuity of care
    Limited provider supervision of regimen
    Shorter duration of subspecialty care
    Negative regimen side effects

Disease Factors. Persons with rheumatic diseases are prime candidates for adherence problems due to the chronicity and fluctuations in their disease activity. This is particularly troublesome when adherence is found to be inconsistently related to disease activity (21). Patients may have few natural incentives, such as symptom relief or improved function, to adhere to prescribed regimens.

Regimen Factors. The list of these factors in Table 2 suggests that regimens for rheumatic diseases induce nonadherence because they are often complex, costly, of significant duration, and provide delayed benefits. Delayed benefits may particularly undermine patient adherence, as in the case of nonsteroidal antiinflammatory drugs in the treatment of JRA requiring at least an 8-week trial (24). How providers manage regimens is also critical; limited supervision, feedback, and comprehensive subspecialty care has been associated with nonadherence (2).

IMPROVING ADHERENCE

Adherence intervention studies are rare in the rheumatology literature (see references 2,6,15,20 for reviews). However, extrapolating from this meager database and a wider database in clinical medicine, some suggestions for improving adherence can be made.

Adherence improvement strategies can be broadly classified as educational, organizational, and behavioral (6). *Educational strategies* rely on verbal and written instructions designed to inform patients and their families about the illness, regimen requirements, and the importance of consistent adherence. The strategies are necessary but not sufficient to improve adherence. *Organizational strategies* address the delivery of health care, including increasing accessibility to health care services, tailoring and simplifying regimens, and increasing provider supervision and feedback. Organizational strategies are promising, particularly those that emphasize greater supervision and feedback to patients and their families. *Behavioral strategies* refer to procedures designed to alter specific adherence behaviors by monitoring adherence, providing feedback and positive reinforcement, and soliciting social support from family members. These behavioral strategies, such as teaching patients and their families to monitor, prompt, and reward themselves for adherence, seem to be the most effective (2,5,6). Behavioral strategies are often combined with educational strategies and can be effectively merged with organizational strategies.

Table 3 provides specific recommendations for improving adherence by type of strategy. Clearly, providers can have a substantial impact on patient adherence. However, adherence does not occur in a clinical or social vacuum. Patients may experience personal and family adjustment problems that need to be addressed in addition or prior to addressing adherence problems (9).

Interventions also need to be tailored to individual patients and families based on their unique circumstances, barriers, and resources as revealed by an individualized assessment (25). One approach is to obtain information about adherence barriers through structured interviews or questionnaires. This information can be used to problem-solve with the patient on ways to overcome specific barriers.

Table 3. Adherence improvement strategies for rheumatic disease regimens.

Educational strategies
  Provide clear verbal and written information
  Make sure patients have the skills to carry out regimens
  Re-educate about treatments and adherence as needed
  Emphasize the importance of adherence, especially when patients are asymptomatic or in remission
  Increase education about rheumatic diseases in the community to foster early diagnosis and referral for subspecialty care
Organizational strategies
  Minimize costs of treatments (e.g., use generic medications)
  Reduce complexity of regimens (e.g., reduce number of exercises)
  Reduce adverse effects of regimens (e.g., use coated medications)
  Address barriers to adherence and sources of patient/family dissatisfaction on a continuing basis
  Link families to resources that can reduce financial and service accessibility barriers to adherence
Behavioral strategies
  Use self-management training to encourage autonomy and self-esteem
  Demonstrate and have patients behaviorally rehearse complex regimens such as exercises
  Increase provider and family member supervision of regimens
  Have patients monitor adherence
  Provide social and tangible reinforcers to increase adherence, especially when treatment benefits are delayed

CONCLUSIONS

Rheumatology providers play an important role in assessing and managing adherence problems. Potentially the most important benefit is that patient care and outcomes will be enhanced. Providers will also be able to more accurately evaluate the efficacy and cost-effectiveness of their therapeutic endeavors.

However, as health care providers, we must only ask patients to adhere to regimens that are likely to be efficacious, congruent with the Hippocratic Oath: "I will follow that system of regimen which, according to my ability and judgment, I consider for the benefit of my patients, and abstain from whatever is deleterious and mischievous" (26).

Patients and their families demand and deserve an active role in their health care. The term "compliance" lost favor in the literature because it implied an authoritative approach to health care that required unquestioned obedience by patients to providers' recommendations (6). It was replaced by the term "adherence," which implied a cooperative partnership between patients and providers as reflected in the following perspective by Cassell (27): "Doctors do not treat chronic illnesses. The chronically ill treat themselves with the help of their physicians; the physician is part of the treatment. Patients are in charge of themselves. They determine their food, activity, medications, visits to their doctor—most of the details of their own treatment."

Finally, as rheumatology providers, we may need to entertain the possibility that failing to adhere to prescribed regimens may be strategic, rational, and adaptive in selected cases (28). As noted by Cousins (29), "The history of medicine is replete with accounts of drugs and modes of treatment that were in use for many years before it was recognized that they did more harm than good." Perhaps, when our patients are nonadherent, we need to closely examine what we are recommending and why. This examination may lead us to evaluate the goals and methods for reaching treatment objectives that more appropriately address the day-to-day quality of life for our patients and their families.

REFERENCES

1. Bradley LA. Adherence with treatment regimens among adult rheumatoid arthritis patients: current status and future directions. Arthritis Care Res 1989;2:S33–9.
2. Rapoff MA. Compliance with treatment regimens for pediatric rheumatic diseases. Arthritis Care Res 1989;2:S40–7.
3. Thompson SM, Dahlquist LM, Koenning GM, Bartholomew LK. Brief report: adherence-facilitating behaviors of a multidisciplinary pediatrics rheumatology staff. J Pediatr Psychol 1995;20:291–7.
4. Haynes RB, Taylor DW, Sackett DL. Compliance in health care. Baltimore: The Johns Hopkins University Press; 1979.
5. Meichenbaum D, Turk DC. Facilitating treatment adherence: a practitioner's guidebook. New York: Plenum; 1987.
6. Rapoff MA. Adherence to pediatric medical regimens. New York: Kluwer Academic/Plenum; 1999.
7. Haynes RB. Introduction. In: Taylor DW, Sackett DC, editors. Compliance in health care. Baltimore: The Johns Hopkins University Press; 1979. p. 1–7.
8. Cramer JA. Overview of methods to measure and enhance patient compliance. In: Cramer JA, Spilker B, editors. Patient compliance in medical practice and clinical trials. New York: Raven Press; 1991. p. 3–10.
9. Rapoff MA, Barnard MU. Compliance with pediatric medical regimens. In: Cramer JA, Spilker B, editors. Patient compliance in medical practice and clinical trials. New York: Raven Press; 1991. p. 73–98.
10. Backes JM, Schentag JJ. Partial compliance as a source of variance in pharmacokinetics and therapeutic drug monitoring. In: Cramer JA, Spilker B, editors. Patient compliance in medical practice and clinical trials. New York: Raven Press; 1991. p. 27–36.
11. Bardare M, Cislaghi GU, Mandelli M, Sereni F. Value of monitoring plasma salicylate levels in treating juvenile rheumatoid arthritis: observations in 42 cases. Arch Dis Child 1978;53:381–5.
12. Rapoff MA, Lindsley CB, Christophersen ER. Improving compliance with medical regimens: case study with juvenile rheumatoid arthritis. Arch Phys Med Rehabil 1984;65:267–9.
13. Cramer JA. Microelectronic systems for monitoring and enhancing patient compliance with medication regimens. Drugs 1995;49:321–7.
14. Urquhart J. Role of patient compliance in clinical pharmacokinetics: a review of recent research. Clin Pharmacokinetics 1994;27:202–15.
15. Kroll T, Barlow JH, Shaw K. Treatment adherence in juvenile rheumatoid arthritis: a review. Scand J Rheumatol 1999;28:10–8.
16. Hays RD, Kravitz RL, Mazel RM, Sherbourne CD, DiMatteo MR, Rogers WH, et al. The impact of patient adherence on health outcomes for patients with chronic disease in the medical outcomes study. J Behav Med 1994; 17:347–60.
17. De Klerk E, van der Heijde D, van der Tempel H, van der Linden S. Development of a questionnaire to investigate patient compliance with antirheumatic drug therapy. J Rheumatol 1999;26:2635–41.
18. Kaplan RM, Simon HJ. Compliance in medical care: reconsiderations of self-predictions. Ann Behav Med 1990;12:66–71.
19. Lorish CD, Richards B, Brown S. Missed medication doses in rheumatic arthritis patients: intentional and unintentional reasons. Arthritis Care Res 1989;2:3–9.
20. Brus H, van de Laar M, Taal E, Rasker J, Wiegman O. Compliance in rheumatoid arthritis and the role of formal patient education. Semin Arthritis Rheum 1997;26:702–10.
21. Belcon MC Jr, Haynes RB, Tugwell P. A critical review of compliance studies in rheumatoid arthritis. Arthritis Rheum 1984;27:1227–33.
22. Ruley EJ. Compliance in young hypertensive patients. Pediatr Clin North Am 1978;25:175–82.
23. Smith M. The cost of noncompliance and the capacity of improved compliance to reduce health care expenditures. In: Improving medication compliance: proceedings of a symposium. Washington (DC): The National Pharmaceutical Council; 1985. p. 35–44.
24. Lovell DJ, Giannini EH, Brewer EJ Jr. Time course of response to nonsteroidal antiinflammatory drugs in juvenile rheumatoid arthritis. Arthritis Rheum 1984;27:1433–7.
25. Kreuter MW, Strecher VJ, Glassman B. One size does not fill all: the case for tailoring print materials. Ann Behav Med 1999;21:276–83.
26. The Oath. In: Adams F, trans. The genuine works of Hippocrates. Vol. 2. New York: William Wood; 1886.
27. Cassell EJ. The nature of suffering and the goals of medicine. New York: Oxford University Press; 1991.
28. Deaton AV. Adaptive noncompliance in pediatric asthma: the parent as expert. J Pediatr Psychol 1985;10:1–14.
29. Cousins N. Anatomy of an illness as perceived by the patient. New York: Bantam; 1979.

Additional Recommended Reading

Cramer JA, Spilker B, editors. Patient compliance in medical practice and clinical trials. New York: Raven Press; 1991.

Drotar D, editor. Promoting adherence to medical treatment in childhood chronic illness: concepts, methods, and interventions. Mahwah (NJ): Lawrence Erlbaum Associates; 2000.

Rapoff MA. Adherence to pediatric medical regimens. New York: Kluwer Academic/Plenum; 1999.

Shumaker SA, Schron EB, Ockene JK, McBee WL, editors. The handbook of health behavior change. 2nd ed. New York: Springer; 1998.

Work Disability

SARALYNN H. ALLAIRE, ScD, CRC

Work disability is commonly defined as cessation of work due to the effects of health conditions before the normal age for retirement. Other definitions include increased sick leave use, reduced work hours, diminished opportunity for promotion, and limitation in ability to work.

WORK DISABILITY RATES

Work disability is a substantial problem for persons with rheumatic diseases and a challenge in terms of social and health policy. Arthritis is the leading cause of work loss and the second leading cause of work disability payments (1,2). In 1991–1993 National Health Interview Survey (NHIS) data, 4.83 million persons reported a work limitation that was at least partially related to a musculoskeletal condition (3).

In clinical samples of persons with rheumatoid arthritis (RA), work disability prevalence rates have varied between 26.3% and 50% after one decade of disease (4–6), increasing to 90% with longer disease duration (4). Work disability prevalence among persons with osteoarthritis (OA) was found to be 13.7% in one study, compared with 3.4% among persons without arthritis and 26.3% among those with RA (6). The prevalences of work disability associated with ankylosing spondylitis and systemic lupus erythematosus appear to be lower than for RA (7). However, the economic effect of work disability in these diseases is enhanced by the generally earlier age of onset in comparison with RA. In U.S. and Canadian studies, slightly more than a quarter of subjects with fibromyalgia received some sort of disability pension (8,9).

Adults with a history of juvenile rheumatoid arthritis (JRA) and other childhood rheumatic diseases appear to be employed at rates only slightly less than peers without illness (10). However, many employed individuals (41%) reported having difficulty doing their jobs, and 21% had resigned from a job due to JRA (11).

Other musculoskeletal conditions, such as back injuries and cumulative trauma disorders, are additional causes of work disability. Back injuries are the leading industrial injury, and at least 2.6 million persons are permanently disabled by back pain (12). Rates for both back injury and cumulative trauma disorders continue to increase.

RISK FACTORS

Risk factors that affect work disability can be useful in determining whether and how disability can be reduced. Risk factors exist at both the individual and the societal level.

Two types of individual factors increase the risk for work disability in all adult rheumatic disease samples studied: health status and the characteristics of work, especially job physical demand (4,13–16). For health status, both the presence of comorbidity and more severe disease increase the risk of work disability. A low level of education or nonprofessional/administrative type of work is a significant factor in some studies, probably because each indicates the physical demand level of jobs. Hand use appears to be particularly problematic for persons with RA, especially women (13,17). Working 40 hours or more per week is also a problem for many persons. Job autonomy—an individual's degree of control over work pace and activities—has been a significant factor in some samples, especially those with higher numbers of blue-collar workers (4,13,14). Other risk factors include older age, greater commuting difficulty, less support from family members or co-workers, depression, and desire to be at home. For adults with JRA, continued disease activity, polyarticular JRA, and female gender are associated with unemployment and lower salaries.

Societal risk factors include economic conditions, attitudinal and architectural barriers, types of jobs available, employer practices, and the characteristics of disability pension plans. When the economy is poor, applications to disability pension plans increase, a reflection of the effect of the unemployment rate on work disability. Discrimination, as well as inaccessible work places, transportation systems, and homes, make it difficult for persons with chronic health conditions to work. Employers may view arthritis less negatively than many other conditions. However, because arthritis is common among older persons, age discrimination may produce a combined discriminatory effect. Gender may be an additional basis for discrimination among women. The physical demand and autonomy characteristics of the jobs available in a national economy influence the number of employment opportunities available to those with health impairments.

The disability management practices used by an employer determine in part the job retention rate among employees with health conditions. Early return to work, temporary light duty, and job accommodation programs promote retention, while early retirement through use of disability pension plans promotes work disability.

Work disability rates are higher in countries where disability pension compensation levels are high relative to wages (up to 100%), compared with the U.S., where the Social Security Disability Insurance program compensates at an average of 45% of salary. Only 25% of U.S. employees are covered by additional employer disability pension plans.

EMPLOYMENT OUTLOOK

There have been many changes in the U.S. national economy in recent years and the current status of employment among persons with arthritis is unknown. The low unemployment rate in the late 1990s and increased use of technologies, such as robots and computers, have expanded work opportunities. Other changes, however, such as increased job turnover, may have had negative effects. It remains unclear whether the rate of employment among persons with disabilities has increased since the passage of the Americans With Disabilities Act (ADA).

Much arthritis-related work disability no doubt occurs among workers aged 55 years and older. Premature work cessation among these persons has been of less concern as they were near the normal age for Social Security retirement benefits. This will change due to the increase in the age for receiving full retirement benefits to 67 years; those retiring at age 62 will receive a lower portion of benefits.

The fact that job physical demand and autonomy are important predictors of work disability suggests that this disability could be reduced through job accommodation in some cases. However, few persons with musculoskeletal conditions have received accommodations, and those supplied appear to have been provided too late to make a difference (18). The reasonable accommodation provision of the ADA may be its chief accomplishment, but few persons with rheumatic diseases are using the ADA at work (19).

ASSESSMENT

Assessment should identify the presence of immediate problems; priority is then given to persons who are currently on sick leave or who indicate that they cannot do their job. Tools are available to help identify patients at greater risk for work disability. These include the Work Limitations Questionnaire (20) and the Work Instability Scale (21), which was developed to assess the need for workplace modifications among employed persons with RA. Adults without immediate employment problems and adolescents need guidance to help them factor in the long-term impact of their disease on employment and to consider appropriate jobs or careers.

The individual's health status should be evaluated, including frequency of acute illness episodes, degree of symptom control, functional status, and scheduling of any surgery. The short- and long-term suitability of the current job can then be examined. Job assessment topics should include the following: 1) difficulty getting to and from work, beginning within the patient's home; 2) physical barriers encountered at the worksite; 3) job physical demand and autonomy, including the number of work hours; 4) relationship of the patient with the employer, including the employer's attitude toward disability; 5) relationships with co-workers; and 6) employer and co-worker awareness of the patient's condition. If employment problems are likely, opportunity for change with the current employer should be evaluated, including factors such as the employee's length of tenure, availability of other jobs, and any job training or educational benefits. Previous work history, educational background, specialized job training, and interests should also be assessed.

It is also essential to evaluate family support and financial need. The beliefs of family members about the ability of the patient to work should be explored. Balancing employment with activities outside of work, such as self-care activities, household work, and recreation, is likely to be an issue for many persons with rheumatic diseases. Assessment should include success in accomplishing these activities as well as the willingness and availability of family members to help or use of paid services.

Currently unemployed patients may have a need or desire for employment. In such cases, evaluation should cover stability of the rheumatic condition, work history to ascertain earning potential, types of benefits received, and possible alternative sources of health insurance.

Areas of assessment for children and adolescents include histories of helping at home and inclusion in educational, social, and recreational activities. Other areas for assessment include summer and after-school work or volunteer experiences, parental beliefs about the child's ability to work, and the child's interests and academic achievement.

INTERVENTION

The overall approach to intervention is to facilitate patient decision-making. This can be accomplished by initiating discussion about actual or potential interactions between the person's rheumatic disease and employment, as well as by active listening, examination of alternatives, and referral for vocational services. To avoid misunderstandings, any communication with employers should be conducted through the patient.

The usual goal is to preserve or facilitate employment, as employment provides important financial, psychological, and other benefits. Goal setting needs to be individualized to each individual's circumstances, however, as employment is not possible or desirable for all. For employed patients, intervening at the primary prevention level is ideal. Unfortunately the potential for work disability often is not addressed until job loss is imminent and intervention is more difficult, if not too late. Chances for return to work diminish as time away from work lengthens.

Primary Prevention for Future Work Disability

Because individuals without current employment difficulties may encounter problems in the future, actions taken to reduce risk of job loss may be preventive. The first step is to promote awareness of potential problems. Persons with energy limitations can be counseled about reducing demands at work, in commuting, and in completing activities outside of work. To some extent this means managing demands more efficiently, although reducing the number of activities in at least some spheres may also be required.

If the individual's job is physically demanding, exploration of future job change options should be initiated. Available resources, including the person's employer, should be exploited early in the disease course when patients are more likely to be employable. Career counseling and vocational testing services of the state–federal vocational rehabilitation program, which exists in all states, should be available at no cost to many persons with rheumatic diseases (Table 1). Private vocational counseling is another alternative. Administrative and professional jobs often are characterized by low physical demand and high autonomy and therefore meet the needs of persons with rheumatic diseases. These positions may be more stressful, but as circumstances dictate, additional training or education needed to obtain such positions is advisable.

Pre-vocational experiences are extremely important for children and adolescents with rheumatic diseases. Parents may need help in obtaining any assistive technology needed for the child to do household chores and other activities. The activities a child enjoys can provide a preliminary guide to future voca-

Table 1. Primary resources for vocational counseling and rehabilitation.

Government-sponsored vocational rehabilitation services
  Although differences in administration of the state-federal vocational rehabilitation program exist among the states, most persons with rheumatic diseases
    should be eligible for the following services:
    Vocational testing
    Vocational guidance and counseling
    Skill and academic training
    Job support services
    Job placement assistance
    Job accommodation assessment and provision
    Restoration services (e.g., physical therapy, vehicle and home modifications)
One-Stop career centers
  One-Stop centers bring together employment and training services for all people, not just those with health impairments, into one place. The location of the
    nearest center (not necessarily called a One-Stop center) can be obtained from the website www.ttrc.dolecta.gov/ETA or from the U.S. Department of
    Labor at (202) 291-0316 (voice).
Independent living centers
  These centers provide advocacy services and services that help persons with disabilities live on their own.
Job accommodations
  The Job Accommodation Network (JAN) is a toll-free consulting service that provides information about job accommodations and the employability of per-
    sons with disabilities; 1-800-232-9675 V/TDD; http://janweb.icdi.wvu.edu/; jan@jan.icdi/wvu.edu
  Americans with Disabilities Act (ADA) Disability and Business Technical Assistance Centers (DBTACS) are regional centers that provide information,
    training, and technical assistance. The DBTACS can make referrals to local sources of expertise in reasonable accommodation; 1-800-949-4232 V/TTY.
  The state-federal vocation rehabilitation program is available in each state; evaluation for and purchase of assistive technology can be provided to eligible
    persons.
  Many states have accommodation-related service projects funded through the Assistive Technology Act of 1998; www.matp.org/f_geninfo.html
  The RESNA (Rehabilitation Engineering and Assistive Technology Society of North America) Technical Assistance Project can refer individuals to projects
    in all states and US territories that offer technical assistance on technology-related services for individuals with disabilities; services may include infor-
    mation and referral centers to help determine what devices may assist a person and centers where a person can try out devices and equipment, assistance
    in obtaining funding and equipment exchange programs; (703) 524-6686 (voice); (703) 524-6639 (TT); www.resna.org
  Some Easter Seals service sites have assistive technology specialists who can provide services related to job accommodation including evaluation, some-
    times at the workplace; www.easter-seals.org
Information
  The Arthritis Foundation has excellent pamphlets about employment challenges available for adults and teenagers, and about Social Security benefits;
    1-800-283-7800
  The National Multiple Sclerosis Society publishes a booklet containing information about how to request a job accommodation entitled "The Win-Win Ap-
    proach to Reasonable Accommodations: Enhancing Productivity on Your Job"; it is available online at www.nmss.org/booklets/win.html
  The US Equal Employment Opportunity Commission has information available about employment aspects of the Americans With Disabilities Act; 1801 L
    Street, NW, Washington, DC 20507

tional interests. The child's inclusion in academic, social, and recreational activities needs to be facilitated to build vocational experience and social skills.

Assistance can be given to adolescents in obtaining summer and after-school work or volunteer experiences. At age 15 (one year prior to eligibility), the teen can be referred to the state–federal vocational rehabilitation program for vocational counseling, transitional services, and, depending on financial criteria, funding of college or other vocational education or training. Early referral is crucial, as eligibility can take time to establish and wait lists may exist. Parents may need education regarding their child's abilities, the value of employment, and possible problems or difficulties that may exist. Career choices that seem unrealistic can be managed by exploring the appeal of the chosen field, encouraging the teen to seek volunteer experience, and helping the teen interview people currently working in the field. Positive attitudes on the part of professionals and parents and attempts to facilitate the child's choice are more successful than ready dismissal.

Secondary Prevention for Current Work Disability

Employed persons currently experiencing work problems need immediate attention to prevent or delay job loss. Nearly all patients with rheumatic diseases have some difficulty with job access or performing job functions, and greater levels of these difficulties are associated with lower job satisfaction (22).

The individual's employer is the first resource, but if the employer is unaware of the person's condition, the pros and cons of providing such information must be weighed. Employees are often surprised at the positive reaction of employers to their health condition, but the possibility of discrimination exists. Repercussions, such as not being considered for promotions, can occur. More positive reactions are ensured if the employee can present ways of managing disease effects that maintain productivity.

Retaining the individual's current job is often the best option. Job accommodation may be needed, but in some cases changes in activities that are not related to work are sufficient, especially if the main problem is fatigue. Ways of reducing energy used in commuting can be sought, such as obtaining a handicapped license plate or placard or accessing special transportation. Working at home, perhaps just one day per week, may be an option for some jobs. Family meetings can result in better management of household work responsibilities. Use of paid household work services can be encouraged.

Job accommodation or modification may be required to enable the person to work more easily and productively. Such accommodations may include job restructuring, use of assistive devices, training for new job duties, provision of a personal assistant, modification of the work environment, and job reassignment. Little is known about what specific kinds of accommodations benefit persons with rheumatic diseases, although working from home, changing job duties, and changing hours have been reported by women with RA or fibromyalgia

(17,23). Rheumatic diseases, RA in particular, often lead to the need for increased time to complete activities of daily living and self-care (24). Energy-saving accommodations therefore may be especially valuable.

Many persons with disabilities are not familiar with the wide range of possible accommodations. Primary resources include the Job Accommodation Network and the state–federal vocational rehabilitation program (Table 1). Employers are often concerned about the cost of accommodations; however, the overwhelming majority of accommodations are inexpensive, and the ADA requires only that an accommodation be adequate to accomplish the job. Also, there are 3 tax incentive programs to help employers cover accommodation costs. If an expensive accommodation is needed, options include cost sharing with the employer, or, in some cases, funding by the state–federal vocational rehabilitation program.

Good management of paid vacation time, accumulated sick leave, and short-term sick leave benefits, when available, can help the individual susceptible to disease flares continue working. A few days of rest when a flare is beginning or during periods of stress can sometimes avert longer periods of disability. The Family Medical Leave Act can be utilized by covered employees to obtain medical leave. For persons currently on sick leave, inquiries should be made about early return-to-work, transitional work, and/or job accommodation programs.

When keeping a current job is no longer possible, the next best option is often a job change with the same employer. A good work history is an asset, and persons with RA who were able to change their jobs within the same employer had a higher job retention rate than those who changed employers (4). Suitable jobs include those with low physical demand, high autonomy, and allowance for periodic change in position, and those that do not involve repetitive physical tasks. Jobs involving communication skills and/or thought processes are good choices. Reduction in salary should be avoided if at all possible, but if unavoidable, the fact that the income is likely to be higher than that from disability programs should be considered. Some employers offer job-training opportunities that can lead to better future jobs. The ADA requires that employees with disabilities be considered for vacant positions for which they are prepared.

When continuing employment with the individual's current employer is not possible or desirable, the remaining employment option is change of employers, possibly including change of job type or career. Referral for government-sponsored or private vocational rehabilitation services should be considered, because physical restoration and vocational training services have been linked to employment gain (25). If the individual prefers, or is minimally impaired, services provided through the One Stop career center program (Table 1) may be adequate. These centers integrate various job programs and are open to all U.S. residents. If disability-related services are required, a referral is made to the state-federal vocational rehabilitation program.

Working at home avoids the energy expenditure of commuting, but it can be socially isolating. Starting a business is appealing to many people, but while this would meet job autonomy needs, the time requirements are often great.

Tertiary Prevention for Return to Work

It can be difficult for persons who have not been employed for an extended period to return to work, but it is possible. Among persons with RA, 10% of those who left the work force returned to work at a later time (4). Trial return-to-work programs are available to persons receiving either Social Security Disability Insurance (SSDI) or Supplemental Security Insurance (SSI) income. The Ticket to Work and Work Incentives Improvement Act of 1999 is the most significant of these, consisting of vouchers to pay for employment, vocational rehabilitation, or other services needed to help the person return to work. Health insurance is an issue for persons interested in returning to work; the Work Incentives provisions of the 1999 act provide for Medicare coverage for up to 6.5 years. Some states may also elect to extend Medicaid coverage to disabled workers who return to work. Persons who return to work and then are forced to stop working again due to impairments are eligible for benefit reinstatement. Persons who are interested in returning to work should be advised to contact their state–federal vocational rehabilitation program for employability evaluation, an independent living center for advocacy services, and their local Social Security office for detailed information about programs.

Stopping Work

Work cessation may be the best, or only, option for some. Persons with severe RA may find that joint symptoms and functional status improve somewhat following withdrawal from work (14). Individuals with health problems that require frequent hospitalization may find that their productivity is lowered by job interruptions. The family and financial circumstances of some patients require and permit a family care rather than employment role. Finally, older workers with long disease duration may find it especially difficult to work, because of both their physical condition and discrimination against older, disabled workers.

For persons who are considering leaving the work force, discussion can focus initially on the benefits of working versus not working. Employment almost always provides greater financial return and, for younger persons, greater future financial security. Other advantages include personal achievement, group health insurance coverage and other employee benefits, and opportunity for socialization. On the other hand, stopping work may provide health advantages, including additional time for self care. Volunteer activities can provide fulfillment.

Individuals under the age of 65 who are unable to engage in substantial gainful activity (a monetary amount that changes annually) because of an impairment expected to last at least 12 months or result in death, and who have contributed sufficiently to Social Security, are eligible to apply for SSDI. Those who have not contributed, including children, but who meet financial need criteria are eligible to apply for SSI. Approval is based primarily on medical disease criteria, such as a positive rheumatoid factor test and x-rays showing joint damage. When such criteria do not exist, approval is based on residual functional capacity and the person's age, education, and prior work experience. For children, approval is based on an individualized functional assessment.

Persons with specific test results are more likely to obtain initial approval. Pain with positive examination findings, such as in fibromyalgia, is an acceptable criterion, but difficulty in obtaining approval on the first review can be anticipated. Several levels of appeal are available, and pursuit of appeal is often fruitful. Persons receiving SSDI or SSI are subject to continuing disability reviews; the timing of reviews (every 6 months to 7 years) depends on the recipient's age and the nature and severity of impairment. Those receiving SSDI are eligible for Medicare benefits after 2 years, while those receiving SSI are immediately eligible for Medicaid. Recipients of SSDI can earn a very limited amount of income from employment without losing benefits.

REFERENCES

1. Yelin E. Arthritis: the cumulative impact of a common chronic condition. Arthritis Rheum 1992;35:489–97.
2. US Department of Health and Human Services. Soc Secur Annu Stat Suppl. Washington (DC): Social Security Administration; 1991.
3. Yelin E, Callahan L, the National Arthritis Data Work Group. The economic cost and social and psychological impact of musculoskeletal conditions. Arthritis Rheum 1995;38:1351–62.
4. Yelin E, Henke C, Epstein W. The work dynamics of the person with rheumatoid arthritis. Arthritis Rheum 1987;30:507–12.
5. Wolfe F, Hawley DJ. The long term outcomes of rheumatoid arthritis work disability: a prospective 18-year study of 823 patients. J Rheumatol 1998;25:2108–17.
6. Gabriel SE, Crowson CS, Campion ME, O'Fallon WM: Indirect and nonmedical costs among people with rheumatoid arthritis and osteoarthritis compared with nonarthritic controls. J Rheumatol 1997;24:43–8.
7. Mau W, Listing J, Zeidler H, Zink A. Standardized employment rates in chronic inflammatory rheumatic diseases [abstract]. Arthritis Rheum 2000;43 Suppl 9:S163.
8. Wolfe F, Anderson J, Harkness D, Bennett RM, Caro XJ, Goldenberg DL, et al: Work and disability status of persons with fibromyalgia. J Rheumatol 1997;24:1171–8.
9. White KP, Speechley M, Harth M, Ostbye T. Comparing self-reported function and work disability in 100 community cases of fibromyalgia syndrome versus controls in London, Ontario: The London Fibromyalgia Epidemiology Study. Arthritis Rheum 1999;42:76–83.
10. Peterson LS, Mason T, Nelson AM, O'Fallon WM, Gabriel SE. Psychosocial outcomes and health status of adults who have had juvenile rheumatoid arthritis: a controlled, population-based study. Arthritis Rheum 1997;40:2235–40.
11. Muney K, Hanson V, Mukamel M, Boone D. Health status and achievement in adult life of patients diagnosed with juvenile rheumatoid arthritis [abstract]. Arthritis Rheum 1987;30 Suppl 4:S200.
12. Chronic back pain. Washington (DC): National Institute on Disability and Rehabilitation Research; 1993. Rehab Brief, Vol. 15 No. 7.
13. Reisine S, McQuillan J, Fifield J. Predictors of work disability in rheumatoid arthritis patients: a five-year followup. Arthritis Rheum 1995;38:1630–7.
14. Allaire SH, Anderson JJ, Meenan RF. Reducing work disability associated with rheumatoid arthritis: identification of additional risk factors and persons likely to benefit from intervention. Arthritis Care Res 1996;9:349–57.
15. Gran JT, Skomsvoll JF. The outcome of ankylosing spondylitis: a study of 100 patients. Br J Rheumatol 1997;24:1171–8.
16. Stein H, Walters K, Dillon A, Schulzer M. Systemic lupus erythematosus—a medical and social profile. J Rheumatol 1986;13:570–6.
17. Mancuso CA, Paget SA, Charlson ME. Adaptations made by rheumatoid arthritis patients to continue working: a pilot study of workplace challenges and successful adaptations. Arthritis Care Res 2000;13:89–99.
18. Yelin E, Sonneborn D, Trupin L. The prevalence and impact of accommodations on the employment of persons 51–61 years of age with musculoskeletal conditions. Arthritis Care Res 2000;13:168–76.
19. Allaire SH, Evans SR, LaValley MP, Merrigan DM. Use of the Americans With Disabilities Act by persons with rheumatic diseases and factors associated with use. Arthritis Care Res 2001;45:174–82.
20. Massarotti E, Reed J, Wester L, Burke T, Lerner D. Reliability and validity of the Work Limitations Questionnaire for patients with osteoarthritis [abstract]. Arthritis Rheum 2000;43 Suppl 9:S163.
21. Gilworth G, Chamberlain MA, Harvey A, Leeds AT. Reducing work disability in rheumatoid arthritis—development of a work instability scale [abstract]. Arthritis Rheum 2000;43 Suppl 9:S164.
22. Allaire SH, Li W, LaValley MP. Work problems reported by employed persons with rheumatic diseases and their association with work satisfaction [abstract]. Arthritis Rheum 2000;43 Suppl 9:S128.
23. Henriksson C, Liedberg G. Factors of importance for work disability in women with fibromyalgia. J Rheumatol 2000;27:1271–6.
24. Kuper IH, Prevoo M, van Leeuwen MA, van Riel P, Lolkema WF, Postma DS, et al. Disease associated time consumption in early rheumatoid arthritis. J Rheumatol 2000;27:1183–9.
25. Straaton KV, Harvey M, Maisiak R. Factors associated with successful vocational rehabilitation in persons with arthritis. Arthritis Rheum 1992;35:503–10.

Additional Recommended Reading

Allaire SH, Partridge AJ, Andrews HF, Liang MH. Management of work disability. Arthritis Rheum 1993;36:1663–70.

Cooper C. Occupational activity and the risk of osteoarthritis. J Rheumatol Suppl 1995;43:10–2.

Greenwald S, Gerber L. The Americans With Disabilities Act. Bull Rheum Dis 1992;41:5–7.

Hernandez B, Keys C, Balcazar F. Employer attitudes toward workers with disabilities and their ADA employment rights: a literature review. J Rehabil 2000;66:4–16.

Kaye HS. Is the status of people with disabilities improving? Washington (DC): US Department of Education, National Institute on Disability and Rehabilitation Research; 1998. Disabilities Statistics Abstract No. 21.

Reisine S, Fifield J. Expanding the definition of disability: implications for planning, policy, and research. Milbank Q 1992;70:491–508.

Straaton KV, Maisiak R, Wrigley M, Fine PR. Musculoskeletal disability, employment and rehabilitation. J Rheumatol 1995;22:505–13.

White PH, Shear ES. Transition/job readiness for adolescents with juvenile arthritis and other chronic illness. J Rheumatol Suppl 1992;33:23–7.

Wolfe F, Ross K, Anderson J, Russell IJ, Hebert L. The prevalence and characteristics of fibromyalgia in the general population. Arthritis Rheum 1995;38:19–28.

Yelin EH. Musculoskeletal conditions and employment. Arthritis Care Res 1995;8:311–9.

SECTION E: CLINICIAN RESOURCES

CHAPTER

43

Clinical Care and the World Wide Web

LAURA RAY, MA, MLS

The Internet is used for communication and education, as well as practice and marketing. Yet, as with all technological tools, it is wise to remember that philosophy and objectives should drive the selection and use of Internet-based technology. The use of this technology in turn provides opportunity for the review and redefinition of philosophy and objectives. Internet-based technology can only be of true value when it assists and enhances objectives.

This chapter assumes the reader has a basic understanding of the structure of the Internet and World Wide Web; how they are accessed; how to use web browsers (i.e., software such as Netscape Navigator, used to access web sites); as well as hypertext and hypermedia links (i.e., annotated documents linked to other documents, graphics, images, or sounds). I will cover searching for information on the web, evaluating web sites and search services, and creating web sites. Numerous web site URLs (Uniform Resource Locators—web "addresses") are provided. Please note that although these URLs are accurate at the time of writing, they may—as any web user knows—change in the future. Searching the medical literature, an important component of evidence-based medical practice, will not be covered in terms of the exact steps to produce a series of related articles. Nevertheless, good basic research practices are described and discussed. Understanding how to use the web is important in terms of getting to medical literature and related topics. This chapter recognizes and addresses the many ways that the web may be used in clinical practice and for clinical practitioners.

INFORMATION SEARCHING AND THE WORLD WIDE WEB

Varying estimates on the size of the web put it at 320 million to 1 billion pages (1). The vast majority of the web is publicly accessible, but a significant minority of "private" sites require fees or authorization to access. Also, despite the obvious enormity of this information bank, "everything" is not on the web. Vast resources of nonelectronic information continue to exist in libraries and other collections. Nonelectronic information searching skills should not be abandoned, and possessing such skills will assist one to develop electronic information searching skills.

Electronic information has obvious information storage, retrieval, and manipulation benefits. Web-based electronic information brings the additional benefits of hypertext and hyper-media annotations, as well as a host of "value-added" services. Web-based mediums are increasingly being used for library catalogs and commercial databases. For access to electronic information not included in library and commercial information banks, one must also know how to effectively and efficiently search the web.

Web Search Directories

The leading web search services claim to index 35 million to over 1 billion pages. Web search services may be divided into *search directories* and *search engines*. With the explosive growth of the web over the last decade, search directories are gaining importance as a way of finding accurate and reliable information. Unlike search engines, search directories use human beings to compile lists of selected web sites classified by subject. Rather than all pages of a site, only the main page is listed. In addition, capitalizing upon their human indexing, search directories provide annotations and evaluations of web sites. Probably the best known search directory is Yahoo (http://www.yahoo.com), which currently includes 1.5-1.8 million web sites. Recently, Open Directory Project (http://dmoz.org) has gained prominence as the search directory of choice, currently including 2.2 million web sites (2,3). Virtually every leading search engine includes Open Directory among its services. Other medicine-related search directories are: Health A to Z: The Search Engine for Health and Medicine (http://www.healthatoz.com), MedExplorer: Health/Medical Internet Search Engine (http://www.medexplorer.com), Medical World Search (http://www.mwsearch.com), and the "Health and Medicine" section of Resource Discovery Network (http://www.rdn.ac.uk). For a list of web sites that provide MEDLINE searching, consult the "Internet MEDLINE Comparison Table" at Medical Matrix (http://www.medmatrix.org).

Web Search Engines

Web search engines use software called "spiders" (or "robots" or "crawlers") to request data from Gopher, FTP (File Transfer Protocol), and HTTP (HyperText Transmission Protocol) servers. FTP allows simple file transfer via the Internet. Gopher allows access to files and data via simple menus. HTTP allows access to web sites. When one uses a search engine, only the information indexed and stored by that search engine is searched. Requests may be subject-specific (seeking data with

Table 1. Key points to consider when evaluating a web site.

History, including creator, authority, affiliation, partners, and sponsor
Purpose or philosophy
Content
Audience, relevance, and uniqueness
Scope, context, and coverage, as well as size and growth rate
Selection criteria, critical thinking, objectivity, and censorship
Accuracy and documentation
Writing quality
Design and presentation format
Stability, consistency, continuity, and maintenance
Currency or updating—frequency and scope
Interface—clarity and speed
Accessibility
Navigation, site index, and searchability
Connectivity or links to other sites
Help information and customer support
Value-to-cost ratio, usefulness, and comparability

Table 2. Key points to consider when evaluating a web search service.

Selection criteria or human involvement in indexing, reviewing, and
    screening
Interface, including clarity, speed, and basic/advanced search capability
Search tips and help information
Boolean logic connectors (e.g., and, or, not)
Proximity searching (e.g., near, adj)
Phrase searching
Case and punctuation sensitivity
Truncation capability
"Field" searching (i.e., limiting a search to a particular portion of a web
    site)
"Stop words" (e.g., to, be)
Results display, including ranking methods and retrieval limitations
Cost or fee

particular keywords) or site-specific (seeking data in particular locations). Once data is located, the software indexes and stores the information it has found. Both the main page and additional pages of a site are indexed. Web pages matching search criteria are retrieved and ranked according to relevancy. When one uses a search directory, there is a reasonable expectation that listed web sites meet academic, professional, or cultural criteria and standards. However, a search engine simply lists web pages that match search criteria.

EVALUATING WEB SITES

Even if one conducts a "good" search and retrieves a manageable list of web pages that include desired information, how can one evaluate a web site? Web sites are relatively easy to create, and peer review is still developing in this area. Table 1 lists some key points to consider when evaluating a web site. Practice publications and current awareness services are increasingly providing reviews of web sites and should be included in one's regular literature review routine. Two web-based review services are Netsurfer Digest (http://www.netsurf.com/nsd) and The Scout Report (http://scout.cs.wisc.edu/report).

EVALUATING WEB SEARCH SERVICES

There are currently thousands of search services on the web, but approximately 30 are recognized as the leaders. Their search speed is nearly equivalent, but their search results can differ widely. Each can cover different, occasionally overlapping, parts of the web—thoroughness means searching with multiple services. Search results routinely include duplicate or invalid URLs. "Popular" sites tend to get indexed more, sites with frames or image maps often have trouble getting indexed, and it can take months for a new site to be indexed. Search services can be affected by partnership constraints and often include distracting advertisements. Most disturbing is the not-uncommon practice of charging for preferential listings in search results. Table 2 lists some key points to consider when evaluating a web search service. Two web-based search service review services are Search Engine Watch (http://www.search-enginewatch.com) and Search Engine Showdown (http://www.searchengineshowdown.com).

SEARCH PRINCIPLES

Research is very personal. Notwithstanding good basic search principles, one finds success and comfort in personally developed search practices. It is always a good idea to physically write down, in a sentence or paragraph, exactly what one is seeking. Note key words and think of synonyms for them. Finally, compose or construct the search statement. This is done in a way that is similar to the combination of concepts or values in deductive logic or algebra. Be as specific as possible at the outset, then broaden the search as needed. A narrow search will result in high relevance and low retrieval, while a broad search will result in lower relevance and higher retrieval.

With web searching, one should consider browsing search directories before using a search engine. Try to have the patience and discipline to use a variety of search directories and engines, as well as new search services as they are created. Eventually most people gravitate to one or two search services of personal choice. Search services operate in very similar manners. Check the service's search tips and help information for specifics on how the service operates.

Keep searches simple; complex searches often lead to the retrieval of much irrelevant information. Be specific, using general terms only when necessary. Enter the most important concepts first. Boolean connectors can be used on many search services, and are usually indicated with upper case text. In front of terms, one generally uses + to indicate "and" (or include this term, even if it is a "stop word") and − to indicate "not" (or exclude this term). If available, proximity searching (i.e., using "near" or "adj" connectors) is particularly good for full-text searching. The truncation symbol is usually *. Phrase searching can be very effective, and phrases are usually enclosed in quotation marks. If available, "field" searching is best when one limits the search to a web site's title and URL. Many search services allow you to limit or refine by searching within a set of search results. If the first 30 hits of a set of search results are not on point, change the search statement and/or consider using a different search service.

Once search results are obtained, evaluate each retrieved web page. If the retrieved page is not the home page of the site, go to the home page to more easily evaluate the site. The home page should reveal the site's purpose, scope of services and information, as well as navigation methods and help information. If available, a site index is particularly helpful for evaluation. Once a web site is identified as appropriate and valuable, "bookmark" that site. Maintaining a well-organized list of

Table 3. Comparisons of 5 leading search engines.

	AltaVista	HotBot	Excite	Google	Northern Light
Creator/ producer	Started in 1995 by Digital Equipment Corp.; now owned by CMGI, which is part of Lycos	Started in 1996 by Inktomi Corp.; now owned by Wired Digital, Inc., which is part of Lycos	Started in 1995 by Excite, Inc.; recently joined @Home Network to form Excite @Home	Started in 1999 by Google, Inc.	Started in 1997 by Northern Light Technology, LLC
Components and features	Engine; directory/index; membership benefits; partner services; news, maps, people/company finder, job listings, etc.	Engine; directory/index; partner services; news, maps, people/company finder, job listings, etc. [No longer signing up members.]	Engine; directory/index; membership benefits; partner services; news, company finder, job listings, etc.	Engine; directory/index; job information	Engine; directory/index; "Special Collection" (25 million documents from 7,000 publications); membership benefits; news, etc.
Coverage	550 million web pages; RemarQ newsgroups; multimedia files	110 million web pages; Usenet newsgroups; multimedia files	250 million web pages; Usenet newsgroups; Usenet classifieds	705 million web pages; 640 million web URLs (See "Other Notes")	350 million web pages; "Special Collection"
General search features	Regular and advanced searching; media/topic searching; "Family Filter"	Simple and advanced searching; image, video, and MP3 searching	Regular and advanced searching; news, photo, MP3, and product searching	Regular searching; "Safe Search"	Regular and "Power" searching; "Business" and "Investext" searching; "Family-Friendly Resources"
Special search features	Boolean *and, or, not*; proximity *near*; phrase; date; upper/lower case; truncation; parentheses; fields; search refinement; help information	Boolean *and, or, not*; phrase; date; upper/lower case; truncation; parentheses; stop words; fields; search refinement; help information	Boolean *and, or, not*; phrase; truncation; parentheses; search refinement; help information	Boolean *and, or*; boolean-type *not*; phrase; truncation; parentheses; stop words; search refinement; help information	Boolean *and, or, not*; phrase; date; truncation; parentheses; fields; search refinement; help information
Languages	25	11	14	35	5
Other notes	In 1999, started policy of "paid placement" in search result list—a web site can purchase a word, thereby having its site appear at the top of a search result list (5).	Search results may also indicate "Top 10 Site Results"—the 10 "most popular" sites.	Excite@Home provides 24-hour access to "advanced personalized services."	Claims to index over 1 billion pages because of indexing 705 million web pages and 640 million URLs (6).	Also organizes search results in "Custom Folders" (i.e., subject classification) Can purchase documents online. Can pay for "alert" (i.e., current awareness) service.
Sample search results*	248 hits	"more than 600" hits	192 hits (cannot date restrict)	491 hits (cannot date restrict)	425 hits (in 292 sources)

* Number of hits resulting from a search seeking information on fibromyalgia patient education programs for adult women.

bookmarks, or favorite web sites, is analogous to creating a personal search directory. Rather than repeatedly going through the entire search and evaluation process, you can return to web sites that have helped in the past.

Excellent current news about, and comparison reviews of, web search services are published in the literature on a regular basis (4). Table 3 notes key points on 5 of the leading search engines, primarily gleaned from their individual web sites: Alta Vista (http://www.altavista.com), HotBot (http://www.hotbot.com), Excite Search (http:www.excite.com), Google (http://www.google.com), and Northern Light (http://www.northernlight.com). Also listed are numbers of hits resulting from a search seeking information on fibromyalgia patient education programs for adult women. The search statement (fibromyalgia AND "patient education" AND women AND adult) was limited to English language in all 5 engines, as well as limited to 1998-present in AltaVista, HotBot, and Northern Light.

In addition to singular search engines, there are metasearch (or "megasearch," "panoramic," or "parallel") search engines. A metasearch engine sends a search statement to several search services, receives the results, deletes duplicates, and displays the results in a single list. Often you can specify the singular services for the metasearch service to use. Searching with one service, rather than connecting to several different search services, can save time and reduce

frustration. However, metasearching is generally best for simple questions. Each singular search service has some unique search methods and options. Metasearch services may not be able to use all the available options of each search service it covers, and a search service may not recognize all options used in a metasearch. For example, you can include boolean operators in a metasearch statement, but the operators will not be applied within a search service that does not support them. One medical metasearch service, Stanford University's MedBot (http://www-med.stanford.edu/medworld/medbot) allows you to select up to 4 indices to search at the same time from a list of 5 directories, 8 search engines, 4 medical index sites, 5 medical education and learning sites, 3 medical news sites, and 2 medical image sites. Table 4 notes key points on 3 other metasearch services: Ixquick (http://www.ixquick.com), QueryServer (http://www.queryserver.com), and Vivisimo (http://vivisimo.com).

One of the emerging search software programs that may have great impact upon the web is the "Intelligent Agent" or "Bot." This software is said to dig through data, adding features such as analysis, filtering, integration, and rapid presentation of information. Much more research and development is needed, but it is anticipated that intelligent agents will be used for routine and repetitive searches, organizing disparate information, and creating new forms of interactivity and informa-

Table 4. Comparison of 3 leading metasearch services.

	Producer	Components	Features
Ixquick	Ixquick.com, Inc.	More than 10 search engines and several directories	"Stars" results ranked high by search engines, 13 languages
Query Server	Open Text Corp.	10 search engines as well as 10 news, 12 medical, 8 financial, and 13 U.S. government sites	Allows results to be "clustered" by content, site, or both content and site
Vivisimo	Vivisimo, Inc.	More than 8 search engines, Open Directory and Yahoo, as well as numerous news, government, and business sites	Spontaneously "clusters" results—classification not predetermined; ranks clusters

tion processing (7). One intelligent agent available for free use is Intelliseek's (http://www.intelliseek.com) "BullsEye" version 2. Consult the BotSpot (http://botspot.com) for additional information on Bots.

PURPOSES FOR WEB SITES

When determining methodologies for achieving an objective, the web may be viewed as one information medium to be considered along with print, audiovisual, and other electronic information media. Beyond information searching objectives, the web provides a vast new medium for information storage, retrieval, and manipulation objectives. Hypertext and hypermedia annotations are bringing dramatic change and capabilities to traditional presentation of electronic information. Virtually every type of organization is using the web for communication, service, operations, practice, marketing, and education. A good web site can help an organization make announcements (e.g., invite participation in a clinical study), provide a forum via discussion lists or chat rooms, augment customer/client service, have a consistent and positive image, identify and describe customers/clients and what those customers/clients want, and target selected groups and generate new business.

A web site can also help organize information for a vast array of practical operations. For example, web-based electronic patient records can allow the practitioner to more easily consult with colleagues and educate the patient at the point of care (8). *Telemedicine* is a rapidly developing field encompassing information provision in support of medical decision-making, as well as practicing medicine at a distance (9). Consult the Telemedicine Information Exchange (http://tie.telemed.org) for additional information.

Perhaps the most exciting developments associated with the web involve education. The production of web-based educational programs can be incredibly time-consuming and demand a significant commitment of development personnel and money. However, the benefits are obvious—a multimedia program through which individual users can proceed as their intellect, interest, and time allow. In addition, web-based educational programs are accepted as "distance learning" by government and corporate leaders, who view such learning as a panacea for a variety of educational and networking logistic problems.

Multimedia education and training has long been recognized as having higher rates of retention and recall in both individual self-study and group settings. The web allows complex information to be conveyed in a structured and universal format virtually anywhere in the world. After successful development, web-based educational programming has relatively low costs with substantial student/customer benefits, including conve-

nience, low cost, and more interesting multimedia and interactive formats. People still like to travel to meetings, but people will also attend a meeting that comes to them.

SERVERS AND HOSTING SERVICES

Good planning is essential for an individual or organization seeking to establish a presence on the web. One of the first questions to be addressed is on what server will the web site be placed? If you simply want to make available lots of HTML (HyperText Markup Language—the continuously evolving standard language of web sites) files, putting them on an existing FTP or Gopher server might be fine. However, data access is slower on FTP/Gopher servers, and web servers have higher capabilities. The real issue is whether to set up your own web server or lease space from an Internet service provider (ISP) or web hosting service (WHS). Beyond the large commercial ISPs, such as America Online, virtually every major metropolitan area telephone book lists ISPs and WHSs. However, not all ISPs provide web hosting services.

Web servers can be run on almost any computer, and server software is available for almost any operating system or platform (10). (For more information, consult Apache Server Project [http://httpd.apache.org] or WebSTAR [http://www.webstar.com] for Mac). In addition to the server, you will need a router (to ensure proper delivery of data), Channel Service Unit/Data Service Unit (CSU/DSU—used to convert phone signals to data understandable by the router), and high-speed leased line connection. Leased lines range from 56 kbps (56 kilobits or 56,000 bits per second; 56K line) to 45 mbps (45 megabits or 45,000,000 bits per second; T3 line).

The advantages of setting up a server are that you only need an ISP to provide a connection to the Internet, usually $1000-$3000 to install and configure. Then you will have complete control of, and flexibility with, the server's features. However, you also have the responsibility of maintaining the server and backing up files.

A very good alternative, if you know enough of the lingo to be dangerous, is to lease space from an ISP or WHS. With this arrangement, there is no need to have a dedicated computer or expensive connection. The ISP or WHS has total control over how the server is used, but also has the responsibility of maintaining the server. An ISP or WHS charges fees for setup ($40-$100) as well as for disk space and bandwidth (usually $50-$1500 per month), but can provide a variety of expertise and such services as marketing for your web site. For the interested beginner or personal site developer, consult one of the following free World Wide Web site services: GeoCities (Yahoo; http://geocities.yahoo.com), Tripod (Lycos; http://www.tripod.lycos.com), or Angelfire Communications (Lycos; http://www.angelfire.lycos.com). Again, ISPs and WHSs are listed in telephone books. You may also want to consult *Leasing a Server* (National Center for Supercomputing Applications List; http://www.hypernews.org/HyperNews/get/www/leasing.html) or *The List*—The Definitive ISP Buyer's Guide (http://thelist.internet.com).

When selecting an ISP or WHS, there are several important questions to ask. What's included in the fee—initial set-up, monthly fee, data storage, bandwidth amount, site usage, and tracking statistics? How many connections do they have to the backbone provider; how many telephone lines do they have, and at what speed do they connect? How are their telephone connections made (e.g., local number, 800 number)? How reliable is their server—what is their guaranteed up-time, server testing time (hopefully not during peak use), and notice of maintenance down-time? Do they provide programming and database support? How do they manage files—what are their procedures for storage size, updates, weeding? What are their backup procedures—are they regular and complete? Is a unique domain name available? What type of interface (e.g., menu) do they have? What are their customer service hours—do they provide 24 hour, 7-day support and maintenance? Is more than one person allowed on the account? Do they have an "Acceptable Use Policy" (e.g., no commercial activity)? In addition, you should look carefully at their web site and other sites they have developed—would you return to these sites? Do they understand your goals and objectives? How established is the ISP or WHS?

WEB SITE PLANNING

Having selected an ISP or WHS, you must now get down to the detailed process of building and maintaining a web site. Unless you are a one-person operation, it is extremely important to get input from everyone involved, particularly front-line customer service. Who is contacting your organization and what information or services do they want? Get the decision-makers to use the web. Provide training and support for the web site team. Keep everyone informed, particularly when positive comments are received and complaints are effectively resolved.

Lynch and Horton describe an excellent comprehensive web site planning process that comprises the following phases: 1) definition; 2) architecture; 3) design; 4) construction; 5) registration and marketing; and 6) tracking, evaluation, and maintenance (11). The definition phase may seem overly detailed, but successful completion of this phase is vital to the achievement of all that follow it. Thorough definition entails understanding of production, technology, server support, budgeting, and funding sources.

Definition

Definition begins with production issues, particularly identifying the purpose of the web site. How will the site support the organization's mission and goals, as well as be integrated with the organization's other resources? What are the site's short- and long-term goals; objectives, strategies, and methods to achieve objectives; and evaluation methods? Who is the site's audience, and how do they use the web? Other production issues concern the web site team. Who will actually produce the site—in-house staff, an outside contractor, or a combination of the two? If you use a contractor, make sure they

understand that they are providing "work for hire"—be very sure to copyright the information on the site, as well as the interface or "look and feel" of the site. Who will liaison with the contractor? Who will manage the production process? Who will be content experts? Who will be the Webmaster?

Definition continues with technology issues. Few members of the web site team will understand the equipment and software, but it is important for everyone to be familiar with the language being used. Basic to everything is the operating system (e.g., Unix) and bandwidth (e.g., Ethernet, ISDN), as well as scripting language, application programming interface, and browser software. Common Gateway Interface (CGI) scripting, supported by almost every web server, is server-side scripting (usually done in Perl programming language), and has an open architecture that allows interactivity from web pages, database integration, user authentication, and information verification. However, its open architecture also means that it is open to abuse—use the safest scripts possible and minimize the number of programs accessible via the CGI (12). Application server-side software (e.g., Cold Fusion) or page server software (e.g., Open Source PHP) may be desired for easier database access and management (13). JavaScript is a client-side scripting language that can add interactivity and conditional behavior to web pages (14).

Beyond the basics, technology issues encompass a wide variety of advanced features. Complementing HTML, XML (eXtensible Markup Language) is the web-based "metalanguage" developed by the World Wide Web Consortium (W3C) that allows customizable markup. Java language (http://java.sun.com) is the object-oriented programming language used to create distributed executable applications (e.g., interactive multimedia). Java Applets are self-contained programs, written in Java language, that can be inserted like a graphic. (See the JavaBoutique at http://javaboutique.internet.com.) Style sheets are analogous to templates, allowing style regulation and consistency. DHTML (Dynamic HTML) is a combination of scripts, HTML tags, style sheets, and distinct file formats (15) that allows the markup of behavior and appearance of HTML-marked content. Many "plug-in" and multimedia software products are also available. PDF (Portable Document File) format, developed by Adobe Corporation (http://www.adobe.com) allows files created with desktop publishing packages to be viewed in their original typed design, and multimedia objects, graphs, charts, and hypertext links can be inserted. Streaming audio/video allows for play to begin almost immediately, and continues to play as it downloads; nonstreaming audio/video must entirely download before it plays. With streaming technology, producers and artists can more easily control copyright because the user never really gets a copy of the file.

Many people use "authoring tools" to create web sites. These are often described as WYSIWYG (what you see is what you get), because you can see what a page will really look like while composing it. Many of these tools are notorious for writing inefficient or ugly HTML code, because they try to reformat HTML to reflect what they consider to be correct. A promising new product is Macromedia's Dreamweaver, which appears to provide clean HTML code as well as shortcuts for creating DHTML, JavaScript, and style sheets. HTML editors allow the simple generation of HTML tags. Examples include HomeSite (http://www.allaire.com/products/homesite), HotDog Professional (http://www.sausage.com), and BBEdit for Mac users (http://www.barebones.com/products/bbedit).

Web site definition concludes with issues surrounding server support, budgeting, and funding sources. Revisit the questions for the ISP detailed above, particularly their backup and disaster recovery plans. Prepare a detailed budget including staff salaries and benefits, hardware and software purchase and support, staff training and support, outsourcing, database maintenance and support, and content development and updating. You may want to consider seeking funding from grants, sponsorships, partnerships, or advertising.

Architecture

Once the web site is defined, its architecture—the content and structural overview of the site—can be planned, including a site map, table of contents, outlines, and thumbnails. Be sure to develop the best possible "help" section and identify how site users will communicate with support. Such communication could be via email, a discussion list forum, or live chat room. Keep in mind the enormous information capacity and multimedia capabilities of a web site. Develop evaluation/selection and maintenance/updating/weeding criteria for documents and services to be offered. Put all documents and services into categories on a hierarchical chart, and create brief informative labels for these categories. Specify the programming or technology supporting the site and its specific features. Develop a timeline, particularly highlighting the implementation schedule for design and construction. Develop prototypes for several pages of the site, as well as sketches of the interface and graphics.

Design

A well-designed site will lead to more effective and efficient use of the site, as well as easier management. The literature is replete with web site design information. Two web sites that may be of assistance are the *Yale C/AIM Web Style Guide* (http://info.med.yale.edu/caim/manual) and the *Style Guide For Online Hypertext* (http://www.w3.org/Provider/Style).

Design for content first, then appearance. Each page should primarily contain information, then graphics/images. Remember that people may view the site using many different browsers. If international use is anticipated, consider providing the site in different languages. The top 6 inches of the site's home page are critical space. This is where one grabs an audience, but attention is not necessarily earned with a flashy graphic that takes a long time to load. It is wise to provide text at the top, which can be read while graphics/images are loading. The home page should state the site name, purpose, scope, and date of last update—this is what a user will want to see to determine if the site is worth reviewing. For maximum user convenience, the home page should also display, in their entirety or as navigation links, the organization's "snail" mail address, telephone and fax numbers, clickable email address, and such legal notices as copyright, disclaimers, and sponsorship.

A web site allows one to "envision" information (16). Develop a theme and create an impression and atmosphere with consistent layout, color, and text. Determine the lowest resolution display used by the intended audience, and make sure the page layout and graphics do not exceed this capacity. Be careful when choosing a background—different browsers may display a background incorrectly. Use understandable and meaningful icons and buttons. Seriously consider whether or not to use frames. Frames can disable a browser's "back" function and cause printing/saving problems; they can also disallow bookmarking of a site, confuse search engines, and necessitate the annoying use of multiple scroll bars.

Be sure to indicate file types, and post documents in standard formats. Edit and proofread all text. Write clearly and concisely. When considering the horizontal space allotted to characters, examine "variable width" (or "proportion") font versus "fixed width" font. Avoid excessive use of capital letters and bold and italic fonts—they are hard on the eye and some browsers have trouble with italics. Use high contrast between text and background. When it comes to color, the 216 colors of the "web-safe" palette (i.e., 6×6×6 color cube—6 shades each of red, green, and blue), are more than adequate. Avoid red/green and blue/green combinations (in deference to color blindness). Remember to use white space effectively.

Do not put vital information within graphics, because it may not get read/indexed by search engines. Provide a "text-only" option for the site, as well as alternative text for graphics/images. Avoid the excessive use of graphics or images, and always state their size. Use thumbnails, and again, state the size of the full images. Consider reducing bit or color depth for faster loading, and consider preloading graphics or images that are used repetitively. The .JPG (or JPEG – Joint Photographic Experts Group) format is best for photos, and .GIF (Graphical Interchange Format) format works best for graphics. You may want to use an *image map* (such as a graphic with areas that are "clickable") instead of a navigation menu, but consider the download time for such graphics. Streaming audio/video is increasingly popular, but requires plug-ins.

The site, and each individual page, should be comfortable and effortless to use. Offer layers of approaches based on the "triple taxonomy" of user experience, field of interest, and site resources (17). Help the user to understand how the site operates. Provide categories, and display the most important or commonly used functions first. Minimize the number of navigation steps, and avoid excessive internal links. A site map is an excellent structural overview and index tool. If allowing site search capability, keep display and search refinement options on the same page as the search page.

Users may access the site at any point, so each page must be capable of standing on its own, use descriptive titles, and provide navigation links back to the home page. It is also a good idea to put the copyright notice on every page of the site. Use headings, lists, and link menus to organize documents. State when a document was created and updated. When considering external links, be courteous. If you want to link to another site, it is a good idea to inform that site's Webmaster.

Web designers are acutely aware of the needs of disabled people using the Internet. In May 1999, the W3C published its recommended Web Accessibility Initiative (WAI) Guidelines (http://www.w3.org/WAI) covering items such as text size (at least 24-point) and the number of times the keyboard is manipulated (18). The Center for Applied Special Technology developed the "Bobby" tool to help analyze whether a site meets WAI guidelines. You may want to consider getting a "Bobby Approved" icon for a site addressing rheumatic disease. Connect to http://www.cast.org/bobby for information.

Construction

After completing the comprehensive design process, the actual site construction can begin. Lynch and Horton offer an excellent checklist for construction stages: 1) HTML (and/or XML) finished for all pages, all page content in place; 2) navigation link structure finished; 3) programming linked to pages, ready for beta testing; 4) database components linked to pages; 5) graphic design, illustration, photography finalized; 6) final proofread of all content; 7) database and programming functionality tested; 8) database reporting features tested and verified; 9) user support tested; and 10) content components, HTML code, programming code, and other development materials archived (11).

Registration and Marketing

The site is now ready for use, and it is time for registration and marketing. As stated above, the information on the site, as well as the "look" and "feel" of the site, should be copyrighted from their inception. Beyond copyright, the site domain (i.e., the URL) must be named and registered. The domain registry system is undergoing changes, with new registrars being approved by the Internet Corporation for Assigned Names and Numbers (ICANN; http://www.icann.com) and new "functional" top level extensions being created (i.e., beyond those of .com, .edu, .net, .org). To see if your desired domain name is available, consult Network Solutions, Inc. (http://www.networksolutions.com) or an accredited registrar. ICANN can provide a list of accredited registrars. Domain registration applications are available from the Internet Network Information Center (http://www.internic.net) and accredited registrars, as well as on the sites of most WHSs and domain-hosting ISPs. Registration fees vary, but are generally $70 for the first 2 years, and $35 annually thereafter. Consider registering under .com, .net, and .org to cover all the bases. It is best to keep the domain name easy to spell and remember—if possible no more than 15 characters. Lower case text is recommended, and unusual characters should be avoided. Obviously, you should avoid another's trademark. If using your own organization's name in the domain name, register it as a trademark. ICANN's "Dispute Resolution Policy" was designed to resolve international domain name disputes (19). The United States' "Anticybersquatting Consumer Protection Act of 1999" indicates further recognition of the problem of domain name trafficking.

Standard marketing methods—direct mailing, press releases and articles, as well as print, radio, and television ads—can be effectively used to market a web site. Put the site address on business cards, letterhead, bills, statements, packaging, promotional materials, and publications. Consider exhibiting at meetings, as well as using kiosks in public spaces. If you are leasing space from an ISP or WHS, get on their "What's New" page. There are also marketing methods unique to the web. As stated above, search engines use software to seek data from sites according to specific subjects or locations. Site pages are retrieved based on the keywords in their section and "Meta tags" in their section. The search software may give higher scores to keywords that come first or that occur more frequently. Thus, creative manipulation of keywords and Meta tags will increase a site's odds of favorable placement in a search results list. Care is needed, however. A keyword may be rejected if it is repeated more than 7 times. Current trends seem to favor words beginning with "a" (e.g., "Arthritis" is likely to appear before "Rheumatology"). In addition, even the best Meta tags will not overcome the growing practice of search engines allowing words to be purchased. To learn more about search engines and Meta tags, see the information under LinkExchange's *Submit It!* (http://www.submit-it.com/subopt.htm).

Registration and marketing information and services are available from numerous sources. Here are some selected sites: Netscape's *!Register-It!* (http://register-it.netscape.com/), Web Ignite Corporation (http://www.web-ignite.com), Gethits.com (http://www.gethits.com), SitePromoter (http://www.sitepromoter.com), *World Wide Web Mailing Lists* (post to the appropriate list, http://www.leeds.ac.uk/ucs/WWW/WWW_mailing_lists.html), Open Directory Project (http://www.dmoz.org/Computers/Internet/WWW/Website_Promotion), and Yahoo (http://dir.yahoo.com/Computers_and_Internet/Internet/World_Wide_Web/Site_Announcement_and_Promotion/). Virtually all of the leading search and metasearch engines also offer free site listing services. Look for the "Add URL" or "Submit Site" link.

Management: Tracking and Evaluation

Having created your web site, you must now be concerned with effective and efficient management of the site. This encompasses tracking, evaluation, and general maintenance. Usage reports greatly assist the demonstration of service. ISPs and WHSs often offer a variety of site usage reporting mechanisms, typically tracking site usage peak hours, content/file usage, navigation methods, and where users are located. Beyond users, keep track of sites that visit one's site. *Cookies* allow a web site to get information about its users, including information about a user's past search sessions and preferences. Cookies are files stored on a site user's computer (usually for short, specified time periods) that are retrieved by the site server at the beginning of subsequent interactions with that user. Data mining is far more complex and entails the use of pattern recognition software capable of answering sophisticated market research questions. Such questions can involve classification/prediction (who will buy, what will they buy, and how much will they buy), segmentation (types of site users), association (relationships between users and site products/services), clustering (hidden groups in data), visualization (distributions and patterns in data), and optimization (how to maximize online presence and desired outcome) (20).

User feedback and evaluation strategies should be used to help guide site adjustments. Review the site's legal notices. Strictly monitor copyright. Investigate all notices that one's site contains infringing material, and promptly remove such material. Test the site on new browser and HTML standards. Sample search the site to test its performance and appearance. Review page content in terms of its information and syntax, as well as site navigation, particularly intrapage links. Review directories and files. Strictly maintain security and privacy. Have confidentiality/security levels to protect file access, and require passwords. Do not allow public access to configuration files, and hide access and error logs. If allowing users to send email, have a predefined address. If using scripts for forms processing, check for loopholes. A web site must virtually "guarantee" the protection of information on its visitors, and failure to do so may result in criminal or civil action.

Firewalls keep unauthorized (and unwanted) traffic from the Internet out of a protected network (i.e., local area or wide area networks), yet still allow that network's users to access the Internet. Most firewalls are routers, filtering incoming datagrams based on the datagram's source address, destination address, higher level protocol, or other specified criteria. More sophisticated firewalls use "proxy servers" (or bastion hosts) that provide direct access to the Internet by internal users, acting as their proxy, while filtering out unauthorized incoming traffic.

Several web sites provide diagnostic tools to help evaluate sites. All of them check HTML code and link validation. They may also suggest Meta tags, assist with image size reduction, and test server performance and reliability. Diagnostic sites include WebSite Garage (http://websitegarage.netscape.com) and W3C's HTML Validation Service (http://validator.w3.org). You may also consult the Web Standards Project (WSP; http://www.webstandards.org), a group of W3C crossover members and web designers. As always, consulting colleagues and experts can be helpful. Consider subscribing to discussion lists such as HTML-Group (listserv@airgunhq.com) or ADVANCED-WEB (listproc@listserver.com), as well as monitoring news groups such as Miscellaneous Web Authoring Issues (Usenet news: comp.infosystems.www.authoring.misc).

REFERENCES

1. Dahn M. Counting angels on a pinhead: critically interpreting Web size estimates. Online 2000;24(1):35–40.
2. Sherman C. Humans do it better: inside the Open Directory project. Online 2000;24(4):43–50.
3. Search Engine Watch. Reviews, ratings & tests: reviews & statistics: directory sizes. Available at: http://www.searchenginewatch.com. Accessed July 30, 2001.
4. Hock R. Web search engines: (more) features & commands. Online 2000;24(3):17–26.
5. Internet search engine update. Online 2000;23(4):16.
6. Internet search engine update. Online 2000;24(5):12.
7. Kirkwood HP Jr. Bookmark central: x marks the BotSpot. Online 1999; 23(4):83–4.
8. Sullivan F, Gardner M, Van Rijsbergen K. An Information retrieval service to support clinical decision-making at the point of care. Br J General Practice 1999;49:1003–7.
9. Chen H-S, Guo F-R, Lee R-G, Lin C-C, Chen J-H, Chen C-Y, et al. Recent advances in telemedicine. J Formosan Med Assn 1999;98:767–72.
10. Zhou J-Z. The Internet, the World Wide Web, library web browsers, and library web servers. Information Technology and Libraries 2000;19(1): 50–2.
11. Lynch PJ, Horton S. Web style guide: basic design principles for creating web sites. New Haven: Yale University Press; 1999, p. 1–10.
12. Mortensen KP. Working the web. Internet Law Researcher 2000;5(4):12.
13. Antelman K. Getting out of the HTML business: the database-driven Web site solution. Information Technology and Libraries 1999;18(4):176–81.
14. Niederst J. Web design in a nutshell: a desktop quick reference. Sebastopol, CA: O'Reilly & Associates; 1999, p. 379.
15. Schmeiser L. The complete website upgrade & maintenance guide. San Francisco: SYBEX; 1999, p. 478.
16. Andres C. Great web architecture. Foster City, CA: IDG Books Worldwide; 1999, p. 45.
17. Quint B. Designing the perfect information portal. Information Today 2000;17(2):7.
18. World Wide Web Consortium. Web accessibility initiative. Available at http://www.w3.org/WAI. Accessed July 30, 2001.
19. Osborne D. Don't take my name in vain! ICANN dispute resolution policy and names of individuals. Communications Law 2000;5(4):127–8.
20. Mena J. Data mining your website. Boston: Digital Press; 1999, p. 10–9.

Additional Recommended Reading

Schlein AM, Flowers JR Jr, Kisaichi SK, Weber P (editors). Find it online: the complete guide to online research. 2nd ed. Tempe, AZ: Facts on Demand Press; 2000.

Harris R. A guidebook to the web. Guilford, CT: Dushkin/McGraw-Hill; 2000.

Ackermann E, Hartman K. Searching and researching on the Internet and the World Wide Web. Wilsonville, OR: Franklin, Beedle & Associates; 2000.

Cohen J. Communication and design with the Internet. New York: W.W. Norton; 2000.

Greenspun P. Philip and Alex's guide to web publishing. San Francisco: Morgan Kaufmann Publishers; 1999.

Powell TA. Web design: the complete reference. Berkeley, CA: Osborne/McGraw-Hill; 2000.

McClelland D, Eismann K, Stone T. Web design studio secrets. 2nd ed. Foster City, CA: IDG Books Worldwide; 2000.

Gordon-Murnane L. Evaluating net evaluators. Searcher 1999;7(2):57-66.

Perle EG, Williams JT, Fischer MA. Electronic publishing and software, part II [on liability issues]. The Computer Lawyer 2000;17(2):15–28.

CHAPTER 44

Links and Organizations

CYNTHIA M. KAHN, MA

Many resources exist specifically for people with rheumatic diseases. Although a variety of national resources provide patient education, most services will vary from community to community and from state to state. A current list of organizations and resources in your area may be compiled through local organization offices, community agencies, and the blue pages in the telephone book (1).

The Internet can also be a valuable resource for information. However, patients should be advised that not all web sites are equal when it comes to medical information. Readers should ask the following questions when evaluating information obtained from the Internet:

- Who is posting the information, and who is sponsoring the site? Nonprofit and government groups, such as the Arthritis Foundation and the National Institutes of Health, are likely to provide reliable information, whereas sites devoted to "miracle cures" should be evaluated with caution.
- Where is the content being developed? This information is usually available in the "Who We Are" or "About Us" link. Look for an advisory board with medical credentials.
- How often is the material updated? Research advances are happening daily. If you're looking at information dated 1996, for example, it's probably no longer completely accurate.

The list of organizations, agencies, associations, and sources provided below is not intended to be comprehensive, but to provide a starting point for patients or professionals looking for more information on a particular topic or rheumatic disease. Finally, the Internet is a dynamic environment; while these resources were all available at the time of publication, their status may change over time.

GENERAL RESOURCES ON RHEUMATIC DISEASES

Arthritis Foundation
P.O. Box 7669
Atlanta, GA 30357-0669
404-872-7100
800-283-7800
www.arthritis.org

The Arthritis Foundation provides excellent patient education materials on a variety of rheumatic diseases. It can also help patients access local resources by referring them to local chapter offices within the U.S. that often sponsor exercise and self-management courses. Some professional education materials are also available.

The Arthritis Society (National Office)
393 University Avenue, Suite 1700
Toronto, Ontario M5G 1E6
CANADA
416-979-7228
800-321-1433
www.arthritis.ca

The Arthritis Society provides education materials and information on Canadian programs and resources for people with rheumatic disease.

National Institute of Arthritis and Musculoskeletal and Skin Diseases
1 AMS Circle
Bethesda, MD 20892
(301) 495-4484
(877) 22-NIAMS
www.nih.gov/niams

NIAMS is a component of the National Institutes of Health that both funds research on rheumatic diseases and disseminates information. They provide fact sheets, brochures, and other educational information. On their web site, patients can conduct searches for medical information and find out about ongoing clinical trials.

Missouri Arthritis Rehabilitation Research and Training Center
130 A P Green, DC330.00
One Hospital Drive
Columbia, MO 65212
www.muhealth.org/~arthritis

The MARRTC is a nonprofit educational institution that has a great web site for people seeking information on arthritis and rheumatic diseases.

On the Web

www.pdr.net/gettingwell/arthritis/consumers.html

The web site of the *Physicians' Desk Reference* has a section for consumers as well as for health professionals, including recent articles on the latest drug treatments for people with arthritis.

GENERAL WEB-BASED HEALTH INFORMATION

www.webmd.com

WebMD provides healthcare information for both consumers and health professionals. Consumers can access health news, articles, research reports, condition-specific centers and communities, and interactive tools and programs.

DISEASE-SPECIFIC RESOURCES

American Fibromyalgia Syndrome Association
6380 E. Tanque Verde, Suite D
Tucson, AZ 85715
520-733-1570
www.afsafund.org

American Juvenile Arthritis Organization
(a council of the Arthritis Foundation)
1330 West Peachtree Street
Atlanta, GA 30309 404-872-7100
www.arthritis.org/communities/about_ajao.asp

Lupus Foundation of America, Inc.
1300 Piccard Drive
Suite 200
Rockville MD 20850
301-670-9292
800-558-0121
www.lupus.org

National Fibromyalgia Partnership, Inc.
140 Zinn Way
Linden, VA
22642-5609
866-725-4404
www.fmpartnership.org

NIAMS Pediatric Clinic
www.nih.gov/niams

The National Institutes of Health has a free pediatric rheumatology clinic at its research hospital on the NIH campus in Bethesda Maryland. The clinic offers diagnosis, evaluation, and treatment for children with arthritis and other chronic rheumatic diseases. For more information, visit the NIAMS web site at www.nih.gov/niams or call 1-877-22-NIAMS.

National Osteoporosis Foundation
1232 22nd Street NW
Washington, DC 20037
202-223-2226
877-868-4520
www.nof.org

National Psoriasis Foundation
6600 SW 92nd Avenue
Suite 300
Portland, OR 97223
503-297-1545
800-723-9166
www.psoriasis.org

Scleroderma Foundation
12 Kent Way
Suite 101
Byfield, MA 01922
978-463-5843
800-722-4673
www.scleroderma.org

Sjogren's Syndrome Foundation
366 North Broadway
Suite PH-W2
Jericho, NY 11753
516-933-6365
800-475-6475
www.sjogren's.org

Spondylitis Association of America
P.O. Box 5872
Sherman Oaks, CA 91413
818-981-1616
800-777-8189
www.spondylitis.org

RESOURCES FOR CHRONIC PAIN

American Chronic Pain Association
P.O. Box 850
Rocklin, CA 95677
916-632-0922
www.theacpa.org

American Pain Foundation
201 N. Charles Street
Suite 710
Baltimore, MD 21201-4111
www.painfoundation.org

American Pain Society
4700 W. Lake Avenue
Glenview, IL 60025
847-375-4715
www.ampainsoc.org

COMPLEMENTARY AND ALTERNATIVE MEDICINE RESOURCES

National Center for Complementary and
Alternative Medicine
NCCAM Clearinghouse
P.O. Box 8218
Silver Spring, MD 20807-8218
http://nccam.nih.gov

The National Center for Complementary and Alternative Medicine, a branch of the National Institutes of Health, conducts and supports basic and applied research and training into CAM therapies. You can receive a free packet of information on alternative therapies by writing to the address above.

American Academy of Medical Acupuncture
5820 Wilshire Boulevard Suite
500 Los Angeles, CA 90036
323-937-5514
www.medicalacupuncture.org

American Dietetic Association
216 West Jackson Boulevard
Chicago, IL 60606-6995
312-899-0040
www.eatright.org

American Massage Therapy Association
820 Davis Street Suite 100
Evanston, IL 60201-4444
847-864-0123
www.amtamassage.org

Association for Applied Psychophysiology
and Biofeedback
10200 W. 44th Avenue
Suite 304
Wheat Ridge, CO 80033-2840
800-477-8892
www.aapb.org

Association for the Advancement of Behavior Therapy
305 Seventh Avenue
New York, NY 10001-6008
(212) 647-1890

Maintains a referrals service that can provide names of therapists trained in cognitive behavioral therapy in your local area.

On the Web

http://vm.cfsan.fda.gov/~dms/supplmnt.html

The United States Food and Drug Administration Center for Food Safety and Applied Nutrition disseminates information regarding health claims of various supplements, as well as warning and safety information.

www.altmednet.com

This is a data source for health professionals interested in remaining current on alternative medicine topics. The site contains full text of all articles published in the monthly newsletter, *Alternative Medicine Alert*, reporting on evidenced-based interventions across the spectrum of medical conditions, in addition to standards, position papers, and organizational links.

ASSISTIVE DEVICES/EQUIPMENT

There are many companies that make assistive devices and equipment for use in the home or office. The following are just a few that can either provide a catalog or let you shop online.

Illinois Assistive Technology Project
1 West Old State Capitol Plaza
Suite 100
Springfield, IL 62701
800-852-5110
217-522-7985
www.iltech.org

This nonprofit organization helps people find assistive devices and maintains lists of companies that sell them.

ABLE DATA
8630 Fenton Street
Suite 930
Silver Spring, MD 20910
800-227-0216
www.abledata.com

An online repository of assistive technology products.

Aids for Arthritis, Inc.
35 Wakefield Drive
Medford, NJ 08055
800-654-0707
www.aidsforarthritis.com

Ergonomic Solutions
129 N. Sylvan Drive
Mundelein, IL 60060-4949
800-755-4950
www.goergo.com

Mature Smart
1788 West Cherry Street
Jesup, GA 31545
800-720-6278
www.maturesmart.com

North Coast Medical
Consumer Products Division
18305 Sutter Blvd.
Morgan Hill, CA 95037
800-235-7054

Sears Home HealthCare
3737 Grader Street
Suite 110
Garland, TX 75041
800-326-1750

Smith and Nephew
P.O. Box 1005
Germantown, WI 53022
800-558-8633
www.smith-nephew.com

RESOURCES FOR HEALTH PROFESSIONALS

American College of Foot and Ankle Surgeons
515 Busse Highway
Park Ridge, IL 60068
800-421-2237
847-292-2237
www.acfas.org

American College of Rheumatology
1800 Century Place, Suite 250
Atlanta, GA 30345
404-872-7100
www.rheumatology.org

The American College of Rheumatology is the professional organization of rheumatologists and associated health professionals dedicated to healing, preventing disability, and curing the more than 100 types of arthritis and related disorders. The ACR provides professional education through scientific meetings, journals, and other materials. Through the ACR Research and Education Foundation, the ACR seeks to increase research in the rheumatic diseases while fostering the careers of young investigators.

American Nurses Association
600 Maryland Avenue, SW
Suite 100
West Washington, DC 20024-2571
1-800-274-4ANA
www.ana.org

American Occupational Therapy Association
4720 Montgomery Lane
Bethesda, MD 20824
301-652-AOTA
www.aota.org

American Physical Therapy Association
1111 North Fairfax Street
Alexandria, VA 22314
703-684-2782
www.apta.org

American Psychological Association
750 First Street NE
Washington, DC 20002-4242
202-336-5500
www.apa.org

American Society for Bone and Mineral Research
2025 M Street, NW
Suite 800
Washington, DC 20036-3309
202-367-1161
www.asbmr.org

Association of Rheumatology Health Professionals
(A Division of the American College of Rheumatology)
1800 Century Place, Suite 250
Atlanta, GA 30345
404-633-3777
www.rheumatology.org

Canadian Physiotherapy Association
2345 Yonge Street, Suite 410
Toronto, Ontario M4P 2E5
800-387-8679
416-932-1888
www.physiotherapy.ca

National Association of Social Workers
750 First Street NE
Suite 700
Washington, DC 20002-4241
800-638-8799
202-408-8600
www.naswdc.org

On the Web

(Please see Chapter 43, Clinical Care and the World Wide Web for additional web-based resources for health professionals.)

www.cochrane.org

The Cochrane Library is dedicated to preparing, maintaining, and promoting the accessibility of systematic reviews of the effects of health care. It also provides a medical database with search category of complementary and alternative medicine listing randomized, controlled trials.

www.ncbi.nlm.nih.gov/entrez

The National Library of Medicine site allows you to search the medical literature and retrieve information on clinical trials from the NLM electronic database using PubMed.

www.mdconsult.com

MD Consult provides medical information service with full text journals and reference books, practice guidelines, medical news, drug information, MEDLINE, and other services. Membership required.

The editors would like to thank Carolyn McGrory, MS, RN, and Judy Sotosky, MEd, PT, for their contribution to this chapter.

REFERENCE

1. McGrory CH, Sotosky JR. Arthritis: common problems and their solutions. A guide to multidisciplinary interventions. Philadelphia: Hahnemann University, 1990.

Subject Index